Published and forthcoming Oxford Handbooks

OXFORD MEDICAL PUBLICATIONS

Oxford Handbook of
Public Health
Practice

Oxford Handbook of
Public Health Practice

Third edition

Edited by

Charles Guest
Senior Specialist, Australian Capital Territory Government
Health Directorate & Australian National University,
Canberra, Australia

Walter Ricciardi
Professor of Hygiene and Preventive Medicine & Director
of the Department of Public Health, Università Cattolica
del Sacro Cuore, Rome, Italy; President of the European
Public Health Association (EUPHA)

Ichiro Kawachi
Professor of Social Epidemiology & Chairman of the
Department of Society, Human Development and Health,
Harvard School of Public Health, Boston, USA

Iain Lang
Consultant in Public Health, NHS Devon & Senior Clinical
Lecturer in Public Health, National Institute for Health
Research Collaboration for Applied Health Research
and Care for the South West Peninsula (PenCLAHRC),
University of Exeter Medical School, Exeter, UK

OXFORD
UNIVERSITY PRESS

OXFORD
UNIVERSITY PRESS

Great Clarendon Street, Oxford, OX2 6DP,
United Kingdom

Oxford University Press is a department of the University of Oxford.
It furthers the University's objective of excellence in research, scholarship,
and education by publishing worldwide. Oxford is a registered trade mark of
Oxford University Press in the UK and in certain other countries

First edition published 2001
Second edition published 2006
Third edition published 2013

Impression: 1

British Library Cataloguing in Publication Data
Data available

Library of Congress Control Number: 2012946418

ISBN 978–0–19–958630–1

Printed in China by
C&C Offset Printing Co. Ltd.

Dedication

Proceeds from the sale of this book will be donated to public health projects undertaken by Oxfam.

The editors hope that this small text will help any reader to leave the health of the public in a better state than you found it.

From CSG, to the memory of my brother James, who needed better health care:

They also serve, who only stand and wait.[1]

From IAL, to GHCL and IJUL, both of whose gestations overlapped with that of this book.

Reference

1 Milton, J. (1999). When I consider how my light is spent. In: Ricks, C, ed., *Oxford Book of English Verse*, p. 168. Oxford University Press, Oxford.

Foreword to the third edition

When tackling day-to-day problems in public health it is easy to forget its spectacular successes. It is also easy to forget that many of the important advances we now take for granted were not immediately accepted or put into practice, even if the preventive strategy was surprisingly simple and highly effective.

A well-known example is Semmelweiss' demonstration that hand-washing with chlorinated lime solution prevented 'childbed fever'. He instigated the practice in an obstetric clinic in Vienna in May 1847 and showed that the monthly maternal mortality rate in the clinic fell from 10–20% in the preceding year to 1–2% in the following year. His findings were dismissed by the medical establishment, a major reason being that there was no known mechanism to explain his findings. Increasingly disheartened by his failure to change practice, Semmelweiss was admitted to an asylum with severe depression in 1861 and died there in 1865. Only years after his death was the importance of hand-washing to prevent the transmission of infections within hospitals widely accepted.

The resurgence of severe hospital-transmitted infections in the last few decades was in part due to a failure to adhere to what Semmelweiss had demonstrated so convincingly more than a century before. However, modern surveillence systems soon identified the emerging epidemic and re-emphasis on hand-washing with anti-bacterial agents in hospitals has much reduced the problem.

Nowadays we take the harmful effects of smoking for granted and anti-smoking campaigns are a core public heath activity. Strong evidence linking smoking to lung cancer and then to vascular and respiratory diseases was first published in the early 1950s. But these findings were also dismissed by the medical establishment, most of whom smoked. It took until about 1970 for there to be widespread acceptance that smoking was a major cause of ill-heath, and only then did concerted actions start in earnest against the use, sale, and advertising of tobacco.

In the 21st century smoking is still a major cause of premature death. In most high-income countries the prevalence of smoking is declining, and smoking-related mortality has also begun to decline. However, in the more populous low-income and middle-income countries smoking rates are rising, and smoking-related mortality is becoming increasingly common.

Despite all that has been achieved there is still a need to convince the medical profession and the general public of the effectiveness of popula-tion-based approaches to disease prevention. In Semmelweiss' time dis-ease causation was often believed to be the result of imbalances in the 'four humors' within the body. Medical texts at the time emphasized that each case of disease was unique, the result of a personal imbalance, and that the main role of the medical profession was to establish precisely each patient's unique situation, case by case. Curiously, the current fashion for 'personalized medicine' has elements of this type of philosophy. Public health practitioners thus need to remind the public of how much better their day-to-day lives are as a result of population-based preventive measures, and that much can still be achieved from such interventions. This handbook will stimulate beginners and experts in public health to improve their practice.

Valerie Beral, DBE, AC, FRS
Professor of Epidemiology
University of Oxford, UK
2012

Foreword to the second edition

At some point in their lives, readers of this handbook have no doubt confronted the same dilemmas that I faced when I chose to retire from clinical practice to embark on a career in public health. At the time I made my choice, my senior colleagues alerted me to the strict hierarchy that exists across the diverse branches of the health sciences. They cautioned that the prestige of any given specialty within the house of medicine is inversely proportional to the size of the object it addresses. Hence, if your chosen field of specialty happens to deal with microscopic objects like chromosomes and genes, you can be assured of high prestige, as well as unlimited access to funding. If, on the other hand, your chosen field happens to deal with the opposite end of the spectrum from genes—that is, the health of entire populations—then you had better resign yourself to a life of chronic under-funding, low prestige, and being ignored by the rest of the world. Treating individual patients (as in clinical practice) lies somewhere between these two extremes. Clinical practice may not be as 'sexy' as genetics, but at least you can be assured of a steady income, as well as the satisfaction of seeing the fruits of your labour on a daily basis. By contrast, the translation of public health knowledge into practice often seems excruciatingly slow, and the results of our interventions are seldom directly observable at the individual level.

As this handbook illustrates, the public health approach has at its disposal a powerful set of practices that can transform the health of populations. Indeed, public health can lay claim to a number of significant victories that have improved the lives of millions. Thomas McKeown considered that the major improvements in mortality from infectious diseases during the last century occurred not through medical advances, but through public health measures, specifically improvements in sanitation and nutrition. The earliest convincing evidence of cigarette smoking as a cause of cancer was published by Ernest Wynder in 1953—the same year as the discovery of the genetic code. Armed with this knowledge (as well as subsequent epidemiological evidence), public health practitioners have helped millions of smokers to quit their habit, as well as prevented millions more from initiating, with the result that countless lives have been saved. It represents a victory on a scale that few in the molecular field could lay claim to—at least so far …

There are dozens of textbooks dealing with advanced epidemiological methods but precious few that focus on the skills needed to practice the art of public health. This handbook provides a valuable antidote to that imbalance.

Ichiro Kawachi
2006

Foreword to the first edition

Originality, practical focus and comprehensive coverage are not qualities normally found together in textbooks in the field of medicine and health care. In public health, the field, at least in Britain, is even thinner.

The editors have pulled off a remarkable feat—meeting these challenges and drawing together a team of diverse talents to do the thinking and writing. From values to decision-making, from organizations to people, from strategy to team-working, the whole of public health practice is conceptualized in a fresh imaginative way.

Readers will see, described in this book, the skills they use day-to-day, but will seldom recognize themselves, they will identify needs and knowledge gaps that they had not previously acknowledged, and they will find inspiration in the examples of good practice …

In the *Oxford Handbook of Public Health Practice* …, you will have found a true soul mate.

Liam Donaldson
Chief Medical Officer
Department of Health
2001

Acknowledgements

We thank the following for assistance of many kinds in the development of this edition.

At Oxford University Press, Michael Hawkes, Anna Winstanley, Beth Womack, and others.

David Pencheon, David Melzer, and Sir Muir Gray, former co-editors of this text, all made helpful suggestions in the development of the third edition.

Sir David Watson and the staff of Green Templeton College, University of Oxford, and the Rockefeller Foundation Bellagio Study Centre, Italy, provided generous hospitality in the later stages of editing.

At the Australian Capital Territory Government Health Directorate, Ranil Appuhamy, Peggy Brown, Mark Cormack, Emm Dale, Susannah Taylor, and colleagues in the Population Health Division, supported this work in many ways.

CSG would like to thank Hilary, Stephanie, and William, for loving consideration during some difficult times in recent years.

Not every idea in this or any book can be traced to its source. We apologize for any omission here, and would be grateful to hear from readers with amendments, corrections, or other suggestions, by mail to:

Dr Charles Guest
Australian Capital Territory Government Health Directorate
GPO Box 825
Canberra ACT 2601
Australia
Or email: charles.guest@act.gov.au

CSG
WR
IK
IAL

Contents

Detailed Contents

Contributors

Jane An
Harvard School of Public Health
Boston MA, USA

Kate Ardern
Ashton, Leigh and Wigan Primary
Care Trust
Wigan
Lancashire, UK

Tar-Ching Aw
Faculty of Medicine and Health
Sciences
United Arab Emirates University
Al-Ain, United Arab Emirates

Gabriele Bammer
National Centre for Epidemiology
and Population Health
Australian National University
Canberra, Australia

Nicholas Banatvala
World Health Organization
Geneva, Switzerland

Alex Barratt
Department of Public Health and
Community Medicine
University of Sydney
Sydney, Australia

John Battersby
Eastern Region Public Health
Observatory
Cambridge, UK

**Dame Valerie Beral DBE,
AC, FRS**
Cancer Epidemiology Unit
University of Oxford
Oxford, UK

Martin Birley
BirleyHIA
Kingston
Surrey, UK

Stefania Boccia
Institute of Hygiene
Università Cattolica del Sacro
Cuore
Rome, Italy

Paul Bolton
Center for Refugee and Disaster
Response
Department of International
Health
Johns Hopkins Bloomberg School
of Public Health
Baltimore, USA

Peter Brambleby
NHS Croydon and London
Borough of Croydon
London, UK

Anne Brice
NHS National Knowledge Service
Oxford, UK

Frederick M. Burkle, Jr
Harvard Humanitarian Initiative
Harvard School of Public Health
Boston MA, USA

Amanda Burls
Department of Primary Health
Care
University of Oxford
Oxford, UK

Hilary Burton
Foundation for Genomics and
Population Health
Cambridge, UK

Martin Caraher
Centre for Food Policy
City University of London
London, UK

Ben Cave
Ben Cave Associates Ltd
Leeds, UK

Charlotte Chang
Labor Occupational Health
Program
University of California, Berkeley
Berkeley CA, USA

Simon Chapman
School of Public Health
The University of Sydney
Sydney, Australia

Paul Cosford
Health Protection Agency
London, UK

Diana Delnoij
Centrum Klantervaring Zorg
Utrecht, The Netherlands

Don Eugene Detmer
American Medical Informatics
Association and
University of Virginia
Charlottesville VA, USA

Anna Dixon
The King's Fund
London, UK

Martin Eccles
Institute of Health and Society
Newcastle University
Newcastle-upon-Tyne, UK

Julian Elston
NHS Cornwall and Isles of Scilly
St Austell, UK

Gene Feder
University of Bristol
Bristol, UK

John Fien
RMIT University
Melbourne, Australia

Julian Flowers
Eastern Region Public Health
Observatory
Institute of Public Health
Cambridge, UK

Sharon Friel
National Centre for Epidemiology
and Population Health
Australian National University
Canberra, Australia

Michael S. Frommer
School of Public Health
The University of Sydney
Sydney, Australia

Steve Gillam
Department of Public Health and
Primary Care
Institute of Public Health
Cambridge, UK

Mike Gogarty
NHS North East Essex
Colchester, UK

Lawrence Gostin
O'Neill Institute for National and
Global Health Law
Georgetown Law School
Washington DC, USA

Caron Grainger
Coventry Primary Care Trust
Coventry, UK

J. A. Muir Gray
Better Value Healthcare
Oxford, UK

Felix Greaves
Imperial College London
London, UK

Chris Griffiths
Barts and The London School
of Medicine and Dentistry
London, UK

Sian Griffiths
School of Public Health and
Primary Care
The Chinese University of Hong
Kong, Hong Kong, People's
Republic of China

Jeremy Grimshaw
Clinical Epidemiology Programme
Ottawa Health Research Institute
Ottawa, Canada

Charles Guest
Australian Capital Territory
Government Health Directorate
and Australian National
University
Canberra, Australia

Malcolm Harrington
The University of Birmingham
Birmingham, UK

Eric Heymann
Global Brigades ASG
London, UK

Alison Hill
South East Public Health
Observatory
Oxford, UK

Richard S. Hopkins
Bureau of Epidemiology
Florida Department of Health
Tallahassee FL, USA

Rebekah Jenkin
School of Public Health
The University of Sydney
Sydney, Australia

Edmund Jessop
National Specialist Commissioning
Advisory Group
UK Department of Health
London, UK

Christine M. Jorm
School of Public Health
The University of Sydney
Sydney, Australia

Marina Karanikolos
European Observatory on Health
Systems and Policies
Brussels, Belgium

Ichiro Kawachi
Harvard School of Public Health
Boston MA, USA

Bernadette Khoshaba
London School of Hygiene and
Tropical Medicine
London, UK

Andrew J. Kibble
Division of Environmental Health
and Risk Management
The University of Birmingham
Edgbaston, Birmingham, UK

Kalyanaraman Kumaran
South West (South) Health
Protection Unit
Exeter, UK

Iain Lang
NHS Devon and PenCLAHRC
University of Exeter Medical
School,
Exeter, UK

Tim Lang
Centre for Food Policy
City University of London
London, UK

David Lawrence
London School of Hygiene and
Tropical Medicine
University of London
London, UK

Katherine Mackay
Australian National University
Medical School
Canberra, Australia

Sara Mallinson
Division of Health Research
Lancaster University, UK

Martin McKee
London School of Hygiene and
Tropical Medicine
University of London
London, UK

Robyn Martin
Centre for Research in Primary
and Community Care,
University of Hertfordshire, UK
School of Public Health
The Chinese University of Hong
Kong, Hong Kong, People's
Republic of China

Alan Maryon-Davis
King's College
University of London,
London, UK

David Melzer
Peninsula Medical School
Exeter, UK

Ruairidh Milne
University of Southampton
Southampton, UK

Rubin Minhas
British Medical Journal Technology
Assessment Group
BMJ Evidence Centre
London, UK

Meredith Minkler
School of Public Health
University of California, Berkeley
Berkeley CA, USA

John Newton
NHS South Central Strategic
Health Authority
Newbury
Berkshire, UK

Don Nutbeam
University of Southampton
Southampton, UK

Sarah O'Brien
Department of Health Sciences
and Epidemiology
University of Manchester
Manchester, UK

Virginia Pearson
NHS Devon and Devon County
Council
Exeter, UK

David Pencheon
NHS Sustainable Development
Unit
Cambridge, UK

Jennie Popay
School of Health and Medicine
Division of Health Research
Lancaster University
Lancaster, UK

Angela Raffle
Bristol North Primary Care Trust
Bristol, UK

Jem Rashbass
Eastern Cancer Registry and
Information Centre
Cambridge, UK

Walter Ricciardi

Professor of Hygiene and Preventive Medicine & Director of the Department of Public Health, Università Cattolica del Sacro Cuore, Rome, Italy;
President of the European Public Health Association (EUPHA)

Thomas Rice

UCLA School of Public Health
Los Angeles CA, USA

Richard Richards

NHS Derbyshire County Primary Care Trust
Derbyshire, UK

Sonia Roschnik

NHS Sustainable Development Unit
Cambridge, UK

P. J. Saunders

Sandwell Primary Care Trust
West Bromwich
West Midlands, UK

Alex Scott-Samuel

Department of Public Health
University of Liverpool
Liverpool, UK

Fiona Sim

London Teaching Public Health Network
London School of Hygiene and Tropical Medicine
London, UK

Don Sinclair

NHS Solutions for Public Health
Oxford, UK

Lauren Smith

Office of the Commissioner
Massachusetts Department of Public Health
Boston MA, USA

Daniel M. Sosin

Coordinating Office for Terrorism Preparedness and Emergency Response,
Centers for Disease Control and Prevention,
Atlanta GA, USA

Chris Spencer Jones

NHS South Birmingham
Birmingham, UK

Nick Steel

School of Medicine, Health Policy and Practice
University of East Anglia
Norwich, UK

Andrew Stevens

Department of Public Health, Epidemiology and Biostatistics
University of Birmingham
Birmingham, UK

Alison Stewart

Foundation for Genomics and Public Health
Cambridge, UK

Roscoe Taylor

Department of Health and Human Services
Hobart, Australia

Barry Tennison

formerly Honorary Professor of Public Health and Policy
London School of Hygiene and Tropical Medicine
London, UK

Kasisomayajula Viswanath

Harvard School of Public Health
Boston MA, USA

Jeanette Ward

Department of Epidemiology and Community Medicine University of Ottawa, Ottawa, Canada

Stuart Whitaker
The Centre for Occupational
Health and Wellbeing Ltd, UK

Gareth Williams
School of Social Sciences
Cardiff University
Cardiff, UK

John Wright
Epidemiology and Public Health
Bradford Teaching Hospitals NHS
Trust
Bradford, UK

Introduction

Since the first edition of this book was published in 2001, international security, health protection, sustainable development, and human rights have all grown as challenges on the global health agenda. Public health practice responds to changing priorities, and to the problems that cannot be predicted. The *Oxford Handbook of Public Health Practice* outlines the methods that will help you to get started, whatever your assignment might be.

Public health problems are challenges to the 'science and art of preventing disease, prolonging life and promoting health through the organized efforts of society.'[1] Basic to the practice of public health are understandings of:

- collective responsibility, with a major role for the state in protecting and promoting the public's health
- preventive activity
- the determinants of health and disease, along a spectrum from socioeconomic determinants to the more immediate concerns of the quality of health care
- multi-disciplinary approaches, with partnerships of many kinds, including the populations served.[2]

The third edition of the Handbook updates a text that should continue to provide an introduction to working methods across this very broad field. Wherever possible, evidence for our approach is cited. Yet there are many activities in public health where the evidence for practice is still lacking. We have encouraged contributors to identify, wherever possible, what is best practice, while the careful reader will find that much still relies on the recommendations of experts. It will be clear that many opportunities for development of evidence in the field of public health remain.

The acknowledgements page lists former co-editors of this Handbook, David Pencheon, David Melzer, and Sir Muir Gray, who have each made helpful suggestions to this third edition. The current editorial group salutes the earlier work for the first and second editions. Our belief that the early development of the Handbook was sound is shown by the essential continuity of structure maintained for this third edition.

Although initially conceived for readers in developed countries, we were delighted that the World Health Organization included this Handbook in its Blue Trunk Library, a collection of essential texts distributed to parts of the globe in greatest need. For example, 100 Blue Trunks have been distributed in Afghanistan: we would be very pleased to learn from readers there how to improve the book for their use in future.

The basic roles for public health practice, as described in the Future of Public Health,[3] of assessment, policy development and assurance, continue. These roles are elaborated in different ways around the world to develop competencies for the local needs of public health practice.

We have reviewed many lists of competencies, and have adapted them in re-developing the table of contents for this edition.

Most topics have witnessed change since the second edition, reflected in the revision of chapters, and re-design of many areas for the book. While the intent of the book has not changed, there are new topics, and new emphases. These include sustainable development (broadly speaking, including climate change), information technology, translating evidence to policy, programme planning, control of expenditure, and the public health workforce. Some chapters explicitly address emerging issues, but this Handbook does not aim primarily to provide comprehensive factual information on new public health problems. We should emphasize that the focus of the book is method, rather than factual content.

Most readers of this book will already have a basic understanding of epidemiology and statistics. We trust that the many applied topics included will complement your understanding of, and capacity to make use of, these disciplines. The contents of the book are now briefly outlined.

Part 1 presents various assessment techniques to help formulate a public health problem. Particularly at the outset, this will often require perspectives from ethics and economics, as well as from health. Part 2 outlines the principles and practice of using data and evidence, to arrive at intelligence and information. Information should be the basis of action, with a wide range of examples in Part 3. Some of the Direct Action described is urgent; all of it is important activity for public health practitioners to understand. All public health practitioners are influenced by, and influence, health policy. How this happens, considering formulation and implementation of policy for public health, is the point of Part 4. Part 5 presents topics at the interface of public health practice and clinical care. Depending on the system you are working in, improvement in the quality and safety of healthcare may form a major part of your responsibilities, while the principles outlined here are generally transferable to a wide range of services that influence public health. We return to some basic personal and organizational issues for Parts 6 and 7. The methods and skills outlined here are essential to build on the assessments and policy elaborated earlier, for public health improvement throughout the health system, and sometimes in other sectors.

We invite your suggestions, on the Reader's comments card, to refine what public health practice can deliver in your country or community though future editions of this Handbook.

One generous review described this Handbook's first edition as the 'public health book of the year, if not the decade.'[4] Ten years later, that can only remain true if readers are also active as our critics. Your constructive engagement in future revisions of this text should add to practice that not only improves health, but also spreads hope and understanding, around the world.

CSG
WR
IK
IAL

References

1 Acheson ED. (1988). *Public health in England*, Report of the Committee of Inquiry into the future development of the public health function. HMSO, London.
2 Beaglehole R, Bonita R. (1997). *Public health at the crossroads*. Cambridge University Press, Cambridge.
3 Committee for the Study of the Future of Public Health (1988). *The future of public health*. National Academy Press, Washington DC.
4 Tiplady P. (2002). *Public Health*, **116,** 384.

Part 1

Assessment

1.1 Scoping public health problems

Gabriele Bammer

Objectives

This chapter aims to help you figure out what you can most effectively do, within the constraints of the resources you have, to address the public health problem you are concerned with.

What does scoping mean?

Scoping is the process of identifying all the aspects of the problem that are important before setting priorities for the approach that we will take to it. This allows us to use available resources most effectively. Aims include making the needs of the problem central (rather than our own expertise), ensuring that contentious issues are recognized and addressed, and focusing beyond individual behaviours to political, social, environmental, business, and other influences.

Scoping is the preparatory stage of a project where we systematically think about what we can best do with the time, money, and people we have at our disposal in order to use those resources most effectively. It involves considering:

- What is most important for addressing the problem?
- What needs to be done to get there?
- Who needs to be on-side?
- What are the likely blocks and how can they be overcome?

Why is scoping an important public health skill?

Scoping is particularly important as it helps us:

- broaden our view of the problem beyond what we know and understand, recognizing and respecting different points of view
- decide if we want to challenge the way in which the problem is generally dealt with, by paying more attention to something society sees as marginal or has excluded
- consider issues of legitimacy
- set boundaries.

A central aspect of scoping is to start by broadening the view of the problem, to move us beyond our own outlook and to help us see the problem through the eyes of others. The aim is to appreciate what various disciplines and stakeholders can contribute. The approach taken is then not limited to what we know. In this way, the problem becomes central, rather than our own expertise.

This process involves recognizing and respecting different points of view, giving us a rich understanding of the problem and an array of possible responses. Interestingly, in controversial areas, paying attention to the range of arguments also often smooths the path to compromise. Views may soften once people feel they have been respectfully heard. In addition, if people know that all reasonable alternatives have been considered, they will usually be more satisfied with the choice that is made. Therefore, starting off with a broad approach can help get people on-side for the action that is eventually decided upon (see Box 1.1.1).

Box 1.1.1 Feasibility of a heroin trial

In the 1990s, I led a major study investigating the feasibility of trialling diamorphine (pharmaceutical heroin) prescription as a treatment for heroin dependence.[1] We took opposition to the trial proposal very seriously, investigating—**and finding ways to respond to**—concerns raised by police, ex-users, the general community, and others. To our surprise, that process turned many opponents into supporters.

In addition, by considering a range of perspectives, scoping helps us decide whether a fresh approach is needed to the problem, perhaps even one that challenges conventional thinking. Are there aspects of the problem that are currently not taken into account or that are on the periphery, which should be more central?

When the status quo is challenged or controversial issues tackled, issues of legitimacy often come into play. Who is funding the project? Which organizations, researchers, and stakeholders are involved? These are important in helping determine whether the project is attempting to be even-handed or is pushing a particular point of view.

The end product of scoping is to consciously set effective boundaries around how we will address the problem. Scoping helps us get to the nub of an issue, rather than tinkering at the margins or reinventing the wheel. There is always a limit to what any project can attempt, but we often do not realize the extent to which we have control over what we undertake. We can decide what is central, what is marginalized and what can be ignored in our project.

This is particularly important when resources are very limited. It helps us plan ahead, so that we can finish the project, rather than running out of money or time halfway through. Scoping may also be able to identify a way to proceed that is most likely to lead to more resources later.

Eight questions useful for scoping

- What is already known about the problem?
- What can different stakeholders and academic disciplines contribute to addressing this problem?
- Which areas are contentious?
- What are the big-picture issues? In other words, what are the political, social, and cultural aspects of the problem?

and

- Why is this problem on the agenda now?
- What support and resources are likely to be available for tackling the problem?
- Which parts of the problem are already well covered and where are the areas of greatest need?
- Where can the most strategic interventions be made?

The first four questions help identify the dimensions of the problem, while the last four help set priorities.

Addressing the scoping questions

Finding out what is already known about the problem

A key issue here is to systematically review the literature about previous research on the problem. 📖 Chapter 2.7 provides guides for how to do this. Other sources of existing information may also be relevant, such as government white papers, non-government organization position papers, and business group statements.

Working with stakeholders and disciplines

In terms of figuring out how existing knowledge might best be built on, liaison with a range of stakeholders and academic disciplines is critical. Key steps include:

- identifying which stakeholders and disciplines are relevant
- finding appropriate representatives
- getting their input
- rewarding them.

It is useful to cast the net widely to identify relevant players. As well as using the review of existing knowledge, we should think laterally and use our contacts and networks. It may be useful to identify two categories of stakeholders—those affected by the problem and those in a position to influence the problem—and to ensure that both are adequately included.

📖 Chapter 3.4 takes us through the issues of representativeness and input from consumers, who are usually those affected by the problem. In terms of those who can influence the problem, representativeness tends to be less of an issue. Instead, targeting the most appropriate decision makers and practitioners may be more critical. For example, there is little point involving local government officials if the decision-making power rests with the national government.

Targetting is also important in terms of disciplinary input, as disciplines are usually quite heterogeneous in terms of what they cover. Finding the right kind of expertise for the problem is therefore the challenge. For instance, a sociologist with ethnographic skills is not particularly useful if a national survey will provide the most pertinent data.

Key questions to ask ourselves before seeking input from stakeholders and disciplinary experts are:

• How can they make a meaningful contribution?
• How can we ensure they will be listened to respectfully?
• Will what they say actually be taken into account?

This will guide how we seek input and is also a critical aspect of reward. Recognition involves being included and taken seriously, as well as being kept informed about how their input was used and, eventually, what outcomes were achieved.

Dealing with areas of contention

While it can be tempting to avoid areas of contention, it is generally advisable to deal with them explicitly and early. It helps greatly to be dispassionate and sincerely open to hearing all arguments, as well as to identify the basis of the controversy—for example, is it a clash of egos, a misunderstanding resulting from poor communication, a conflict of interests, or a difference in values? This helps us think about how we want to position our approach to the public health issue and if we want to try to resolve the disagreement.

There are a number of participatory methods that can help people understand why others think differently.[2] In general, people respond positively if they feel confident that their views are being heard and taken seriously. Then, even if they disagree with the final approach that is taken, they will often think it is fair.

Legitimacy particularly comes into play here (see Box 1.1.2). Taking a dispassionate stance only works if it is genuine and demonstrable.

Box 1.1.2 Legitimacy of the World Commission on Dams

The World Commission on Dams aimed to provide a balanced assessment of how effective large dams had been in providing irrigation, electricity, flood control, and water supply, and at what cost, especially in terms of country debt burden, displacement and impoverishment of populations, and disturbance of ecosystem and fishery resources. Legitimacy came through its origins in a workshop hosted by the World Conservation Union and the World Bank, which was attended by representatives of pro- and anti-dam interests. It systematically furthered its legitimacy by striving for balance between these interests among its 12 commissioners and its 68 member stakeholder forum, as well as its broad funding base drawing on 53 public, private and civil society organizations.[3]

What can we do if we are not disinterested, but are pushing for a particular outcome? Read the chapters on advocacy and activism (📖 Chapters 4.5 and 6.8)! The issue becomes one of understanding the opposition and being able to counter it—both through being able to draw on a wide range of allies and being able to effectively frame our argument.

Tackling big-picture issues

Tackling the big picture issues is specifically linked to the stakeholders who can influence the problem. The point here is to move beyond considering the problem just in terms of individual behaviours to also take into account, for example, the influence of government policy, advertising, and business practice. Changes here can be more far-reaching and effective.

On the one hand, we should view these perspectives as we would those of any other stakeholder, i.e. something that we need to respectfully take into account. Steps include finding out who the key actors are, if there is any formal level of co-ordination, and what level of authority the actors and the co-ordinating group carry. We should attempt to involve players who can represent big-picture issues and not just assume that they will not be interested. They may well be aware of the problem and welcome an opportunity to be involved in dealing with it.

On the other hand, we need to recognize the power imbalance and that the key players may not see the problem under consideration as being of any consequence or may not wish to legitimize our activity by participating in it, especially if it threatens their interests. We must exercise extra caution, so that these stakeholders do not hijack the agenda, bog the process down or stymie action.

Setting priorities

The same processes of discussions with key players and lateral thinking are also key to setting priorities. Understanding the big-picture context of the problem is particularly useful for figuring out why the problem is on the agenda now and the points of strategic intervention. Clarifying what is already known about the problem will point to what is well covered and give some ideas about the areas of greatest need. The latter will be enhanced by discussions with a wide range of disciplinary experts and stakeholders. Such discussions will also highlight the level of support available for tackling the problem and possibly identify additional resources.

An iterative process

An iterative, rather than a linear, process in addressing the eight scoping questions will most probably work best and reduces the danger of getting bogged down, especially when charting unfamiliar territory.

The judicious use of experts is crucial to saving time and maintaining momentum. The challenge is to discern what is needed to put together an understanding of the problem, what we know and don't know, and who to bring in to fill the gaps. As new players are brought into the picture, their contributions may lead us to revisit our understandings of what is known or the areas of disagreement or the priorities. We must be open to this, but we also need a clear sense of direction so that we are not diverted by less relevant agendas which other players may have.

Back-to-back spirals are illustrative of the process—the outward expansion of the top spiral indicates the build-up of knowledge and perspectives, whereas the inward direction of the second shows the knowledge and perspectives being used to set priorities (Figure 1.1.1). The loops illustrate revisiting what is known, bringing in other people who might have a useful perspective, and so on. As the figure illustrates, the starting point may be somewhat off centre; in other words, our own knowledge and expertise may be limited, but the end point of scoping is an action plan that addresses central issues.

'Reality testing' can profitably be undertaken at several points. The aim here is to find holes in the knowledge base or the arguments on which priorities are based and, from this, to highlight where further data gathering or consultation is required. This is where advisory and reference groups can be invaluable, as they can be asked to comment along the way.

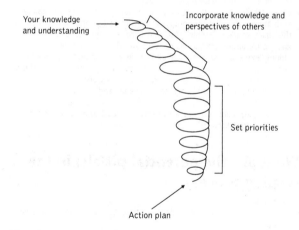

Your knowledge and understanding

Incorporate knowledge and perspectives of others

Set priorities

Action plan

Figure 1.1.1 Broadening, aligning, and focusing perspectives.

What are the competencies needed for effective scoping?

Key competencies include:
- integrity (including being clear about whether or not we are dispassionate)
- credibility in terms of acknowledged expertise about the problem and/or the scoping process
- possession of a wide-ranging network of contacts, so that we know the key players or an intermediary who can provide access to them
- skill in facilitating meetings and interactions, including encouraging open debate and the challenging of ideas, handling negotiations and conflict, and creating a positive atmosphere
- management skills
- an open mind to ideas from others
- the ability to think laterally and creatively
- understanding the 'cultures' of different stakeholders and the ability to empathize with different concerns, without being captured by them
- the ability to identify which disciplines are relevant and enough knowledge about the disciplines to know what they can offer, to identify experts, and to involve experts in working on the problem
- understanding the relevant policies and other big-picture issues, their history, the key players, and the political sensitivities
- the ability to integrate a range of knowledge and expertise, to cut through to the essentials, and to lead a priority-setting process
- the ability to build alliances with those we need to have on-side in order to move forward.

What are the potential pitfalls in the scoping process?

Potential pitfalls include:
- *Not having enough resources*: including time, to undertake an adequate process
- *No real commitment*: by those in a position to act to understanding and dealing with the problem. For example, a process can be set in train for reasons of political expediency and the plug may be pulled as soon as the political heat dies down
- *Not being the right person for the job*: for example, if we are not interested in this process, not experienced enough to keep control, or if we cannot deal with a diverse range of views respectfully
- *Getting bogged down*: losing momentum and timeliness can be fatal. Beware of wallowing in factual detail, meetings without a clear purpose, and red herrings. We should not feel that we have to be on top of all the material, but instead rely on experts who understand the stakeholder or disciplinary perspectives.

- *Choosing inappropriate representatives of stakeholders:* involving people in a process helps legitimize their point of view and we should think carefully about including fringe groups. If people who are not well-regarded are included in the process, respected players may pull out or not participate fully
- *An inappropriate balance:* the problem has to be seen in perspective, so that the process involves an appropriate mix of stakeholders and academic disciplines, the powerful and the powerless, and, for a dispassionate approach to contentious issues, different points of view
- *Avoiding the contentious issues:* ignoring particular groups in an attempt to avoid controversial issues will often backfire, with their exclusion providing them with additional opportunity to further their cause and even undermining the outcomes of the process
- *Exhausting key players:* stakeholder representatives and experts from particular disciplines usually have a substantive job to do and they may get no recognition or credit for being involved in our scoping process. Use their time wisely, sparingly, and efficiently
- *Promoting conflict:* scoping processes that involve contentious issues usually seek to find compromise, but if the players are not chosen carefully and the process is not handled appropriately, conflict can be escalated, rather than reduced
- *Not showing leadership:* if we do not show leadership when we are in charge of the scoping process, it is open to being hijacked by the more powerful participants. This can also be a factor in the promotion of conflict
- *Avoiding decisions:* never underestimate the temptation not to make a decision when the problem is difficult or contentious. Yield not to temptation!
- *Not being prepared to combat the wrath of the powerful:* when scoping processes involve challenging entrenched power bases, provoking a reaction could well be a measure of success. The challenge is not to be naïve and to be prepared to counter these forces
- Not learning from our mistakes
- *Inexperience:* this can be overcome by finding mentors, powerful allies, and supportive colleagues.

How will you know when you have been successful?

Markers of success are an approach to the problem that has:

- broad-based support
- clear and implementable steps for increasing understanding and moving to a solution
- commitment from the key players and the stakeholders they represent to stay involved in seeking a solution
- respect between opponents.

For issues where a major power base has been challenged and where the power base is seeking to protect its interests, measures of success include:

- a coalition that includes people of influence, which will stand up to the power base and continue to fight for the solution
- openings for negotiation.

A successful scoping process lays a strong foundation for effectively tackling a problem, and increases the chances of developing a solution on budget and on time.

Further resources

Arksey H, O'Malley L. (2005). Scoping studies: towards a methodological framework. *International Journal of Social Research Methodolgy*, **7**, 19–32.

Executive Office of the President, Council on Environmental Quality (1981). *Memorandum for general counsels, NEPA liaisons and participants in scoping*. Available at: ℘ http://ceq.hss.doe.gov/nepa/regs/scope/scoping.htm (accessed 19 August 2010).

Mulvihill PR. (2003). Expanding the scoping community. *Environmental Impact Assessment Review*, **23**, 39–49.

Wood G, Glasson J, Becker J. (2006). EIA scoping in England and Wales: practitioner approaches, perspectives and constraints. *Environmental Impact Assessment Review*, **26**, 221–41.

References

1 Bammer G. (1997). The ACT heroin trial: intellectual, practical and political challenges. The 1996 Leonard Ball Oration. *Drug & Alcohol Review*, **16**, 287–96.

2 McDonald D, Bammer G, Deane P. (2009). *Research integration using dialogue methods*. Australian National University E Press, Canberra. Available at: ℘ http://epress.anu.edu.au/dialogue_methods_citation.html.

3 World Commission on Dams. (2000). *Dams and development: a new framework for decision-making*. Earthscan, London. Available at: ℘ http://pubs.iied.org/pdfs/9126IIED.pdf

1.2 Priorities and ethics in health care

Sian M. Griffiths, Robyn Martin, and Don Sinclair

Objectives

As a result of reading this chapter you will be able to:
- understand the language of ethics and the role ethics plays in public health
- recognize ways in which public health ethics differ from bioethics
- understand the principles of priority-setting within a constrained budget
- appreciate how ethics should underpin public health interventions
- appreciate the importance of ethics-based public health policy-making

Definitions

- *Ethics* constitute a coherent and consistent system of morality, values, virtues, and responsibilities that guide issues such as who should make health decisions, how those decisions are made and the principles that should underpin health decisions. Ethics serve as 'a beacon to warn of the danger and to show the way—as a lighthouse . . .'.[1] In summary, 'ethics' refers to a variety of techniques for understanding the moral life, i.e. how an act is judged to be right or wrong.[2]
- *Public health ethics* constitute the system of morality, values, virtues, and responsibilities that guides decision-makers with responsibility for the health of populations. Such a system may be implicit or explicit, but in a democracy, where legitimacy ultimately derives from the people, it may be highly desirable to codify the principles that are used to justify decisions. This allows the people to understand and possibly challenge the process by which decisions are taken.
- *Public health ethics differ from the body of bioethics:* bioethics govern the relationships between healthcare providers and consumers of health services. This distinction becomes particularly evident when considering that a provider of healthcare generally has a direct duty of care to each individual patient, whether this duty is defined by national statute or regulation, or by a local commissioning agreement, such as may be made between a hospital and a commissioner. In private healthcare, the duty to provide care for a patient is typically defined by an individual's personal contract with a provider or by the terms of an insurance policy.

- Unlike bioethics, *public health ethics recognize that there will be circumstances where the health of the wider population justifies overriding the autonomy and rights of the individual.* The decision-maker with responsibility for the health of a population may be required to balance the needs of different individuals or groups within this population and to allocate resources between them, even if this disadvantages some individuals compared to others.
- *Priority setting* describes a process by which an explicit decision is made to provide some health services, rather than other services. Such decisions may directly compare two or more services, or may evaluate one service against a set of criteria, and recommend that it be provided if it meets certain thresholds (e.g. sufficient clinical benefit for an acceptable cost). It is relatively straightforward to compare the clinical- or cost-effectiveness of two treatments that are used for the same disease. If both produce the same clinical benefit it may be sensible to provide the less expensive. If one provides greater clinical benefit than the other, it may be necessary to compare the cost-benefit ratios for each treatment in order to recommend the more cost-effective treatment. Sometimes a health service commissioner may not be able to provide a treatment that would otherwise be regarded as cost-effective, because the overall cost would be prohibitive.
- *Ethics should underpin decisions about health care priorities*: the distinction between the ethical responsibilities of healthcare providers and those of public health decision-makers is not always clear cut. For example, a healthcare provider may be required to offer a scarce resource (e.g. intensive care beds) to those patients most likely to benefit from this resource, rather than to other patients. This situation is most likely to arise in response to a major local or national disaster (e.g. pandemic influenza) when health service capacity is overwhelmed. Judgements must then be made on which patients should or should not receive this scarce resource.
- *Ethics theories* are statements of principles that can be used to justify certain actions[3]. Such theories may provide a rational basis for decision-making, which is itself open to consultation and debate. Certain theories of ethics have assumed particular importance both for policy formulation and specific decision-making at various times in the history of the NHS. Currently, there is an intense focus on cost-containment across the system, while promoting individual choice of provider.
- *The prevailing (and sometimes opposing) ethics theories* that are used to justify particular decisions about the future of the NHS, as well as specific decisions about funding particular treatments include:
  - *utilitarianism*[4]—making decisions that result in the greatest good for the greatest number
  - *communitarianism*—making decisions that arise from the values and traditions of local communities and populations
  - *liberal individualism*—based on rights theory (emphasizing the freedom of individuals to pursue their own ambitions, but recognizing that one person's entitlement might constitute another's obligation)

- *principle-based common morality theory*—where the set of values shared by members of a society give rise to principles of obligation e.g. recognition of individual rights and autonomy, obligations of beneficence and non-maleficence and justice—the fair distribution of benefits and risks.
- There has been increasing emphasis on improving the health of local communities and increasing their involvement in both public health and health service decision-making. This has included a degree of explicit communitarianism in that local government has been required to form partnerships with a variety of other local organizations to jointly assess the needs of the population for health improvement and make plans to improve health and reduce local inequalities. In England this process is called Joint Strategic Needs Assessment, and is still being supported during the current reorganization signalled in 2010.[5]

From 2001 an entire set of NHS reforms occurred in response to the NHS Plan[6]—based on the principles of autonomy (more patient involvement in service planning), utilitarianism (seeking to reduce management costs in order to improve investment in front-line services) and communitarianism (promoting local community involvement and oversight of health service decisions). The autonomy principle has influenced much of the recent market reforms in the English NHS, with the requirement for patients to be offered a wide choice of providers for most health services. The English NHS now faces further reform based on market principles with localism and less central regulation.

Why is ethics important for public health?

Making best use of limited resources—whether it is called rationing or priority setting—is a fact of life. Limited resources need to be made to go as far as possible. This means saying 'No' to some people, whilst others benefit. This is not a comfortable thing to do, but one in which many people in public health are necessarily involved. Competition for resources may be the result of a new treatment becoming available, demand growing for treatment because of increased patient awareness or because more people in an ageing population need the treatment. The pressures of innovation, public participation, patient expectation, person-focused care, political policies, and socioeconomic factors make priority setting a vital part of public health practice in ensuring the health of the local population.

All health services have their different ways of organizing healthcare delivery and of making choices about which services will be provided within budgets set by funders; be they through taxation, insurance, or personal out-of-pocket spending. With limited resources comes the necessity to make difficult choices and the need to ensure best value for the finances available.

In England the process for determining which services will be provided to a local population will depend on GP-led primary care-based organizations commissioning those services.

In Wales and Scotland, these decisions are made at national level. In not-for-profit organizations, contracts will be negotiated according to funders guidelines, and in private sector organizations they may be made by Boards of Directors.

Whatever the mechanism for deciding priorities, funders are faced with a host of service demands and difficult decisions. Mechanisms for deciding which new investment or disinvestment decisions should be made need to be founded on ethical principles and made within a transparent policy framework that not only clinicians and managers understand, but local people agree and accept.

Ethics serve an important role in providing a framework for public health policy and practice. This framework helps public health policy makers and practitioners to make difficult public health decisions, but also constrains policy-makers and practitioners from undertaking over-zealous interventions that potentially intrude unnecessarily into private lives.

Ethics also make transparent the assumptions and values underlying health decisions so as to enable open challenge and debate of those assumptions and values. It is particularly important to address the apparent conflict between the values of clinicians (who are trained to consider the needs of individual patients generally without explicit reference to the competing needs of other patients) and the values of commissioners (who are responsible for planning and procuring health services for entire populations and must balance the needs of different groups of patients). In order to bring both sets of values into the decision-making process, health service commissioners have been increasingly engaging clinicians in the commissioning process (clinical engagement).

Over the next few years, the current reorganization of the NHS in England will hand responsibility for commissioning most health services to groups of primary care clinicians (clinical leadership). It is anticipated that this will ensure the needs of local patients are addressed, but it will emphasize the potential conflict between the needs of individuals and the needs of the local population. It also increases the likelihood that access to services will vary across the country.

Box 1.2.1 Key questions

- How can we be fair when making rationing decisions?
- How do we account for our decisions?

Ethics are essential when applying the requirements of national programmes to commission services for local populations. The NHS in England is continually striving for greater efficiencies in order to better serve the public (see Box 1.2.1).

There is an ongoing programme to improve service quality while delivering greater efficiency. This is known as 'Quality, Innovation, Productivity and Prevention' (QIPP). The underlying premise is that clinicians can lead the process of providing (or commissioning) better services in a more cost-effective way if they take responsibility for developing better ways to make services available to patients, and cut out any unnecessary obstacles or waste in the system. The QIPP programme takes the view that new ways of working (innovation)—sometimes including new processes or even new technologies—can help patients receive care more effectively or more quickly, thus improving both quality (for the patient) and productivity (for the NHS).

Preventing ill-health or preventing complications (such as re-admission to hospital) also lead to better quality and more efficient use of resources. The QIPP programme has a number of national work streams focusing, for example, on long-term conditions, urgent care and end-of-life care, and aiming to improve quality and productivity across care pathways. QIPP is also supported by systematic sharing of good practice. It is easy to assume that there could be few challenges to the aims of QIPP, but its implementation in local populations can give rise to the sort of conflicts in values that require attention to ethics.

Healthcare commissioners have been examining situations where their populations have been receiving higher rates of some services than the national or local average. They have sought to understand whether this is the result of higher local need, or the result of more active providers seeking to increase their own work (and, hence, income). This has led to conflict between commissioners and providers over what is the appropriate level of activity for these services compared with local need. The resulting discussions are best informed by attention to an agreed ethics framework (see Box 1.2.2).

Box 1.2.2 Guidelines to clinicians

1. If you want something outside your current fixed envelope of resource, can it be done by substituting a treatment of less value?
2. If demand for your service is increasing, what criteria are you using to agree the threshold of treatment?
3. If you do not believe that it is possible to either draw thresholds of care or substitute treatment then within a fixed budget which service might you give a smaller resource to in order for you to enlarge yours?

Legislation and professional regulation already provide some policy and practice frameworks, but these more rigid frameworks are not always up-to-date, are not always appropriate to situations where urgent decisions need to be made, and are slow to amend where new public health threats emerge.

Ethics frameworks

These are codes of practice that can be applied to the process of decision-making to ensure consistency with an agreed set of values (e.g. autonomy and equity). They provide assistance in the gaps left by legislation and professional regulation, and can be useful tools for helping decide which populations have the greatest need for services or which services provide the best outcomes within available resources (Box 1.2.3).

> **Box 1.2.3 Example of the use of an ethical framework in practice**
>
> In 1997, Oxfordshire Health Authority developed an explicit priority-setting process to decide whether to invest in or disinvest from particular health services. It was based on three main principles:
> * Evidence of clinical effectiveness (and cost-effectiveness)
> * Fairness (treating patients fairly, avoiding discrimination, and reducing inequalities)
> * Patient choice (respecting patients as autonomous individuals and seeking to maximize their control over their own healthcare)

Ethics frameworks can be developed in consultation with communities and tested against the values of these communities. They can also be updated as necessary to reflect changes in community values or changes in the types of decision that need to be made.

It is important to see the use of ethics and tools (such as ethics frameworks) based on ethics principles as practical resources to help make consistent, transparent decisions that make sense within the context of community values. It is therefore appropriate to consider the criteria that may determine how a community considers a decision to be reasonable. In this context, a decision may be judged to be reasonable if it involves an appropriate group of people considering an appropriate question, using a process that is itself deemed reasonable. In the following section, two examples illustrate how this triumvirate of person, question, and process may operate at national or local level.

How do ethics assist in policy and practice governing the commissioning of hospital services?

English context

Within the English national health system, Parliament votes on departmental spending and therefore sets the overall budget for the Health Service. The Department of Health sets national priorities and allocates money to local decision-makers. Similar processes exist in the other countries within the UK. At a national level, the National Institute for Health and

Clinical Excellence (NICE) makes recommendations on whether certain services or technologies should be available throughout England and Wales. Whether decisions are made at national or local level, they are made in the context of a fixed amount of available resource. Investment in treatments for some groups of patients reduces the opportunity to fund treatments for other patients.

National decision-making

The National Institute for Health and Clinical Excellence (NICE) considers whether the NHS should invest in particular technologies in England and Wales. The questions (i.e. which technologies should be considered for use in which group of patients) are initially identified by expert committees, then tested with a group of stakeholders, including patients, healthcare providers, commissioners, and manufacturers.

The finalized questions are then considered by Government Ministers who provide a national policy perspective. Those questions deemed by Ministers to be appropriate for appraisal by NICE receive an expert assessment of the evidence and are considered in detail by appraisal committees whose members include representatives from a wide range of stakeholder groups (e.g. patients, carers, experts, professional bodies, providers, commissioners, and manufacturers). The committees hold part of their meetings in public (allowing a degree of transparency) and publish the documentation that is not deemed confidential (for commercial or academic reasons).

The appraisal committees have a defined process for considering evidence of clinical and cost-effectiveness, and for giving weight to certain groups of patients. There is a process for consulting the public where decisions are likely to lead to significant restrictions of the availability of a technology. Finally, there is a process by which a limited set of stakeholders can appeal against NICE's recommendations. From time to time, NICE undertakes public consultations to update its procedures.[7]

Under the current NHS reforms, the role of NICE is set to expand. Although it will continue assessing technologies, it will take on responsibility for determining the standards for health and social care that will apply throughout England and Wales. NICE will also have an increased role in making recommendations about public health interventions.

As local government takes on more direct responsibility for health improvement, NICE will produce guidelines to assist the commissioning of preventative and health-promoting services. It is likely that NICE will need to develop new ways to value the benefits of such services compared with the clinical services with which it is familiar. It may also be required to make decisions based on very different forms of evidence. Most new clinical technologies are proposed on the basis of evidence collected from clinical trials, the majority of which are intervention studies. To assess the effectiveness and cost-effectiveness of health promotion interventions delivered in natural communities may depend on more observational studies.

Local decision making (Box 1.2.4)

Box 1.2.4 Case study: using a framework of ethics in making difficult choices: experience from Oxford

An ethics framework was structured around three main components:

Evidence of effectiveness
- Consider:
  - Is there good evidence that the treatment is not effective?
  - Is there good evidence that the treatment is effective?
  - Is there a lack of good evidence either way?
- It is desirable to obtain good quality evidence about effectiveness, and research aimed at obtaining such evidence should be encouraged. However, when evidence is poor, then a judgement about the likely effectiveness has to be made in the knowledge that good quality evidence is not available.

Equity
The basic principle of equity (fairness) is that people with similar needs should be treated similarly. This principle should be applied consistently at different times and in different settings, with no discrimination on grounds that are irrelevant to the need for healthcare.

In developing the principles on which equity is based, two broad approaches can be taken:
- maximizing the welfare of patients within the budget available (a utilitarian approach), often expressed in terms of the cost-effectiveness of different health services
- giving priority to those in most need (a rights approach).

Patient choice
Respecting patients' wishes and enabling patients to have control over their healthcare are important values (the principle of autonomy based on liberal individualism). Within those healthcare interventions that are purchased, patients should be enabled to make their own choices about which treatment they want to receive. It is a matter of fundamental respect that patients should always be treated as much as autonomous individuals as possible. This is one of the stated reasons for the active promotion of patient choice of provider that is a feature of recent health service reforms in England.

When considering the principle of patient choice, it is important to recognize that the principle of effectiveness is usually addressed by considering the best available evidence from well-conducted published studies. These studies normally consider the effectiveness of a treatment in a large group of patients. Sometimes the evidence suggests that a treatment generally provides insufficient benefit (or is too expensive) to be provided. However, each patient is unique and there may be a good reason to believe that a particular patient stands to gain significantly more from the treatment than most of those who formed the study group in the relevant research. Evidence that this individual patient has significantly different circumstances compared with most patients may be used to demonstrate *exceptional circumstances*. This may justify such a patient receiving treatment that is not normally provided.

This ethics framework was used in the process of making decisions to:

- Structure discussion and ensure that the important points were properly considered
- Ensure consistent decision-making, over time and with respect to decisions concerning different clinical settings
- Enable articulation of the reasons for decisions that are made.

Since 2002, Primary Care Trusts (PCTs) were responsible for commissioning most health services in England. In an effort to rationalize and strengthen their decision-making processes, nine PCTs in central South East England (responsible for health services for 4.2 million people) merged the processes they had developed for choosing how or whether to commission certain specific interventions. This led to the creation of a single shared process for selecting the questions to be addressed, and a single process for reviewing evidence, consulting local clinicians, and preparing documentation. Two Priorities Committees were established (out of four predecessor committees) where patients, clinicians, and managers representing both commissioning and provider organizations consider the evidence against the criteria contained in a common ethical framework.[8] This shared ethical framework is based on the principles of utilitarianism (effectiveness, cost-effectiveness, and affordability), autonomy (individual need and the ability to make decisions), and communitarianism (needs of the community). It specifically includes provision for addressing horizontal equity (attributing the same value to people with the equivalent needs) and vertical equity (giving priority to people who have greater needs in order to reduce inequalities). The Priorities Committees base their decisions on a thorough review of available published evidence, together with comments from local clinicians (requiring effective clinical engagement). They do not meet in public, but their recommendations are made to the PCTs, which choose, in their public board meetings, whether to adopt them as formal policies, thus affording a degree of public scrutiny. As the current Health Service reforms intend to abolish PCTs in 2013, it remains to be seen whether the new General Practice Commissioning Consortia will seek to maintain a common prioritization process.

How do ethics assist in policy and practice governing the treatment of patients in general practice?

General practitioners (GPs) are usually independent practitioners contracted to provide NHS services to registered patients. In general, their contracts require them to provide services that they deem 'necessary and appropriate' for individual patients. These contracts do not take account of any duty to balance resources between different patient groups, but increasingly GPs are being asked to make collective decisions about prescribing drugs or commissioning services based on the needs of populations. This conflict between the needs of individuals and the needs of populations will become more apparent as GPs take on responsibility for commissioning hospital services under the latest NHS reorganization.[5] There will be direct conflict between the principles of autonomy (as expressed by 'patient choice') and utilitarianism, which seeks to use resources to obtain the greatest good for the population (even if this means that some individuals do not receive the best care available to them).

If the current NHS reforms are to successfully deliver clinically-led commissioning, with groups of GPs acting collectively to secure the best care for their patients, it will be necessary for legislation to address these conflicts between duties to the individual and the population. An ethics framework would be a useful tool to assist such decision-making. If the local population and other stakeholders are involved in its development, this should add legitimacy (by the principle of communitarianism) to the decision making process and provide transparency (respecting the principle of autonomy).

How do ethics assist in policy and practice governing the prevention and control of communicable diseases?

Medical science has provided many solutions for the threat of communicable diseases through the development of vaccinations, antivirals, and antibiotics. However, not all diseases can be controlled by vaccination and drugs. This is particularly the case where disease carriers and contacts refuse to co-operate with medical practitioners, and where new diseases emerge for which no treatments or vaccines have yet been developed. Public health legislation often provides powers of isolation, quarantine, exclusion from public places, and in some cases compulsory screening, treatment, and vaccination (see Boxes 1.2.5 and 1.2.6). Even when legislation provides these powers, it tends to leave to the discretion of the public health practitioner when to implement them. Ethics assists in decisions on when to exercise powers that potentially infringe autonomy and rights.

Box 1.2.5 Case A: should you detain against his will someone with multidrug-resistant resistant tuberculosis (MDR-TB) who refuses to remain in voluntary isolation?

There may be good public health arguments to justify long-term detention of the patient to prevent the spread of MDR-TB to others who come into contact with him. Legislation in most states provides powers to detain in these circumstances. However, a 'power' implies exercise of discretion. If there were no discretion there would be a duty to detain, rather than a power.

What ethics principles govern the exercise of this power? A utilitarian approach suggests that a coercive measure, such as detention might be taken where the overall benefit to society resulting from detention outweighs the overall loss to society.[9] How do you measure such benefit and loss? You need to undertake a risk assessment in relation to the patient, based on available scientific evidence about the disease: How infectious is this condition? How much contact does the patient have with others? How responsible is he in his health behaviours?

Evidence is also needed on the consequences of imposing coercive measures. Will other patients go underground to avoid detention? Will detention discourage ill persons from seeking diagnosis? What will be the economic and social consequences to the patient and his family of detention? Does detention pose the risk of discrimination, stigma, and marginalization? Are there any other alternatives to detention that might work better for the patient? Would you choose to detain other patients in the same situation or is there something about this patient that leads to you treating him differently?

Duties of beneficence and non-maleficence tell you that you need to do what is best for the patient and to do him no harm, so arguments that it is for the good of society to detain him will need to be convincing to override the patient's right to autonomy and private life.

The need for a professional risk assessment imposes duties on the public health community to develop an evidence base to underpin such risk assessments, and a duty on individuals working in public health to keep up to date on evidence. Any such measure should only be taken where there is a demonstrable public health benefit to be achieved.

Box 1.2.6 Case B: in case of a disease pandemic, for which there are limited health resources, who should have priority access to those resources?

This is an issue unregulated by legislation, and provides an example of a situation in which ethics must step in the fill the gaps left by law. There will be conflicting ethical obligations in such a case. Healthcare providers owe duties of beneficence to all patients, suggesting a duty to provide healthcare to every patient who needs health resources. Where resources are limited, however, duties of beneficence do not assist in choices between patients.

Triage principles will suggest that resources should be given to those most likely to benefit from treatment, underpinned by ethics arguments that limited resources should be used as efficiently and effectively as possible. A utilitarian approach will support the view that priority should be given to those persons who will be essential to the functioning of society during the pandemic. This would suggest that health care workers themselves, as well as other essential service workers should be prioritized over other patients. It may justify priority for mothers of families with small children, or other carers within society. Utilitarianism will also support the view that priority should be given to the treatment that is most effective in reducing the spread of disease to others.

Other ethics theories, particularly theories of ethics of care, will support prioritizing for treatment those persons with the longest productive life years ahead of them. Opposing ethics arguments might criticize these approaches as discriminatory and suggest that a lottery for resources, or a first-come-first serve approach would be fairer.

Ethics debate will not produce a clear and convincing answer to an ethical 'hard case' such as this. However, an ethics framework will provide language and tools for debate, and demand transparency in relation to the values and virtues underpinning choices.

How do ethics assist in policy and practice governing the prevention and control of non-communicable diseases?

The ethics of public health interventions in the case of non-communicable diseases are more complex. Whereas communicable disease infringements of the private behaviour of individuals can be justified on the basis of prevention of the spread of disease to the wider population, non-communicable diseases, in most cases, result from individual life choices and most directly affect the persons making those choices (see Boxes 1.2.7 and 1.2.8).

Box 1.2.7 Case C: should the state intervene to prevent an individual from smoking in a public place?

Mill's 'harm principle' states that 'the only purpose for which power can be rightfully exercised over any member of a civilized community, against his will, is to prevent harm to others. His own good, either physical or moral, is not a sufficient warrant'.[10]

The harms of first- and second-hand tobacco smoke are well documented.[11] In the case of smoking in a public place, we can begin by arguing that we are prohibiting smoking to protect other people at risk of being affected by tobacco smoke, in which case the ethics issues are similar to those in the case of communicable disease. What if all the other persons in the room are consenting adults who are themselves smoking, or if the smoker is sufficiently far from any other person such that any risk is negligible? Then we will need to look for other less direct harm to justify intervention, such as the social costs to the family and friends of the smoker if he should suffer smoking harms, and the cost to society of resulting health care.

Our ethics arguments may also to turn to the extent to which the smoker or his companions are autonomous persons making informed decisions on their own health, for Mill's harm principle is premised on the autonomy of the individual. Has the smoker made a free and non-manipulated informed choice to smoke? We can argue, using the science of behavioural psychology, that influences such as tobacco advertising, smoking in the media and peer pressure have distorted the smoker's ability to make a free and informed choice and caused him to put his health at risk by smoking.[12] Ethics arguments would then suggest that public health institutions have a responsibility at least to counter the malign influences so as to restore the autonomy of the individual. Similar arguments apply to the state's duty to address obesity harms by limiting advertising and misleading labelling of high fat, salt and sugar products.

Box 1.2.8 Case D: should the state impose taxes on the purchase of alcohol to limit alcohol-related harms?

Excessive alcohol use causes health harms to individuals, and social and economic harms to family and society.[13] Evidence suggests that, because it is price sensitive alcohol consumption can be manipulated by the pricing of alcohol[14] increasing alcohol taxes serves both to reduce alcohol harms and to increase government revenues to support health care and other public goods. This suggests the state has a public duty to use taxation as a tool to the benefit of the public's health.

However, as with smoking restrictions, alcohol taxation serves to restrict the liberty of the individual to make a lifestyle choice. We can argue that reducing alcohol levels will benefit the health of drinkers, although these arguments are not as strong as they are in relation to tobacco unless drinking is excessive. However Mill's harm principle suggests that this is not sufficient to warrant intervention. People choose to drink alcohol because it gives them pleasure even when they are aware of the risks posed to their health.

We can justify countering alcohol industry advertising with health messages to restore autonomous decision-making, but it is more difficult to justify interfering with the choice to drink alcohol. We may also justify interventions into excessive drinking, though it is arguable that even here we are interfering with autonomy. The difficulty lies in interventions that affect careful and sensible consumption of alcohol.[15]

It can also be argued that taxation of products operates in a discriminatory manner, in that an increase in alcohol prices will affect the choices of the less well off more significantly than those of the better off. Arguments that have been used to support tobacco taxation, given the inherent harmfulness of tobacco, are not as persuasive here. Nor is alcohol the only product, not harmful in itself, but only in excessive use, willingly and widely consumed.

We might argue that we should also impose high taxes on food stuffs, sweets, and snacks that, when consumed in excess, can cause dental and health harms, and which result in significant economic costs to society. Any state initiative that is not transparent and evidence-based will be contrary to ethics, regardless of the benefit of the outcome. The end does not justify the means. Hence, the ethics of alcohol taxation are complex, and dependent on a solid scientific evidence base. There will always be counter-arguments. Once again, the language and theories of ethics will serve as a useful framework to facilitate transparent debate.

How do ethics assist in policy and practice governing the prevention of unintentionally harmful acts?

As demonstrated above, legislation may be used in a number of ways to restrict the autonomy of individuals both for their benefit and for wider societal benefits. When considering potentially harmful acts, it is useful to consider the balance of harms and benefits, and how these are distributed in society.

Legislation requiring that most car drivers wear seatbelts is an infringement of individual autonomy. It is paternalistic in that the state has chosen to intervene on behalf of the citizen, possibly against the wishes of the citizen. However, it is justified by the reduction in fatalities and particular forms of injuries suffered by car drivers. As such, it appears that the harms and benefits affect the same people, i.e. drivers. However, there are additional benefits to the rest of society in that the reduction in harm to drivers is associated with a reduction in health care costs to the NHS (and thus to the general public). This leaves more resources available for other patients, and the restriction of drivers' autonomy can therefore be justified by the principles of utilitarianism.

It is salutary to remember that when the compulsory seatbelt legislation was being debated, there were many opponents who not only saw this as an infringement of civil liberties, but also posed counter arguments e.g. the belief that drivers would be more likely to drive recklessly if they wore seat belts and therefore considered themselves protected. As in the case for alcohol taxation, it is necessary to consider evidence and rational argument very carefully and to balance the respective ethics principles when formulating policy.

Responding to changing policy

The model developed in Oxford (Box 1.2.4), England, was driven by the market culture of the mid-1990s, and in particular the contract culture and extra-contractual referrals. The election of a new government in 1997 brought with it changes in political philosophy, as well as policy. The mode of choice and decision-making changed. However, with the election of the Coalition government in 2010 emphasis has once more shifted to a more libertarian and free market philosophy.

The role of public health in supporting decisions about priorities for health and health care for a population will be crucial, although mechanisms for providing this support as yet remain unclear. Changing structures continue to pose a challenge. NHS providers will become Foundation Trusts and will compete with a diverse supply of 'any willing 'providers in the public and private sectors for referrals without geographic constraint. Underlying these policies is the political strategy to devolve choice, and the funding to support it, to the front line, monitored through the regulatory frameworks of the National Commissioning Board. The tension between individual and population decision-making underscores the need for a mechanism to discuss questions such as:

- How much will local decision-making be able to take into account the needs of the population not just for elective health care, but for prevention or long-term care?
- What values will underline these decisions. For example, it is easier to calculate the cost of a quality-adjusted life year (QALY) for a new drug than for a night-sitting service in palliative care, but which is of greater value to the patient dying of cancer?
- How should one value lifestyle drugs compared with counselling in general practice?
- What is the value of prescriptions for exercise?

Whatever national systems develop, the need remains for local systems of priority set within the context of overall guidance.

Role of public health practitioners and teams

Within health economies and organizations, public health provides the support to take an overview across the community and to balance external needs of local communities. This may involve balancing issues concerning community safety or domestic violence, with needs specific to the health service, such as balancing competing hospital priorities.

The skills of needs assessment, critical appraisal, application of evidence-based care and management of risk that are key to public health are all needed to develop this role.

Whatever changes occur to the structure of the health services, local clinicians will continue to make decisions on a patient by patient basis, guided by accepted good practice guidelines. The difficulty of balancing resources can be assisted by clear processes and common ethics values, with the development of appropriate decision-making frameworks within which trade-offs can be made. To do this requires open and mature debate.

References

1 Miké V. (2003). Evidence and the future of medicine. *Evaluation and the Health Professions,* **26**, 127.
2 Beauchamp T, Childress J. (1994). *Principles of biomedical ethics*, 4th edn. Oxford University Press, Oxford.
3 Griffiths S, Jewell T, Hope T. (2006). Setting priorities in health care. In: Pencheon D, Guest C, Melzer D, Muir Gray JA, eds, *Oxford handbook of public health practice*, 2nd edn, pp. 404–10. Oxford University Press, Oxford.
4 Mill J. (1969). Utilitarianism. In: *Collected Works of John Stuart Mill*, Vol 10. University of Toronto Press, Toronto.
5 Department of Health (2010). *Equity and excellence: liberating the NHS*. HMSO, London.
6 Department of Health (2000). *The NHS plan: a plan for investment, a plan for reform*. HMSO, London.
7 National Institute for Health and Clinical Excellence (2012). *How we work*. NICE, London. Available at: ✆ www.nice.org.uk/aboutnice/howwework/how_we_work.jsp
8 Solutions for Public Health (2012). *Resources*. SPH, Oxford. Available at: ✆ www.sph.nhs.uk/sph-psu/resources
9 Coker R, Thomas M, Lock K, Martin R. (2007). Detention and the threat of tuberculosis. Evidence, Ethics and Law. *Journal of Law and Medical Ethics*, **35**, 609–15.
10 Mill JS (1869/2002) *On Liberty*. Dover Publications, Mineola.
11 World Health Organization (2005). *Framework Convention on Tobacco Control*. WHO, Geneva.
12 Hatsukami D, Slade J, Benowitz N, *et al*. (2002). Reducing tobacco harm: Research challenges and issues. *Nicotine & Tobacco Research*, **4**, 89–101.
13 Rehm J, Mathers C, Popova S, Thavorncharoensap M, Teerawattananon Y, Patra J. (2009). Global burden of disease and injury and economic cost attributable to alcohol use and alcohol-use disorders. *Lancet*, **373**, 2223–33.
14 Wagenaar A, Salois M, Komor K. (2009). Effects of beverage alcohol price and tax levels on drinking: a meta-analysis of 1003 estimates from 112 studies. *Addiction*, **104**, 179–90.
15 Walker T. (2010). Why we should not set a minimum price per unit of alcohol. *Public Health Ethics*, **3**, 107–14.

1.3 Assessing health status

Julian Flowers

Objectives

Assessing population health is a fundamental element of most public health activity. We cannot improve health and measure success without being able to conduct health assessments. These may be components of, for example:
- measuring burden of disease
- needs assessment
- assessing health equity and health inequality
- resource allocation
- planning
- health impact assessment
- service evaluation.

This chapter is intended to identify key principles involved in assessing the health of a defined population, rather than individual health status. It should help identify some techniques and approaches that can be applied in practice. Good health assessments require skills in epidemiology and information management and analysis; synthesis of information and opinion from a range of sources; leadership, political and partnership working, and persistence. A successful health assessment should influence decision making–something should change as a result, for example:
- a service should be commissioned
- further work could be undertaken
- a decision to undertake a health policy or programme should be informed.

A typology of health assessments

There are a range of approaches to health assessment depending on the objective. Health assessments often have both quantitative and qualitative elements. They synthesize a range of information and views from a range of sources. A few common approaches are listed below:
- *Health needs assessment (HNA)* (📖 see Chapter 1.4): starts with a population and identifies key health issues to aid prioritization, development of health programmes and commissioning of services.

- *Health impact assessment (HIA) (*☐ *see Chapter 1.5):* starts with a policy or programme and tries to identify and weigh the health benefits or disbenefits, which might accrue . If has been defined as 'a combination of procedures, methods and tools by which a policy, program or project may be judged as to its potential effects on the health of a population, and the distribution of those effects within the population'.[1]
- *Health equity audit:* starts with defined sub-populations and tries to identify health inequalities and inequities of service provision.[2]
- *Health care needs assessment:* starts with a defined population at risk of receiving an intervention and attempts to quantify the number who might benefit and the magnitude of that benefit.
- Other types of health assessment include health economic evaluation, environmental impact assessment and health technology assessment.

Key steps of health assessment

Health assessments are often an iterative process
(Figure 1.3.1)
Key steps include:
- Being clear about why you are conducting the assessment, who it is intended for and what you hope to achieve.
- *Defining your population clearly:* e.g. the adult population (aged 18 and over) in such and such area. Patients on general practice registers with chronic obstructive pulmonary disease.
- *Population health relative to whom:* assessments usually include a comparative element. The choice of comparator may depend on the audience; for example:
  - a regional health officer may be interested in comparison with other regions and also variation within their region
  - a national policy maker may be more interested in international comparison and a local practitioner may be more interested in peer comparison of similar organizations
  - the choice of comparator can be political, as well as scientific and may affect acceptance of the assessment.
- *What aspects of heath are you considering?* Specificity is generally helpful.
- *Who needs to be involved?* There is often a 'desk-based' element to health assessments which can be done in isolation, but usually assessments are joint efforts and partnership working is important. For example, in England a joint strategic needs assessment process has been introduced (see Box 1.3.1). Working out who you need to involve is a key step which will depend on the objective of the assessment. For example, if you are trying to determine key health priorities for a community it will be important to involve key informants or the public directly through surveys or focus groups. If the assessment relates to a health care intervention, clinicians and patient representative groups maybe important.

- *Perspectives on health:* professionals, the public. and their representatives and policy makers often have different perspectives on health and health priorities.
- *Identify and assemble data, facts and other information:* can you use what is routinely available or do you need to collect data especially for the assessment?
- How will you communicate the results of your assessment?
- How will you evaluate success?

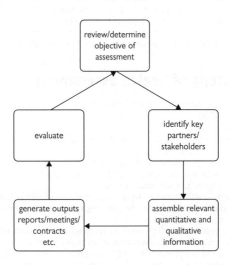

Figure 1.3.1 Health assessments can be thought of as cyclical, iterative processes.

Box 1.3.1 **Joint strategic needs assessment**

Joint strategic needs assessment (JSNA) was introduced as a statutory needs assessment in England in 2008. It requires local government to work together with health care commissioners (PCTs) and describes a process that identifies current and future health and wellbeing needs in light of existing services, and informs future service planning taking into account evidence of effectiveness. JSNA identifies 'the big picture' in terms of the health and wellbeing needs and inequalities of a local population. Since introduction JSNAs have been conducted across England. They have varied in their style, content and effectiveness across the country, but as a process they have fostered strong partnership working across the health and local government sectors. Some have been data dense, others have been more action focused and strongly linked to commissioning, but a testament to their success is the survival of the process through the major health reforms in England in 2010.

Further information

Department of Health (2007). *Joint strategic needs assessment*. HMSO, London. Available at: ◌
   http://www.dh.gov.uk/en/PublicationsandstatisticsPublications/PublicationsPolicyAndGuidance
   /DH_081097

Association of Public Health Observatories (2008). The Joint Strategic Needs Assessment
   (JSNA) core dataset. HMSO, London. Available at: ◌ http://www.dh.gov.uk/en/
   Publicationsandstatistics/Publications/PublicationsPolicyAndGuidance/DH_086676

Assembling relevant information

The essence of all assessment is to:
- assemble relevant information on a particular issue
- determine if there is a problem and if so the priority and magnitude of that problem(s)

and
- determine what (if anything) to do about it.

Some general principles for assembling data
- *Be systematic:* there is usually more than one source of data or potential set of health indicators (summary measures of health)
- *Have a framework:* broad health assessments might include 'domains' such as:
  - sociodemographic characteristics of the population for example age and sex, socio-economic factors such as income, social class, deprivation
  - broad health status
  - life expectancy and summary measures of population health (see pp. 32–33)
  - *cause specific mortality rates*—often heart disease, cancer, stroke, age-specific and premature mortality rates
  - burden of disease measurements such as disease prevalence
  - lifestyle or health behaviour

- *health inequalities*—variation or differences in health status measures between sub sections of the populations such as ethnic or racial groups, socioeconomic groups or age and sex.

Or follow well known frameworks such as Dahlgren and Whitehead.

An examples of the domains used in English health profiles is shown in Table 1.3.1.

Table 1.3.1 Domains and indicators in health profiles

Domains	Examples of indicators
Community	Deprivation, violence
Children and young people	Childhood obesity, breast feeding, teenage pregnancy
Adult health and lifestyle	Adult smoking, obesity
Disease	Disease prevalence, cancer incidence, TB rates
Life expectancy and causes of death	Life expectancy, mortality from cardiovascular disease and cancer, death rates from injury

Measuring health status and summary measures of population health

Health as a concept is difficult to measure directly and we often make inferences about population health status from other measures such as mortality and morbidity. However, there is good evidence that asking people to rate their health on a simple scale from excellent to bad is predictive of mortality and health services utilization.[3,4]

Increasingly, measures of health or disability are being combined with life expectancy to produce summary measures of population health. There are two variants:
- health expectancies
- health gaps.

Figure 1.3.2 attempts to illustrate these. It shows population survivorship against age. The overall area of the figure illustrated an idealized life-span of 100 years lived in perfect health until a sudden death at age 100.

Curve C represents actual survivorship, and curve A that which is lived in good health. Area A represents a measure of health expectancy, whereas area B, which is the difference between idealized and actual health, is a health gap.

Examples of each in routine use include:
- *Health expectances:* healthy life expectancy (HLE), disability-free life expectancy (DFLE), health active life expectancy (HALE).
- *Health gaps:* years of life lost (YLL), disability-adjusted life years (DALYs), healthy life years (HeaLYs).

Whilst these measures have a strong appeal in assessing health, they have several drawbacks:
- *Availability of data:* all these measures rely on some population estimates of health or disability which can be difficult to obtain, particularly sub nationally. DALYs rely on estimates of disease prevalence and duration and severity of disability which are rarely available.
- *Uses:* although in countries with well-developed systems for monitoring mortality it may be possible to monitor death rates and life expectancy, lack of systematic measurement of relevant morbidity measures reduce the usefulness of summary measures of public health in monitoring health over time although they are useful in comparative health assessment.
- Complexity of calculation.
- Reliability of self-reported health status.

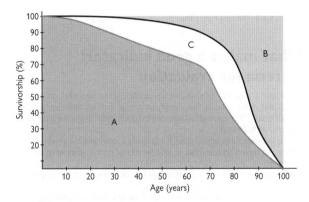

Figure 1.3.2 Summary measures of population health.

Sources of data

There is a wealth of data available for health assessments, and the availability and quality of data is increasing all the time. Data is available for international, national, regional, and local comparison. Good sources include:
- *International:* country wide from WHO, Gapminder
- European
- *Country wide:* EUROSTAT
- *Health regions:* Project ISARE
- Local
- Health observatories
- Other health observatories of similar projects.

The data cube (Figure 1.3.3) provides a useful framework for thinking about the kinds of data that can be helpful.

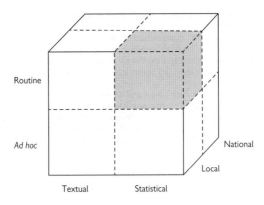

Figure 1.3.3 The data cube (After Stevens & Gillam, 1998).[5]

What makes a good indicator? Criteria for evaluation

With such a plethora of data and limited resources for conducting assessments we need criteria for identifying those metrics that we genuinely should track. There are good sources for such criteria and a framework is outlined as follows:[6,7]

- Are the measures actionable? If so, at what level and by whom?
- Are the measures sensitive to interventions? If so, within what time frame?
- Are the measures easily understood by collaborating organizations, policy makers, and the public?
- Is the meaning of an increase or decrease in a measure unambiguous? It should be clear whether a high values is desirable or undesirable and what direction of change we are trying to achieve.
- Do the measures stand alone or are they aggregated into an index or summary measure? Summary measures of health can be useful, but sometimes it is not obvious and the indicator should be deconstructible into its core components
- Are the measures uniform across communities? Comparison and comparability are important.
- To what extent do measures address inequalities, as well as overall burden?
- Can unintended consequences be tracked? Often people manage the system to indicators and there can be unintended consequences (gaming) or knock-ons.
- Do the available data correspond to the geographic level of the intervention? Data should be available at the level required for action
- How timely are the data? They should be as timely as possible.

- Are the measures reliable and valid? Are they reproducible, repeatable, and have face, criterion, and construct validity as far as possible.
- Can the measures be produced for population subgroups? The ability to calculate indicators for subpopulations allows us to address health inequalities, inequality, and variations.
- Are indirect methods of estimation appropriate? If we can't obtain direct measures of the issue of interest, often we can estimate or infer from other sources.
- Should data reporting be part of an incentive-based population health improvement system? If we can't get the data we need it could be required or mandated as part of the system through contracts, or commissioning processes.

Presenting and communicating data for health assessment

There is no shortage of information and data that can be collated as part of a health assessment, but succinct and accurate communication is key. Over the last few years, presentational techniques have improved and the evidence base for methods of communication has been growing. These include social marketing techniques which use segmentation to match the communication channels and methods with the audience.

One approach, developed by Public Health Observatories and common across a range of quantitative health assessments in the UK, is the use of graphical health profiles (Figure 1.3.4). These present health indicators in 'spine chart|' format that compares for an area, each indicator against the national average. It also scales and shows the overall distribution of each indicator and includes a measure of statistical significance represented by the colour of the 'blobs', which show the indicator value for that area. In this example (Figure 1.3.4), we show an area with a wide range of health problems (relative to England)—the area has more socioeconomic deprivation, violence, dental problems, teenage pregnancy, high levels of mortality, more tuberculosis, and so on.

Data sharing and transparency

Data transparency is increasing access to public data (see, for example, www.data.gov and www.data.gov.uk) indicating a new 'relationship' of the state and public sector with the public and taxpayers. However:
- Care needs to be taken to avoid disclosing data which could potentially identify an individual?
- Data should be presented in forms that people can use and accompanied by sufficient explanatory information (metadata) to encourage appropriate interpretation.

● Significantly worse than England average
○ Not significantly different from England average
● Significantly better than England average
○ No significance can be calculated

England Worst ◇ Regional average* · England Average · England Best

25th Percentile — 75th Percentile

*In the South East Region this represents the Strategic Health Authority average

Domain	Indicator	Local No Per Year	Local Value	Eng Avg	Eng Worst	England Range	Eng Best
Our communities	1 Deprivation	37812	23.2	19.9	89.2		0.0
	2 Children in poverty	9267	27.1	22.4	66.5		6.0
	3 Statutory homelessness	413	5.93	2.48	9.84		0.00
	4 GCSE achieved (5A*-C inc. Eng & Maths)	929	40.6	50.9	32.1		76.1
	5 Violent crime	3576	21.9	16.4	36.6		4.8
	6 Carbon emissions	1316	8.1	6.8	14.4		4.1
Children's and young people's health	7 Smoking in pregnancy	434	15.7	14.6	33.5		3.8
	8 Breast feeding initiation	1980	71.6	72.5	39.7		92.7
	9 Physically active children	15767	58.4	49.6	24.6		79.1
	10 Obese children	199	9.2	9.6	14.7		4.7
	11 Tooth decay in children aged 5 years	n/a	1.6	1.1	2.5		0.2
	12 Teenage pregnancy (under 18)	171	53.0	40.9	74.8		14.9
Adult's health and lifestyle	13 Adults who smoke	n/a	27.0	22.2	35.2		10.2
	14 Binge drinking adults	n/a	19.7	20.1	33.2		4.6
	15 Healthy eating adults	n/a	30.0	28.7	18.3		48.1
	16 Physically active adults	n/a	8.3	11.2	5.4		16.6
	17 Obese adults	n/a	24.1	24.2	32.8		13.2
Disease and poor health	18 Incidence of malignant melanoma	17	10.8	12.6	27.3		3.7
	19 Incapacity benefits for mental illness	2800	27.5	27.6	58.5		9.0
	20 Hospital stays for alcohol related harm	3502	1970	1580	2860		784
	21 Drug misuse						
	22 People diagnosed with diabetes	7115	4.34	4.30	6.72		2.69
	23 New cases of tuberculosis	37	23	15	110		0
	24 Hip fracture in over-65s	156	517.7	479.2	843.5		273.6
Life expectancy and causes of death	25 Excess winter deaths	82	18.4	15.6	26.3		2.3
	26 Life expectancy - male	n/a	76.8	77.9	73.6		84.3
	27 Life expectancy - female	n/a	81.0	82.0	78.8		88.9
	28 Infant deaths	15	5.26	4.84	8.67		1.08
	29 Deaths from smoking	232	218.5	206.8	360.3		118.7
	30 Early deaths: heart disease & stroke	144	89.9	74.8	125.0		40.1
	31 Early deaths: cancer	176	110.2	114.0	164.3		70.5
	30 Road injuries and deaths	103	63.1	51.3	167.0		14.6

Figure 1.3.4 A spine chart presentation of a population health profile.

Further resources

Cavanagh S, Chadwick K. (2007). *Health needs assessment.* NICE, London. Available at: 🕮 http://www.nice.org.uk/media/150/35/Health_Needs_Assessment_A_Practical_Guide.pdf

Network of Public Health Observatories. *Health profiles* (Hone page). DoH, London. Available at: 🕮 http://www.apho.org.uk/default.aspx?RID=49802

Universtiy of Birmingham. *Health care needs assessment.* Available at: 🕮 http://www.hcna.bham.ac.uk/three.shtml

West Midlands Public Health Observatory. *Health impact assessment gateway.* Available at: 🕮 http://www.apho.org.uk/default.aspx?RID=40141

Data sources

International

WHO. Available at: 🕮 www.who.int
Gapminder: Available at: 🕮 www.gapminder.com

European

ISARE. Available at: ℘ http://www.i2sare.eu/

EUROSTAT. Available at: ℘ http://epp.eurostat.ec.europa.eu/portal/page/portal/region_cities/regional_statistics

European Commission. *Public health indicators.* Available at: ℘ http://ec.europa.eu/health/indicators/policy/index_en.htm

Association of Public Health Observatories. Available at: ℘ http://www.apho.org.uk/default.aspx?QN=HP_INTERACTIVE

References

1 Mindell J. (2003). A glossary for health impact assessment *Journal of Epidemiology Community Health*, **57(9),** 647–51. Available at: ℘ http://jech.bmj.com/cgi/doi/10.1136/jech.57.9.647

2 Health Development Agency. (2005). *Understanding the barriers to completing health equity audit in PCTs.* NHS, London. Available at: ℘ http://www.nice.org.uk/nicemedia/documents/understanding_barriers.pdf

3 Kyffin RGE, Goldacre MJ, Gill M. (2004). Mortality rates and self reported health: database analysis by English local authority area. *British Medical Journal*, **329,** 887–8.

4 Miilunpalo S, Vuori I, Oja P, Pasanen M, Urponen H. (1997). Self-rated health status as a health measure: the predictive value of self-reported health status on the use of physician services and on mortality in the working-age population. *Journal of Clinical Epidemiology*, **50,** 517–28. Available at: ℘ http://www.ncbi.nlm.nih.gov/entrez/query.fcgi?cmd=Retrieve&db=PubMed&dopt=Citation&list_uids=9180644

5 Stevens A, Gillam S. (1998). *Needs assessment: from theory to practice*, BMJ series 3 **316:** 1448–51. Available at: ℘ http://www.bmj.com/content/316/7142/1448

6 Bilheimer LT. (2010). Evaluating metrics to improve population health. *Preventing Chronic Disease*, **7(4),** A69. Available at: ℘ http://www.ncbi.nlm.nih.gov/pubmed/20550827

7 Pencheon D. (2008). *The Good Indicators Guide: understanding how to use and choose indicators.* Available at: ℘ http://www.apho.org.uk/resource/item.aspx?RID=44584

1.4 Assessing health needs

John Wright and Ben Cave

Objectives

HNA is a systematic method of identifying the unmet health and health-care needs of a population and recommending changes to meet these unmet needs. It is used to improve health and other service planning, priority setting, and policy development. HNA is an example of public health working outside the formal health sector and presenting back to colleagues. Successful HNAs will also ensure that non-health agencies benefit from their findings.

This chapter will describe why HNA is important and what it means in practice. Professional training and clinical experience teaches that a health professional must systematically assess a patient before administering any treatment that is believed to be effective. This systematic approach is often omitted when assessing the health needs of populations.

Box 1.4.1 shows what can happen when a HNA is conducted systematically—both health outcome and service delivery were improved.

Box 1.4.1　TB service in a rural African hospital[1]

- *Setting:* a rural district hospital in South Africa.
- *Problem:* increasing overcrowding in the hospital due to the rising incidence of TB resulting from human immunodeficiency virus (HIV)/acquired immune deficiency syndrome (AIDS). Concerns by staff about high levels of treatment failure.
- *Methods:* review of TB register information on detection rates and outcomes. Review of current clinical practices. Interviews with health professional and patients to determine views of TB care.
- *Results:* case detection rate of TB had increased by 90% over a period of 4 yrs. Patients were admitted to hospital for the 2-month intensive phase of treatment creating major problems of overcrowding. Haphazard follow-up in any local clinic led to poor data on outcomes. Outcome data indicated only 27% (n = 66) of patients were cured or completed treatment and 43% (n = 160) were lost to follow-up. Major gaps in patients' understanding about TB and its relationship to HIV/AIDS were identified.

- *Action:* new guidelines were developed for the region to allow home-based treatment. A community-based treatment service was established using village health workers to support treatment in patients' own homes. An outreach team was set up to co-ordinate care, promote community awareness, and train and support village and clinic health workers. Within 12 months care and completion rates had improved to 86% with patients having to stay for days, rather than months in hospital.

Defining need

Need, in the sense used in this chapter, implies the capacity to benefit from an intervention. 'To speak of a need is to imply a goal, a measurable deficiency from the goal and a means of achieving the goal'.[2]

HNA is *not* the same as population health status assessment (see 📖 Chapter 1.3). HNA incorporates the concept of a capacity to benefit from an intervention. It therefore introduces an assessment of the effectiveness of relevant interventions to supplement the identification of health problems. Thus, the researcher does not start with a blank sheet but with a theory to test or a technology to apply—HNA is not a value-free examination of a population, but starts from a specific point. HNA should also make explicit what benefits are being pursued by identifying particular interventions.

The capacity to benefit is always greater than available resources and so HNA should incorporate questions of priority setting through considering the cost-effectiveness of the available interventions (see 📖 Chapters 1.2 and 1.6).[3]

Thus, at different times HNA is used to define:
- the goal (improved health outcomes and improved health equity)
- the deficiency (poor health outcomes, inequities in health)
- the means of achieving the goal (effective intervention).

Approaches to needs assessment

A number of approaches to needs assessment have been suggested,[4] including:
- *'Epidemiologically based' needs assessment:* combining epidemiological approaches (specific health status assessments) with assessment of the effectiveness and possibly the cost-effectiveness of the potential interventions.
- *Comparative:* comparing levels of service receipt between different populations.
- *Corporate:* canvassing the demands and wishes of professionals, patients, politicians, and other interested parties.

In this chapter an epidemiological approach to determining priorities is explored. This incorporates clinical effectiveness, cost-effectiveness, and patients' perspectives.[5] It incorporates qualitative and quantitative information. While comparisons of health service usage are commonly used as indicators of need, population-based usage rates typically vary markedly between areas, often for unexplained reasons. In addition, the link between usage rates and improved health outcomes is often hard to demonstrate.

The distinction between individual needs and community needs is important to consider. Some needs will be shared across communities, while some needs will be specific to smaller subsets or to individuals. HNA should be sensitive to these differences.

HNA involves the active, explicit, and systematic identification of needs, rather than a passive, *ad hoc*, implicit response to demand. The assessment of health needs can be clarified by differentiating between needs, demands, and supply (see Box 1.4.2) and by remembering that health needs are not necessarily restricted to health-*care* needs. Ideally, HNA will identify both met and unmet need. Health needs include wider social and environmental determinants of health, such as deprivation, housing, diet, education, and employment. Health needs should ideally be appropriately addressed ('met'), but these needs are too often unmet (e.g. poor housing, poor access to primary care, health illiteracy, undiagnosed hypertension, ignored moderate depression) or 'over met' (e.g. prescribing antibiotics for sore throats).

Box 1.4.2 Different aspects of health needs

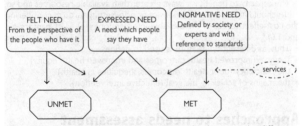

This figure does not engage with the relationship between the different types of need. A need is shown as a claim for service.

Health and social care services cater for normative needs. By definition they do not cater for unmet normative needs. HNA should ensure that normative needs, met and unmet, are catered for. The HNA process should ensure that normative needs adequately reflect felt and expressed needs and the best scientific evidence.

Definitions of need are adapted from Spicker P. *Social need*. Available at: ℬ www2.rgu.ac.uk/publicpolicy/introduction/needf.htm

HNA provides the opportunity for:

- profiling/examining the population's health status, describing the patterns of disease in the local population and the differences from district, regional, or national disease patterns
- learning more about the needs and priorities of patients, and the local population
- highlighting areas of unmet need and providing a clear set of objectives to work towards to meet these needs
- deciding rationally how to use resources to improve the health of the local population in the most effective and efficient way
- influencing policy, interagency collaboration, or research and development priorities.

Importantly, it also provides a method of monitoring and promoting equity in the provision and use of health services and addressing inequalities in health (see Box 1.4.3 for the case of addressing the health needs of older people after an earthquake; and Box 1.4.4 for the case of health services needs assessment among patients with coronary heart disease).[6]

Box 1.4.3 Health needs of older people after earthquake

- *Objective:* to compare the differences between rural and urban health needs and the utilization of services of older people after the 2005 (October) earthquake in Kashmir.
- *Setting:* the Neelum Valley of Kashmir, Pakistan, 4 months after the earthquake.
- *Methods:* a comparative, descriptive study to examine rural and urban health needs and to compare ways in which older people used services after the earthquake. Semi-structured interviews were conducted to collect information regarding demographic background, medical and drug history, self-reported health status, health care access and utilization, and social/financial concerns. Clinical records were reviewed. Physical indicators for older patients also were collected on site.
- *Results:* the health profile, access to health care, service availability, and prevalence of non-communicable diseases was found to differ between urban and rural settings. The greatest gap, at all sites, was that non-communicable disease management was inadequate during non-acute, post-earthquake medical care. Health service utilization varied by gender: in conservative rural areas older, traditional women were less likely to receive medical services while older men were less likely to access psychological services in all sites.
- *Conclusion:* findings highlight specific health needs and issues related to long-term, chronic disease management. It is important to strengthen capacity to respond appropriately to medical disasters, which includes preparedness for treating the health needs of older people.[7]

Box 1.4.4 Epidemiologic health needs assessment—coronary heart disease[8,9]

- *Objective:* to assess whether the use of health services by people with coronary heart disease reflected need.
- *Setting:* a health district in the United Kingdom with a population of 530,000.
- *Methods:* the prevalence of angina was determined by a validated postal questionnaire. Routine health data were collected on standardized mortality ratios, admission rates for coronary heart disease, and operation rates for angiography, angioplasty, and coronary heart disease. Census data were used to calculate Townsend scores to describe deprivation for electoral wards. The prevalence of angina and use of services were then compared with deprivation scores for each ward.
- *Results:* angina and mortality from heart disease were more common in wards with high deprivation scores. However, treatment by revascularization procedures was more common in more affluent wards which have low deprivation scores.
- *Conclusion:* the use of revascularization services was not commensurate with need. Steps should be taken to ensure that health care is targeted to those who most need it.

A framework for assessing the health needs of a population

Box 1.4.5 summarizes the questions or steps involved in a formal HNA process. This seldom follows a simple linear progression through the steps—needs assessments often develop from several steps concurrently. HNA can be approached in much the same way as doing a jigsaw, so that different pieces are put together to give a full picture of local health requirements and potential interventions.

Box 1.4.5 Questions to be answered in a formal HNA process

- *What is the problem?* Identify the health problem to be addressed in the defined population.
- *What is the size and nature of the problem?* Carry out a health status assessment for the population, covering the relevant areas of ill-health and/or potential health gain.
- *What are the current services?* Identify the existing services and interventions being delivered, focusing where relevant on quality, effectiveness, and efficiency.
- *What interventions do patients, professionals and other stakeholders want?* Consult with these groups.

- *What interventions does scientific knowledge recommend?* Identify interventions by reviewing the scientific knowledge. What are the most appropriate and cost-effective solutions? Find and appraise.
- *What are the resource implications?* Choose between competing ways of meeting needs (competing interventions) and decide on competing priorities—resources are always limited.
- *What are the recommendations and the plan for implementation?* What agencies need to take action and by when?
- *Is assessing need likely to lead to appropriate change?* Identify expected health gains and how the effect of subsequent actions can be monitored.

Needs assessment requires careful preparation

Undertaking needs assessment involves identifying the right issue, using the right technical methods, and managing the process effectively. Start with attention to defining the problem. Objectives should be clarified and should be as simple and focused as possible. Care should be taken not to raise unrealistic expectations. The right team should be convened, with all relevant stakeholders, including (as relevant to the issue) the service funders, the clinicians, and the users (public involvement) (see 📖 Chapters 3.4 and 6.8). Leadership is important (see 📖 Chapter 6.1), as is clear and effective communication during the process, especially if there is multiagency involvement. Access to relevant information and informants should be sought at an early stage.

What is the health problem?

The focus of the needs assessment exercise should be clearly identified. A health problem may come to attention from many sources, including the results of a population health status assessment, input from patients or stakeholders, government priority setting, or the scientific and professional literature.

An initial clarification of the issues can be valuable. A first step in clarifying the definition of the problem is a search of the health and social science databases for the topic. A review of the published health literature will provide a national and international perspective about the health topic and provide methods and results (for example, case definitions, disease incidence and prevalence, current provision of health services) that may be applicable to the local population.[4,6] Where access to journals is limited then search engines such as PubMed, Google, and Google Scholar can provide useful evidence. A search of grey literature sources (for example, public health professional bodies and government health department databases) can provide models and information.

After initial clarification, it should become apparent whether the problem justifies a full and systematic needs assessment.

What is the size and nature of the problem?

With a working definition of the health problems in mind, relevant health status data can then be collected. This should aim to establish:

- the number of people in the studied population who are likely to be suffering from the target condition or conditions
- their characteristics
- the extent to which they are already receiving appropriate interventions.

Accurately estimating how many people would benefit from each of the potential interventions is desirable but often difficult. Graham[10] challenges public health to look to the future: populations and health needs change, especially in the context of a changing climate, whereas health status data is usually historic. HNAs should identify a timescale. Previous chapters provide a guide to sources of information.

What are the current services?

There are several sources of data on health care in a locality. Hospital activity data can provide information on hospital admissions, diagnoses, length of stay, operations performed, and patient characteristics. Clinical indicators can provide information on the comparative performance of hospitals and health authorities.

Health care provision (e.g. numbers of family doctors per capita, number of operations per capita) is often compared with national or international norms, although there is rarely evidence of a link between provision and health outcome.

What do professionals, patients, and other stakeholders want?

Consult a wide range of stakeholders to describe local health needs. Local health professionals in primary and secondary care will have valuable contributions to make about the health needs of their local community. Other stakeholders, such as health authorities, local government agencies, and voluntary groups are also important contributors, not only for their knowledge and beliefs, but also so as to engage them in the assessment, and encourage ownership and eventual implementation of the results.

Consult users, carers, and the public (see 📖 Chapters 3.4 and 6.8). Historically, health services have been weak at involving users and the public in decision-making about local health care. Best practice now recognizes the importance of obtaining greater public involvement: various methods for ensuring public input to health service planning are summarized below.[11]

- *Citizens' juries*: local people who are representative of the population are selected to sit on a jury for a specified period of time. Members are presented with information from different experts on health topics and debate the issues surrounding them.
- *Health panels*: standing panels of local people representative of population. These can be large (more than 1000 people) panels, which are surveyed at regular intervals about key health issues, or smaller panels where the members meet and discuss different topics. Members are replaced at regular intervals.

- *Focus groups*: groups of 6–12 participants with a facilitator who encourages discussion about health topics, which is recorded on tape or by an observer.
- *Interviews*: interviews with randomly or purposefully selected individuals to canvass their views and opinions. Users, carers, or other stakeholders (e.g. community leaders) can all be valuable contributors.
- *Questionnaires*: these allow structured information to be collected from a large sample of local people on one or more health topics. Such surveys can provide information on user satisfaction, perceived needs, and use of health services. Other generic health measures such as quality of life scores,[12] or disease-specific measures can also be included.
- *Specific planning methodologies*: for example, meta-planning, 'Planning for Real', 'open space' events. These are all approaches to planning which use specific techniques to promote the involvement of local communities and stakeholders.

What are the most appropriate and cost-effective interventions?

An essential part of a HNA is the review of the clinical effectiveness and cost-effectiveness of interventions that can address the identified health needs. Evidence about the effectiveness of health interventions or services can be found in databases of good-quality systematic reviews such as the Cochrane Library,[13] or publications such as the *Effective Health Care Bulletins*.[14] The United States Agency for Healthcare Research and Quality[15] and the UK National Institute of Health and Clinical Effectiveness[16] can also be good source of information on effectiveness and on professional consensus on treatment. Where there is limited evidence of effectiveness of interventions then professional consensus about best practice may have to be relied on.

What are the resource implications?

Economic appraisal, including cost-effectiveness, should be considered if health needs are to be met optimally with limited resources. At a practical level this involves:[17]

- determining how resources are currently spent (programme budgeting—see 📖 Chapter 7.2);
- defining options for change (marginal analysis) by specifying alternatives:
  (a) identify potential services requiring additional resources
  (b) identify services which could be provided at the same level of effectiveness, but at reduced cost, releasing resources for (a);
  (c) identify services that are less cost-effective than those identified in (a)
- assessing the costs and benefits of the principal options;
- decide on the best option, aiming to increase investment in (a) and reduce investment in services identified in (b) and (c).

The third example in this chapter (see Box 1.4.6) shows how the needs assessment process can help plan services, using generalizable research and local surveys involving users.

Implementation

The information collected in the needs assessment must be clearly collated, analysed, and presented. This will usually be in a written report. A summary of key findings is useful in communicating the results to the decision-makers and those who will be affected by the decisions.

Reporting the results, however, is not the end of the process. The HNA should develop a plan for action. Building agreement to a practical implementation plan for meeting the unmet needs is an essential part of needs assessment.

Does assessing need create change?

Factors that will increase the likelihood of needs assessment leading to change are:
- consideration of the potential resource implications of the assessment from the beginning (discussion between commissioners and assessors)
- methodological rigor to ensure that the results are valid and believed
- ownership of the project by relevant stakeholders from the start and effective involvement during the work
- effective dissemination of the results (see 📖 Chapters 6.4 and 6.5) the existence of a practical plan for implementing the necessary actions to partly or fully meet the identified unmet needs.

Box 1.4.6 Health needs assessment in an English prison [18]

- *Objective:* to quantify the need for alcohol interventions in a prison population and to make recommendations.
- *Setting:* a large prison in the south of England.
- *Methods:* epidemiological data from national prison surveys were applied to the prison population, taking into account age, gender, ethnicity, and sentence/remand status. Expected incidence and prevalence of alcohol problems was compared with data from prison records of alcohol interventions. Semi-structured interviews were carried out with a sample of prison staff, service providers and some prisoners. Information on national policy, the impact of alcohol and evidence of effectiveness was also used to highlight issues for attention.
- *Results:* dependent drinkers were very likely to be identified and treated appropriately. However, there were substantial gaps in services for people with less severe problems (particularly identification and brief advice as recommended nationally). Alcohol services provided relatively little monitoring data and there were questions about value for money of some interventions. Recommendations for improvement were made.
- *Conclusion:* prison staff were keen to make improvements and recognized that, despite the damage it causes, alcohol misuse receives little attention when compared with drug services. The project helped to quantify service requirements and opened a dialogue about the re-alignment of alcohol services.

HNA starts from the health of a defined population and results in proposals (for policy, programmes, strategy, plans. or other developments). Health Impact Assessments (HIAs); see 📖 Chapter 1.5) start from proposals and compare how they may affect population health and health inequity. Table 1.4.1 shows the similarities between these two approaches. HNAs can be useful inputs to HIAs.

Table 1.4.1 Comparison of HNA with HIA

	HNA	HIA
Starting point	Population	Proposal (policy, plan. programme or project) within or outside the health sector
Primary output	Inform decisions about strategies, service priorities, commissioning, and local delivery plans, and inform future HIAs	Recommendations to maximize beneficial, and minimize adverse, effects on health. These are made with reference to a specific proposal and are made to inform decision-making.
Does each approach take account of inequalities and aim to improve health?	*Yes:* describe health needs and health assets of different groups in local population	*Yes:* identify how proposals may affect the most vulnerable groups in population.
Involve stakeholders	Ideally (dependent on resources)	Ideally (dependent on resources)
Involve sectors outside health sector	Sometime	Always
Based on determinants of health	Sometime	Always
Use best available evidence	Always	Always

Conclusion

HNAs should, ideally, be an expression and analysis of community need. Care should be taken over the dissemination and storage of these reports. They will contain valuable information about local communities and so confidentiality may be an issue. They will also be of great use to local communities and to other services and so the results should be shared. It must also be acknowledged that health needs are not static: assessments provide snapshots of the needs of the local population. Health needs and the health and social care services that try to address them are always changing. It is important to ensure that the assessment work is reviewed and updated and that service delivery is in line with current and projected health needs for all groups and individuals within any given community.

Further resources

Hooper J, Longworth P. (2002). *Health needs assessment workbook.* had, London.

Murray SA. (1999). Experiences with 'rapid appraisal' in primary care: involving the public in assessing health needs, orientating staff, and educating medical students. *British Medical Journal*, **3,** 440–4.

National Health Service Management Executive (1991). *Assessing health care need.* Department of Health, London.

Wright J. (1998). *Health needs assessment in practice.* BMJ Books, London.

References

1 Wright J, Walley J, Philip A, *et al.* (2004). Direct observation for tuberculosis: a randomised controlled trial of community health workers versus family members. *Tropical Medicine & International Health* **9**, 559–65.

2 Wilkin D, Hallam L, Dogget M. (1992). *Measures of need and outcomes in primary health care.* Oxford Medical Publications, Oxford.

3 Donaldson C, Mooney G. (1991). Needs assessment, priority setting, and contracts for health-care: an economic view. *British Medical Journal*, **303**, 1529–30.

4 Stevens A, Raftery J (eds). (1997). *Health care needs assessment*, 2nd series. Radcliffe Medical Press, Oxford.

5 Wright J, Williams DRR, Wilkinson J. (1998). The development of health needs assessment. In: Wright J, ed., *Health needs assessment in practice*, pp. 1–11. BMJ Books, London.

6 Rawaf S, Bahl V. (1998). *Assessing health needs of people from minority ethnic groups.* Royal College of Physicians, London.

7 Chan EY, Griffiths S. (2009). Comparison of health needs of older people between affected rural and urban areas after the 2005 Kashmir, Pakistan earthquake. *Prehospital. & Disaster. Medicine*, **24**, 365–71.

8 Jacobson B (2002). Delaying tactics. *Health Service Journal*, **112,** 22.

9 Payne N, Saul C. (1997). Variations in use of cardiology services in a health authority: comparison of coronary artery revascularisation rates with prevalence of angina and coronary mortality. *British Medical Journal*, **314,**: 256–61.

10 Graham H. (2010). Where is the future in public health? *Milbank Quarterly*, **88(2)**, 149–68.

11 Jordan J, Dowswell T, Harrison S, Lilford R, Mort M (1998). Whose priorities? Listening to users and the public. *British Medical Journal*, **316**, 1668–70.

12 Bowling A (1997). *Measuring health: a review of quality of life measurement scales*, 2nd edn. Open University Press, Buckingham.

13. Cochrane Library summaries. Available at: ℘ http://summaries.cochrane.org/ (accessed 24 May 2012).

14 Royal Society of Medicine Press. *Effective health care bulletins.* Available at: ℘ http://www.york.ac.uk/inst/crd/ehcb_em.htm (accessed 24 May 2012). [Effective Health Care Bulletins are bi-monthly publications for decision-makers, which examine the effectiveness of a variety of health care interventions. They are based on a systematic review and synthesis of research on the clinical effectiveness, cost-effectiveness, and acceptability of health service interventions. This is carried out by a research team using established methodological guidelines, with advice from expert consultants for each topic. The bulletins are subject to extensive and rigorous peer review.]

15 The United States Agency for Healthcare Research and Quality. Available at: ℘ http://www.ahrq.gov/ (accessed 30 June 2005).

16 National Institute of Health and Clinical Effectiveness. Available at: ℘ http://www.nice.org.uk (accessed 14 January 2006).

17 Scott A, Donaldson C. (1998). Clinical and cost effectiveness issues in health needs assessment. In: Wright J (ed.). *Health needs assessment in practice*, pp. 84–94. BMJ Books, London.

18 Brotherton P, Withers M. (2010). *Health needs assessment in an English prison.* Unpublished case study prepared for OUP.

1.5 Assessing health impacts

Alex Scott-Samuel, Kate Ardern, and Martin Birley

Objectives

By reading this chapter you will become familiar with:
- the background and policy context of health impact assessment (HIA)
- current and emerging concepts and methods of HIA
- the impact of HIA
- an approach to conducting rapid and comprehensive prospective HIAs on major public policies, programmes, and projects.

Definition and scope

HIA is 'a combination of procedures, methods and tools by which a policy, programme, or project may be judged as to its potential effects on the health of a population, and the distribution of those effects within the population'.[1] HIA also identifies appropriate actions to manage those effects. It may focus on projects such as a new factory, housing development, or health centre, programmes such as crime reduction or urban regeneration, or policies such as an integrated transport strategy or a youth unemployment policy. On a broader scale, HIA can be employed to assess global public policies in areas such as international trade, war, and human rights.

HIA builds on the fact that a wide range of economic, social, psychological, environmental, and political influences determines a community's health. It is important to try to estimate these influences on health *prospectively* and so HIA ideally precedes the start of the project, programme, or policy concerned.

The aims of prospective HIA are:
- to systematically assess the potential health impacts, both positive and negative, intended and unintended, of projects, programmes, and policies
- to improve the quality of public policy decisions by making recommendations that are likely to enhance predicted positive health impacts and minimize negative ones.

The key output of an HIA is a set of evidence-based recommendations for beneficially modifying a proposal so that its overall health impacts are enhanced and any potential health inequalities are minimized.

The importance of health impact assessment

HIA is an important public health method because it:

- promotes equity, sustainability, and healthy public policy in an unequal and frequently unhealthy world
- improves the quality of decision-making in health and partner organizations by incorporating into planning and policy-making the need to address health issues
- emphasizes social and environmental justice (it is usually the already disadvantaged who suffer most from negative health impacts)
- involves a multidisciplinary approach
- encourages public participation in debates about public health, planning, and other public policy issues
- gives equal status to qualitative and quantitative assessment methods
- makes values and politics explicit and opens issues to public scrutiny
- demonstrates that health is far broader than health care issues.

HIA is used in public policy decision-making in a wide and rapidly increasing range of economically 'developed' and 'less developed' countries throughout the world. HIA has had a high profile in countries of the South since the 1980s.[2] The remainder of this section documents more recent developments in the North.

Europe

The UK,[3,4] The Netherlands, and Sweden were the first countries in Europe to establish HIA programmes. In The Netherlands, HIA became government policy in 1995, following which a screening programme on new policy and legislation was introduced. In Sweden, HIA has been used since 1998 at local government level to assist in achieving local public health targets. The World Health Organization's (WHO) European Centre for Health Policy, together with other European partners, initiated a project in 1999 to bring together available experience and try to reach a consensus on how HIA can best be used to improve health policy development. The most important outputs of this project have been the Gothenburg consensus statement[1] and the generally raised levels of awareness of HIA both in European countries and in the European Commission (EC).

There has been considerable interest in the European Union (EU) in incorporating HIA into the development of EU policy. In 2001 the EC Directorate General for Health and Consumer Protection (DG Sanco) commissioned the development and piloting of a methodology for HIA of European policy. The resulting European Policy Health Impact Assessment (EPHIA) guide was published in 2004.[5]

The EC has also implemented a system of integrated impact assessment (IIA) of all EU policy. IIA implies the relatively superficial impact assessment of policies on a number of different dimensions. This was partly a response to the range of assessments, for example, environmental, health, gender, economic, being carried out on new European policies. The EC system has however been criticized for the undue influence of the corporate sector on its operation.[6]

United Kingdom

There has been strong national support for HIA in the UK, where both central government and the devolved governments in Scotland and Wales have commissioned substantial HIA programmes. The Greater London Assembly has carried out HIAs on London's culture, urban renewal, transport, energy, housing, and waste management strategies. HIAs have been undertaken as part of the planning process for major capital developments within the National Health Service. The UK Faculty of Public Health has included HIA as a core competency for all public health professionals.

The UK's HIA Gateway[7] has enabled the sharing of good practice and lessons learned from undertaking HIA and provided an evidence base for HIA theory, practice, and evaluation.

North America

In Canada, health has featured within environmental impact assessments (EIAs) since the 1980s. HIA as a separate procedure was first incorporated into the legislative framework of British Columbia in 1993, although this pioneering initiative subsequently lapsed. HIA has since been introduced in a number of Canadian provinces, including Nova Scotia and Quebec.

In the USA, while health considerations have similarly played a role within EIA, HIA was slow to emerge. Pioneering late 1990s projects were undertaken in California (San Francisco and Los Angeles) and in Minnesota. In 2002 a meeting at the Harvard School of Public Health assessed the possibilities for HIA within the USA.[8] The change of government in 2008 led to increases in the profile of and the funding for HIA.[9,10]

Australasia

Both Australia and New Zealand developed health-focused EIA in the 1990s. More recently, in 2004, the New Zealand government launched a policy tool for HIA.[11] In the same year an Australian–New Zealand collaborative project developed and piloted an equity-focused HIA approach.[12]

Globally

At a global level, the WHO has a HIA adviser at its Geneva headquarters, and has published a special issue of its *Bulletin*[13] on HIA. The WHO has also played a major role in promoting the consideration of health within strategic environmental assessment (SEA). SEA is concerned with the strategic impact of policies and has been the subject of policy and legislation by the EC and by the UN Economic Commission for Europe.

The potentially important role of health impact assessment in global public policy is beginning to be recognized.[14,15] HIA is increasingly used by global agencies such as the World Bank and by transnational corporations, especially the oil and gas and mining and minerals sectors. The Equator Principles[16] are a set of benchmarks used by lending banks for managing environmental and social issues in development project finance globally. They have become the global standard for banks and investors on how to assess major development projects and are used by over 60 major financial institutions around the world.

A key influence on the globalization of HIA during the next decade will be the report of the WHO's Commission on Social Determinants of

Health.[17] The report proposed widespread adoption of and capacity building for 'health equity impact assessments' of economic, trade and other key public policies.

The HIA process

Advantages
As the number of HIA studies grows, accumulating evidence shows that HIA can draw attention to potential health impacts in a way that permits constructive changes to be made to project or policy proposals. This has potentially enormous benefits for major developments, which are costly or propose significant change to existing service provision or organization.

Disadvantages
However, potential drawbacks to the adoption of HIA as a routine part of planning include the limited capacity and capability to undertake HIA. Therefore, whilst this chapter describes a comprehensive approach to HIA, we appreciate that time and resources may dictate a more condensed approach. There has been considerable interest in the use of 'rapid HIA' and a range of tools is available.[5,7,18]

In both comprehensive and rapid HIA, it is important to distinguish between *procedures* and *methods* for HIA (see Figure 1.5.1):
- procedures are frameworks for planning and implementing HIAs
- methods are the systems for carrying them out.

Procedures **Methods**

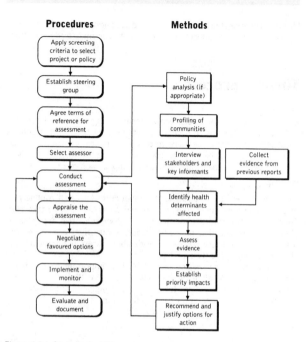

Figure 1.5.1 Stages in the HIA process.

Managing a health impact assessment: procedures

There are four procedures in the HIA process:
- screening
- steering group, terms of reference, and scope of HIA
- negotiation of favoured options
- implementation, monitoring, and evaluation.

Screening

The issues on which the selection of candidates for HIA is based are listed in Box 1.5.1. Potential projects, programmes, or policies should be rapidly assessed with regard to their likely performance in relation to each of these issues. While the procedure is necessarily crude, it can give a useful indication of how resources for HIA can be most effectively deployed. For the remainder of the sections describing procedures and methods, the term 'project' is used to refer to projects, programmes, or policies.

Box 1.5.1 Health impact assessment screening procedure:

- Economic issues:
  - the size of the project and of the population(s) affected
  - the costs of the project, and their distribution.
- Outcome issues:
  - the nature of potential health impacts of the project
  - the likely nature and extent of disruption caused to communities by the project
  - the existence of potentially cumulative impacts.
- Epidemiological issues:
  - the degree of certainty (risk) of health impacts
  - the likely frequency (incidence/prevalence rates) of potential health impacts
  - the likely severity of potential health impacts
  - the size of any probable health service impacts.

During HIA screening, there is a general need to give greater priority to policies than to programmes, and to programmes than to projects, all other things being equal. This is due to the broader scope—and hence potential impact—of policies compared with programmes and to projects. Another strategic consideration is that HIA should be prospective wherever possible. Timing may be affected by planning regulations and other statutory frameworks, such as whether the project requires an EIA. The relevance of the HIA to local decision-making is another key concern.

Steering group, terms of reference, and scope

Following screening and project selection, a multidisciplinary steering group should be established to agree the terms of reference (ToR) of the HIA, and to provide advice and support as it develops. Its membership should include representatives of the commissioners of the HIA, the assessors carrying it out, the project's proponents, affected communities, and other stakeholders as appropriate. Members should ideally be able to take decisions on behalf of those they represent.

The ToR provide a quality assurance procedure for the HIA. They are project specific, but should always include:

- steering group members' roles, including those of chair and secretary
- the nature and frequency of feedback to the steering group
- the HIA methods to be used
- the form of the project's outputs and any associated issues, e.g. ownership, confidentiality, and copyright
- *the scope of the HIA:* what is to be included and excluded, and the boundaries of the HIA in time and space
- an outline programme, including any deadlines
- the budget and source(s) of funding.

Negotiation of favoured options (following the identification and prioritization of impacts)

Consideration of alternative options does not conclude the process. Even when there appear to be clear messages regarding the best way forward, it cannot be assumed that these will automatically be adopted. Achieving agreement on options for mitigating or enhancing predicted health impacts requires skillful negotiation on the part of those involved.

Implementation, monitoring, and evaluation

To some extent, a HIA is analogous to an audit cycle in which the results of subsequent monitoring and evaluation in turn influence the continuing operation of the project. The indicators and methods proposed for monitoring depend on the nature and content of the project, and on the perceived importance of this stage of the assessment.[19]

In HIA, outcome evaluation is constrained by the fact that negative impacts that have been successfully avoided (or weakly positive ones that have been successfully enhanced) due to the modification of the project will clearly not be identifiable. In practice, things are rarely this perfect and it may be possible to construct and compare notional and actual outcomes relating to the originally proposed and actual post-HIA projects. Multi-method assessments of specified outcomes (*triangulation*) should be undertaken where feasible, in order to increase validity.

Process evaluation involves the assessment of HIA procedures and methods against the terms of reference initially agreed by the steering group; impact evaluation—arguably the most important evaluation element—involves the assessment of the extent to which the agreed recommendations of the HIA were successfully implemented.

A consistent finding of a number of studies is that undertaking HIA has produced unpredicted beneficial outcomes such as improved local partnerships, raising the profile of health issues on the political agenda, reducing social exclusion, empowering and engaging local communities, and improving and informing the quality of local decision-making.

Methods for assessing health impacts

The range of methods used for HIAs should reflect the nature and complexity of the subject matter. It is important to use all methods and involve all disciplines that may contribute to the overall task, commonly:
- policy analysis
- profiling of affected areas/populations
- identification of potential positive and negative health impacts
- assessment of perceived health risks
- quantification and valuation of health impacts
- ranking the most important impacts
- consideration of alternative options and recommendations for management of priority impacts.

Before looking at these methods, we will discuss the key area of participation.

Participation in HIAs

The process of HIA requires broad participation if a comprehensive picture of potential health impacts is to be established. Public participation
throughout the HIA is essential, both to ensure that local concerns are
addressed and for ethical reasons of social justice. The cooperation and
expertise of a wide range of stakeholders and key informants will be
needed, including:

- those involved at all levels in the project
- those likely to be directly affected by the project
- others who have knowledge or information of relevance to the
  project and its outcomes, e.g. local shopkeepers or service providers,
  community groups
- local or outside experts whose knowledge is relevant to the project
- relevant professionals, e.g. family practitioners, public health nurses,
  social or community workers
- voluntary organizations.

Barnes[20] has identified the importance of using robust and well-planned
methods of community participation in adding value and credibility to HIA
recommendations. She also highlights the need for HIA practitioners to
understand and record people's health experiences which underlie routinely collected statistics. Exclusive reliance on quantitative methods may
oversimplify the complexity of real-life situations.

Policy analysis

HIAs of policies will require initial policy analysis to determine key aspects
that the HIA will need to address; this may build on or use material already
available from earlier policy development work.[5] Key aspects include:

- content and dimensions of the policy
- socio-political and policy context
- policy objectives, priorities, and intended outputs
- trade-offs and critical sociocultural impacts which may affect its
  implementation.

Profiling of affected areas/populations

A profile of the areas and populations likely to be affected by the project is
compiled using available socio-demographic and health data and information from key informants across the public and non-statutory sectors. The
profile should cover groups whose health could be enhanced or placed at
risk by the project's effects. Vulnerable and disadvantaged groups require
special consideration.

Identification of potential positive and negative
health impacts

The range of potential health impacts identified in a HIA depends on the
definition of health that is employed. Like most governments and the
World Health Organization, we recommend using a socio-environmen-
tal model that features a wide range of linkages by which projects can
impact upon health, and a causal model of health impact in which a project changes the prevalence of health determinants and this, in turn, may

change the health status of the affected population groups. Table 1.5.1 presents the health determinants most often encountered in HIA.

Methods for identifying the potential health impacts of a project will vary according to the human and financial resources available. Clearly, a short workshop discussion involving a group of stakeholders around a table will employ different methods from a comprehensive assessment. Ideally, impact identification should involve qualitative fieldwork (typically interviews, focus groups and/or workshops, and sometimes Delphi studies or scenarios) and quantitative studies, such as mathematic modelling of project outcomes, surveys, and economic analysis.

Respondents will include relevant experts and purposive samples of key informants, including affected subpopulations. Literature searches are also employed in impact identification. The essential aim, whichever methods are used, is to systematically consider the range of potential changes to health determinants and outcomes likely to result from the development/ construction and operation of the project.

Assessment of perceived health risks

Perceptions of risk are, when possible, recorded at the time of identification of potential impacts. In some instances existing evidence will permit precise assessment of risk. In many cases, however, risk assessment will be based on subjective perceptions. Assuming adequate sampling, such subjective risk data are arguably no less valid or important than are more precise technical data—particularly where sensory perceptions (such as increased noise or smell, or deterioration of outlook) or experiences (such as discrimination) are concerned. Petts et al.[21] have produced a useful guide to understanding what influences people's assessment of risk.

Risk perceptions can be recorded using simple scales of measurability (potential impacts are characterized as qualitative, estimable, or calculable) and of likelihood of occurrence (definite, probable, possible or speculative). The temptation to quantify such scales should be resisted—such numbers could not be compared or manipulated with validity and would carry a spurious authority.

Quantification and valuation of health impacts

It may prove possible to assess the size of quantifiable (estimable/calculable) impacts at the time they are identified by informants; in other cases this will need to be done separately, e.g. through reviews of previously published evidence. The same applies to valuation—although evidence on the resource implications and opportunity costs of potential impacts will often prove hard to come by. However, such data can in principle be made comparable using QALYs or DALYs, or other such cost–utility measures. Some authors have described mathematic modelling methods used to quantify health impacts, particularly in relation to environmental impacts on health, such as air pollution, road accidents, and methods of waste disposal. The Foresight Vehicle Initiative HIA undertaken for the UK's Department of Trade and Industry[22] used modeling, and health and transport economic forecasting to quantify the health impacts of innovations in road transport technology.

Table 1.5.1 Health determinants encountered in HIA

Categories of health determinants	Examples of specific health determinants
Biological factors	Age, sex, genetic factors
Personal and family environment	Family structure and functioning, primary/secondary/adult education, occupation, unemployment, income, risk-taking behaviour, diet, smoking, alcohol, substance misuse, exercise, recreation, means of transport (cycle/car ownership)
Social environment	Culture, peer pressures, discrimination, social support (neighbourliness, social networks, isolation), community/cultural/spiritual participation, crime
Physical environment	Air/water quality, noise, smell, view, housing conditions, working conditions, public safety, civic design, shops (location/range/quality), communications (road/rail), land use, waste disposal, energy, local environmental features
Public services and public policy	Access to (location/disabled access/costs), quality of primary/community/secondary health care, child care, social (security) services, housing, leisure amenities, employment, public transport, law and order, other health-relevant public services, non-statutory agencies and services, equity/democracy in public policy.

Ranking the most important impacts

Encourage informants to prioritize/rank the potential impacts that they identify. Once all the initial evidence has been collected, a priority-setting exercise should be carried out. Because of different perceptions of risk there will rarely be complete consensus; criteria may need to be agreed so that the views of all informants are adequately reflected and valued. Such criteria are likely to include the frequency with which potential impacts are identified, the probability of occurrence, severity/importance, and public and political opinion.

Consideration of alternative options and recommendations for management of priority impacts

Unless there is total consensus, a series of options for providing the optimum health impact of the project being assessed should be defined and presented. The ultimate result will be an agreed set of recommendations for modifying the project such that its health impacts are optimized—in the context of the many and complex constraints that invariably constitute the social, material, and political environment in which it will be undertaken.

Communicating with key stakeholders is critical to the success or otherwise of an HIA. There are often political and organizational systems that require formal feedback such as local authority committees, health service boards, and local strategic partnerships. A HIA that is submitted to a planning enquiry will sometimes require a nominated senior officer to give evidence.

Recommendations

If HIA is going to be a worthwhile exercise it is crucial that it is able to demonstrate both effectiveness and efficient use of resources. Therefore it follows that any recommendations resulting from HIA studies should:
- be practical
- aim to maximize health gain and minimize health loss
- be socially acceptable (a degree of pragmatism may be inevitable)
- consider the cost of implementation
- consider the opportunity cost
- include preventive as well as curative measures
- be prioritized in terms of short-, medium-, and long-term objectives
- identify a lead agency or individual
- identify the drivers and barriers to change
- be acceptable to the lead agency
- be capable of being monitored and evaluated.

The list given above is, of course, not definitive and as HIA develops other criteria will be added. Too often, however, recommendations are of a general, rather than a specific nature, which makes monitoring difficult if not impossible. Also, if there was poor teamwork the recommendations may only reflect one person's viewpoint and may fail to appreciate the logistics of implementation. It will also mean that key agencies do not feel that they have ownership of the recommendations.

The impact of HIA

HIA has been applied to a wide range of policies, programmes, and projects and has had significant influence on policy making and planning. Examples of its effectiveness in the UK include the Finningley airport study[23] which resulted in the incorporation of an independent airport health impact group into the regulatory framework for an airport, and the Greater London Assembly's HIA programme,[24] which modified a range of London's socioeconomic and environmental strategies. A series of 17 European case studies documented many examples of positive impacts of HIAs in a range of European countries.[25] However, systematic documentation of the impacts of HIAs remains the exception; it needs to become the rule if the future of HIA is to be guaranteed.

Some conceptual and methodological issues

Science or art?

HIA is a decision support process that draws on a scientific knowledge base. Each HIA is specific to a location in time, space, and local conditions, although its evidence base can be evaluated, and the rigor with which procedures and methods are implemented can (and should) be assessed.

Uncertainty

Uncertainties encountered during the undertaking of HIAs frequently dictate the need to make assumptions: these are often acceptable, but should be declared explicitly.

Timing

HIA should take place early enough in the development of a project to permit constructive modifications to be carried out prior to its implementation, but late enough for a clear idea to have been formed as to its nature and content.

Cost and depth

The financial and opportunity costs of undertaking HIA dictate the need both to screen candidate projects and also to have available a range of methods according to the depth of analysis required.

Climate change and peak oil

The world is entering a new epoch dominated by climate change and oil scarcity. These twin challenges are likely to amplify existing health risks and inequalities.[26] As a consequence, projects that are designed today will have to operate in an energy regime that uses at least 80% less oil. Oil usage and greenhouse gas emissions will have to be reduced significantly in project inputs and outputs—and in HIA recommendations.

Politics

Although HIA is itself part of the political process, external political imperatives may sometimes inappropriately determine the outcome of the decision being assessed. Disagreements or power inequalities between different stakeholder factions may be similarly important. Health impact assessments will often be taken out of context to justify pre-set political positions. None of this 'policy-based evidence making' should deter us from continuing to use this innovative approach to promote healthy public policy.

References

1 WHO European Centre for Health Policy. (1999). *Health impact assessment: main concepts and suggested approach*, Gothenburg consensus paper. ECHP, Brussels.

2 Birley MH. (1995). *The health impact assessment of development projects*. HMSO, London.

3 Will S, Ardern K, Spencely M, Watkins S. (1994). *A prospective health impact assessment of the proposed development of a second runway at Manchester International Airport*, written submission to the public inquiry. Manchester and Stockport Health Commissions, Manchester.

4 Scott-Samuel A. (1996). Health impact assessment—an idea whose time has come. *British Medical Journal*, **313**, 183–4.

5 Abrahams D, den Broeder L, Doyle C, et al. (2004). *EPHIA—European policy health impact assessment: a guide*. IMPACT, University of Liverpool, Liverpool. Available at: ℗ http://www.liv.ac.uk/ihia/IMPACT%20Reports/EPHIA_A_Guide.pdf (accessed 26 August 2010).

6 Smith KE, Fooks G, Collin J, et al. (2010). Is the increasing policy use of impact assessment in Europe likely to undermine efforts to achieve healthy public policy? *Journal of Epidemiology and Community Health*, **64**, 478–87.

7 Association of Public Health Observatories. (2007). *The HIA Gateway*. Available at: ℗ http://www.apho.org.uk/default.aspx?QN=P_HIA (accessed 26 August 2010).

8 Krieger N, Northridge M, Gruskin S, et al. (2003). Assessing health impact assessment: multidisciplinary and international perspectives. *Journal of Epidemiology and Community Health*, **57**, 659–62.

9 Collins J, Koplan JP. (2009). Health impact assessment: a step toward health in all policies. *Journal of the American Medical Association*, **302**, 315–17.

10 Robert Wood Johnson Foundation, The Pew Charitable Trust. *Health Impact Project*. Available at: ℗ http://www.healthimpactproject.org (accessed 26 August 2010).

11 Public Health Advisory Committee (2004). *A guide to health impact assessment: a policy tool for New Zealand*. Public Health Advisory Committee, National Advisory Committee on Health and Disability, Wellington. Available at: ℗ http://www.nhc.health.govt.nz/publications/phac-pre-2011/guide-health-impact-assessment-2nd-edition (accessed 24 May 2012).

12 Mahoney M, Simpson S, Harris E, Aldrich R, Stewart Williams J. (2004). *Equity focused health impact assessment framework*. Australasian Collaboration for Health Equity Impact Assessment, Newcastle. Available at: ℗ http://www.hiaconnect.edu.au/files/EFHIA_Framework.pdf (accessed 26 August 2010).

13 WHO. (2003). Special issue on HIA. *Bulletin of the World Health Organization*, **81(6)**. Available at: ℗ http://www.who.int/bulletin/volumes/81/6/en/ (accessed 26 August 2010).

14 Scott-Samuel A, O'Keefe E. (2007). Health impact assessment, human rights and global public policy: a critical appraisal. *Bulletin of the World Health Organization*, **85**, 212–17.

15 O'Keefe E, Scott-Samuel A. (2010). Health impact assessment as an accountability mechanism for the International Monetary Fund: the case of Sub-Saharan Africa. *International Journal of the Health Service*, **40**, 339–45.

16 Equator Principles (2006). *The Equator Principles*. Available at: ℗ http://www.equator-principles.com (accessed 26 August 2010).

17 Commission on Social Determinants of Health. (2008). *Closing the gap in a generation: health equity through action on the social determinants of health*. WHO, Geneva.

18 Harris P, Harris-Roxas B, Harris E, Kemp L. (2007). *Health impact assessment: a practical guide*. Centre for Health Equity Training, Research and Evaluation (CHETRE), University of New South Wales, Sydney.

19 Parry JM, Kemm J. (2005). Criteria for use in the evaluation of health impact assessments: recommendations from an European workshop. *Public Health*, **119**, 1122–9.

20 Barnes R (2004). HIA and urban regeneration: the Ferrier Estate, England. In: Kemm J, Parry J, Palmer S, eds, *Health impact assessment. Concepts, theory, techniques and applications*, pp. 299–307. Oxford University Press, Oxford.

21 Petts J, Wheeley S, Homan J, Niemeyer S. (2003). *Risk literacy and the public. MMR, air pollution and mobile phones*. Department of Health, London. Available at: ℗ http://www.dh.gov.uk/asset-Root/04/07/40/99/04074099.pdf (accessed 26 August 2010).

22 Abrahams D. (2002). *Foresight Vehicle Initiative Comprehensive Health Impact Assessment. Executive summary*. IMPACT—International Health Impact Assessment Consortium, University of Liverpool, Liverpool. Available at: ℗ http://www.liv.ac.uk/ihia/IMPACT%20Reports/FVI_Comprehensive_-_Summary.pdf (accessed 26 August 2010).

23 Abdel Aziz MI, Radford J, McCabe J. (2000). *Health impact assessment, Finningley Airport*. Doncaster Health Authority. Available at: ℗ http://www.doncasterhealth.co.uk/documents/finningley/finningley_report.html (accessed 26 August 2010).

24 Taylor L, Gowman N, Quigley R. (2003). *Evaluating health impact assessment.* Health Development Agency, London. Available at: ✒ http://www.iaia.org/publicdocuments/pubs_ref_material/Evaluating%20HIA%20pdf.pdf (accessed 26 August 2010)

25 Wismar M. Blau J. Ernst K, et al. (eds). (2007). *The effectiveness of. health impact assessment.* European Obserrvatory on Health Systems and Policies, WHO, Copenhagen. Available at: ✒ http://www.euro.who.int/__data/assets/pdf_file/0003/98283/E90794.pdf (accessed 26 August 2010).

26 Costello A, Abbas M, Allen A, et al. (2009). Managing the health effects of climate change: Lancet and University College London Institute for Global Health Commission. *Lancet,* **373,** 1693–733.

1.6 Economic assessment

Peter Brambleby

Objectives

This chapter will help the reader to:
- understand the tools, techniques and approaches of health economics
- apply a health economics way of framing a discussion when the need arises in management situations
- pose better questions when important choices are apparent and when the help of a professional health economist is involved.

What is health economics?

Health economics is concerned with managing scarcity, supporting decisions and evaluating results, where resources are deployed in health and health care (see Box 1.6.1). All professional health care activity involves making choices. This can be particularly challenging in promoting health, preventing disease and treating ill health since:
- the outcome may be attributable to multiple interventions
- the outcome may not be evident for several years
- resources are insufficient to meet all the need (ability to benefit from an intervention) and demand (what patients or the caring professions ask for)
- the evidence base on outcomes and resources is often incomplete.

The practitioner often has to make, or advise others on making, choices such as:
- deciding whether or not to introduce a new intervention or service
- deciding how one could go about comparing many bids for new money when only a few of the bids could be funded
- deciding the best way to find how to take money out of a service.

Whether one is involved with the planning or the delivery of health care, the job involves many complex choices. In predominantly publicly-funded systems (such as the UK's NHS), or public/private mixed economies (such as most of continental Europe), there is the added dimension of having to be publicly accountable for stewardship of scarce resources. The techniques of health economics help to expose the trade-offs between the options and make the decision-taking process open to scrutiny and participation.

Box 1.6.1 Health economics

Health economics is a discipline that brings a systematic approach to the management of issues of scarcity and choice in health care.

Despite its name, economics is not primarily about 'making econo-mies' nor even about money. Money is just one type of resource. Other resources include people, time, and buildings. Costs can be tangible and easy to ascribe a monetary value to, such as medicines, staff, or journeys to hospital, or they can be intangible, such as pain and disability. All types of cost are potentially relevant, though are some are set aside in particular applications. Economic appraisal is about relating costs to outputs and outcomes. It is about return on investment in health and health care. It is therefore just as concerned with evidence of effectiveness as it is with resources.

The steps of economic appraisal often follow this sequence:
- What are we trying to achieve?
- What are the different ways of achieving this (the options)?
- How do these options compare with each other, taking adverse effects into account as well as benefits?
- What costs are involved for each option, taking not only health-care factors and intangible costs into consideration, but other factors such as costs to social services or to the patient?

Similarly, if a service might be stopped, the considerations are:
- What are we trying to achieve?
- What are the different ways of achieving this (options)?
- What benefits will be lost with each option?
- What resources will be released with each option?
- If resources might be redeployed, what is the net gain and net cost (or saving)?

Health economics provides a means of handling these decisions. It can be regarded as a way of framing the discussion (a shared perspective on problem-solving that decision-makers find useful), and as a particular set of tools and techniques to articulate the costs, benefits, and trade-offs.

Health economics as a way of thinking

Health economics is not a substitute for thought, but a way of organiz-ing it.[1] It is not a technical fix that tells you precisely what to do.[2–7] The approach is *utilitarian*—trying to get the greatest good for the greatest number, and concerned with *efficiency*—getting the greatest outcome from a fixed amount of resource.

Although these are the health economist's starting points, they need not necessarily be adopted as the deciding criteria when decisions are taken. The gulf between what is possible and what can be afforded (by the individual or the state), and the inevitability of having to choose, is the starting point for economic appraisal. Health economics recognizes the existence of trade-offs inherent in any system. Choice involves sacrifice. It is perfectly legitimate to trade-off some efficiency for the sake of other considerations, such as equity. Equity can be described as the willingness to give a protected 'fair share' to a particular group in society in need, even if that does not maximize total outcomes from the available resources for the population as a whole. It serves to emphasize that choices are not free—there is an *opportunity cost* (benefit foregone) once resources are committed. In other words, once resources have been committed, the real cost is not the monetary value, but the best alternative use to which that resource could have been put. Just like many other disciplines that contribute to the practice of public health (e.g. epidemiology and sociology) economic appraisal is concerned with whole populations and not just individuals.

Economic evaluations

Economic evaluations deal with the relationships between costs and outcomes when choices have to be made between competing options. Sometimes the outcomes are the same and the issue is simply 'which option consumes least resources, taking all costs into consideration?' In this situation the appropriate tool is *cost minimization analysis*.

More often the costs and outcomes are both different, but the units in which the outcomes are measured are the same (for example, years of life added for choices between cancer treatments; peak expiratory flow rates for choices between asthma treatments; or successful live births in choices between infertility treatments). In such cases the appropriate tool is *cost-effectiveness analysis*.

Sometimes the choice is between very different types of outcome, measured in very different units, and with very different costs. An example would be deciding whether to put some additional resources into cancer care, orthopaedics, or diabetes. The issue is one of finding a common set of units such as QALYs to allow a 'cost per QALY' comparison on a like-for-like basis. The term given to appraisals that convert different sorts of outcome into these common 'utility' units is *cost–utility analysis*. The great advantage of this approach, despite the limitations of ascribing QALY units, is that it allows comparisons between very different interventions, and that is helpful to policy makers in pursuit of allocative efficiency (see Box 1.6.1).

Sometimes it is simply a question of weighing up whether the costs of a new intervention outweigh the benefits or not, and whether it should go ahead at all. Costs and benefits are both ascribed a monetary value in order to make the comparison. This is *cost–benefit analysis*. (Note that 'cost–benefit analysis' has a precise meaning and is not a blanket term for all comparisons of costs and outcomes—a better phrase to describe these techniques collectively is *economic appraisal*.)

The tools for addressing these situations are shown in Box 1.6.2.

Box 1.6.2 Forms of economic evaluation

- *Cost minimization analysis:* when the outcomes (benefits) of alternative interventions are the same in terms of volume and type, the cheapest programme should be chosen on the grounds of efficiency. For example, choosing between a branded and a generic antibiotic to treat a streptococcal infection.
- *Cost-effectiveness analysis:* when both the costs and outcomes of alternative interventions are *different*, then the efficient choice is that intervention, which costs least to produce a unit of outcome (such as a life saved), for example, choosing between two interventions of different cost and effectiveness that both lower blood pressure in people with hypertension.
- *Cost–utility analysis:* when the outcomes from alternate interventions are *not* the same, then a 'common outcome currency' (such as a QALY) is used as a measure of benefit to enable comparisons to be made between interventions. Choice of intervention will then depend on the cost of producing a unit of the chosen currency (e.g. the cost per QALY), for example, choosing between hip replacements, coronary artery bypass grafts, and haemodialysis for the next year's investment.
- *Cost–benefit analysis:* the preceding evaluative methods all leave the outcome/benefit side of the equation in 'natural' units (clearing infection, lowering blood pressure, QALYs, etc.). Cost–benefit analysis places monetary values on these benefits (to enable direct comparison between the inputs and the outcomes. This analysis can help to decide whether to do something at all or not (for example, if the value of the input is greater than the output it might be better not to do it), or when choosing between options to assess which gives the greatest ratio of outcome to input. An illustration of this application might be whether or not to invest in installing crash barriers along a 10-mile stretch of road to avoid road traffic deaths and injuries (where deaths and injuries are ascribed a monetary value).

Additional concepts

The appraisal tools described above are a simplification of the decision-guiding process. A health economist will also apply an annual percentage '*discounting*' to costs and benefits that fall at some time in the future to give them all a present-day value (this could be of the order of, for instance, 6% per annum). A benefit in the future is valued less highly than a benefit today (hence, the value of a benefit only available at some time in the future is 'discounted').

A *sensitivity analysis* would also be done to several values, rather than single point estimates, since data on costs and outcomes are seldom precise. This yields a range of estimates to assist decision-makers.

Priority setting through programme budgeting and marginal analysis

A pioneer of programme budgeting and marginal analysis (PBMA) was Professor Alain Enthoven, who took it from its application to the American armed forces and applied it to health care planning (or purchasing) at the population level. He endorsed its use in the UK NHS in his 1999 Rock Carling Fellowship review.[8]

An entire issue of *Health Policy*[9] was devoted to articles on this topic. Table 1.6.1 gives an outline of PBMA.

The UK Department of Health, with parallels in other parts of the UK NHS, has been exploring PBMA. This was promised by the 1997 Labour government in its first major policy document on health *The New NHS: Modern, Dependable* (London, 1997):

- *Para 6.22:* 'Partnerships between secondary and primary care physicians and with social services will provide the necessary basis for the establishment of 'programmes of care', which will allow planning and resource management across organisational boundaries.'
- *Para 9.18:* 'Efficient use of resources will be critical to delivering the best for patients. It is important that managers and clinicians alike have a proper understanding of the costs of local services, so that they can make appropriate local decisions on the best use of resources.'

Another significant strand of policy was the creation of the NICE, now emulated in many other countries around the world, which appraises evidence of effectiveness and cost-effectiveness and publishes technology appraisals and clinical guidance (see ℘ http://www.nice.org.uk/).

Is *health* economics different from conventional economics?

From the conventional point of view of economics, health care is unusual.[10] Standard economic ideas of supply and demand are often difficult to square with the reality of how health-care systems actually function. In virtually all countries demand for health care is mediated through a medical professional—consumers are not sovereign as in a typical market model. Patients need the help of a clinician to identify what their state of health really is, what their health-care needs are, and what interventions are appropriate to address them. This is known as the *agency role* of the health professions.

Both supply and demand for health care, especially secondary health care, are heavily regulated and managed. Complex insurance markets—run by the state, the independent sector, or a mixture of the two—have grown up in response to the inherent uncertainties of illness and the costs of treatment. Governments can play a significant part in health-care regulation, from setting rules about practitioner qualifications through to resource allocation, standard setting, and direct control of provision.

Table 1.6.1 Programme budgeting and marginal analysis (PBMA)

Action	Comments
Define health care programmes	Break down the priority setting process into more manageable and meaningful programmes (e.g. client groups, specialties, disease groups) and define health care objectives and outputs for each
Establish programme management groups	Management groups (clinicians, managers, user representatives) are responsible for priority setting within their programme
Understand the chosen programmes	Identify current spending on, and broad outputs from, each programme.
Define subprogrammes of care (if it helps)	Identify further breakdowns in programmes, with estimates of spending and defined objectives
Focus on marginal change	Most priority setting concerns changes to existing services, i.e. changes at the margin. Therefore, most attention can be paid to changes *within*, rather than *between* programmes. However, do not be afraid to look across programmes for a population, perhaps spread across several providers, and examine marginal changes between programmes. Just bear in mind that the management challenge of shifting resources between programmes is considerable, and needs agreement in principle at the outset.
Identify incremental 'wish lists' (and decremental 'hit lists')	Given extra (or fewer) resources, what services should be expanded (or reduced) to deliver a closer fit with the programme's stated objectives?
Make proposals based on relative benefits generated by changes in spending	What would be implemented from the wish lists if specific amounts of money were made available or taken away?
Consider equity and policy implications	The steps above focus on efficiency—getting more health care/healthiness for each unit of resource—but check against other considerations such as 'fair shares', local strategy and national policy.
Consult	Out of necessity 'point estimates' of cost and outcome are used in PBMA. If you can, conduct a sensitivity analysis. Do not let the veneer of scientific precision blind you to the underlying value judgements. PBMA helps clarify and organize thought. It is imperative to check the assumptions with those most affected
Choose where to invest and where to disinvest; evaluate results and share the learning	Having identified new patterns of spending based on clinical and economic evidence, decisions need to be taken to implement changes and then evaluate them. Share the learning by disseminating your experience.

The importance of the margin

Another important concept in health economics is that of the *margin*—the cost of the *next* (or one additional) unit of input or the benefit of the *next* unit of output. The importance of this is that in health care many choices are made about relatively small incremental changes in service (either to increase or decrease), rather than whole-scale strategic shifts. The issue is often described thus: 'What is the extra cost over and above what we pay now, and what is the extra benefit?' (The reverse applies for disinvestment decisions: 'What resources do we release and what benefits do we lose?')

A related concept is the *stepped cost*.

Examples

Suppose a cardiac surgery unit is built, staffed, and equipped to deal with 900 patients a year and funded accordingly. This would mean all the costs—'fixed costs' (like buildings), 'semi-fixed costs' (like staff salaries), and 'variable costs' (like medicines)—were covered. Suppose that with this complement of buildings, the staff and equipment could actually cope with a further 50 patients. The additional (marginal) cost of each extra patient up to 50 would be relatively small, and chiefly reflect the 'variable costs'. However, a point would come when, to accommodate just one more patient, extra staff would have to be taken on or a new ward built—that would be a substantial 'stepped cost'.

To see the relevance of this, imagine you are a health care purchaser with 200 extra patients requiring cardiac surgery and three cardiac centres within reasonable travelling distance for your population. It would be in everyone's interest to try and spread that additional workload between all three centres if that would enable them all to work closer to capacity, but if that were not possible, then it might be better to make a single strategic investment (stepped development) at just one.

The same applies to benefits. Suppose an immunization programme reaches only 80% of the child population. An additional £50,000 might enable a further 10% to be reached, but the addition of a yet another £50,000 on top of that might only enable a further 5% to be reached. In common parlance this is 'the law of diminishing returns'; to the economist it is known as 'diminishing marginal benefit'.

The important points to remember are that *average* cost and benefit (*total* cost divided by *total* benefit) can differ substantially from *marginal* cost and benefit. Marginal cost and marginal benefit do not increase (or decrease) in a smooth linear fashion, they tend to go in steps.

A further important point is that harm arising from unintended consequences and known adverse effects of powerful therapeutic interventions tends to rise in linear fashion or accelerate, rather than diminish. There may come a point where increasing inputs lead to net added harm and past the point of *optimal* health investment.

Ethics and equity

The ethical stance of health economics is sometimes questioned by clinicians because the utilitarian approach can seem to be at odds with the 'Hippocratic' ethic of doing the very best for the individual in a trusting doctor–patient relationship. (Economics is not known as the 'dismal science' for nothing!) However, an economist would justify the pursuit of efficiency on the grounds that the true cost of inefficiency is borne in terms of pain, disability, and premature death by those waiting for treatment. In a publicly-funded health care system, where policy making, funding, and provision are all controlled largely by the state, the primary objective of trying to ensure the greatest good for the greatest number is legitimate. One could extend this and argue that it is better to have a system where everyone gets access to a service that meets basic standards, even if those are not the very best possible, if the alternative means that some should go without altogether.

Efficiency (allocative versus technical)

In general terms, health care policy makers and those who 'commission' are primarily concerned with '*allocative efficiency*'—trying to maximize the population health gain from a fixed allocation of resources. (One is trying to reach a position where no one waiting for treatment has a greater ability to benefit than anyone who is already being treated.)

Health care 'providers' are more often concerned with *technical efficiency*—achieving a desired objective at the least cost. Many of the objectives are set for them: numbers to be treated, waiting times, and so on. Allocative efficiency is about doing the right things. Technical efficiency is about doing things right.

Since the 1990s, in an attempt to address both types of efficiency, the NHS in England has experimented with a market model whereby the funds are held by 'commissioners' and devolved, ostensibly according to population need, to 'providers' who deliver the care. This was an attempt to harness 'market forces' to drive up quality and drive out inefficiency. Although introduced by a Conservative administration, the Labour administration that followed it in 1997 perpetuated many elements of the model, especially the separation of purchasing and providing roles. For a lucid analysis of the strengths and weaknesses of the market models in the NHS see Enthoven.[8]

Conclusions

Everyone concerned with health care can benefit from a familiarity with health economists' ways of thinking, language, and some of the tools in the toolkit. Health economics gives a structured approach to decision-making in health care where resources are always scarce, need appears almost limitless, and choices are inevitable. It is not a formulaic approach that bypasses critical appraisal, but it can greatly improve the rigor and transparency of the decision-making process.

Further resources

Donaldson C, Bate A, Brambleby P, Waldner H. (2008). Moving forward on rationing: an economic view. *British Medical Journal*, **307**, 905–6.

Mitton C, Donaldson D (2001). Twenty-five years of programme budgeting and marginal analysis in the health sector, 1974–1999. *Journal of Health Service Research Policy*, **6**, 239–48.

Ruta D, Mitton C, Bate A, Donaldson C (2005). Programme budgeting and marginal analysis: bridging the divide between doctors and managers. *British Medical Journal*, **330**, 1501–3.

UK Department of Health. National Programme Budget Project—publications and resources guidance manual, spreadsheets, case studies, discussion forum and contacts. Available at: http://www.dh.gov.uk/programmebudgeting (accessed 7 September 2010).

www.healthknowledge.org.uk/interactivelearning/index_margins.asp (accessed 24 May 2012).

References

1 Drummond MF, O'Brien BJ, Stoddard GL, Torrance GW. (1997). *Methods for the economic evaluation of health care programmes*, 2nd edn. Oxford University Press, Oxford.

2 Robinson R. (1993). Economic evaluation and health care (a series of six articles in the BMJ). What does it mean? *British Medical Journal*, **307**, 670–3.

3 Robinson R. (1993). Costs and cost minimisation analysis. *British Medical Journal*, **307**, 726–8.

4 Robinson R. (1993). Cost effectiveness analysis. *British Medical Journal*, **307**, 793–5.

5 Robinson R. (1993). Cost utility analysis. *British Medical Journal*, **307**, 859–62.

6 Robinson R. (1993). Cost benefit analysis. *British Medical Journal*, **307**, 924–6.

7 Robinson R. (1993). The policy context. *British Medical Journal*, **307**, 994–6.

8 Enthoven A. (1999). *Rock Carling Fellowship 1999. In pursuit of an improving National Health Service*. Nuffield Trust, London.

9 *Health Policy*. (1995). Special issue devoted to programme budgeting and marginal analysis. **33**.

10 McGuire A, Henderson J, Mooney G. (1988). *The economics of health care: an introductory text*. Routledge, London.

11 Mooney G, Gerard K, Donaldson C, Farrar S. (1992). *Priority setting in purchasing: some practical guidelines*, Research Paper 6. National Association of Health Authorities and Trusts (NAHAT), Birmingham.

Part 2

Data and information

2.1 Understanding data, information, and knowledge

Barry Tennison

Objectives

The aim of this chapter is to help the public health practitioner to:
- Appreciate the subtleties of the varied forms of information about the health of a population and related matters
- Develop a toolkit for thinking about the complexity of information and its uses
- Orientate themselves positively towards the decisions and actions needed, applying wisely and with good judgement the information and knowledge available
- The classification (taxonomy) of types of information given in this chapter should help the public health practitioner to:
  - assess the relevance, timeliness, accuracy, and completeness of available information
  - decide which types of information are most appropriate for a particular public health task
  - make optimal use of information that is not ideal, and assess the effects of its departure from perfection.

The use of the words 'data' and 'information'

Some people are purists. They will use the word 'data' (singular or plural) for raw numbers or other measures, reserving the word 'information' for what emerges when data are processed, analysed, interpreted, and presented. This has the virtue of making clear the sequence of steps that are involved in turning observations about the world into a form that is useful to those who wish to draw conclusions, and to act. This always involves the use of judgement in assessing the information as a source of evidence (alongside other evidence), and combining this judiciously with accepted best practice to arrive at usable knowledge. This process is summarized in Figure 2.1.1.

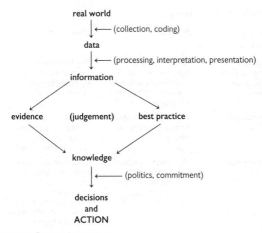

Figure 2.1.1 From reality to action.

In practice, many people use 'data' and 'information' more or less inter-changeably, perhaps on the grounds of the greyness of some of these distinctions and steps. However, in assessing the value of what emerges as information from these steps, the practitioner must bear in mind the fundamental issues which affect the quality of the data:

- *Validity:* are the data capturing the concept or quantity the practitioner intends? Are the definitions and methods of data collection explicit and clear?
- *Selection bias:* where the data mislead because they are not representative of the population or problem being considered, for example because of poor sampling.
- *Classification bias:* where there is a non-random effect on putting data into groupings, for example in non-blind assessments of health outcome.
- *Statistical significance:* where, although differences seem apparent, analysis shows that they are reasonably likely to have occurred by chance (see, for example, Marshall and Spiegelhalter[1]).
- *Precision:* is the sample size sufficient to estimate the prevalence of disease (say) with precision? How wide are the 95% confidence intervals surrounding the estimate?

What kinds of data sources are there?

In most countries, there are many different sources of information on the health of the population.[2] Different types of information vary in their 'CART': Completeness, Accuracy, Relevance (and/or Representativeness), Timeliness.

Data sources also vary in the ease with which a 'base population' can be identified, for use in the denominator, or for calculating rates. Typical data sources for local areas are summarized in Table 2.1.1.

Table 2.1.1 Data sources

Source	Strengths	Weaknesses
1. Routine data sources		
Population estimates. Census or population registers	Usually reasonably accurate, especially if complemented by local authority (UK) or other government data	May be problems with small area estimates, especially between censuses
Birth/abortion notifications	Reasonably accurate—often several possible data sources	No complete data on spontaneous abortions. Sometimes non-standard coding used
Mortality records	Most reliable health data as death tends to be unequivocal. Total mortality reliable	Insensitive measure of health. Physician's cause of death specification often inaccurate/incomplete. Non-fatal disease not reflected in mortality figures
Morbidity measures: infectious disease notifications (see 📖 Chapter 2.4)	Certain diseases notifiable (mandatory). Generally adequate for monitoring trends	Often incomplete, sometimes inconsistently incomplete
Morbidity measures: disease registers (see 📖 Chapter 2.7)	Key group identified. Often do not cover whole country	May miss people due to no contact or non-identification
Impairment, disability and handicap	Functional status often more relevant than disease status	Usually available from surveys only
Health services data: access and supply, utilization, costs	May be potentially relevant especially if condition almost always results in health care use, e.g. fractured femur	Likely to be incomplete. Data tend to identify health service activity and settings rather than receipt of (effective) interventions. Data quality may be poor
Data from other agencies—social care, housing, environmental risks, etc.	May be relevant	May be poor quality. May be incomplete. Categories and definitions may be incompatible with other data

(Continued)

Table 2.1.1 Contd.

Source	Strengths	Weaknesses
2. Surveys (see 🕮 Chapter 2.8)		
National surveys, or surveys from other countries	Available. May be authoritative and highly relevant	Require 'modelling' to local population characteristic. May not be generalizable to local population. Quality variable
Previous local surveys	Relevant and usually appeal to a local audience	Quality variable
Local surveys to be commissioned	Can be tailor-made	Often expensive
3. Qualitative data		
Local descriptive accounts of environmental or social factors	May give a good understanding or stimulate research	The scale of health impact of identified problems may be difficult to assess
People's perceptions of how health problems affect them	May give a good understanding of what really affects people	Qualitative data can need careful handling, as details of context, background, and question wording can result in unstable responses

A 'population health information' system can help in assembling data sources on a population. Such systems often involve a partnership between different agencies involved with a population, and can allow coordination of health information activities. A comprehensive population health information system would ideally record both:

- *Personal health events:* health-related occurrences or states pertaining to an identified person (examples are myocardial infarction or smoking status).
- *Population health factors:* health-related features or occurrences that apply to a population defined by some combination of person, time, and place (examples are exposure of a defined population to a health risk like a toxic spill or prevalence of smoking in teenage girls in a specified locality, derived from a survey).

Such a system would also allow both routine and *ad hoc* analyses in such a way that both events and factors are linked.

What does the information describe?

Information about the health of a population can cover:

- *Demography:* the basic characteristics of the population, such as age, sex, geographic distribution, and mobility.

- *Health-related characteristics or risk factors:* such as measures of deprivation, living conditions, employment, housing, or more medical factors or physiologic measurements (e.g. blood glucose levels).
- *Health need data:* such as the distribution of the indications for an intervention such as hip replacement[3] or the distribution of different thresholds for intervention.
- *Mortality:* the death experience of the population, including causes of death and variation according to the dimensions of person, place, and time.
- *Morbidity:* the health or illness experience of the population, including prevalence and incidence of diseases.
- *Health service use data:* such as diagnoses, interventions, and procedures, and health outcomes of interventions; it may be useful to distinguish patient interactions with *agents*, such as nurses or doctors from their use of *settings*, such as hospital, day hospital, health centre, or home in using the health service.
- *Health economic data:* often concerning the costs of interventions, and the distribution of activity and costs at marginal or average levels.

Clarity and judgement are needed about when one of these types of data is being used as a *proxy* for another. For example, where mortality data are firm and morbidity data poor in quality, with care, mortality may be seen as a good proxy for morbidity—this might work well for certain kinds of heart disease or cancer, but very poorly for most mental health problems. Similarly, care is needed in moving from burden of disease (mortality, morbidity, or even more carefully, health service use) to health *need*.

In terms of how it is collected, assembled, and made available, information can be either:

- *Routine:* collected, assembled, and made available repeatedly, according to well-defined protocols and standards; such data are usually part of a *System of data collection by which information is:*
  - made available at regular intervals
  - intended to allow tracking over time
  - codified according to national or international standards (for example, using the International Classification of Diseases (ICD[4])).
- *Specially collected:* for a particular purpose, without the intention of regular repetition or adherence to standards (other than those needed for the specific study or task); such data are usually:
  - aimed at a specific, time-limited study or task
  - codified according to the task in hand and the wishes of the investigators (sometimes in ignorance of the availability of suitable standard codes and methods)
  - difficult to compare (between times, places, and people) with routine data and other specially collected data.

Most of the data published in medical journals fall in the category 'specially collected'.

Table 2.1.2 gives important examples of information according to these dimensions. Note that these are only *examples*, but the table may help to see where an existing, new, or proposed data source sits, and the corresponding opportunities and drawbacks.

Table 2.1.2 Information collected according to the dimensions 'routine' and 'specially collected'

	Routine data	Specially collected data
Demography	Census counts, birth registration	Survey of homeless, roofless, and rough sleepers
Risk factors	Census details, such as housing conditions	Survey of ethnicity and coronary risk factors. Local survey of tobacco use
Mortality	Death registration, coroner's records, medical examiner's records	Some cohort studies which capture deaths search for deaths probably due to suicide, using multiple sources
Morbidity	National health surveys (such as the Health Survey for Eng-land[5] or the National Health Interview Survey in the USA[6]). Disease notifications and registers	Case finding for an outbreak. Survey to establish prevalence of a specific dis-ease. Most cohort studies
Health need	(mainly proxies)	Survey of prevalence of indications for specific intervention, such as hip re-placement
Service use	Use of in-patient beds. At-tendances at out-patient department, emergency room, or physician's office	Observational study of use of a hospital department. Follow-up study of out-comes of hip replacement
Economic	Accounts of health service organizations. Cost and price tables[7,8]	Costing of an existing or proposed service

Classification of intrinsic types of data

It is sometimes useful to categorize data as hard or soft (Table 2.1.3). In fact, there is a spectrum from 'hard' to 'soft' data: data are never completely hard or soft.

Harder data tend to be:
• precise (or intended to be precise)
• often numerical; if not, then coded according to a firm protocol
• reproducible, and likely to be similar even if the data collectors or individuals studied are varied.

Softer data tend to be:
• qualitative, attempting to capture some of the subtlety of human experience

- often narrative or textual in form, at least as they are collected
- imbued with some subjectivity, due to the complexity of the personalities of the data collectors and the individuals studied.

Table 2.1.3 Examples of data considered to be harder or softer

	Harder	Softer
Demography	Ethnic breakdown of a population according to a given ethnic classification. Proportion of houses with a specific amenity (e.g. a bath)	Narrative account of nature and composition of a neighborhood
Risk factors	Blood pressure. Proportion of smokers, non-smokers, and ex-smokers (according to precise definitions)	Patient experience of symptoms. Smoking 'careers' of teenagers
Mortality	Numbers dying of a specific disease. Survival data after specific interventions	Impact of deaths on the survivors
Morbidity	Prevalence of disease in a population at a moment in time. Numbers of admissions to a particular hospital	Reasons why a family doctor refers patients to hospital. Reported quality of treatment given by a particular hospital

(Note that some people will use the term 'soft' when they wish to imply that the data have inherent tendencies to imprecision, even if they are 'hard' in the sense of being numeric or strongly coded.)

Neither hard nor soft data are intrinsically better than the other. The utility of the information (in terms of better decision-making) often comes from combining the two:

- harder data usually allow more precise analysis and comparisons, but may fail to capture subtleties of human experience and preferences
- softer data usually capture more of the 'truth' about the world, but often at the expense of emphasizing the uniqueness of circumstances, rather than aiding comparisons and conclusions.

The important thing to assess is *fitness for purpose*: are the existing or proposed data fit for the purpose for which they are intended, the conclusion to be drawn, the decision to be made, or the action to be taken? For example, for deciding the allocation of resources, one requires relatively hard data to obtain a degree of precision and transparency, so that the judgements involved are explicit. On the other hand, soft data may be useful in deciding on a change in the pattern of services provided, for example when a client population (such as teenagers) seems to make poor use of current services: a well-designed qualitative survey may reveal some of the reasons, and a potential service configuration response. Softer data are also essential when capturing patient preference[9] or professional experiences.[10,11]

Absolute and comparative information

Often data about one location, one time, or one population are difficult to interpret in isolation; or worse, seem to beg obvious conclusions when, in fact, *comparison* with similar data elsewhere, previously, or in another population suggests a different conclusion or decision.

Comparative data are available on a local, regional, national,[12-14] or international[15] level. The WHO publishes comparative data between countries, for example on comparative performance of health systems.[16]

Assessing the appropriateness and usefulness of particular information

Experience shows the truth of the adage that the information you think you want is seldom the information you actually need; and the information you have seldom matches either need or want [often attributed to Finagle: in full, Finagle's law is often quoted thus 'The information you have is not what you want; the information you want is not what you need; the information you need is not what you can get; the information you can get costs more than you want to pay' (or a variation thereof)]. The pragmatic public health practitioner must learn to cope with what is possible, not to set impossible standards, and to make the appropriate allowances, professionally, for shortcomings of the available information. Above all, public health practitioners must not allow themselves or others to despair and to declare tasks impossible without the necessary information (which is, in fact, unavailable or unfeasible).

Box 2.1.1 is a checklist of issues to consider when assessing data or a data source for fitness for purpose. None of these issues is absolute, and the balance of advantage and disadvantage must be assessed using judgement.

Conclusion

All too often, when faced with a decision, there is a call for more information (or worse, a new information system). Frequently, either the available data are in fact, with care and interpretation, fit for the purpose for the decision needed; or the costs (including money, skills, burden of effort, and delay) of the new information or system is not commensurable with the problem faced. The above checklist, and this chapter, should help the practitioner to find a pragmatic, but wise balance between what is needed and what is feasible and adequate.

Box 2.1.1 Checklist for assessing appropriateness and usefulness of data and data sources

Technical issues
- Are the definitions sufficiently clear and appropriate?
- Are the target and study populations sufficiently clear?
- Are the data collection methods sufficiently clear and sound?
- How complete, accurate, relevant, and timely are the data? How much does this matter?
- Do any differences that appear reach statistical significance, and what are the confidence limits or intervals? (Consider the use of a Bayesian approach[17]).

Issues relating to the conclusion or decision involved
- Is the study population sufficiently representative of the target population for the purpose of the decision or proposed action?
- Do we need absolute or relative estimates to make the best decision?
- What precision is needed for the decision (taking into account confounding factors, random variation, and the influence of external factors such as resource availability, professional opinion, and politics)?
- Would a simpler or existing data source suffice, for example by using comparative data; by extrapolating or interpolating, with care; or by transferring data from a similar or analogous situation?
- Would qualitative information suffice (or be best), when habit automatically suggests quantitative data?

Further resources

Health Canada Online. ℘ http://www.hc-sc.gc.ca/english/ (accessed 29 March 2005).
Rigby M. (ed.) (2004). *Vision and value in health information.* Radcliffe Medical Press, Oxford.
UK National Electronic Library for Health. ℘ http://www.nelh.nhs.uk/ (accessed 29 March 2005).
US Department of Health & Human Services. ℘ http://www.os.dhhs.gov/ reference/index.shtml (accessed 29 March 2005).

References

1 Marshall EC, Spiegelhalter DJ. (1998). Reliability of league tables of in vitro fertilization clinics: retrospective analysis of live birth rates. *British Medical Journal*, **316**, 1701–5.
2 Detels R, McEwen J, Beaglehole R, Tanaka H. (eds) (2002). *Oxford textbook of public health.* Oxford University Press, New York.
3 Frankel S, Eachus J, Pearson N, *et al.* (1999). Population requirement for primary hip-replacement surgery: a cross-sectional study. *Lancet*, **353**, 1304–9.
4 World Health Organization. *The WHO family of international classifications.* Available at: ℘ http://www.who.int/classifications/en/ (accessed 20 March 2005).
5 Department of Health. Health Survey for England. Available at: ℘ http://www.dh.gov.uk/PublicationsAndStatistics/PublishedSurvey/HealthSurveyForEngland/fs/en (accessed 20 March 2005).
6 National Centre for Health Statistics. National Health Interview Survey (NHIS). Available at: ℘ www.cdc.gov/nchs/nhis.htm (accessed 20 March 2005).
7 Department of Health. Reference costs. Available at: ℘ http://www.dh.gov.uk/PolicyAndGuidance/OrganizationPolicy/FinanceAndPlanning/NHSReferenceCosts/ (accessed 21 January 2006).

8 Centres for Medicare & Medicaid Services. *Cost reports.* Available at: ℬ http://www.cms.hhs. gov/CostReports/ (accessed 21 January 2006).

9 Silvestri G, Pritchard R, Welch HG. (1998). Preferences for chemotherapy in patients with advanced non-small cell lung cancer: descriptive study based on scripted interviews. *British Medical Journal*, **317**, 771–5.

10 Jain A, Ogden J. (1999). General practitioners' experiences of patients' complaints: qualitative study. *British Medical Journal*, **318**, 1596–9.

11 Dowie R. (1983). *General practitioners and consultants: a study of outpatient referrals.* King Edward's Hospital Fund for London, London.

12 National Statistics, Official UK statistics. Available at: http://www.statistics.gov.uk (accessed 20 March 2005).

13 Statistics Canada, Canadian statistics. Available at: ℬ http://www40.statcan.ca/z01/cs0002_ e.htm (accessed 8 September 2005).

14 National Centre for Health Statistics, US statistics. Available at: ℬ http://www.cdc.gov/nchs/ (accessed 21 March 2005).

15 World Health Organization. *WHO Statistical Information System (WHOSIS).* Available at: http://www.who.int/whosis/ (accessed 21 March 2005).

16 World Health Organization. *Health systems performance.* Available at: ℬ http://www. who.int/ health-systems-performance/ (accessed 21 March 2005).

17 Spiegelhalter DJ, Myles JP, Jones DR, Abrams KR. (1999). Methods in health service research: an introduction to Bayesian methods in health technology assessment. *British Medical Journal*, **319**, 508–12.

2.2 Information technology and informatics

Don Eugene Detmer

Objectives

After reading this chapter you should be able to:
- identify the emerging sub-disciplines within biomedical and health informatics that are critical to the skillful use of health information and communications technology in the health sciences
- appreciate how informatics is applied to public health, clinical medicine, and research and that its roles are in rapid evolution.

Introduction

Informatics relating to health encompasses significant applications in public health, clinical care, and biomedical research. Despite the relative youth of the scientific discipline, biomedical and health informatics are recognized widely as essential to competent practice as a health professional (see Box 2.2.1). This is due primarily to the limits of human cognition and the growth in the knowledge base of medicine. The limitations of natural human memory cannot match the capacity of relevant knowledge managed through computer systems. This is as true for public health and population health management as it is for 'just in time' patient-specific decision support at the point of care. Indeed, with the addition of genomics and proteomics, all patients acquire the equivalent of orphan diseases since each have unique biology and differing life experiences. Plus, the explosive growth of information and communications technology allows an infrastructure capable of supporting this trend. It is anticipated that continued evolution of learning health care systems consisting of adaptive evidence-based decision support systems will assure far greater efficiency, effectiveness, quality, safety, and integration of new knowledge resulting in better outcomes for individuals and populations.

The field will expand to include informatics applications to traditional care plus primary prevention, health education, and computer-based therapies, including robotic surgery and self-administered programmes for cognitive psychological therapy. Models for all of these dimensions exist today. Development of computer-based public health and population's records has lagged behind patient and personal health records in many nations, but this is likely to change dramatically over the next decade as the repositories of person-specific health data become more and more accessible to health system managers and researchers.

Definition

While there is no formally accepted nomenclature or taxonomy for informatics relating to health today, one can identify 7 overlapping yet somewhat distinct domains:
- *Translational bioinformatics:* computing for genomics, proteomics, epigenetics and management of the knowledge bases these fields generate.
- *Clinical informatics, or informatics for use in patient care:* electronic medical records of three types: patient, personal, and population.
- *Public health informatics*, or informatics relating to the health of populations, including populations with special needs.
- *Computer methods*, semantics, and ontologies for health applications.
- *Consumer health, or e-health informatics:* including links to patients and professional caregivers.
- Health information policy.
- *Health information networks:* local, regional, national, and global.
- *Knowledge management:* utilizing structured databases such as results of randomized clinical drug trials.
- *Adaptive evidence-based decision support systems:* computer-based software that offers expert advice as guidelines and protocols and the capacity to determine whether or not the advice proves to be good for the patient's health status or a population of generally similar people.

Some fields with which informatics integrates:
- computer science, information and telecommunication science, cognitive science, statistics, decision science, and management/organizational science
- library science
- bioscience and biomedicine
- knowledge management, decision support
- evidence-based medicine, knowledge bases such as Medline
- public and populations health sciences–biostatistics, epidemiology, health services research
- health policy and management, organization behaviour, risk management, quality and safety.
- Health values and bioethics.[1]

Using informatics in health care

Early use focused disproportionately upon primary care settings in Europe and administrative functions and laboratory results reporting in North America, but attention was also given to improving decision-making through clinical alerts and diagnostic supports. Widespread adoption of electronic medical record systems has been slower than desired due to a number of factors amongst which are perverse financial incentives, clinician resistance, awkward user interfaces, legal, and cultural barriers.[2]

Robust systems are of necessity complex and they require a mixture of hardware, software, and maintenance. Relevant legal and policy infrastructures are essential to handle such issues as authentication, security, and confidentiality. Further, evolutionary standards are essential to enhance interoperability, refinement, and utility of data emerging from biomedical, clinical, and public health care, and research into relevant knowledge banks. Recently, a number of developed economies have embarked upon national health information infrastructures and global efforts to collaborate on standards are underway.[3] The rise of the Internet linked to the above components will totally change the practice of health care. For example, personal health records that allow patients to interact with their clinicians and the patient's own medical record whenever and wherever they wish, offer the potential to greatly improve performance and outcomes of a variety of chronic illnesses including home monitoring.[4] De-identified data from these records and other sources can then be used for a host of public health investigations including bio surveillance and community health.[5] Public policy relating to privacy can conflict with the need for access to person-specific data for a variety of types of biomedical and public health research.[6]

Implementation of computer systems into clinical environments typically involves substantial change in work processes; change management and an understanding of organizational behaviour as well as ongoing tailoring of software programmes to local circumstances is involved. Complex adaptive systems theory is particularly useful to supporting implementation and gaining major improvements in performance, particularly for safety and quality of care.[7]

Evidence on IT systems improving care processes and outcome

A growing body of evidence reveals that computer-based health records systems (incorporating decision support) can improve the safety of care, particularly with respect to medications.[8]

Research is still needed, but there is evidence that IT systems and communication technology can result in better care, better outcomes, and more informed patients.[9,10] Evidence of the usefulness of Health Information and Communications Technology (HICT) for public health is needed. While more research would be helpful, the bulk of evidence today reveals that better informed patients are less anxious, begin treatment earlier, are more satisfied with their care, follow advice better, opt for lower risk interventions, and reduce health care costs through greater self-management and a more efficient use of resources.

IT and public health

Global epidemics such as HIV/AIDS or SARS offer real evidence that IT systems can be extremely important in determining the spread of a disease, analysing patient care data for clusters of symptoms to help understand the nature of the disease, and evaluating programmes that seek to manage the disease effectively. As the population health record matures during this decade, benefits are likely to become more impressive with on-going surveillance critical for wellness programmes, community health, environmental risks, disease control, and potentially bioterrorism.[5]

What should you look for in a health care IT system that will deliver better quality and outcomes?

Capabilities in IT systems that are likely to improve patient safety, quality and outcomes include electronic prescribing, continuity of care records that offer a concise summary of key patient data and can be accessed from a variety of clinical settings, decision support for medications that incorporate such capabilities as clinical alerts, reminders for preventive care, dosage calculation support, 'just-in-time' knowledge service, integrated evidence-based clinical pathways that allow for over-riding by the clinician, and personal health records that capture records added by the patient that include alternative medications not typically listed by patients in ordinary paper-based settings, and the capacity to aggregate performance data on clinical practice for both clinician and statistical analysis.

If one is 'shopping' to purchase a clinical IT system for use in either a primary care or institutional setting, it is important to visit sites that are actively using the system to determine its functionality in real world terms. The more complex the system the more important it is for a team to visit to assure that all key users' needs will be met. The capacity of systems to interoperate with other systems outside the core setting is of increasing importance. Ease of implementation, cost, and built-in decision support are other factors worthy of evaluation.[12] A key challenge for complex institutions is assuring that the entire enterprise can cross communicate. Dedicated systems for individual specialties may keep one set of consultants happy, but greatly limit the capacity to achieve major gains in productivity across the institution.

Public health informaticians have recently generated a list of competencies for this discipline (see public health competencies website). Readers interested in a personal assessment of their informatics capabilities should find it helpful.

Further resources

There are far too many websites available to do justice to the issues raised here, but what follows will give the reader some sense of the scope of issues involved.

Public Health Informatics Competencies

℘ http://www.cdc.gov/InformaticsCompetencies/ (accessed 13 April 2011).

Medical Knowledge Bases

Biomed Central ℘ http://www.biomedcentral.com/ are open access web-based repositories for scientists and the public (accessed 13 April 2011).

Clinical Trials are biomedical research databanks relating to clinical trials of medications. ℘ http://www.clinicaltrials.gov/ (accessed 13 April 2011).

GenBank is a biomedical research databank at the National Center for Biotechnology Information (NLM, NIH). ℘ http://www.ncbi.nlm.nih.gov/ (accessed 13 April 2011).

Medline Plus is a website with range of consumer health information. ℘ http://medlineplus.gov/ (accessed 13 April 2011).

Public Library of Science ℘ http://www.plosmedicine.org/home.action

PubMed Central is a free continually updated source for access to the medical literature at the US National Library of Medicine. ℘ http://www.ncbi.nlm.nih.gov/pmc/ (accessed 13 April 2011).

Unbound Medicine ℘ http://www.unboundmedicine.com/, Map of Medicine ℘ http://www.mapofmedicine.com/,

Up-to-Date ℘ http://www.uptodate.com/home/index.html offer PDA and computer-based knowledge support for busy clinicians (accessed 13 April 2011).

Standards, vocabulary, and terminology

Health Level 7 is a major standards development group. ℘ http://www.hl7.org/ (accessed 13 April 2011).

SNOMED-CT is a systematized nomenclature of medicine (SNOMED) that incorporates universal health care terminology. ℘ http://www.ihtsdo.org/ (accessed 13 April 2011).

Standards Standard is a periodic web journal maintained by AMIA to give readers an update of the activities of major international standards organizations. ℘ http://www.amia.org/standards-standard (accessed 13 April 2011).

Unified Medical Language Systems is a compendium of knowledge sources for medicine. ℘ http://www.nlm.nih.gov/research/umls/ (accessed 13 April 2011).

National Health Information Infrastructures

Australia. ℘ http://www.ehealth.gov.au/internet/ehealth/publishing.nsf/content/home (accessed 3 September 2012).

Canada ℘ http://www.infoway-inforoute.ca/ (accessed 13 April 2011).

NCVHS. http://www.ncvhs.hhs.gov/ (accessed 13 April 2011).

United Kingdom ℘ http://www.connectingforhealth.nhs.uk/ (accessed 13 April 2011).

USA ONCHIT ℘ http://healthit.hhs.gov/portal/server.pt/community/healthit_hhs_gov__home/1204

References

1 Shortliffe EH, Cimino JJ. (2006). *Medical informatics: computer applications in health care and biomedicine*, 3nd edn. Springer, New York.

2 Berner ES, Detmer DE, Simborg D. (2005). Will the wave finally break? A brief view of the adoption of electronic medical records in the united states. *Journal of the American Medical Informatics Association*, **12**, 3–7.

3 Detmer DE. (2003). Building the National Health Information Infrastructure for Personal Health, Health Care Services, Public Health, and Research. *BMC Medical Informatics and Decision-Making*, **3**, 1–40.

4 Detmer DE, Bloomrosen M, Raymond B, Tang P.(2008). Integrated personal health records: Transformative tools for consumer-centric care. *BMC Medical Informatics and Decision-Making*, **8**, 45–72.

5 Friedman DJ, Parrish RG. 2nd (2010). The population health record: concepts, definition, design, and implementation. *Journal of the American Medical Informatics Association*, **17**, 359–66.

6 Nass SJ, Levit LA, Gostin LO. (2009). *Beyond the HIPAA privacy rule: enhancing privacy, improving health through research.* National Academy Press, Washington, DC.

7 Institute of Medicine. (2001). *Crossing the quality chasm: a new health system for the 21st century.* National Academy Press, Washington, DC.

8 Bates DW, Gawande AA. (2003). Improving safety with information technology. *New England Journal of Medicine*, **348**, 25–34.

9 Chaudhry BD, Wang JD, Wu SD. (2006). Systematic review: impact of health information technology on quality, efficiency, and costs of medical care. *Annals of Internal Medicine*, **144**, 742–52.

10 Black AD, Car J, Pagliari C, *et al.* (2011). The impact of eHealth on the quality and safety of health care: a systematic overview. *PLoS Medicine*, **8**, e1000387. doi:10.1371/journal.pmed.1000387.

11 Blue Ridge Academic Health Group. Advancing Value in Health Care (2008). *The Emerging Transformational Role of Informatics*, Report. Blue Ridge Academic Health Group, Atlanta.

12 Lorenzi NM, Kouroubali A, Detmer DE, Bloomrosen M. (2009). How to successfully select and implement electronic health records (EHR) in small ambulatory practice settings. *BMC Medical Informatics and Decision-Making*, **23**, 9–15.

2.3 Qualitative methods

**Sara Mallinson, Jennie Popay, and
Gareth Williams**

Objectives

After reading this chapter you should be able to:
- to introduce key features of qualitative research
- to outline how different qualitative methods can be used to answer
  different types of research question
- to describe some of the most widely used qualitative methods
- to explain key issues in the analysis of qualitative data and common
  features of the analysis process
- to outline the importance of qualitative research in a public health
  context.

Principles of qualitative research

The aim of qualitative research is to develop concepts and theories that
help us understand social phenomena. This often means asking questions
about behaviour/action, sometimes referred to as '*agency*', and its relationship to *social structure*. Using a range of qualitative research methods,
social scientists explore the meanings people attach to their experiences
and how these are shaped by different contexts.

Most qualitative research is underpinned by a social constructivist philosophy that assumes the phenomena being studied are the product of
subjective interpretations. These interpretations are informed by perceptions, beliefs, and experiences and are rich, diverse, and shifting. To
understand how social phenomena are constructed, and how they might
shape action, qualitative research focuses on the perspective of members
of a particular group or setting. A range of study designs and data collection methods can be deployed to capture peoples' perspectives, but
an interview or a focus group is not treated as a 'slice of reality'. It is
regarded as a process of contextually bounded 'meaning-making' between
the researcher and the researched.

Reflexivity about the constructed nature of data is important to the
qualitative research process. The researcher (their interests, background
and theories), the study design (the sampling, the data collection method,
the analysis), and the context (where and how the study is conducted)
impacts the outcome of the research. Instead of trying to control all these
factors (which is impossible in naturally occurring settings), there is an
increasing effort to account for all possible influences. This 'transparency'
at all stages of the research process *should* improve quality by surfacing

the strengths and weaknesses of a piece of work. Unfortunately, qualitative research is not always done well, so an awareness of quality markers is important for those doing and using qualitative research.[1]

The uses of qualitative research

Though qualitative health research has been used to address a wide range of questions it is possible to group these into four broad types concerned with:

- the meanings different social groups attach to particular phenomena and how these interact with agency
- perceptions about the needs of different social groups and how these needs can be met
- barriers to and enablers of effective implementation and/or uptake of new policies/interventions/practices
- how understandings of subjective experience and meanings can help to explain results of larger quantitative studies.

In describing the type of knowledge produced by qualitative research addressing these questions and the general approaches used we draw on examples of research involving people living in disadvantaged circumstances because of the significance of this work to public health practice. However, it is important to recognize that qualitative research has also been used to illuminate the social, cultural, and organizational factors shaping the behavior of professional groups such as doctors and public health practitioners.[2]

The meanings different social groups attach to particular experiences/behaviours

Questions about the meanings individuals attach to phenomena and how these shape human 'agency' in the context of social structures are the core concern of qualitative research and underpin all the other types of questions. However, much of this research is primarily concerned to increase empirical and/or theoretical understanding about social life rather than explicitly to inform policy and/or practice, although the results can have important implications for both. These studies are often stand-alone, but some are linked with larger quantitative studies. Many use a single method of data collection, typically semi- or unstructured interviews. Others use multiple methods combining individual and group interviews or including observations.

This body of research includes studies of the meanings attaching to health-damaging behaviour (see Box 2.3.1) and of the experience of living in disadvantaged places (see Box 2.3.2). These studies highlight the need to contextualize risk factors, such as smoking, diet, alcohol, lack of exercise, and drug taking, by reference to the wider material and environmental conditions in which risks are embedded. They also reveal that 'lay knowledge' about the causes of ill health and health inequalities is complex and multifaceted. This type of research can contribute to the planning and delivery of more appropriate interventions. Without the understanding it offers public health practice may inadvertently reduce disadvantaged groups to unthinking bearers of various assets, deficits and risks.

Box 2.3.1 **Smoking and coping with poverty**
Hilary Graham's study of smoking amongst women in the UK included secondary analysis of existing quantitative data on smoking prevalence amongst different groups and a qualitative study based on semi-structured interviews with a small sample of poor white mothers bringing up young children. In her analysis of the qualitative data Graham developed the concept of smoking as a coping mechanism demonstrating how women caring for children whilst living in poverty relied on a cigarette to help them manage very stressful situations. Later research suggested that this relationship did not hold for mothers from South Asian and African Caribbean backgrounds.[3]

This body of research includes studies of the meanings attaching to health-damaging behaviour (see Box 2.3.1) and of the experience of living in disadvantaged places (see Box 2.3.2). These studies highlight the need to contextualize risk factors, such as smoking, diet, alcohol, lack of exercise, and drug taking, by reference to the wider material and environmental conditions in which risks are embedded. They also reveal that 'lay knowledge' about the causes of ill health and health inequalities is complex and multifaceted. This type of research can contribute to the planning and delivery of more appropriate interventions. Without the understanding it offers public health practice may inadvertently reduce disadvantaged groups to unthinking bearers of various assets, deficits and risks.

Box 2.3.2 **Understanding people, place, and health inequalities**
A mixed method study in four contrasting urban areas consisted of: analysis of routine health data at local authority ward level; a household survey of perceptions of place and subjective heath status in smaller neighbourhoods in these wards; and a longitudinal qualitative study using in-depth interviews with a small sample of adults drawn from the household survey. The findings of the qualitative study highlighted multiple pathways between the material, social, and psychological dimensions of place, health related behaviours and health outcomes. People living in difficult circumstances acknowledged the differential impact of social and economic conditions on health, but also emphasized 'strength of character' as a way of coping with these. The researchers argued that this was a form of resistance to the moral judgements made about poor people's failure to cope and their unhealthy behaviours.[4,5]

Subjective perceptions about the needs of different social groups and how these needs can be met
Qualitative health research addressing this type of question aims to contribute to the development of more appropriate/effective ways of preventing ill-health and/or promoting health. One approach is to undertake a

stand-alone qualitative study and then use the findings to develop a more appropriate intervention and evaluate it (see Box 2.2.3). Another is to embed qualitative research into a Health Impact Assessment (HIA). HIA can be particularly useful to inform decisions in contested circumstances where official and community views could be in conflict (see Box 2.3.4). These studies provide a more holistic picture of the phenomenon under investigation, by incorporating the perspectives of different stakeholders and combining different types of knowledge/evidence. HIAs may also use participative qualitative approaches involving the group targeted by a proposed intervention in the design and conduct of the research.

Box 2.3.3 Developing new policies and practices

An in-depth interview based study of thirty-six people attending TB clinics in rural Pakistan explored the impact of TB on people's lives and the relative importance of factors associated with individuals, care processes, and the cultural context on help seeking behaviour. The researchers concluded that deficiencies in provision were the most important influences on treatment uptake and compliance and they used these findings to design new service delivery strategies and evaluated these in a RCT.[6,7]

Box 2.3.4 Health impact assessments

A recent HIA of plans to demolish sub-standard housing in a South Wales community included a qualitative study (involving individual in-depth interviews and focus groups) alongside public meetings and secondary analysis of existing data about the locality. Although in theory the plan could be seen to be positive with clear health benefits the qualitative findings revealed that despite recognizing housing problems residents and local professionals were ambivalent and uncertain about the developments because of the potential disruption to social and family networks.[8]

Barriers and enablers to effective implementation and/or uptake of interventions and/or services

Qualitative research is a common element of process evaluations the aims of which are to understand the strengths and weaknesses of new policies, interventions or practices and to identify the factors that impinge on successful implementation. Process evaluations are typically mixed method and the qualitative element is usually not an identifiable separate study. They may focus on a single 'case' or involve a series of case studies as with the process evaluations of healthy school initiative.[9] Process evaluations involving integrated qualitative elements or separate qualitative studies can also be embedded in impact evaluations using experimental or quasi-experimental designs (see Box 2.3.5).

Box 2.3.5 Qualitative research and process evaluations

A trial aimed at reducing smoking in early teenage years through a 'peer-led' intervention, used qualitative methods as part of a process evaluation that aimed to understand the strengths and weaknesses of the intervention design.[10]

A randomized controlled trial (RCT) of the installation and use of domestic smoke alarms included an embedded qualitative study which used semi-structured interviews to explore people's perceptions of the risk of fire and barriers and enablers to the installation and maintenance of domestic smoke alarms.[11]

Understanding subjective experience/meaning to explain results of larger quantitative studies

The findings of the process evaluations described in Box 2.3.5 were used to understand the results of the RCTs in which they were embedded. For example, the qualitative study of smoke alarm use found that people disabled alarms because they went off when they were cooking. Qualitative research conducted independently of a larger quantitative study can also be used in this way. For example, Noyes and Popay[12] conducted a systematic review of qualitative research on help seeking behaviour in an effort to explain the diverse results of multiple trials of TB treatment interventions.

Qualitative designs and methods

There are a range of study designs used in qualitative research (sometimes referred to as methodology) and within these designs different methods of data collection can be used. A study design should be tailored to answer a particular research question. Choices about scope, ethics and access, feasibility and timing, sample size, sampling strategy, data collection method and analysis technique should all be addressed at the planning stage. Qualitative research can be unexpectedly time consuming. A poorly planned project will usually produce poor quality results. Below the most common types of design are briefly described. More details can be found in the texts listed in the bibliography.

Study designs

Ethnography

Studies of communities or groups of people in their naturally occurring settings using a range of methods. The focus is on developing a holistic, in-depth, understanding the social context and 'way of life' of the community or group through immersion in and understanding of social milieu. Participant observation is a key element of most ethnographies alongside other data collection methods. A classic ethnography in the health field is Goffman's[13] 1961 study of a single mental hospital for which he posed as a member of staff for over a year. This work has had profound impact on mental health policy and practice around the world.

Case-study

Generally case study designs involve the systematic study of an individual, a group, or an event with a view to understanding why something happens in a particular context. There is less emphasis on members' tacit knowledge than in ethnography, though it can incorporate a similar range of data, collected from different sources.

Action-research

A combination of action and research (usually in cycles) in which the researcher and participants perform an action, reflect upon it, and then use this knowledge to perform the next action. The emphasis is on the development of practices.

Grounded theory

A methodology where data collection and analysis are conducted at the same time in an interactive process with the one informing the other. Data analysis produces theoretical insights and these are used to collect new data through theoretical sampling to 'test' the theoretical ideas further. This process continues until categories and relationships are 'saturated', i.e. new data does not lead to new developments in the theory developed in the analysis. Thus, the theory generated is 'grounded' in the data.

Data collection methods

While ethnographies and case-studies will often use more than one type of data collection to get different perspectives, it is also acceptable to use just one method to collect data. Some common methods are:

Observation

The researcher attempts to immerse themselves in a study context to watch 'everyday' activities and practices in their natural context. Observers may be participant (fully active members of the context) or non-participant (maintaining distance from the context by not having a formal role in the activities there). The ethical challenges of being an observer have been a source of debate (covert observation, of the kind commonly used in journalism, is particularly delicate and is not often undertaken). The legitimacy of non-participant observation has been questioned as researcher presence may change the context under investigation. Most observation studies use field diaries to record data. Occasionally video and audio recording may be used.

Interviews
Individual interviews are conducted with respondents often selected purposively because of their experience of phenomena of interest (e.g. a health condition, an intervention, a place). Sample sizes can vary, but typically include 20–30 interviewees. Interviews can be unstructured (e.g. oral history or life-history) or guided by a topic guide which highlights topics to be discussed with each interviewee rather than formal questions. Interviewees are encouraged to express ideas and experiences in their own words. The interviews are usually taped and transcribed for analysis.

Focus group discussion
A small number of subjects are brought together to discuss the topic of interest (ideally 6–8 people). Care is taken with the composition of the group to ensure members do not feel intimidated, but can express opinions freely. A topic guide is usually used to focus the discussion and the researcher moderates the group to ensure group dynamics are managed and that a range of aspects of the topic are explored. The discussion is frequently tape-recorded, and transcribed for analysis.

Diaries/auto-biographies
Participants keep a diary for a set period focusing on key events they judge to be memorable. The method is particularly good for longitudinal data collection where recall may be a challenge, and where repeated interviews are not feasible. Diaries may be more or less structured and may be paper-based, computer based, or online blogs. The data are likely to be analysed in the same way as an interview transcript.

Analysing qualitative data

Qualitative analysis is the point at which data and theory are brought together to try and generate new understandings and explanations of social phenomena. Done well, it is a time-consuming and intellectually challenging process and new researchers will frequently under-estimate the time required for an analysis phase. Two elements in the analysis process can be distinguished:
● the purpose (what is being sought)
● the practice (how it is done).

These are briefly discussed below and more details can be found in the resources listed at the end of the chapter.

The purpose of data analysis
As we have already said, the purpose of a research project (defined by the research questions) should shape the study design and methods for data collection (for example, whether interviews or observations have been conducted). This purposeful data collection should also shape how questions are asked and the extent to which something like an interview, for example, is guided by the researcher (as in a traditional topic guided interview) or left to run with as little intervention as possible (for example, in life-history work). How data are analysed will be driven by these interests.

For example, one might perform a narrative, life-history, discourse, or conversation analysis on the same extract from an interview, hence the importance of surfacing researcher standpoint and the theory driving a particular piece of research. Some examples of different approaches to analysis are summarized below.

Narrative analysis

Looks at the way a person constructs a 'story' in the light of the audience and their purpose for giving the account. There is a focus on language, imagery, metaphor, and rhetorical purpose in the story being told.

Content analysis

Looks at the way themes and issues arise across texts (including interview transcriptions). Analysis may focus on the context, frequency, and/or how themes are patterned by, e.g. gender or ethnicity. This is a descriptive level of analysis.

Conversation analysis (CA)

Focuses on the structure of communication and conversation management such as turn taking, grounding, pause with the aim of revealing how *meaning* is constructed in interaction. CA is very specialized and marks both words spoken and how conversation proceeds (for example intonation).

Discourse analysis

Explores the way knowledge is produced in particular contexts through the use of specialized language or theories and through performances, interaction and rhetorical devices used to persuade. A range of texts can be analysed (interview transcripts, video, letters, policy documents).

The practice of data analysis

There are different approaches to qualitative data analysis (QDA) underpinned by different theories, but some common elements can be identified. In the broadest terms QDA involves identification of themes and concepts and categories in order to develop ideas or 'theories' about the data and relationships within it.

Most researchers begin by getting to know their data, for example, by mapping instances of events and themes before moving on to more abstracted and theoretical analysis. However, if grounded theory is being used rudimentary and emergent theoretical categories would be introduced at a very earlier stage to inform further data collection.

Thematic analysis involves sifting and reducing raw data to an accessible summary of 'themes' identified in the data about the nature of whatever topic is being researched, whether it is living through urban regeneration, experiencing depression, doing public health work, or being incontinent. One approach to thematic analysis is to use a 'code and retrieve' system. This involves devising a system of codes and applying these across the whole data set (e.g. all interview transcripts) to maximize opportunities for exploring emerging themes and areas of difference or non-conformity. This is a useful process of immersion, although it can be time consuming. While manually indexing transcripts is feasible, many qualitative researchers use computer-aided qualitative data analysis software (CAQDAS) to facilitate the process. Whether done manually or with software, the system for thematic analysis should:

- order and sort raw data into a manageable form
- ensure that analysis is rigorous and transparent
- allow within and across case searching to identify recurring categories and typologies
- allow easy movement from categories and themes back to raw data to check that the link between analysis and data is maintained during abstraction
- allow for revision and additions to be made as ideas are 'tested'.

While computer software can help with various stages of analysis, it will not perform analysis. The intellectual work of devising coding schemes and developing theories about the data is the responsibility of the researcher. Software is simply a tool that can help with the systematic sorting of data, if appropriately applied.

Conclusion

This chapter aims to introduce the reader to some of the most common approaches to qualitative work, the importance of ensuring that qualitative research remains sensitive to the constraints of data and context, and the value of qualitative research for public health practice. Issues around ethical research practice and governance are important features of good quality qualitative research and all research must be planned and executed with appropriate protection for the participants involved (public or professionals).

We acknowledge that this is a brief review and only touches lightly on a range of complex issues. The references below provide more detailed discussion of qualitative methods, analysis, and study appraisal. While training and excellent books and papers on qualitative methods are available to those wishing to explore qualitative research, seeking out qualitative expertise for research teams is essential. Fully embracing the contribution of qualitative data and qualitative thinking in a field like public health, which is dominated by quantitative approaches, requires an openness of perspective, but bringing together qualitative and quantitative research will enhance the public health evidence base. Science cannot develop if it remains trapped within dualisms which cut it off from the insights and understandings provided by qualitative forms of social science.[14]

Further resources

Bourgault I, Dingwall R, De Vries R. (2010). *Qualitative methods in health research.* Sage, London.
Denzin KN, Lincoln YS. (2005.) *The Sage handbook of qualitative research*, 3rd edn. Sage, London.
Hammersley M, Atkinson D. (1983). *Ethnography: Principles in Practice.* Tavistock, London.
Morgan D. (1996). *Focus Groups as qualitative research.* Sage, London.
Pope C., Mays N. (2006). *Qualitative Research and Health Care.* Blackwell Publishing, Oxford.
Ritchie J, Lewis J. (2003). *Qualitative Research Practice.* Sage, London.
Ruben H, Ruben I. (2005). *Qualitative interviewing: the art of hearing data.* Sage, London.
Silverman D. (2006). *Interpreting qualitative data*, 3rd edn. Sage, London.
Yin RK. (2008). *Case study research: design and methods.* Sage, London.

References

1 Seale C. (1999.) *The quality of qualitative research.* Sage, London.
2 Mallinson S, Popay J, Kowarzik U. (2006). Developing the public workforce: a 'communities of practice' perspective. *Policy and Politics*, **34**, 265–85.
3 Graham H. (1993). *When life's a drag: women, smoking and disadvantage.* HMSO, London.
4 Graham, H (1994). Surviving by smoking. In: Wilkinson S, Kitzinger C (eds) *Women and Health: Feminist Perspectives.* Taylor and Francis, London.
5 Popay J, Thomas C, Williams G, *et al.* (2003a). A proper place to live: health inequalities, agency and the normative dimensions of space. *Social Science and Medicine*, **57**, 55–69.
6 Popay J, Bennett S, Thomas C, *et al.* (2003b). Beyond beer, fags, egg and chips? Exploring lay understandings of social inequalities in health. *Social Health and Illness*, **25**, 1–23.
7 Khan A, Walley J, Newell J, Imdad N. (2000). Tuberculosis in Pakistan: social-cultural constraints and opportunities in treatment. *Social Science and Medicine*, **50**, 247–54.
8 Williams G, Elliott E. (2010). Exploring social inequalities in health: the importance of thinking qualitatively. In: Bourgeault I, De Vries R Dingwall R, eds, *Handbook on Qualitative Health Research.* Sage, London.
9 Mukoma W, Flisher AJ. (2004). Evaluations of health promoting schools: a review of nine studies. *Health Promotion International*, **19**, 357–68.
10 Campbell R, Starkey F, Holliday J, *et al.*(2008). An informal school-based peer-led intervention for smoking prevention in adolescence (ASSIST); a cluster randomized trial. *Lancet*, **371**, 1595–602.
11 Roberts H, Curtis K, Liabo K, *et al.* (2004). Putting public health evidence into practice: increasing the prevalence of working smoke alarms in disadvantaged inner city housing, *Journal of Epidemiology and Community Health*, **58**, 280–5.
12 Noyes J, Popay J. (2007). Directly observed therapy and tuberculosis: how can a systematic review of qualitative research contribute to improving services? A qualitative meta-synthesis, *Journal of Advanced Nursing*, **57**, 227–43.
13 Goffman E. (1961). *Asylums: essays on the social situation of mental patients and other inmates.* Doubleday/Anchor, New York.
14 Midgley M. (2001). *Science and Poetry.* Routledge, London.

2.4 Epidemiological approach and design

Walter Ricciardi and Stefania Boccia

Objectives

- Understand epidemiological thinking and approaches in a public health context.
- Use the most appropriate measures of disease occurrence.
- Measure the association between an exposure and a health event by using a two-by-two table.
- Measure the impact of a certain disease at the population level.
- Identify the main epidemiological studies.

For more detailed discussion on epidemiologic understanding refer to a standard textbook.[1]

Thinking epidemiology

Epidemiology is the core science of public health, and may be defined as 'the study of the occurrence and distribution of health-related states or events in specified populations, including the study of the determinants influencing such states, and the application of this knowledge to control the health problems'.[2] One of the first examples of an epidemiological approach within a public health context comes from London, 1854, where John Snow first proposed the mechanism for the transmission of cholera. He did this by systematically collecting data regarding the affected individuals, in doing so he discovered an association between cholera diffusion and a local public water pump. Prior to the discovery of bacteria, Snow pushed the local health authorities to close the water pump, eventually resulting in the end of the epidemic.

Modern epidemiology starts in late 1940s, with a more systematized body of principles for the design and evaluation of epidemiological studies. The largest formal human experiment ever conducted was the Salk vaccine field trial in 1954, the results of which laid the foundation for the prevention of paralytic poliomyelitis. In recent years, epidemiologic research has steadily attracted public attention, with the news media boosted by increasing social concern on about health issues. Examples are H1N1 influenza, hormone replacement therapy and heart disease, the effectiveness of mammography screening in the prevention of breast cancer, and many others.

Measuring disease occurrence

Three key measures of disease occurrence are: *risk*, *incidence rate*, and *prevalence* (Box 2.4.1).

Box 2.4.1 The 2 × 2 table, with details of occurrence, associations and impact according to the study design

	Disease		
		Present	Absent	Total
Exposure	Present	a	b	a+b
	Absent	c	d	c+d
	Total	a+c	b+d	N

Cross-sectional study
- Prevalence of disease = $a+c/N$
- Prevalence of disease in exposed = $a/a+b$
- Prevalence of disease in unexposed = $c/c+d$

Cohort studies
- Risk of disease in exposed $(R_1) = a/a+b$*
- Risk of disease in unexposed $(R_0) = c/c+d$*
- Relative risk $(RR) = R_1/R_0$
* denominators change if the study has an active follow-up so that person-time can be calculated:
- Incidence rate of disease in those exposed $(IR_1) = a/PT_1$,
- Incidence rate in those unexposed $(IR_0) = a/PT_0$
- Rate ratio $(RR) = IR_1/IR_0$.

Case-control studies
- Odds of disease among exposed = a/b
- Odds of disease among unexposed = c/d
- Odds ratio = $a/b/c/d = axd/bxc$

Measures of impact
- Attributable Fraction $(AF) = (R_1-R_0)/R_1 = 1-(1/RR) = (RR-1)/RR$

Attributable Fraction for the population
  $(AFp) = AF \times$ proportion of exposed cases in the population.

Risk **or incidence proportion**
This is calculated as the proportion of individuals developing a certain disease during a time period divided by the number of subjects at risk to develop the same disease followed for a defined period of time. It can be interpreted as the probability that a person will develop a certain disease in the time period considered. Calculation of risks implies that the entire denominator does not change during the study period, however unless the time is very short, populations usually change over time. As such, it is always advisable to use the:

Incidence rate
The rate at which new events occur in a population. The numerator is the number of new events that occur in a defined period or other physical span. The denominator is the population at risk of experiencing the event during this period, sometimes expressed as person-time (PT); it may instead be in other units, such as passenger-miles.

Prevalence is a measure of disease occurrence
The total number of individuals who have an attribute or disease at a particular time divided by the population at risk of having the attribute or disease at that time or midway through the period.
- *Period prevalence:* the proportion of individuals with a disease or an attribute at a specified period of time.
- *Point prevalence:* the proportion of individuals with a disease or an attribute at a specified point in time.

Prevalence depends on the incidence and the duration of the disease (Prevalence = Incidence × Duration), it is a measure of disease burden, or the extent of the health problem.

Prevalence data are used to plan health services and allocate resources.

Risk and incidence rates, on the other hand, are useful for predicting the risk of a disease, to identify causes and treatment of the disease, to *describe trends* over time, and for evaluating the effectiveness of preventive programmes.

Practical examples are shown in Box 2.4.2.

Other occurrence measures commonly used in health care are:
- *attack rate* – the proportion of a group that experiences the outcome under study over a given period (e.g. the period of an epidemic).
- *death rate* = an estimate of the portion of a population that dies during a specified period. The numerator is the number of persons dying during the period; the denominator is the number in the population, usually estimated as the midyear population.

Box 2.4.2 Measures of occurrence, impact and association
- *Risk:* assume you wish to measure the annual occurrence of measles in a population of 450 school children. At the beginning of the study 20 children had previously contracted measles, and 30 children had been vaccinated against measles. During the year study period, 12 measles cases were detected, so that the annual risk of measles is 12/400 = 0.030 (or 3%), in the susceptible population.
- *Incidence rate:* suppose that during the annual study period 2 of 400 children initially at risk died, and that 4 children left the school and were no longer traceable. All of these 6 children left the study 6

months after the study commenced, i.e. 6 children contributed only 6 months of follow-up, with the loss of 3 person-years. Suppose again that the 12 cases of measles arise all after 1 month, so that these 12 cases contribute each to 1 month person-time at risk. Therefore the remaining 11 months for each of the 12 cases cannot be considered as time at risk in the denominator, and should be removed, 12 persons × 11 months = 132 person months = 11 person years. Therefore, the denominator for the incidence rate is 400−3−11 = 386 person-years. Thus, incidence rate = 12 cases/386 person-years = 0.031 cases/person-years, or 3.1 cases for 100 persons followed for 1 year.

- *Point prevalence:* the prevalence of nosocomial infection in a hospital on 30 January 2010 = the number of nosocomial cases of infection diagnosed that day, divided by the number of individuals hospitalized that day.
- *Period prevalence:* the prevalence of asthma measured during a 12-month period in a large population of children = the number of all the asthma cases measured during the 12 months (old and new diagnoses) divided by the mean population of children (this number can change from the beginning of the study to the end).
- *Measures of association:* suppose a study aims to measure the risk of measles infection among children, 'exposed' at school A, 'unexposed' at school B. Remember we had 12 cases of measles out of 400 children at risk from school A, while at school B, 6 cases occurred from 300 children at risk. Without person-time at risk, we can only calculate the Risk Ratio = 1.50 $[(a/a+b)/(c/c+d)]$. Alternatively, in a case-control study, the appropriate measure of association would be the Odds Ratio = 1.51 $(a{\times}d/b{\times}c)$. These similar results show that there is an excess of risk of measles associated with being in school A.

	Disease			
		Present	Absent	Total
Exposure	Present (School A)	12	388	400
	Absent (School B)	6	294	300
	Total	18	682	700

- *Attributable fraction (AF):* assume that the incidence rate (IR_1) of cardiovascular diseases (CVD) is = 84/2,916 person-years among smokers, compared with IR_0 ((non-smokers) = 87/4,913 person-years. IR_1-IR_0 = 11.1 × 1,000 person-years (0.028–0.0177), while AF would be 38% [(0.028-0.0177)/0.028].
- *Interpretation:* 38% of CVD among smokers is attributable to smoking habits (implying that other causes of CVD operate additional to smoking).
  - If the proportion of smokers in the overall population where the CVD risk = 20%, then AFp= 0.38 × 0.20 = 0.076 × 100 = 7.6%.
  - *Interpretation:* in the entire population, we could avoid 7.6% of CVD if smoking was eliminated.

Measures of association

Measuring the effect of a certain exposure/intervention on health status is a key objective of epidemiologic research. There are several approaches to measure associations depending on the type of study design adopted. Consider the two-by-two table (Box 2.4.1), reporting the absolute frequency of individuals according to the two main dichotomous characteristics under investigation, disease, and exposure.

Two main different measures of association are commonly used, according to the study design that generates the data. These are the *relative risk* and the *Odds ratio* (formulas in Box 2.4.1, examples in Box 2.4.2):

- *Relative Risk (RR):* the ratio of the risk of an event among the exposed to the risk among the unexposed; this usage is synonymous with risk ratio.
- *Odds Ratio (OR):* estimates the RR when this cannot be calculated directly. What we compare are not risks, but *Odds* of disease among exposed and unexposed, where the Odds are the ratio of the probability of occurrence of an event to that of nonoccurrence.

How to interpret a relative risk?

RR is equal to 1 when the exposure does not affect the disease's onset, while it is higher than 1 if the exposure increases the risk for the studied disease, or lower than 1 if the exposure decreases the risk for that disease. A RR can vary between 0 and ∞. The RR indicates the *relative effect* of the exposure against the non-exposure. If the Relative Effect is $= R_1 - R_0$ (also called *risk difference, RD*) divided by R_0, this can be easily rewritten as RR-1. E.g. if we have a RR of 2.50, the relative effect of the exposure is to increase the risk of disease by 1.5 (sometimes expressed as 50%) compared with those unexposed. If an effect is described as a 10% increase in risk, it will correspond to a RR of 1.1. A protective exposure (e.g. vaccination) may lead to a RR of 0.8, a reduction in risk among the exposed of 20%.

Measures of impact

When we measure the association between a certain exposure and a disease, we may also wish to take into account the burden of that disease at the population level. These further measures are 'Attributable Fraction' and 'Attributable Fraction for the population' (Box 2.4.1).

- The *Attributable Fraction (AF)* (or attributable proportion) is the proportion of the cases that can be attributed to a particular exposure. In other words, it is the proportion by which the incidence rate of the outcome among those exposed would be reduced if the exposure were eliminated. It is estimated by subtracting the risk of the outcome among the unexposed from the risk among the exposed individuals, divided by the incidence rate in the group.
- The *Attributable Fraction for the population (AFp)* incidence rate is the proportion by which the incidence rate of the outcome in the entire population would be reduced if the exposure was eliminated.

Epidemiological study designs

The simplest studies estimate a risk, an incidence rate or prevalence, while 'analytical' studies examine putative causal relationships. Epidemiological studies may be classified as in Figure 2.4.1.

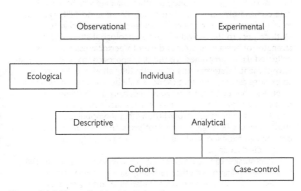

Figure. 2.4.1 Types of epidemiological study.

In *experimental studies* (intervention studies) the investigator intentionally alters one or more factors and controls the other study conditions in order to analyse the effects of so doing. These include:

- *Randomized Controlled Trials (RCT):* epidemiological experiments in which subjects in a population are randomly allocated into groups, usually called *study* and *control* groups, to receive or not to receive an experimental preventive or therapeutic procedure or intervention (e.g. effectiveness of statins vs. placebo in preventing cardiovascular diseases among hypercholesterolemic patients).

- *Field trials:* conducted outside the laboratory, in the general population, in primary care; often, as opposed to studies in academic, tertiary care settings (e.g. effectiveness of vaccination with HBV in a certain high-risk population for the prevention of HBV infection), and the *community intervention trials,* in which the unit of allocation to receive a preventive, therapeutic, or social intervention is an entire community or political subdivision (e.g. effectiveness of fluoridation of potable waters for the prevention of dental caries). A key issue in experimental studies is the comparability of the groups under treatment, which is obtained by a randomization process (See 🔲 Chapter 2.5).

- *Observational studies:* do not involve intervention (experimental or otherwise) on the part of the investigator.

Among them we have:

- *Ecological studies:* are studies in which the units of analysis are populations or groups of people rather than individuals. Usually data comes from updated current statistics, e.g. mortality rate data from national bodies or tumour incidence data from registers. With respect to the individual studies, ecological studies have the strengths of being economic and easy to perform using routinely collected data; sometimes are the only approach that can investigate environmental determinants of health; they allow the researcher to explore associations that cannot easily be done at the individual level (e.g. the relationship between mortality and income[3]); and finally they allow the effect of exposures that strongly vary between populations to be studied, but little within the population. Ecological studies are useful to generate hypotheses on a certain relation between an exposure and a disease, which is usually tested later using individual data.

- *Individual studies:* can be classified into *descriptive studies* and *analytical studies,* depending on whether the study aims to simply describe the distribution of a disease in a population according to some covariate(s), or to study the association between a disease and a postulated risk factor, respectively.

- *Descriptive studies (cross-sectional studies or prevalence studies):* concerned with and designed only to describe the existing distribution of variables without much regard to causal relationships or other hypotheses. These studies find broad applications in public health, e.g. investigating the seroprevalence among specific subgroups of population (e.g. HCV seroprevalence among blood donors[4]), 'knowledge, attitude, and practice' studies (e.g. investigating the public health practitioners knowledge of systematic review and meta-analyses[5]) and to quantify a certain health condition in a subgroup of population to plan screening programmes (e.g. colon cancer prevalence among subjects at high risk[6]). In *cross-sectional studies* a critical issue is sampling in a population that is truly representative of the entire population that we wish to describe.

- *Analytical studies:* allow causal inference, so are also often called aetiological studies.
- *Cohort studies:* measure the occurrence of disease in individuals (grouped in one or more cohorts) followed over time. Typically we have two groups, one exposed to a certain risk factor, the other not exposed. They allow calculating risks/incidence rates and RR. Examples:
  - *The Framingham Heart Study*[7]—the first to investigate the role of lifestyle and related factors in the risk of CVD. At its inception in 1948, thousands of citizens without CVD from Framingham (a small US city) were enrolled and data from extensive physical examinations and lifestyle interviews were collected. Subjects were then followed for many years to study CVD incidence.
  - *For investigating diseases with short induction*—e.g. food-borne infections. Individuals who ate foods at one or more meals over a short period are identified as a cohort. Among them, some might have eaten certain contaminated foods and some not. We study the risk of infection among those exposed to particular foods, compared with those who did not eat those foods.[8]
  - *Occupational health studies*—where employees exposed to a certain risk factor (e.g. asbestos) are followed over time (prospective or retrospective) to trace the incidence of disease (e.g. mesothelioma[9]), and then compared with cohorts of unexposed subjects (e.g. employees from the same company with different duties, or another company).
- *Case-control studies:* aim to achieve the same goal as cohort studies, but more efficiently, using sampling, frequently adopted when the disease is not common. In order to measure the association between a postulated risk factor and a disease we compare the experience of diseased subjects with control individuals (e.g. physical activity and head and neck cancer), defined as subjects who are free from the disease at the time of enrolment.[10] Case-control studies do not allow the direct calculation of risk, as there is no follow-up of the studied population. The OR, however, should be a good estimate of the RR.

References

1 Rothman KJ, Greenland S, Lash TL. (2008). *Modern epidemiology*, 3rd edn. Lippincott, Williams, & Wilkins. Philadelphia.

2 Porta M, Last JM. (2008). *Dictionary of Epidemiology*, 5th edn. Oxford University Press, Oxford.

3 Auger N, Zang G, Daniel M. (2009). Community-level income inequality and mortality in Québec, Canada. *Public Health*, **123**, 438–43.

4 La Torre G, De Vito E, Langiano E, et al. (2003). Epidemiology of hepatitis C virus antibodies in blood donors from the province of Latina, Italy. *European Journal of Epidemiology*, **18**, 691–4.

5 De Vito C, Nobile CG, Furnari G, et al. (2009). Physicians' knowledge, attitudes and professional use of RCTs and meta-analyses: a cross-sectional survey. *European Journal of Public Health*, **19**, 297–302.

6 DiSario JA, Foutch PG, Mai HD, et al. (1991). Prevalence and malignant potential of colorectal polyps in asymptomatic, average-risk men. *American Journal of Gastroenterology*, **86**, 941–5.

7 ✍ http://www.framinghamheartstudy.org/risk/coronary.html (accessed 26 March 2011).

8 Schmid D, Schandl S, Pichler AM, et al. (2005). *Salmonella enteritidis* phage type 21 outbreak in Austria. *European Surveillance*, **11**, 67–9.

9 Hansen J, de Klerk NH, Eccles JL, et al. (1993). Malignant mesothelioma after environmental exposure to blue asbestos. *International Journal of Cancer*, **54**, 578–81.

10 Nicolotti N, Chuang SC, Cadoni G, et al. (2011) Recreational physcial activity and risk of head and neck cancer: a pooled analysis within the international Head and Neck Cancer Epidemiology (INHANCE) consortium (2011). *European Journal of Epidemiology*, **26**, 619–28.

2.5 Statistical understanding

Kalyanaraman Kumaran and Iain Lang

Objectives

In public health practice you are likely to use statistics for two purposes:
- to summarize information about populations (descriptive statistics)
- to make inferences from data derived from research or other analysis (inferential statistics).

The objective of this chapter is to help you (a) to understand when statistical analysis would be useful, and (b) to interpret correctly the statistics you encounter. It also contains an outline of how to use standardization to compare two populations.

Why is this an important public health skill?

Statistics are important to public health practice, but most public health practitioners are not statisticians. Because statistics are widely used in public health to present and summarize information you need to be confident in interpreting what they mean.

We use statistics to get away from the vagueness of words ('very common', 'quite risky', 'highly unlikely', and so on) in place of which we use numbers: proportions (such as percentages), ways of comparing risks (such as odds ratios), and so on. You will typically want to achieve the best estimate of a value or effect size while having an eye to the extent to which your estimate is likely to approximate the truth. An important part of understanding statistics is recognizing when you need to use statistics (see Box 2.5.1).

> **Box 2.5.1 When do you need to use statistics?**
>
> - To summarize, in numbers or in graphical form, quantitative information using *descriptive statistics*. Terms you may come across are averages (mean, median, and mode) and deviation (variance, standard deviation); range, interquartile range, and outlier; histograms, bar charts, and scatterplots.[1]

- To infer general rules or relationships based on observed or gathered data using *inferential statistics*. When you use inferential statistics in public health practice you will often be doing one of two things: estimating a value (such as a proportion or a risk), and quantifying the uncertainty around that value (for example by using confidence intervals). Some of the practical, conceptual, and epistemological details of being able to draw appropriate inferences are discussed in 📖 Chapter 2.6.

When should you consult a statistician?

The short answer is that you should consult a statistician whenever you are in doubt about using statistics. Public health practice covers a lot of ground and few public health practitioners would claim a high level of expertise in all areas. As a result, you will need to consult experts on particular topics when you do not have the skills needed to tackle a particular problem. Statistics is a highly technical discipline and in certain situations there are right and wrong ways to approach your data. If in doubt, approach a statistician for advice earlier rather than later. This avoids the situation statisticians encounter all too often: a dataset with poor measures or uncontrolled confounding or inappropriate sample size and the question 'What can I do now?'—when the real question is 'What should I have done at the start?' Even worse, it avoids having your final findings questioned by someone who points out statistical errors, casting doubt on the whole project. Befriend a statistician, or group of statisticians, and enrol their help whenever you can. They will often add value in unexpected ways!

Probability

If you read about probability in elementary statistics textbooks you will typically find it introduced using simple examples with simple answers: What are the chances that a coin will land heads, rather than tails if you flip it once? What are the chances of getting two 6s if you throw two six-sided dice? However, when faced with complex real-world situations in public health both the questions and the answers will be complex and may relate, for example, to the expected number of cases of a disease in a population, the likelihood a particular exposure has led to an observed health outcome, or the assessment of your organization's performance when benchmarked against similar organizations. To describe and deal with probability—which we may come across in relation to risk (see 📖 Chapter 6.5)—it is useful to know some of the statistical ways in which it is conceptualized: in terms of distributions, and using p values and confidence intervals.

Distributions

Distributions have to do with the way in which the values of something that has been measured (a 'variable') are distributed in a population.

For example, are they all the same (everybody has one head), split into two groups (most people think of themselves as either male or female), or do they come with a broad range of values (people are of different heights)? The most commonly referred to is the normal distribution—this has a 'bell-shaped curve' when plotted, indicating that there are many cases with values in the middle of the range and then a decreasing number with values farther away from the middle.

This distribution often occurs in physiological measurement (such as blood pressure) or in standardized tests (such as IQ tests). Figure 2.5.1 shows an example of approximately normally distributed data—in this case the data represented in the histogram are BMI scores, based on self-reported weights and heights, of women in India who responded to the WHO's World Health Survey. The smooth line shows the normal distribution—you will see that the actual values correspond closely, though not exactly, to this distribution.

Like all statistical distributions—and there are many—the normal distribution has specific statistical characteristics (which you can look up for yourself if you are interested).

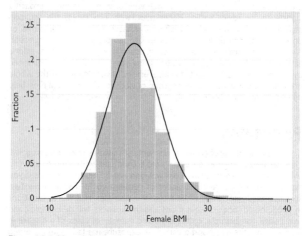

Figure 2.5.1 Normal distribution.

P values

Short for 'probability value', a P value is helpful in assessing whether a given value (or difference) is likely to have arisen by chance. In simple terms, the lower the P value, the less likely it is the thing you are interested in happened by chance. The cut-off value for statistical significance is conventionally set at $P = 0.05$ (though lower values are sometimes used), meaning that P values of less than this are considered statistically significant: meaning that the probability that the effects observed could be due to chance alone is 1 in 20 (or less) if they occurred purely randomly. The smaller the p value, the less likely your results is due to chance alone. Bear in mind, however, that 1 in 20 is an arbitrary figure used by the scientific community to indicate statistical significance.

Confidence intervals (CIs)

The ranges within which you can be confident, to a specified level, that the true value you are estimating lies. In this way they provide a measure of the robustness of results. The most commonly used CI is 95% and you will see something like '28.3 (95% CI 27.1–29.5)', which means an estimated value (point estimate) of 28.3 and a 95% likelihood that the true value is somewhere between 27.1 and 29.5. Another way to think about it is to assume that if you repeat the same study 100 times, the results would lie within the estimated confidence intervals 95 times out of the 100.

You should bear in mind that uncertainty in estimates is mostly determined by sample size—the larger the sample, the greater the likelihood that the sample value is closer to the true population value. It also follows that a narrow confidence interval indicates a large sample and therefore a more precise estimate of the true population value. Box 2.5.2 contains an example of how to interpret confidence intervals and *P* values.

Box 2.5.2 Interpreting confidence intervals and p values

Imagine you want to compare the effects of two interventions, Ashit and Buttout, that each aim to help people quit smoking. You have gathered some data and ask a statistician to help you analyse the results. She tells you the following:
- the successful quit rate with Ashit is 71.5%
- the successful quit rate with Buttout 61.5%
- the difference in quit rates between Ashit and Buttout is 10% (this is the 'mean' difference in effect) and the 95% CI for this difference is 8 to 12, with a p value of 0.003.

What do these numbers mean? In this case the CI is the range of values between which the mean difference would lie on 95 occasions if the study was done 100 times. Put another way, you can be 95% confident that the true difference at population level is between 8 and 12%, i.e. Ashit may be as much as 12% more effective than Treatment B or as little as 8% more effective).

The p value is the probability that a result of this magnitude would occur by chance alone if there were really no difference in effect between the two treatments, i.e. the likelihood of such a result occurring due to chance alone is only 3 in a 1000.

In this case, it seems likely that Ashit is more effective than Buttout and that the difference is about 10%.

Standardization

You will often want to compare mortality or disease incidence between two or more populations—for example, between your region and a neighbouring one, or between your local population and the national average. The comparison of *crude* mortality or incidence rates can be misleading if the populations differ in terms of basic characteristics such as age and gender (which are potential confounders—see 📖 Chapter 2.6). Standardization is a technique used to account for potential confounding variables when comparing two or more population groups, and is most commonly used to adjust for differences in age structure between populations.

Two main techniques are used, direct standardization and indirect standardization, and it is important you understand the differences between them.

- In *direct standardization* the age-specific rates in the populations of interest are applied to age-specific bands in a reference population thereby allowing direct comparison of the two populations. The main advantage of this approach are that it can be used to compare rates across various geographical areas and time and that it allows comparison of the relative burden of different diseases and causes of death within a population. Its main disadvantages are that age-specific rates may not be available for the population of interest as well as not being very reliable or stable for small number of events.

- In *indirect standardization* the observed pattern is compared with what would be expected if the population had the same age-specific rates as in a defined reference population, i.e. the number of actual events is compared with the number of expected events. This produces a ratio called a standardized ratio (e.g. SMR or standardized mortality ratio; SIR or standardized incidence ratio). The standardized ratio for a reference population is always 100 and therefore a value of less than 100 indicates lower rates than the reference population and a value of greater than 100 indicates a higher rate than the reference population. Box 2.5.3 contains a worked example of how to use both forms of standardization.

Box 2.5.3 Direct and indirect standardization

Imagine you are interested in comparing mortality rates in two regions, A and B. The table below shows the number of deaths occurring in each age band in the two populations, the number of people in each band and the calculated death rate in each age band (for simplicity only four age bands have been used).

Age band	Region A			Region B		
	Number of deaths	Population	Rate (per 100000)	Number of deaths	Population	Rate (per 100000)
0–14	2	100,000	2.0	3	110,000	2.72
15–44	19	150,000	12.66	18	130,000	13.84
45–74	196	140,000	140.0	330	250,000	132.0
75+	1480	110,000	1345.45	3560	260,000	1369.23
Total	1697	500,000		3911	750,000	

The crude death rate (number of deaths divided by population) in Region A is 339.4 and in Region B is 521.5 so it appears Region B has a higher death rate A. There are, however, differences in the age structure of the two populations—in Region B more than two-thirds of the population is aged 45 or over, but in Region A less than half the people are that age—and most deaths happen in older age groups.

You can compare the two Regions by direct standardization using a standard reference population. Assume the standard population here has 150,000 people aged 0–14, 300,000 aged 15–44, 400,000 aged 45–75, and 250,000 aged 75+.

If you apply the age-specific rate in each county to the standard population:

The age-standardized death rates—360.5 in Region A, 363.4 in Region B—are very similar suggesting the difference in crude death rates is due to the differences in the age distributions.

Age band	County A			County B		
	Rate (per 100000)	Population	Expected number of deaths	Rate (per 100000)	Population	Expected number of deaths
0–14	2.0	150,000	3	2.72	150,000	4
15–44	12.66	300,000	38	13.84	300,000	42
45–74	140.0	400,000	560	132.0	400,000	528
75+	1345.45	250,000	3364	1369.23	250,000	3423
Total		1,100,000	3965		1,100,000	3997

You can compare the death rates in the two populations using indirect standardization, i.e. applying the age-specific death rates in a standard or reference population to the two counties. Assume the age-specific death rates in the standard reference population are 3 in people aged 0–14, 13 in people aged 15–44, 135 in people aged 45–74, and 1350 in people aged 75+. You can apply these rates to the age bands in the two Regions:

	Region A			Region B		
Age band	Rate (per 100000)	Population	Expected number of deaths	Rate (per 100000)	Population	Expected number of deaths
0–14	3	100,000	3	3	110,000	3
15–44	13	150,000	20	13	130,000	17
45–74	135	140,000	189	135	250,000	338
75+	1350	110,000	1485	1350	260,000	3510
Total		500,000	1687		750,000	3868

SMR = Observed events × (100/Expected events)

SMR (Region A): 87.73   SMR (Region B): 101.11

If the mortality rates in the two populations were similar to that of the reference population their SMRs would be 100. These figures suggest Region A has a lower rate than Region B, but further examination is needed to determine if this is a real difference or just due to chance.

Potential pitfalls

Statistics are tools and like any tools can be misused.

- *Using arbitrary cut-points:* cutpoints at 0.05 for P values and 95% for CIs present the problem that 1 in 20 times they will be wrong: that is, one in twenty times the true value being estimated will fall outside the bounds of a 95% CI, and 1 in 20 times a P value of more than 0.05 will be assigned to a difference that is, in fact, statistically significant. The use of 0.05 and 95% is conventional and other values can be used. It is unclear what the difference is, for example, between a difference with a P value of 0.049 and one with a P value of 0.051: in conventional terms one is statistically significant and the other is not, but in practice there is little difference between them.

- *Drawing faulty conclusions from results that are not statistically significant:* when a P value is above 0.05 you cannot conclude that there is no difference just that you have not found one. This may occur for a number of reasons—often because the sample size is too small. Remember that absence of evidence is not evidence of absence!

- *Prioritizing statistical over practical significance:* establishing statistical significance is useful, but people can become too attached to it and you must always consider clinical or other practical significance. For example, a study reports a new intervention reduces systolic blood pressure by 0.2mmHg and that the reduction is statistically significant ($P < 0.001$). Great—but what does that mean in practice? A change in blood pressure of that size is unlikely to make a difference to any individual patient and even on a population level is not likely to be discernible. It would be easy, if reviewing the evidence, to seize on the low P value and clear statistical significance of this finding and to ignore the practical significance, but it is important you always consider statistics in context and use your professional judgement to interpret what is going on.

- *Forgetting the limitations of statistics in summarizing:* a useful demonstration of this is known as Anscombe's quartet.[2] This shows graphs of four datasets, each with different x and y values and a different overall shape, which nevertheless share key descriptive statistics.(see Figure 2.5.2) In each of the datasets the following values are all identical or very close: the number of observations (11), the mean of the x's (9.00), the variance of the x's (11.00), the mean of the y's (7.50), the variance of the y's (4.1), the correlation between x and y (0.816), and the linear regression line ($y = 3 + 0.5x$). Despite these similarities, the distribution of the values is obviously different in each case. This example highlights the value of graphing data as well as the importance of identifying outliers; more generally, it should remind us to be cautious in assuming that we know everything that is happening in a situation based solely on the use of some summary statistics.

- *Relying on frequentist approaches:* the way of dealing with statistics described here is called a frequentist approach and many statisticians feel this is inferior to a Bayesian approach.[3] It is beyond the scope of this chapter to deal with this but, briefly, the difference relates to how you use existing information about a situation and how you modify this in light of new information received.

- *Thinking you know too much:* it is possible to go wrong with statistics, particularly because the rules that apply in one situation may not apply in others. You should seek the input of a dedicated statistician when in doubt, and do so earlier rather than later—see p. 117.

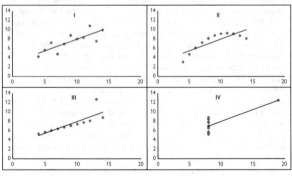

Anscombe's quartet								
I		II		III		IV		
x	y	x	y	x	y	x	y	
10	8.04	10	9.14	10	7.46	8	6.58	
8	6.95	8	8.14	8	6.77	8	5.76	
13	7.58	13	8.74	13	12.74	8	7.71	
9	8.81	9	8.77	9	7.11	8	8.84	
11	8.33	11	9.26	11	7.81	8	8.47	0.38345
14	9.96	14	8.1	14	8.84	8	7.04	
6	7.24	6	6.13	6	6.08	8	5.25	
4	4.26	4	3.1	4	5.39	19	12.5	
12	10.84	12	9.13	12	8.15	8	5.56	
7	4.82	7	7.26	7	6.42	8	7.91	
5	5.68	5	4.74	5	5.73	8	6.89	

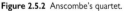

Figure 2.5.2 Anscombe's quartet.

How will you know when/if you have been successful?

You will know you have a good grasp of statistics and their application in public health practice when you find other people approaching you for help with their statistical problems!

Further resources

Campbell MJ. (2006). *Understanding modern statistical applications in medicine*, 2nd edn. BMJ Books, London.

Campbell MJ. (2009). *Statistics at square one*, 11th edn. BMJ Books, London.

Kirkwood B, Sterne J. (2003). *Essential medical statistics*, 2nd edn. Wiley-Blackwell, Harlow.

Rothman KJ. (2008). *Modern epidemiology*, 3rd edn. Lippincott Williams & Wilkins, London.

Tufte ER. (1983). *The visual display of quantitative information*. Graphics Press, Cheshire.

References

1 Porta M, Last J. (2008). *Dictionary of epidemiology*, 5th edn. Oxford University Press, Oxford.

2 Anscombe FJ. (1973). Graphs in statistical analysis. *American Statistician*, **27**, 17–21.

3 Spiegelhalter DJ, Abrams KR, Myles JP. (2004). *Bayesian approaches to clinical trials and health-care evaluation (Statistics in practice)*. Wiley Hoboken, New York.

2.6 Inference, causality, and interpretation

Iain Lang

Felix qui potuit rerum cognoscere causas
(Fortunate is he who can understand the causes of things)[1]

Objectives

Understanding causality and interpreting evidence in public health practice can be challenging. This chapter describes some of the key concepts involved, including association, causation, bias, confounding, and error. Although understanding the causes of things is a key public health skill, just as important are being aware of the limits to our understanding of what causes things, being able to communicate these limits to other people, and being able to make decisions even when the information we have is incomplete or inconclusive. This chapter will help you become familiar with some of the main concepts in this area, to understand how the inferences we can draw from evidence are shaped, and give you some insight into the limits of our understanding based on the available evidence. You may find it useful to read this chapter alongside 📖 Chapters 2.1, 2.4, 2.5, 2.7, and 6.5.

Why is this an important public health skill?

Being able to assess evidence and understand what it represents in terms of cause and effect, or what it might represent, or what it definitely does not represent, is crucial to practicing public health. If you lack the skills and understanding to do this you could find yourself adrift in a sea of claim and counter-claim, unable to differentiate association from causation or confounding from true effect.

When it comes to understanding the causes of things, the 'things' we are concerned with in public health are usually diseases or other harmful conditions (the causes of which we want to identify in order to reduce or prevent them) or successful positive outcomes (the causes of which we want to identify in order to stimulate or promote them).

We may need to understand the causes of things in relation to a piece of formal evidence, such as a critical appraisal of a peer-reviewed study, or in a range of other settings: an article in a newspaper, a letter or email from a concerned individual or group, or a public challenge in a meeting.

Definitions

- *Inference:* is the process of passing from observations and axioms to generalizations. Making causal inferences from observational data is an important aspect of epidemiology and public health practice.[2] When we make inferences we are typically concerned with the interpretation of evidence in light of our prior understandings to reach conclusions about what has occurred (or what will occur).
- *Causation:* is the act of causing something, and *causality* is the relationship between cause and effect. As *The Dictionary of Epidemiology* notes, most 'clinical, epidemiological, and public health research concerns causality'.[2] *Association* between two things means that they co-occur, or that a change in one has been observed to happen alongside a change in the other, In statistics, association means dependence between two or more events or characteristics.[2]
- A *mechanism:* is the way a particular event or outcome occurs and is often described in terms of agents or steps involved.[2] Although the name suggests a physical or mechanical understanding of how things work, in public health a mechanism may be biological, social, cultural, or of some other type or combination of types.
- *Causes* are sometimes referred to as *necessary* or *sufficient:* if a cause is necessary for an outcome then the outcome will not arise unless that cause is present. If a cause is sufficient for an outcome then the outcome can arise if that cause is present and no other cause is needed. If a cause is both necessary and sufficient for an outcome then the cause by itself can bring about the outcome and the outcome cannot occur without the cause. If a cause is neither necessary nor sufficient for an outcome then the outcome can occur without the cause: the cause by itself is not enough to bring about the outcome and other factors are needed. In public health we rarely come across causes that are both necessary and sufficient—that is, single causes with single outcomes. An individual cause is typically neither necessary nor sufficient and we have to consider combinations of causes as well as the importance of context (see below).
- *Confounding* or *confounding bias:* refers to distortion of the measure of the effect of an exposure on an outcome because of the association of both the exposure and the outcome with another factor or factors.[2]
- *Error:* is a false or mistaken result and classified into two types:
  - *Random error*—refers to variation in measurement or results with no apparent connection to other measurements or variables and thought of as being due to chance
  - *Systematic error* or *bias*—refers to variation in measurements or results that is consistently wrong in a particular direction, often because of an identifiable source.[2]

Association versus causation

The difference between association and causation is important and you may hear the warning 'association does not equate to causation.' Two things may occur closely together (in time or in space) and be described as associated, but this does not necessarily mean that one caused the other; they may both be consequences of some third event or there may be no relationship between them. For example, on a population level we might observe an association between having grey hair and cancer: the more grey hair a person has, the more likely they are to receive a cancer diagnosis.

These two things are associated, but this does not mean that one causes the other—having grey hair does not make you more likely to have cancer and having cancer does not make your hair turn grey. In this case, association does not imply causation. (A more reasonable explanation is that both grey hair and likelihood of cancer diagnosis are related to age—though even here the causal relationship is not straightforward and we would not say age causes cancer.)

A noteworthy text on causation in public health contains 'the Bradford-Hill criteria' and presents as a series of viewpoints 'we should especially consider' when thinking about whether an observed association involves causation. The nine points are summarized in Box 2.6.1.

> **Box 2.6.1 Austin Bradford Hill's criteria for identifying an association likely to involve causation[3]**
>
> - *Strength of association:* how strong is the relationship?
> - *Consistency:* is the cause always followed by the supposed outcome, or only sometimes?
> - *Specificity:* does the outcome only follow this cause or does it occur in other ways too?
> - *Temporal relationship:* does the cause precede the outcome?
> - *Biological gradient:* is there a dose-response relationship, i.e. does more of the cause lead to more of the outcome?
> - *Plausibility:* does it make sense that the outcome and the cause are related, biologically or otherwise?
> - *Coherence:* does the apparent relationship between cause and outcome make sense in relation to what we already know on this or related topics?
> - *Experiment:* is the evidence from experiments or quasi-experiments to support the relationship?
> - *Analogy:* are there comparable relationships that would support the idea that this association is a causal one?

Some epidemiologists have pointed out that Hill did not use the word 'criteria' and that these points are not suitable as a checklist to differentiate association from causation.[4]

You will soon realize that it is hard, in a public health context, to talk about 'causes'. Does smoking cause lung cancer? Yes, in a sense, but there are plenty of people who smoke and never develop lung cancer, and of course people who develop lung cancer who have never smoked. Often it is easier to talk about risks and say, for example, that smoking increases the risk of lung cancer (see also 📖 Chapter 6.5).

Confounding and other complications

For something to be classed as a confounder it must satisfy three conditions:
- it must be associated with the suspected cause
- it must be associated with the outcome
- it must not be on the causal pathway between the two—so if *a* causes *b* and *b* causes *c* then we would not call *b* a confounder.

Some examples may help here. If we found lung cancer was more common in people who consumed alcohol than those who did not we might infer alcohol causes lung cancer. However, this would be an incorrect inference and the confounder here is smoking; those who drink alcohol are more likely to smoke, smokers are more likely to get lung cancer, and it is not the case that alcohol consumption causes smoking which causes lung cancer. All three conditions are satisfied so we can identify smoking as a potential confounder of the relationship between alcohol and lung cancer.

To take another example, if we found heart attacks were more common in obese people we might infer that obesity causes myocardial infarctions (heart attacks). A factor that is *not* a confounder in this case is high blood pressure. Obesity is associated with high blood pressure and high blood pressure with myocardial infarctions, so the first two conditions are satisfied, but people who are obese are more likely to have high blood pressure and those with high blood pressure are more likely to experience a myocardial infarction. High blood pressure is not a confounder, in this case, because it is on the causal pathway between obesity and myocardial infarction. (Although there may, of course, be other confounders present.)

In epidemiological studies, confounding can be controlled to some extent through study design (by using matching or randomization) or through statistical analysis (through stratification or modelling), but these approaches depend on being able to identify confounders.[5] A big problem relates to unidentified confounding, that is those situations in which we fail to recognize the presence of one or more confounders. In the example of alcohol, smoking, and lung cancer, if we did not realize smoking was playing a role (i.e. failed to identify it as a confounder) we might wrongly conclude alcohol causes lung cancer (see Box 2.6.2).

Another complication relates to interaction, which occurs when the combined effects of two or more exposures on an outcome are different

Box 2.6.2 Causal diagrams on confounding and interaction

An apparent association between alcohol consumption and lung cancer is confounded by cigarette smoking, which is associated both with alcohol consumption and lung cancer, but not on the causal pathway linking them.

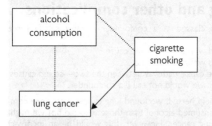

Here, high blood pressure is associated with both obesity and myocardial infarctions, but is not a confounder because it is on the causal pathway: obesity leads to increased blood pressure which can cause myocardial infarctions.

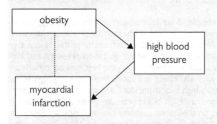

Interaction is said to occur when the combination of two or more factors leads to different outcomes. This could reduce the magnitude or likelihood of the outcome or increase it: here, the combination of long-term exposure to asbestos and cigarette smoking is more likely to cause lung cancer than either of those exposures alone.

from the effects we would expect from each when considered separately. This may reduce or increase the magnitude or likelihood of an outcome. A well-known example relates to the combined effects of smoking and asbestos exposure on lung cancer: the chances of developing lung cancer in those who both smoke and are exposed to asbestos are greater than we would expect based on the chances of developing lung cancer associated with each exposure by itself. Other forms of interaction are apparent in relation to gene-environment interactions: for example, the *APOE* gene is a predictor of late-onset Alzheimer's disease, and various lifestyle factors increase the risk of Alzheimer's disease, but those who have both specific alleles of *APOE* and risky lifestyle behaviours have a magnified risk of dementia.[6] (See also 📖 Chapter 3.7).

Random and systematic error

All measurements are imprecise on some level—measurements to the nearest kilometre are imprecise in terms of meters, measures to the nearest meter are imprecise in terms of centimetres, and so on—so random error is present in any measurement. In public health information one possible source of random error relates to sampling from populations. No single sample, random or otherwise, is fully representative of the population from which it is taken. This means that, for example, the mean of a sample will differ from the mean of the population from which the sample has been drawn. Ways of reducing the random error include drawing a larger sample or drawing multiple samples from the same population.[7]

The important difference between random error and bias is the 'systematic' element of bias such that measured values not only differ from true values, but do so as the result of an underlying factor or factors that affect all the differences in a specific way. As an analogy, think of two archers aiming at a target. One of them is not a good aim and tends not to hit the bulls eye, but to scatter her shots around the target. The other always aims too far to the left and so her shots always land to the left of the target. If the target was removed after they had fired, but you could see where the arrows had landed you might be able to guess where the first archer had been aiming by picking somewhere in the middle of the holes—but this tactic would not work with the second example (unless you knew she always aimed to the left) and you would tend to misidentify where the target had been. In the same way, with random error present we can infer approximately where the true value lies, but with systematic error we risk making an incorrect inference unless we are aware of the type and size of the bias.

Many forms of bias have been described and some of the more common are set out in Table 2.6.1. Biases can be addressed, though not necessarily fully, in either the design or the analysis of a study. RCTs involving random allocation and blinding represent one of the best ways of minimizing bias, but even RCTs can be subject to bias.[8] A well designed RCT is likely to contain the strongest evidence we can obtain from a single study, but we still need to consider the extent to which its results may be generalized (see 📖 Chapter 2.4).

Table 2.6.1 Common types of bias

Type of bias	Source of bias	Example
Selection	Systematic differences between individuals participating in a study and those who do not. This can arise because of self-selection or other aspects of the study selection procedure.	People in households with higher socioeconomic status were more likely to allow measurements of magnetic fields in the home to be taken, but less likely to live close to sources of magnetic fields than those in lower socioeconomic status households.[9]
Reporting	People may be selective about the way they report information. Certain types of information are particularly likely to be misreported, e.g. about levels of alcohol consumption or sexual history.	Women who have experienced abortions may be inhibited about telling researchers about them, leading to systematic under-reporting.[10]
Recall	Individuals wrongly remember and report information about past events, for example because certain events or experiences are particularly memorable	In retrospective studies, mother's reports of gestational age at birth differ depending on whether the delivery was at term or preterm.[11]
Detection	Different assessment or diagnostic techniques tend to be better or worse at detecting particular conditions, or to be applied differently in different settings	In RCTs, knowledge of the arm to which a participant has been assigned can influence assessment of outcome.[12]

What do we do when the evidence is not good enough?

These considerations—of causation versus association, of causes and con-founders, of bias and error—are central to the formal critical appraisal of study findings. As public health practitioners keen to ensure our practice is appropriately evidence-based and to ensure we get the outcomes we want and avoid those we do not, you may also wonder how we can achieve anything, and make any decisions, when there are so many caveats about causes and inferences and the information you have in front of you is less than conclusive. What do you do when the evidence is not good enough?

You might begin by reflecting on the fact that the evidence is never good enough—or at least, not often. For some core public health activities, like vaccination, the evidence available is strong, but for others, like eating five pieces of fruit and vegetables a day, it is less compelling than you might imagine. On some topics RCTs are impractical or unethical and in these situations we are reliant on observational studies. On such topics—including, for example, the health effects of environmental toxins,[13] the long-term consequences of behaviours,[14] or population-level patterns of health[15]—we must rely on data that are suggestive, rather than conclusive.

In the end you will have to make decisions and recommendations and simply declaring the existing evidence is inconclusive is not likely to be helpful (unless you are making the case for conducting research or evaluation). A useful theoretical orientation on this is provided by work on realistic evaluation and evidence-based policy making.[16] This approach to evidence and decision-making is in contrast to the standard focus on weight of evidence and depends instead on the basic realist formula of causation:

mechanism + context = outcome

In this understanding, causes (or mechanisms) do not exist in a vacuum, but operate, and must be understood, in complex social and organizational environments. This implies that what works in one setting will not always work in another and is one reason to be cautious about assuming what has been shown to work in an RCT, for example, will produce the same outcomes when put in place else-where; the context of a trial is different from the 'real' context in which we each work so even if the mechanism is the same, the outcome may be different. Approaches to evaluation that identify it as a social practice rather than as scientific testing can also usefully inform our understanding of how evidence is created and interpreted—all these things occur in complex social and organizational environments.[17]

Once you have realized the evidence is typically not going to be as strong as you would like it to be, you will probably proceed on a pragmatic basis—making the best decision you can based on the best evidence that is available, what you know about the local situation, your prior experience of related issues, and the advice and input of colleagues or partners. In such contexts the more inclusive notion of knowledge-based practice may be more useful than thinking in terms of pure evidence-based practice.[18]

Conclusion

Being able to appraise the strengths and weaknesses of evidence is crucial to effective public health practice. Knowing what is meant by inference, association, causation, bias, and confounding is crucial to shaping our understanding of what can and cannot be inferred from the information available to us. In practice, our decisions and actions will be shaped by combining this understanding with our knowledge of complex local factors and politics.

Further resources

Bonita R, Beaglehole R, Kjellström T. (2007). *Basic Epidemiology*, 2nd edn, pp. 83–97. WHO, Geneva. . Available online at: ℘ http://libdoc.who.int/publications/2006/9241547073_eng.pdf

References

1 Virgil, Georgics, no 2, l 490 quoted in Wilson J. (2008). *Inverting the Pyramid*. Orion, London.

2 Porta M. (ed.) (2008). *A dictionary of epidemiology*, 5th edn. Oxford University Press, Oxford.

3 Hill AB. (1965). The environment and disease: association or causation? *Proceedings of the Royal Society of Medicine.*, **58**, 295–300.

4 Rothman KJ. (2002). *Epidemiology: an introduction*. Oxford University Press, Oxford.

5 Rothman KJ, Greenland S, Poole C, Lash TL. (2008). Causation and causal inference. In: Rothman KJ, Greenland S, Lash TJ, eds, *Modern epidemiology*, 3rd edn, pp. 5–31. Lippincott Williams & Wilkins, Philadelphia.

6 Kivipelto M, Rovio S, Ngandu T, *et al.* (2008). Apolipoprotein E ε4 magnifies lifestyle risks for dementia: a population-based study. *Journal of Cellular and Molecular Medicine*. **12**, 2762–71.

7 Levy PS, Lemeshow S. (2008). *Sampling of populations: methods and applications*, Wiley Series in Survey Methodology, 4th edn. Wiley, Hoboken.

8 Jüni P, Altman DG, Egger M. (2001). Systematic reviews in health care: assessing the quality of controlled clinical trials. *British Medical Journal*. **323**, 42–6.

9 Mezei G, Kheifets L. (2006). Selection bias and its implications for case-control studies: a case study of magnetic field exposure and childhood leukaemia. *International Journal of Epidemiology*, **35**,397–406.

10 Jones EF, Forrest JD. (1992). Underreporting of abortion in surveys of U.S. women: 1976 to 1988. *Demography*, **29**, 113–26.

11 Yawn BP, Suman VJ, Jacobsen SJ. (1998). Maternal recall of distant pregnancy events. *Journal of Clinical Epidemiology*,. **51**, 399–405.

12 Noseworthy JH, Ebers GC, Vandervoort MK, I (1994). The impact of blinding on the results of a randomized, placebo-controlled multiple sclerosis clinical trial. *Neurology*, **44**, 16–20.

13 Lang IA, Galloway TS, Scarlett A, *et al.* (2008). Association of urinary bisphenol A concentration with medical disorders and laboratory abnormalities in adults. *Journal of the American Medical Association, B* **11**, 1303–10.

14 Lang IA, Guralnik J, Wallace RB, Melzer D. (2007) What level of alcohol consumption is hazardous for older people? Functioning and mortality in U.S. and English national cohorts. *Journal of the American Geriatrics Society*, **55**, 49–57.

15 Lang IA, Llewellyn DJ, Hubbard RE, Langa KM, Melzer D. (2011). Income and the midlife peak in common mental disorder prevalence. *Psychological Medicine*, **41**, 1365–72.

16 Pawson R, Tilley N. (1997). *Realistic evaluation*. Sage Publications, London.

17 Greenhalgh T, Russell J. (2010). Why do evaluations of eHealth programs fail? An alternative set of guiding principles. *PLoS Medicine*, **7**, e1000360.

18 Glasby J. (2011). *Evidence, policy and practice: critical perspectives in health and social care*. Policy Press, Bristol.

2.7 Finding and appraising evidence

Anne Brice, Amanda Burls, and Alison Hill

Objectives

Making good public health decisions requires integrating good *information* (much of it routine; see 📖 Chapters 2.1, 2.7 and 2.8) with good *research evidence*. However, there is a vast quantity of research evidence available, much of it poor quality. This chapter aims to help you find and appraise research evidence efficiently, so the best, most relevant research evidence is used to improve health.

Finding research evidence

What sort of evidence do you need?

Before searching for evidence, you need to know what sort of evidence to look for. To do this you need to:
- have a clearly formulated question
- know what study design would best answer the question you have.

To formulate your question you need to specify, for the context of your decision, the:
- population (to whom is the decision being applied)
- exposure (an intervention if the question is about effectiveness, or a risk factor if the question is about harm)
- comparator
- outcome(s)
- time (period or time horizon you are interested in).

This is the acronym PECOT.[1] Another well-known acronym is PICO (Population or participant, Intervention or indicator, Comparator or control, Outcome) which is frequently used for clinical questions.

Table 2.7.1 shows the best primary research design for different questions. If an appropriate study design has not been used then the study is unlikely to provide information of value to your decision. If available, a good quality up-to-date systematic review of studies of the appropriate design will give the best overview.

Table 2.7.1 Best primary research design for different questions

Type of question	Study design
Effectiveness	Randomized controlled trial
Etiology and risk factors	Cohort and case–control studies
Harm	Cohort and case–control studies
Prognosis	Inception cohort/survival studies
Diagnosis	Diagnostic test study (or randomized controlled trial)
Patient experience (e.g. of illness, treatment or service)	Qualitative studies, e.g. questionnaires, focus groups, interviews,
Incidence and prevalence	Cohort or cross-sectional
Value for money	Economic evaluation (e.g. cost-effectiveness study or cost–benefit study)

The question you have formulated, and the best study design to answer the question, will help to shape your search for evidence, and we explain the process in the section below.

Finding the evidence

It can be difficult to find the best research evidence, and to know when you have found it. Developments in technology, particularly on-line databases, mean that you can access a huge range of resources (See Box 2.7.1). However, you need a systematic and reproducible approach to avoid wasting time, missing relevant literature, or having to wade through large quantities of irrelevant citations. Searching techniques need to be *sensitive* (to get as much of the information you *do* need as possible) and *specific* (to minimize the amount of retrieved information that you *do not* need).

Box 2.7.1 Google

Many people use Internet search engines, such as Google, to find health information, particularly when they need it quickly. However, the information you find is more likely to be biased, as there are fewer controls for quality, compared to other sources. For instance, search engines may include paid-for advertisements, it may be difficult to determine who the authors of the information are, and the information you find may not be reliable or up-to-date, and may even be harmful.

You can use a checklist, such as the LIDA tool (www.minervation. com, accessed 29 March 2011), or look for a quality mark such as the Information Standard (www.theinformationstandard.org accessed 29 March 2011), or the HON code (www.hon.ch accessed 29 March 2011) to help ensure that you are using good quality resources.

Searching for scientific literature is not a linear process. Search strategies may need to be refined in the light of citations retrieved in order to improve the identification of relevant papers—often called 'iterative searching'.

Sources of information

Evidence can be found in a wide range of sources. There are between 20,000 and 30,000 biomedical journals, and about 17,000 new biomedical books are published every year. Therefore you need a clearly defined question and knowledge of which source to search.

Sources include guidelines, the Cochrane Library, Medline/PubMed, Embase, Scopus, and many others, plus primary and secondary journals, grey literature, and textbooks. These resources can be accessed in a number of ways, for example via specific databases or via national/international portals [e.g. NHS Evidence (www.evidence.nhs.uk accessed 28 March 2011) in the UK].

Selecting sources

Deciding which sources to search and the nature of your strategy will depend on many factors, including the purpose of your search and the time available. Using a protocol can help you plan your approach and ensure that the search is reproducible. A sample protocol is included in Figure 2.7.1. Other useful resources can be found on the website of the Centre for Evidence-Based Medicine (www.cebm.net, accessed 28 March 2011)

Doing the search

When creating a search strategy it is essential to go back to your carefully formulated question. This will help you identify relevant terms on which to base your search, and to build the blocks of your search strategy. Start with a broad, or sensitive, search. This will find a lot of material, much of which may not be relevant. It is important not to limit or narrow the search too quickly as this may exclude vital evidence from your search results. For example, in order to search as broadly as possible in Medline we need to know how to:

• perform a MeSH (Medical Subject Heading) search
• perform a text word, or free-text search.

For each concept within the search identify the relevant MeSH terms, and also keywords and synonyms to search as free text. Using techniques such as:

• exploding the thesaurus terms
• applying all subheadings
• using truncation and wild cards will help ensure that useful evidence is not excluded.

The search can always be refined later if the results are not as expected. As indexing quality is variable, it is important to build a search strategy using a combination of both MeSH terms and text words, and combine the results using Boolean logic 'operators' such as 'AND' and 'OR' and 'NOT'.

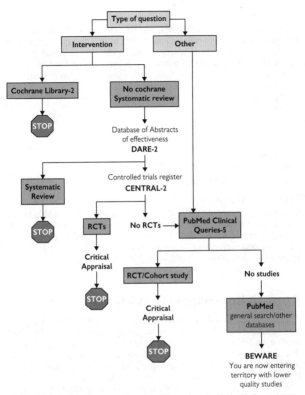

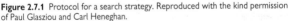

Figure 2.7.1 Protocol for a search strategy. Reproduced with the kind permission of Paul Glasziou and Carl Heneghan.

Searching for quality

To narrow a search, and increase its specificity, requires systematically excluding the least useful articles. The most useful criterion on which to search for quality papers is to look at the methods being used. Look for the use of GRADE (Grading of Recommendations Assessment, Development and Evaluation) (⊛ http://www.gradeworkinggroup.org/publications/index.htm accessed 28 March 2011), an internationally recognized system for assessing the quality of evidence. Reporting checklists for a range of different study types are available through the EQUATOR (Enhancing the Quality and Transparency of Health Research) (⊛ http://www.equator-network.org/accessed 28 March 2011).

Using search filters
Search filters are tried and tested literature search strategies that provide a more effective way of refining your search to find high-quality evidence appropriate to your type of question. They can be used to identify systematic review and randomized controlled trial literature on Medline, and in other databases. There are also methodological search filters which will help you retrieve sound clinical studies that deal with:

- diagnosis
- prognosis
- therapy
- etiology
- guidelines
- treatment outcomes
- evidence-based health-care methods.

These are built into PubMed and Clinical Queries.

Search strategies

Search strategies should be explicit and reproducible. Start with a broad search, and then narrow by quality filters. Remember to match the search strategy to the question, and that searching is an iterative process. For more help and instructional videos in searching for evidence go to Health Knowledge (http://www.healthknowledge.org.uk/interactive-learning/fae/finding-the-evidence accessed 28 March 2011).

Appraising research evidence

Critical appraisal is the systematic assessment of research evidence. No research is perfect. The purpose of appraising a study is not to find fault because it is less than ideal, but rather to identify what, if anything, is of value that could help inform your decision. You might find it helpful to think of the word critical as meaning to find value (i.e. critique), rather than just considering a more common interpretation of the word (to find fault/criticize).

When critically appraising any study you need to be able to tell:
- what question the researchers set out to answer (concise, answerable question in full)
- whether they used an appropriate study design (methods—the right methods done correctly)
- what they did
- what they found (results—in numbers and words)
- the implications of the findings in your context (relevance—so what?).

Screening questions for any study

Given the vast number of potential studies available, you need to triage papers for their potential usefulness. Thus, the first question to ask is 'Is a clear question being addressed?' You need to ensure here that you can identify all the components of the question (PECOT, see 🕮 Finding research evidence). If the answer is no, or you cannot tell, then the paper is unlikely to be useful (in fact, it is likely to be positively unhelpful—it might support your prior belief and thus you ascribe it too much value, and find it difficult to forget).

The next question is 'Did the researchers use an appropriate study design for the question they were asking?' Remember it is usually only worth proceeding to appraise a study in more depth if it has a clear question and appropriate study design.

Appraising the validity of studies of different designs

We use studies to inform our decision making. Thus we need to know to what extent a study's findings are likely to reflect the 'truth'. For example, if a study finds the death rate in those treated with a new treatment is half that in patients given the standard treatment, we would like to be convinced that this is because the new treatment actually halves the death rate and was not simply due to the way study was done. Systematic

---

Box 2.7.2 Randomized controlled trials (RCTs) (see 📖 Chapter 2.4)

- Was the allocation of patients to treatments randomized?
- Was this allocation concealed?
- Were the groups similar at the start of the trial, in terms of factors that might affect the outcome such as age, sex, and social class?
- Were patients, health workers, and study personnel 'blind' to treatment?
- Apart from the experimental intervention, were the groups treated equally?
- Were all of the patients who entered the trial properly accounted for at its conclusion?
- Were patients analysed in the groups to which they were randomized?

See also the validated scale for assessing the quality of an RCT.[2]

Box 2.7.3 Systematic reviews and meta-analyses

To be valid, a review should systematically identify and evaluate all appropriately designed studies that address the question being considered and, where appropriate, combine their results. If this is not done properly there is the potential for bias and the results will not be trustworthy even when the included papers were well conducted.

- Did the reviewers try to identify all relevant studies?
- Did the reviewers assess the quality of the included studies?
- If the results of the studies have been combined, was it reasonable to do so?

See also the validated scale for assessing the quality of a meta-analysis.[3]

Box 2.7.4 Cohort and case-control studies

- Was the cohort recruited in an acceptable way?
- Was the exposure accurately measured to minimize bias?
- Was the outcome accurately measured to minimize bias?

- Have the authors identified all important confounding factors?
- Have they taken into account the confounding factors in the design and/or analysis?
- Was the follow up of subjects complete enough?
- Was the follow up of subjects long enough?

See also the validated scale for assessing the quality of non-randomized studies.[4]

Box 2.7.5 Economic evaluations (see 📖 Chapter 1.6)

- Was a comprehensive description of the competing alternatives given (i.e. can you tell who did what to whom, where, and how often)?
- Was there evidence that the programme's effectiveness had been established?
- Were all important and relevant consequences and costs for each alternative identified?
- Were consequences and costs measured accurately in appropriate units (for example, hours of nursing time, number of physician visits, years of life gained) prior to valuation?
- Were consequences and costs valued credibly?
- Were consequences and costs adjusted for differential timings (discounting)?
- Was an incremental analysis of the consequences and costs of alternatives performed?
- Was a sensitivity analysis performed?

Box 2.7.6 Diagnostic tests

- Did all patients get the diagnostic test and the reference standard?
- Could the results of the test of interest have been influenced by the results of the reference standard?
- Is the disease status of the tested population clearly established?
- Were the methods for performing the test described in sufficient detail?

Box 2.7.7 Qualitative studies

- Was the recruitment strategy appropriate to the aims of the research?
- Were the data collected in a way that addresses the research issue?
- Has the relationship between researchers and participants been adequately considered?
- Have ethical issues been taken into consideration?
- Was the data analysis sufficiently rigorous?

deviation of results from the truth because of the way a study is conducted is known as *bias*.

An important element of critical appraisal is to check that potential biases were both identified and minimized. Since different study designs are prone to different biases, there are specific questions you need to focus on to check their validity. We provide the following checklists as an *aide-mémoire* for the important biases you need to check for when appraising studies of different designs. Where there are specific validated scales these are referenced in the checklists.

Learning critical appraisal skills requires practice and experience, therefore resources that can help with further learning are provided at the end of the chapter.

Making sense of results

One should not waste time looking at the 'results' of a study where the methods lack sufficient validity because it will not be possible to know if an apparent finding is a real effect or simply due to bias because of the way the study was conducted. However, even if the study methods are trustworthy, it is important to consider the results critically. Also consider the way the results are expressed as this might influence the reader's interpretation and subsequent decision-making (see Box 2.7.8).

What are the results?
- How were the outcomes expressed [e.g. odds ratios, risk ratios, risk differences, numbers needed to treat (NNTs), or, in a diagnostic test study, likelihood ratios]?
- If these results are only expressed as a relative risk such as the risk ratio or odds ratio, is there sufficient information to calculate the absolute risk (such as a risk difference or NNT)?
- What was the bottom-line or estimate for each outcome?

Could they have occurred by chance? (see 📖 Chapter 2.5)
- How likely is it that this result occurred simply by chance? (The p value estimates how frequently a result, or a more extreme result, would be seen by chance if there is no true effect.)
- CIs also indicate how much uncertainty due to chance surrounds an estimate. (This is known as precision.) In an unbiased study, the CIs can be interpreted as telling you the range in which the true effect lies

Box 2.7.8 Example of communicating the same evidence with different emphasis . . .

Consider the following results. If nicotine replacement therapy increases the 6-month quit rate from 10% to 17%, there are at least two ways of communicating these results. On the one hand it nearly doubles the quit rate, and on the other hand, because the NNT is about 14 [i.e. 1/(0.17–0.1)], then for every 14 people who take nicotine replacement therapy, 13 of them gain no additional benefit (approximately 2 out of the 14 quitted, although about one would have quit anyway . . .).

with a certain degree of confidence (conventionally 95%). If the 95% CIs of an estimate of relative risk do not cross 1, or the 95% CIs of an estimate of risk difference do not cross 0, then the result is 'statistically significant'.

What do they mean?

- How important is this result for the patient or policy decisions? It is important to consider other ways of expressing the results as the way in which results are expressed can influence how important they appear. For example, try to calculate the NNT if results are reported as relative risks or, in diagnostic test studies, the likelihood ratios where results are expressed as sensitivity and specificity.
- Were all important outcomes considered? (E.g. did the study explicitly consider adverse events?).

Can the results be applied to the local population?

You need to consider whether there are any important differences between the local population or setting and the study population or setting that would mean that the results would be likely to be different locally.

Are the benefits worth the harms and costs?

This is usually not explicitly considered in individual studies. However, the bottom-line is that the probable benefits of a decision need to outweigh the probable harms and costs. To make these judgment public health practitioners will usually need to draw on their wider experience and background knowledge. Bear in mind that, when making policy decisions this usually requires a consideration of the opportunity cost as well.

Further resources

Publications

De Brun C, Pearce-Smith, N. (2009). *Searching skills toolkit: finding the evidence*. Wiley-Blackwell, Chichester.

Glasziou P, Del Mar C, Salisbury J. (2003). *Evidence-based medicine workbook, finding and applying the best evidence to improve patient care*. BMJ Books, London.

Gray JAM. (2009). *Evidence-based health care and public health: how to make decisions about health services and public health*, 3rd edn. Churchill Livingstone, London.

Guyatt G, Rennie D, Meade M, Cook D. (2008). *Users' guides to the medical literature: essentials of evidence-based clinical practice*, 2nd edn. JAMA & Archives Journals, Chicago.

Straus S, Richardson S, Glasziou P, Haynes B. (2005). *Evidence-based medicine: how to practice and teach EBM*, 3rd edn. Churchill Livingstone, London.

Websites

Critical Appraisal Skills Programme. Available at: ℘ http://www.caspuk.net (accessed 29 March 2011) This site gives you the checklists that were developed by the Critical Appraisal Skills Programme (CASP) to help with the process of critically appraising articles for a range of different types of research studies.

Health Knowledge. Finding and appraising the evidence. Available at: ℘ http://www.healthknowledge. org.uk/interactive-learning/finding-and-appraising-the-evidence (accessed 29 March 2011) This is a set of modules take you through the process of how to find the evidence and then how to assess the validity and reliability of the published research in order to provide effective and efficient healthcare.

NHS Evidence Available at:. ℘ http://www.evidence.nhs.uk (accessed 29 March 2011). NHS Evidence provides free access to clinical and non-clinical information - local, regional, national and international. Information includes evidence, guidance and government policy. NHS staff who have an Athens account can also get free access to paid for journals.

Cochrane Collaboration Webliography Available at:. http://www.cochrane.org/about-us/evidence-based-health-care/webliography/ (accessed 29 March 2011). A webliography produced by the Cochrane Collaboration which presents an overview of the most important print and online resources for evidence-based health care and medicine. The site contains listings for a wide range of resources, and includes recommendations for books, articles and online resources browseable by speciality, such as epidemiology, statistics, literature appraisal, reporting guidelines, and more.

PubMed Tutorial. Available at: ℘ http://www.nlm.nih.gov/bsd/disted/pubmed.html (accessed 29 March 2011). A range of tutorials and quick tours relating to searching PubMed, produced by the National Library of Medicine.

References

1 Jackson R, Ameratunga S, Broad J, et al. (2006). The GATE frame: critical appraisal with pictures. *Evidence Based Medicine*, **11,** 35–8.

2 Jadad A., Moore R, Carroll D, et al. (1996). Assessing the quality of reports of randomized clinical trials: Is blinding necessary? *Controlled Clinical Trials*, **17,** 1–12.

3 Wells G, Shea B, O'Connell D, et al. *The Newcastle-Ottawa Scale (NOS) for assessing the quality of non-randomized studies in meta-analyses.* Available at: ℘ http://www.ohri.ca/programs/clinical_epidemiology/oxford.asp (accessed 29 March 2011)

4 Shea B, Grimshaw J, Wells G, et al. (2007). Development of AMSTAR: a measurement tool to assess the methodological quality of systematic reviews. *BMC Medical Research Methodology*, **7,** 10.

2.8 Surveillance

Daniel M. Sosin and Richard S. Hopkins

Disclaimer: The findings and conclusions in this report are those of the authors and do not necessarily represent the official position of the Centers for Disease Control and Prevention or the Florida Department of Health.

Objectives

Effective use of health data is a foundation of public health practice. Surveillance produces an ongoing stream of data that, when appropriately analysed, supports and directs public health action. This chapter provides an introduction to the purposes, design, methods, and uses of public health surveillance systems. Public health programme managers and staff, decision makers, epidemiologists, and students of public health can use this information to assure effective implementation of public health surveillance systems.

What is surveillance?

Public health surveillance is 'the ongoing, systematic collection, analysis, interpretation, and dissemination of data about a health-related event for use in public health action to reduce morbidity and mortality and to improve health'.[1] Thus public health surveillance is a continual process of monitoring health and health indicators and is important for improving health status across a wide range of acute and chronic conditions. Examples of health-related events include episodes of illness or injury, diagnoses of chronic conditions, risk behaviours for adverse health outcomes (e.g. tobacco use or non-use of seatbelts), or completion of a health-care procedure (e.g. Pap smear or measles immunization). The principles of public health surveillance are the same for communicable and non-communicable diseases; however, experience has been more plentiful with communicable diseases.

Historically, infectious disease surveillance has depended upon legally mandated disease reporting by health-care providers, laboratories, and health-care systems. Increasingly, surveillance for both infectious and non-communicable disease events relies on surveys and on data collected for other purposes where public health benefits are secondary (e.g. administrative data, electronic medical records, vital registration). The European Centre for Disease Prevention and Control (ECDC) espouses a comprehensive model of surveillance referred to as Epidemic Intelligence, which combines traditional surveillance methods and goals with expanded methodologies with the intent to identify and characterize emerging threats.[2]

Electronic management and submission of data to public health agencies afford the possibility of instantaneous identification, reporting and review of disease, injury and health indicator data, including laboratory results, very close to the time they are recorded by the provider. Effective use of such near-real-time health data would transform the practice of surveillance for improving public health and medical care.

Syndromic surveillance is an approach where health department staff, assisted by automated data acquisition and generation of statistical signals, monitor disease indicators continually to detect outbreaks of disease earlier and more completely than might otherwise be possible with traditional methods for reporting disease, and to monitor trends and risk variations as they unfold.[3] Efficiency of outbreak detection by these methods needs further investigation, but they have demonstrated benefit for monitoring trends in widespread outbreaks, such as the recent pandemic of influenza A (H1N1).

Surveillance should be conducted in a standardized and consistent manner over time and space and should be designed to support public health action.

Why conduct surveillance?

Public health surveillance is used to support interventions in individual cases; detect and monitor outbreaks; understand the natural history of a disease or injury; estimate the magnitude of disease and risk factors in a target population; identify patterns and changes in agents, conditions, and practices; support treatment guidance, policy development, or programme planning and evaluation; conduct exploratory research; and identify research gaps. These purposes of surveillance systems can be classified into three main categories: case management, outbreak detection and management, and programme management. Individual cases of diseases of public health interest (e.g. tuberculosis) are routinely reported to public health authorities to ensure proper disease management for both the individual and the community (e.g. investigation to locate and treat exposed contacts to an infectious disease or toxin). Public health authorities use surveillance data to detect, track the course and extent of, and manage outbreaks (e.g. severe bloody diarrhoea and secondary haemolytic uraemic syndrome due to ground beef contaminated with *Escherichia coli* O157:H7, or birth defects due to introduction of a new medication, or cancers due to a new occupational hazard). They also use surveillance data for the planning and continuous evaluation necessary to ensure that programmes to prevent and control disease at the community level are effective (e.g. immunizations to prevent infectious diseases, or 'back to sleep' campaigns to prevent sudden infant death syndrome, or interventions to improve quality of clinical care).

Designing a surveillance system

The first step in designing a surveillance system is to state its purpose clearly. The relative importance of many system attributes depends on the purpose (Table 2.8.1). For example:

- A system that is sufficiently timely to support programme planning with a several-year time horizon may not be sufficiently timely for outbreak recognition or immediate control measures.
- When resources are scarce, an automated alarm system for outbreak detection may need to be set with low sensitivity and high positive predictive value (PPV). For case management and programme management, PPV reflects the probability that a case in the database is one being sought by the system and negative predictive value (NPV) reflects the probability that persons not in the database do not have the condition under surveillance. For outbreak detection, PPV reflects the probability that a system signal identifies an outbreak of the type being sought, and NPV reflects the probability that no signal from the system means that no outbreak is occurring.
- If reassurance that an outbreak is not occurring when there is no signal is an important desired feature of the system, a high NPV for outbreaks is important.
- Data quality needs to be particularly high when medical treatment decisions will be made on the basis of data in the system. When surveillance is used as a screening tool to detect events requiring further investigation, lower data quality may be tolerated. Costly

Table 2.8.1 Relative importance (5-point scale) of surveillance system performance attributes that vary by purpose of surveillance

Attribute	Case management	Outbreak detection and management	Programme planning and evaluation
Timeliness	****	*****	*
Sensitivity	****	****	***
Positive predictive value	****	***	****
Negative predictive value	**	*****	***
Data quality	*****	***	****
Representativeness	**	**	****
Flexibility	***	****	*
Stability	****	*****	***

investments in prevention programmes also demand high-quality data for planning and evaluation purposes.

- Flexibility reflects the ability of a system to change as needs change. Outbreak detection systems particularly require flexibility to adapt to changing threats and levels of risk over time.
- Stability, reflected by the resilience of the system to external changes and consistency in operation over long periods of time, is more important in systems for outbreak detection.

System characteristics

System characteristics also vary with the primary purpose of the system (Table 2.8.2):

Data sources

These are most diverse for programme management and least diverse for case management where individual treatment and case management decisions require a follow-up with personal identifiers. Outbreak detection can often be done with data that do not contain personal identifiers, yet timely investigation of cases that may be part of an outbreak may require that identifiers be accessible. Cultural norms and governmental rules for use and protection of personal data for public health purposes can vary by jurisdiction. At any time when personally identified data are collected for public health purposes, utmost care must be taken to meet ethical and legal standards and ensure privacy and confidentiality of the data. Data that are not needed should not be collected.

Data collection

Data collection may be manual or electronic. The point in development of a collection system at which switching from manual records to automated ones makes sense will depend on the level of technology and of trained staff realistically available as well as on the volume of reports and the timeliness needed. In most settings, surveillance data are collected at the most local level in the system and gradually aggregated as they are passed up the chain to surveillance units responsible for larger areas (e.g. county, district, province, or country). More recently, technologic advances have permitted a reversal of this flow. When the data source for surveillance is inherently centralized, data may be collected in a central office and be made available promptly to local public health units.

Analysis

Analysis of surveillance data should be appropriate to the task at hand. Localized acute disease surveillance may need no more than line lists of cases, cases plotted over time (i.e. epidemic curves), and simple mapping. Systems with many streams of data, especially case-based data with demographic detail (e.g. age, race, sex, ethnicity, occupation, and location of residence) may benefit from automated aberration detection and from more complex.

Displays

Increased availability of highly detailed molecular subtyping of organisms causing disease (e.g. PulseNet) also creates a need for software to identify

Table 2.8.2 Surveillance system design characteristics by purpose of surveillance

System design characteristic	Case management	Outbreak detection and management	Programme planning and evaluation
Data sources	Case reports from clinicians, health care facilities, schools, or laboratories	Case reports; electronic health records; administrative healthcare data; highly specific lab data (e.g. PulseNet and other molecular methods); news reports; environmental and workplace monitoring for hazards and exposures; poison center records; sales of over-the-counter or prescription drugs; calls to nurse hot lines; population surveys; countermeasure producers and suppliers	All previous plus: repeated population-based surveys (e.g. Behavioral Risk Factor Surveillance System in the US); vital registration; Census data; social services data; public safety data; registries; periodic evaluation data collections from programme delivery sites
Collection method	Reports by mail, phone, fax, e-mail, web-site, electronic lab reporting (ELR); infection control practitioners and health care organizations	Case reports; direct electronic acquisition and web entry of records coded by ICD10-CM, chief complaint, or other early diagnostic information; ELR; supply of medical treatments	All; personal report; observation (e.g. seat belt use)
Collection frequency	Reported on a set interval after a case is identified at a reporting source (e.g. 24 hours or 1 week)	Case reports as they occur, or batch reporting on a frequent (e.g., daily) or continuous (real-time) basis	Extended periodic interval (e.g. annually)

Data processing	Limited (tabulation and sorting for case investigation and follow-up)	Automated steps for organizing and detecting aberrations	Extensive cleaning and updating of data
Statistical and epidemiologic analysis	Standard and simple measures of central tendency and time plots; direct action case by case; line lists and histograms	Complex analytic routines for pattern recognition; stratified analysis for risk groups; combination of data from mutiple sources; modeling for forecasting acute trends	Routine tables and more advanced modeling/projections (e.g. time series, complex stratified and cluster models)
Reporting and dissemination	Case managers (public health); clinicians; case reporters	Public health and medical practitioners at local, state, federal levels; emergency responders; business; news media; public	Programme managers; policy makers; news media; public

similar isolates and identify apparent time or space clustering among a multitude of cases.

Descriptive and analytic epidemiology

For example, calculations of rates by subgroups and time intervals, mapping of cases and rates, age adjustment, and calculation of relative risks) is useful in all surveillance activity, but especially in support of programme planning and evaluation.

Other data

Surveillance data, summaries, analyses, and recommendations should be *disseminated* regularly to suppliers of data, those with a need to know for clinical and public health purposes, and the general public.

Public health informatics

Public health informatics has been defined as 'the systematic application of information and computer science and technology to public health practice, research, and learning'.[3,4] Modern surveillance systems increasingly acquire electronic data and rsely on information and computer science to optimize the collection, storage, and use of these data. As more clinical records are computerized using standardized electronic health record, messages (e.g. HL-7) and vocabulary standards (e.g. LOINC and SnoMED), rapid and complete transfer of such data into surveillance systems is becoming more feasible. Informatics expertise should be engaged early in the design of surveillance systems. More general information on public health informatics is available in 📖 Chapter 2.1.

Evaluating a surveillance system

Surveillance systems should be evaluated regularly and modified promptly as needed. Evaluations of all types of surveillance systems can be guided by the 'Updated guidelines for evaluating public health surveillance systems'.[1] Systems designed for outbreak detection have some specific characteristics that need attention during evaluation, as indicated in the 'Framework for evaluating public health surveillance systems for early detection of outbreaks'.[2] Evaluations should be undertaken in consultation with system stakeholders, to whom results should also be disseminated.

Table 2.8.1 shows performance attributes assessed in surveillance system evaluation that are likely to vary by purpose. Additional attributes that are common to all surveillance systems are also important. Acceptability—the willingness and authority of participants to contribute to data collection, analysis, and use—is important in all systems that require timely and high-quality data. Cost is always important, but thresholds for acceptable costs will differ based on the condition and on the purpose/use of the data. Ultimately, the performance of a surveillance system depends on whether it accomplishes its stated purpose. To the extent possible, usefulness should be assessed by whether prevention and control actions are taken as a result of analysis and interpretation of data from the system.

General principles for effective surveillance systems

The key contributions of public health professionals to establishing, running, and quality assurance of surveillance systems are to understand the strengths and limitations of the data for the intended purpose of the system and to analyse the data frequently so that utility and quality can be assured. The following principles should be diligently applied:

- Have clear objectives and design the system to meet those objectives.
- Collect only the data needed to meet the explicit objectives.
- Collect direct measures of the condition of interest (e.g. office visits for respiratory disease) before indirect markers (e.g. absenteeism, over-the-counter drug purchases).
- Value and build personal relationships, as well as laws, rules, and technology.
- Demonstrate the public health uses of the data to those who report them.
- In systems that depend on case reports, provide authoritative consultation to reporters, as this will increase reporting.
- Identify and remove barriers to rapid reporting of cases in systems built on case-reporting.
- Build redundancies to minimize the impact of temporary failure of a system.
- Analyse and interpret data by time, place, and person routinely and frequently.
- Integrate the analysis and interpretation of data across all the systems your organization manages.
- Convey confidence about the value of surveillance, epidemiology, and public health practice.

Further resources

Lee LM, Teutsch SM, Thacker SB, St Louis M. (eds) (2010). *Principles and practice of public health surveillance*, 3rd edn. Oxford University Press, New York.

References

1 Centers for Disease Control and Prevention (2001). Updated guidelines for evaluating public health surveillance systems: recommendations from the guidelines working group. *Morbidity and Mortality Weekly Report*, **50(RR-13),** 1–35. Available at: ℗ http://www.cdc.gov/mmwr/preview/mmwrhtml/rr5013a1.htm (accessed 21 June 2010).

2. Paquet C, Coulombier D, Kaiser R, Ciotti M. (2006). Epidemic Intelligence: A new framework for strengthening disease surveillance in Europe. *European Surveillance*, **11,** pii–665. Available at: ℗ http://www.eurosurveillance.org/ViewArticle.aspx?ArticleId=665 (accessed 21 June 2010).

3. Centers for Disease Control and Prevention. (2004). Framework for evaluating public health surveillance systems for early detection of outbreaks; recommendations from the CDC Working Group. *Morbidity and Mortality Weekly Report*, **53(RR-5),** 1–13. Available at: ℗ http://www.cdc.gov/mmwr/preview/mmwrhtml/rr5305a1.htm (accessed 21 June 2010).

4. O'Carroll PW, Yasnoff WA, Ward ME, Ripp LH, Martin EL. (eds) (2003). *Public health informatics and information systems*. Springer-Verlag, New York.

2.9 Investigating clusters

P.J. Saunders, A.J. Kibble, and A. Burls

Objectives

This chapter aims to describe the problems in investigating allegations of environmentally related disease clusters appropriately and effectively. We present recommendations to inform the local decision to investigate such allegations, and a structured approach to carrying out these studies.

Introduction

Community anxieties about the health effects of environmental contamination on public health have increased in recent years. This chapter describes methods conventionally used to investigate alleged clusters of disease, a number of contemporary methodological developments and makes recommendations for an effective public health response. There are over 30,000 chemicals in commercial use,[1] a historical legacy of contaminated sites in industrial regions; a pattern being repeated in developing countries.[2] Major chemical releases receive considerable publicity and several countries have formal mechanisms for the surveillance of, and response to, such events reducing their potential for public health impact.[3,4] However, much less is known about the effects of community exposure to low levels of chemicals. While a dramatic effect on public health is unlikely, the potential for exposure is real as is the toxicity of many chemicals involved and the genuine nature of the concerns of local populations.

Community suspicions about unusual diseases or levels of disease can be easily raised. A person with a disease may be looking for a cause and focus on a local environmental issue. This understandable reaction can readily lead to a campaign raising awareness and recruiting further cases which, of course, may be entirely unrelated. These campaigns can be extremely difficult to respond to effectively. Community concerns must be taken seriously and treated professionally. Not only could the campaign be right, but the fact that people are so animated to take action at least implies some degree of community and individual dissatisfaction with their quality of life.

While advances in statistical methods, data quality, and the power, and utility of Geographical Information Systems (GIS) have all facilitated the analysis of clusters[5] such studies are notoriously prone to error. Clusters of cases may occur purely by chance, and with few exceptions, there is actually little scientific or public health purpose to investigating in detail every individual disease cluster.[6] However, to concerned lay people these clusters can be remarkable and confirm their suspicions of a major health scare. Allaying these concerns without seeming to avoid the issue is a major challenge. Deciding whether to investigate is the first important step in a successful response.

Unless this is done rationally, investigations may be carried out unnecessarily or be refused inappropriately. Doing nothing is not an option. It is important that public health practitioners have the confidence to employ the correct method at the right time and the confidence and justification, when appropriate, not to conduct a study.

Given the importance of these responsibilities, a number of countries require these studies to be conducted. In the UK, for example, guidelines require the surveillance of both sources of environmental contamination and potentially environmentally related diseases.[7,8] In the US, the Center for Disease Control provides a centralized coordinated response service for cancer clusters.[9] Several agencies have produced guidance addressing some of these issues, but none specifically deals with all.[9–15] All these guidelines share some common themes, including the importance of treating complaints about unusual disease distribution with care and caution and generally endorsing an incremental approach, i.e. begin with relatively simple, but robust methods and only proceed to more sophisticated analyses if positive results are obtained that justify further study.

Before the investigation

Intelligence on potential sources of environmental contamination

There has been a significant shift in the approach of environmental law from one of response to an incident to one of prior control and approval. In many countries data on existing and historic sources of potential environmental contamination can be accessed through prior authorization of industries, local air quality review and assessment, chemical incident surveillance systems, inventories of contaminated land, and site emergency plans, etc. Such information can provide useful background information to any site-specific investigations (e.g. identifying potential environmental confounders) and can provide an indication of the sort of hazards existing and the appropriate resources necessary to respond to them.

Point of contact/responsible individual

There should ideally be a nominated individual acting as a first point of contact. This person must have appropriate training in dealing with the public and be supported by a system that ensures the recording and release of appropriate details. This can be achieved through the use of standardized pro forma which should be retained for audit purposes. The first contact should also be used to make an initial assessment of the level and direction of concern.

Review committee

A review committee should be developed to act as an expert forum for investigations. Access to an expert group to offer advice in difficult cases (perhaps even arbitration in disputes) is essential. Placing this responsibility outside the remit of any one particular agency will also lend validity to the decision and will incorporate some degree of both validation (important scientifically) and independence (important in dealing with the media and public) to the investigation.

Initial response (stage 1)

Reported health problem

When the agency is alerted to a community concern by individual member(s) of the public, it is important that as much relevant information as possible is obtained on first contact. This will enable an early assessment and ensure that the response is treated professionally. The symptoms reported must be clearly and consistently documented, e.g. are people reporting the same type of symptoms, are conditions self-reported or clinically confirmed? Allegations from individuals do not necessarily mean that the whole community is worried about potential health effects of contamination. Self-appointed pressure groups do not necessarily represent the views of the community. Unfounded concern can lead to property blight and the wider community may actually want an agency to reassure others that there is no public health concern.

Plausibility

This stage requires assessing whether the reported relationship makes sense given what is known about biology and the mechanisms of health and disease, and the temporal and spatial relationships between the disease and the putative source. Is there any evidence that the alleged exposure will result in the effect reported? There is little point initiating a study if the pollutant under investigation cannot cause the effect reported. However, for most diseases, environmental risk factors are poorly understood and in many cases the concerns will be about disease(s) in general rather than specific disease/exposure linkages. For many diseases, there is a latency period between the point of first exposure and the development of clinical disease. For some cancers this could be decades. Therefore, the address on diagnosis is not necessarily the address at the time of exposure and the investigator must decide whether the effect reported is plausible in terms of the likely period and extent of exposure. Some basic assessment of the geographic relationship between cases and alleged source can also be made at this stage of the investigative process.

Exposure verification

There is a range of information sources (see 📖 Stage 2), which can be assessed for any evidence of a real or potential exposure. A preliminary investigation of the putative source can reveal whether it has been the subject of previous complaints, regulatory action, or could be the source of relevant environmental pollution. However, such a judgment can be extremely difficult to make, e.g. reported symptoms will often be generalized and may not provide any meaningful information on the plausibility of chemical exposure. It is important to establish the number, characteristics, distribution, and timing of complainants. Further assessment of the source is not warranted at this stage.

Environmental hazard

The existence of viable source–pathway–receptor relationships should be considered. Each component needs to be identified and evaluated in order to assess risk. A toxic substance has to be present and there has to be a viable exposure pathway(s) to a target or receptor. If no pathway exists, the contamination may well be a hazard (i.e. there could be an intrinsic toxicity), but it will not present a risk (i.e. the chemical cannot come into contact with a vulnerable target). This is particularly important where specific chemical/disease relationships are being alleged. Again the issue of biological and temporal plausibility will need to be considered when examining any viable source–pathway–receptor relationships.

Apparent excess of cases

If the plausibility criteria are met it may be possible at this stage to ascertain whether the number of cases reported is excessive. For example, region-wide rates of various diseases can be used as an initial screening tool.

Scoping review

At this early stage an initial scoping literature search will provide useful background information on the nature of the process, toxicologic mechanisms, biologic plausibility, and the volume and quality of the literature, and help refine the potential research question.

The decision to continue

By now it should be possible to make some initial judgments. If the referral is clearly unfounded or even malicious in nature then it would be appropriate to stop any further investigation and document the concern for future reference. If a health-based or environmental standard has been exceeded at the site of interest, the appropriate industry regulator should take action. In the case of no apparent disease excess and no environmental standard being exceeded, the investigation should stop. If there is an apparent excess of cases (as reported by the complainant) and a plausible link with an environmental hazard then it would be appropriate to move to stage 2. However, in many cases there will be few, if any, environmental data available. In these cases, if the type of site means that contamination was, or is, feasible then the investigation should proceed to stage 2 particularly if there are concerns that the alleged exposures occurred some time ago. If there is no possibility of prior exposure and data indicate that there is no relevant environmental contamination, the investigation can stop. For example, there would be little need to continue if the only possible source/hazard is a landfill site known to contain inert materials. In this case, the investigator should stop and report back to the community. In the event of no plausible exposure, but a potential excess of disease, the issue should be considered by the agency and, if necessary, referred to the review committee.

Verification of cases and potential excess (stage 2)

Introduction

The aim of this stage is to determine whether a detailed environmental and epidemiological assessment is justified. Appropriate spatial and temporal boundaries should be developed. This will require consideration of factors including meteorological conditions, operational conditions, emissions, land use change, possible period of exposure, and latency period.

Detailed environmental monitoring or modelling is not required at this stage, but the investigator should obtain sufficient information to decide whether the source of the contamination is biologically, spatially, and temporally plausible given the health problems reported. Wherever possible, multisite studies should be considered.

Verification of cases

Case details including any evidence of exposure should be obtained and diagnoses confirmed. The latter may need the input of primary care, hospital departments, and routine data sources such as cancer registration systems.

This is particularly important when dealing with investigations carried out by pressure groups or concerned individuals that purport to show an excess of disease. An active surveillance system for potentially environmentally related diseases would provide valuable *a priori* intelligence.

Literature review refined

The literature search should now be refined and papers obtained at this stage. This should be carried out in a systematic way focusing on the peer-reviewed literature, but should also include good quality grey literature if possible. The review committee should be able to provide support.

Test for excess cases

An observed/expected (O/E) analysis using a suitable reference population is appropriate at this stage. The simplest method of analysis is to choose a study area and compare the observed number of cases in that area with the number of cases that would be expected if the area had the same incidence rate as a larger reference area or population. This analysis, while relatively simple, still requires good quality data and there are methodological issues that need to be considered when interpreting the results. Two methods are commonly used—indirect and direct standardization—although indirect has become the standard methodology.

An O/E comparison might show differences. However, if the prevalence of the condition is related to age or deprivation, an increase in disease levels could be due to large numbers of elderly or poor people in that population. Analysis should take account of such factors as age and gender, and where necessary other factors which may (but not always) need controlling, for example deprivation. It is important to recognize the risk of over-adjustment for social class (any association with environmental factors may be 'adjusted away', since deprived people also are typically more exposed to environmental hazards). A clear explanation of the computation of the expected number is given in a number of reference works.[16]

Another potentially useful method is the statistical control chart which will identify those areas with levels of disease outside of expected variability. This method has been used for decades as a quality control tool in industry and has increasingly been applied to public health research.[17]

Problems and limitations

People living in areas in the vicinity of a source of pollution (e.g. a factory) can identify themselves as being under risk and it may often be tempting to initiate studies in order to clarify the cause of these apparent risks. By their very nature, these studies are *post hoc* since they were prompted by complaints of apparent 'clusters' of ill-health. *Post hoc* hypotheses may lead to bias by focusing on narrow time bands and specific areas where an excess risk has been observed. Other potential weaknesses with this type of analysis include small numbers, multiple testing, inadequate control for confounders, and, almost invariably, absence of exposure measures.[6,18,19] Advice on methodological issues is available from a number of sources.[9,10,13,19–24] If an association is suggested, the investigation can move to stage 3, otherwise stop, document, and report back to the community.

Environmental and exposure assessment (stage 3)

Monitoring and analysis

Ideally it is important to have some direct measurement of exposure, but this can often be extremely difficult.[25] This can present a major issue as a good measure of exposure is a key requirement for drawing conclusions of causality from epidemiological investigations of health outcome. Studies of disease clusters typically involve poor or missing exposure measures.

If the population under consideration is currently being exposed, then biological monitoring may be helpful in establishing exposure or estimating dose levels. Biomarkers can help demonstrate that exposure has occurred and can be used to identify exposed populations for investigation, e.g. urinary thioether assays can be used as biomarkers for chemicals such as polycyclic aromatic hydrocarbons. Biomarkers can also provide an estimate of past exposure providing the pollutant under investigation has a long half-life in the body and is relatively easy to detect (e.g. dioxins).

In the absence of biological measurements or personal air monitoring, exposure has to be indirectly estimated through some other method. Typically these are through the use of proximity to the potential source as an indicator of exposure, environmental measurements such as ambient air monitoring or through the use of computer models such as atmospheric dispersion modelling.

The use of distance from the source is a common and easy to use approach. This approach assumes that exposure decreases with increasing distance from the source. However, the sole use of proximity as an indicator of exposure is wholly unreliable. It is an approach that makes no consideration of the influence of meteorological conditions or process characteristics such as stack height, efflux velocity, plume temperature, etc. Exposure zones may often be several kilometres beyond the site or point of release, introducing considerable exposure misclassification and possibilities for confounding co-exposures from other industries. It is inevitable that these zones will include a large degree of variability of exposure and may include people who are not exposed at all. This may dilute any effect that may be estimated and might result in a true greater effect downwind of the point source being missed. Individuals will also move within and outside these zones and many people will not reside within the zone for most of the day (work, school, etc.).

It is preferable to have some direct measurement of exposure. If an active industrial site is being investigated as a source, emission data may provide an indirect measure of exposure and can be extremely useful in identifying the pollutants emitted. Such data will be readily available as industrial releases are required to meet mandatory limits. However, they are of limited value in terms of a direct measure of exposure since most point sources will release pollutants at a considerable height above ground level.

Many countries have ambient air monitoring networks such as the Automatic Urban and Rural Air Quality Monitoring Network (AURN) in the UK. Such networks can provide useful data on background levels of air pollution and 'hotspot' monitoring at urban roadsides and, occasionally, around point sources. However, many monitoring sites may not be located near the area or source under investigation or do not measure the specific pollutants of concern. As a result it may be necessary to commission environmental monitoring to help identify exposed communities. For example, analysis of soil and vegetation down-wind of a point source can often prove to be a good indication of exposure. Following the release of a large quantity of dioxin from an accident at a pesticide plant in Seveso, Italy, the extent and level of dioxin contamination in soil in the prevailing wind direction was used to identify the most exposed populations.[26] Subsequent analysis of dioxin levels in the plasma of people from these affected areas showed that body burden was closely correlated with levels of environmental contamination.

If monitoring reveals that if the concentrations of pollutants are below a recognized standard, the nature of the investigation should be reconsidered. This does not necessarily mean it should be stopped, as many standards are relatively old or under review, and there are very few chemicals which have actually been evaluated for their health risk. A toxicologic input will be particularly important in the interpretation of the environmental data.

Another approach is to use computer models to predict exposure. Advances in environmental modelling have produced models that can be very helpful in estimating exposure. Air dispersion models are a widely accepted method for regulating emissions to atmosphere from major industry and many commercially available models can predict the worst case ground-level concentration over the short and long-term around industrial sources including concentrations within the nearest area of housing. However, the accuracy of any model is heavily dependent on the quality of the input data which can often be poor or not directly applicable to the case under investigation.

Most studies tend to use a combination of proximity and environmental measurements. In a review of 45 epidemiological studies of air pollution around point and non-point sources, 29% determined exposure solely on proximity measures and most used a combination of proximity and environmental measurements.[27]

Whilst it is important to obtain as much accurate information on potential exposure, poor quality monitoring and modeling can be equally as damaging. A site visit can be helpful to confirm details of potential sources and confirm the plausibility of an exposure pathway. Detailed exposure assessment should not be undertaken unless the health concerns are properly defined and there is some element of biological plausibility. Any monitoring or modelling must focus on compounds that could produce the effects under investigation. Poor quality data can raise expectations in the local community and may incur unnecessary costs.

The decision to continue

If there is evidence of a potentially significant chemical exposure (chemical, level, pathway, spatial, and temporal plausibility) and the health effect is plausible, proceed to stage 4. Otherwise consider referral to the review committee or stop and document.

Epidemiological assessment (stage 4)

Boundaries

It is useful to engage the concerned community in confirming the most appropriate spatial and temporal boundaries. This can help engender a real sense of being involved in the design of the study. It can also provide the researchers with pre-defined boundaries. The areas of concern may not necessarily reflect the realities of exposure assessment. The investigators should consider how meteorological, operational, and technical factors may affect exposure and whether additional environmental sampling and modelling may be necessary to refine the area of exposure. The area of interest may also be manipulated to assess whether there is a risk with proximity, e.g. examining areas at different distances from a putative source.

Identifying all cases within the spatial and temporal boundaries

Appropriate case finding techniques should be employed. If the study is relying on routine data sets, the investigators must assure themselves of the data quality and be aware of the limitations of each data source used.

This may have significance in determining the spatial boundaries of the study, e.g. cancer registration may only be available for a specific period.

Agree an appropriate method

If there are no resources available, such as academic units, to assist in developing an appropriate method the review committee should provide advice. At its simplest this may be a refinement of the O/E analysis performed in stage 2 and/or the use of a dispersal model to identify exposed populations more accurately. It may be more appropriate to use a more sophisticated analysis such as Bayesian mapping or link the study to a larger multisite study. A number of new innovative methods are being developed and deployed such as kernel density contouring[28] and methods that account for residential history.[29,30] If this stage still shows an apparent excess of disease the issue should be referred to the review committee to assess the quality of the study and to determine the need and method for more sophisticated epidemiological or other research studies. Biomarkers of exposure may also be considered appropriate in some circumstances.

Communication strategy

The statutory agencies should seek the involvement of the affected or concerned communities. It is not enough to simply make information available for use by the public. When conducting investigations, involving the community must be an integral part of the process and should be planned for. Worry and concern can lead to stress or anxiety which can exacerbate existing conditions or result in an increase in the reporting of symptoms including those which do not have a toxicologic basis. Openness with the community can alleviate community and individual concerns and help generate a more positive working relationship with the community. If the result of the study shows no significant excess of disease, this information needs to be communicated effectively. Guidance is available from a number of sources including the Department of Health[31] and the ATSDR.[32]

References

1 Royal Commission on Environmental Pollution. (2003). *Chemicals in products: safeguarding the environment and human health*, 24th Report of the Royal Commission on Environmental Pollution., Royal Commission on Environmental Pollution, London.

2 World Health Organization Sustainable Development and Healthy Environments. (1999). *Environmental health indicators: framework and methodologies*, Protection of the Human Environment Occupational and Environmental Health Series. WHO, Geneva.

3 Agency for Toxic Substances and Disease Registry. (2010). National Toxic substances Incidents Program (NTSIP). Document on Internet. ✆ http://www.atsdr.cdc.gov/ntsip/index.html (accessed 17th August 2010).

4 Health Protection Agency. (2005). Chemical Incidents in England and Wales. HPA, Chilton.

5 Elliott P, Wartenberg D. (2004). Spatial epidemiology: Current approaches and future challenges. *Environmental Health Perspectives*, **112**, 998–1006.

6 Rothman KJ. (1990). A sobering start for the cluster busters' conference. *American Journal of Epidemiology*, **132(Suppl.1)**, S6–13.

7 NHS Management Executive. (1993). *Health Service Guidelines HSG(93)38: arrangements to deal with health aspects of chemical contamination incidents*. Department of Health, Health Aspects of the Environment and Food Division, London.

8 NHS Management Executive. (1993). *Health Service Guidelines HSG(93)56: Public health responsibilities of the NHS and the roles of others*. Department of Health, Health Aspects of the Environment and Food Division, London.

9 Alexander FE, Cuzick J. (1996). Methods for the assessment of disease clusters. In: Eliott P, Cuzick J, English D, Stern R, eds, *Geographical and environmental epidemiology methods for small-area studies*, pp. 238–50. Oxford University Press, Oxford.

10 Alexander FE, Boyle P. (1996). *Methods for investigating localized clustering of disease*, IARC Scientific Publication No. 135. International Agency for Research on Cancer, Lyon.

11 Centers for Disease Control. (1990). Guidelines for investigating clusters of health events. *Morbidity and Mortality Weekly Report.* **39**(RR-11): 1–23.

12 Department of Health. (2000). *Good practice guidelines for investigating the health impact of local industrial emissions*. Department of Health, London.

13 Leukaemia Research Fund. (1997). *Handbook and guide to the investigation of clusters of disease*. Leukaemia Research Fund Centre for Clinical Epidemiology, University of Leeds, Leeds.

14 Rothenberg RB, Thacker SB. (1996). Guidelines for the investigation of clusters of adverse health events. In: Eliott P, Cuzick J, English D, Stern R, eds, *Geographical and environmental epidemiology methods for small-area studies*, pp. 264–77. Oxford University Press, Oxford.

15 Kingsley BS, Schmeichel KL, Rubin CH. (2007). An update on cancer cluster activities at the Centers for Disease Control and Prevention. *Environmental Health Perspectives*, **115**, 165–71.

16 Kirkwood BR. (2003). *Measures of mortality and morbidity. Essentials of medical statistics*, 2nd edn. Blackwell Scientific Publications, Oxford.

17 Mohammed MA. (2004). Using statistical process control to improve the quality of health care. *Quality Safe Health Care*, **13**, 243–5.

18 Neutra R, Swan S, Mack T. (1992). Clusters galore: insights about environmental clusters from probability theory. *Science and Total Environment*, **127**, 187–200.

19 Urquhart J. (1996). Studies of disease clustering: problems of interpretation. In: Eliott P, Cuzick J, English D, Stern R, eds, *Geographical and environmental epidemiology methods for small-area studies*, pp. 278–85. Oxford University Press, Oxford.

20 Elliott P, Wakefield JC, Best NG, Briggs BJ. (2000). *Spatial epidemiology—methods and applications*. Oxford University Press, Oxford.

21 Hills M. (1996). Some comments on methods for investigating disease risk around a point source. In: Eliott P, Cuzick J, English D, Stern R, eds, *Geographical and environmental epidemiology methods for small-area studies*, pp. 231–7. Oxford University Press, Oxford.

22 McNally RJ, Alexander FE, Vincent TJ, Murphy MF. (2009). Spatial clustering of childhood cancer in Great Britain during the period 1969–1993.*International Journal of Cancer*, **124**, 932–6.

23 Catelan D, Biggeri A. (2008). A statistical approach to rank multiple priorities in environmental epidemiology: an example from high-risk areas in Sardinia, Italy. *Geospatial Health*. **3**, 81–9.

24 Cook AJ, Gold DR, Li Y. (2007). Spatial cluster detection for censored outcome data. *Biometrics*. **63(2)**, 540–9.

25 Kibble A, Harrison R. (2005). Point sources of air pollution. *Occupational Medicine*, **55**, 425–31.

26 Bertazzi PA, Consonni D, Bachetti S, *et al.* (2001). health effects of dioxin exposure: a 20-year mortality study. *American Journal of Epidemiology*, **153**, 1031–44.

27 Huang YL, Batterman S. (2000). Residence location as a measure of environmental exposure: a review of air pollution epidemiology studies. *Journal of Exposure and Analytic Environmental Epidemiology*, **10**, 66–85.

28 James L, Matthews I, Nix B. (2004). Spatial contouring of risk: a tool for environmental epidemiology. *Epidemiology*. **15**, 287–92.

29 Cook AJ, Gold DR, Li Y. (2009). Spatial cluster detection for repeatedly measured outcomes while accounting for residential history. *Biometrical Journal*. **51**, 801–18.

30 Vieira V, Webster T, Weinberg J, Aschengrau A. (2009). Spatial analysis of bladder, kidney, and pancreatic cancer on upper Cape Cod: an application of generalized additive models to case-control data. *Environmental Health: A Global Access Science Source*, **8**, 3.

31 Department of Health. (1997). *Communicating about risks to public health pointers to good practice*. EOR Division, Department of Health, London.

32 Agency for Toxic Substances and Disease Registry. A primer on health risk communication principles and practices. Document on Internet. ℘ http://www.atsdr.cdc.gov/HEC/primer.html (accessed 17th August 2010).

2.10 Health trends: registers

Jem Rashbass and John Newton

Objectives

The objectives of this chapter are to enable you to:
- understand disease registers in general
- understand cancer registries in particular
- use them efficiently
- be aware of the traps for the unwary
- appreciate the future of disease registers.

Introduction

A disease register is a file of data on all cases of a particular disease or health condition, limited to a defined population. There is a wide range of registries each focused on specific health issues. One recent count in England identified around 250 specific disease registers.[1]

This chapter aims to provide:
- a brief overview of registers and how to get best use of them
- a more detailed account of one of the most comprehensive: the cancer registries.

Registries (the organizations that support registers) arrange systems to collect, collate, and quality assure data on new cases of the condition of interest; they may also collect follow-up (longitudinal) data on identified cases. The resulting records are intended to be permanent, and the data are periodically analysed, tabulated, and reported.

Epidemiological registers can be based on:
- disease, e.g. cancer, psychiatric illness, coronary heart disease, and diabetes
- risk factors, e.g. specific exposures (for example radiation industry workers or genetic factors, including twin status)
- interventions or treatments, for example cochlear implants or renal transplants.

Registers can also be oriented toward service provision rather than epidemiology, but can nevertheless be useful for public health purposes. For example, 'at risk' registers for children might be used to ensure adequate protection for such children, and registers of disabled people run by local authorities have a similar purpose. Communicable disease notification provides an analogous function. However, registers of patients seen or treated in a particular hospital or clinical setting, that are not population based, can be difficult to use for general epidemiological purposes. They may be used as a source of cases for case–control studies[2]—although selection biases are common. In general, clinical databases that are not population-based are more useful for technology assessment and quality improvement than for epidemiological purposes.

The data collected by registries vary widely, but often include personal identifiers, socio-demographic information, disease status (possibly including stage and severity), details of treatments and other interventions, and eventual outcomes.

A registry must establish systems to:

- maintain a reliable notification or identification of cases within the studied population
- ensure comparability of inclusion criteria onto the register: for a diagnosis, strict rules are needed to identify the studied condition, within an agreed classification
- minimize under-coverage—cases not being included when they should be
- ensure that duplication of cases within the register does not occur
- keep the register updated—removing those who have recovered, died, or moved out of the area.

Most registers require patient consent to collect and hold the data. However, in the UK, legislation has allowed cancer registries (and some others) to collect identifiable patient information without prior informed consent (Section 251, NHS Act 2006)—this important caveat is currently subject to annual review by the National Information Governance Board (NIGB) in England and Wales. Any research use of the registry data can only occur with the appropriate ethical approval, especially if identifiable data are held or shared with outside researchers.

Maintaining a register is time and labour intensive and can be expensive. Maintaining motivation and interest is essential and often depends on the person organizing the register. Registers tend to get out of date quickly, and a rigorous process of quality assurance must be in place if the data are to be of high quality.

Many registries are likely to change significantly as health records become electronic and patients can be identified with minimal ambiguity with a unique identifier (for example the UK NHS number). Electronic records improve data accessibility and timeliness, while the unique identifier facilitates linkage to other data sets. Electronic data are not necessarily more accurate than paper records, and may conceal other errors, but they are easier to collect. It pays to remain skeptical of data quality and look for evidence of validity.

How can registers help?

If case ascertainment is high, prevalence, and incidence rates can be computed. Analysis of risks and etiology can be explored, using individual as well as area characteristics. With follow-up data, outcomes can be measured, e.g. survival rates for cancer. If registers are maintained over time they can produce evidence of change in, for example, epidemics or in the effectiveness of interventions.

Registers can be used to assist in the management of chronic disease in clinical settings, triggering follow-up care for people with, for example, diabetes or asthma within a primary care practice. Registers can also form the basis for clinical audit and quality improvement efforts.

An example of a disease register: a cancer registry

The cancer registration system is a unique world-wide resource, there being regional cancer registries covering between 1 and 15 million people in most countries in the world. Each registry is essentially a detailed list of all the cancers that have occurred since each registry was established (e.g. in the UK this was usually around 1970).

Cancer registries in Europe work together through the European Network of Cancer Registries. World-wide, the International Association of Cancer Registries coordinates registry activities. The entire population is covered in the UK and Republic of Ireland, Scandinavia, The Netherlands and Germany (from 1999), Canada and nearly so in the USA. Registries in other countries have complete coverage for subpopulations. Others are hospital based. International details can be found in *Cancer Incidence in Five Continents*.[3]

Important features

Three important features of cancer registries should be remembered:
- Cancer registries contain details of *diagnosed* cancers: they cannot tell you about cancers that we take to our grave without diagnosis
- The record starts at diagnosis and collects details of the patient and the tumour (stage and grade) at that time: there is increasingly information on treatment in the first 6 months
- Most are population based: they provide a denominator for numbers of tumours in relation to the population of which the patients were members.

What is on the register?

Registries differ very slightly, but the minimum content is nationally defined. In the UK, for example, the registry includes details of:
- *The patient:* name, address, postcode, date of birth, sex, their doctors, NHS number.
- *The tumour:* site, histological type, and possibly grade and stage at diagnosis (how advanced the tumour is).
- *Date of diagnosis.*
- *Treatment:* during the first 6 months after date of diagnosis and cause of death.

Many registries will keep extra data on each patient and tumour, and there will be links between multiple tumours in the same patient. The NHS number allows linkage to other datasets where a patient is identified by their NHS number.

In the UK the Office for National Statistics compiles mortality statistics which refer to date of death and residence at death. Survival data refer to place and date of diagnosis.

What the data can be used for?

For each type of tumour and type of patient, it is possible to analyze:

- *Incidence:* of cancer, and trends in incidence. These can be used to make projections in demand and to help judge the effectiveness of preventive strategies. Given the knowledge of the population size, migration, and all-cause mortality, projections of incidence are fairly reliable for up to 10 years.
- *Survival:* of people with cancer, and trends in survival. Trends in survival can be used to make projections and to help judge the effectiveness of treatment.
- *Linkage analysis:* since all cancer registry data now contain a unique patient identifier, the NHS number, records can be linked to any other data set that uses this identifier. For example, hospital episode statistics (HES) data from the UK Department of Health can be used to track in-patient events for patients diagnosed with cancer. In the future, it will be possible to link to any data held within the complete health record (for example, medication, co-morbidities, lifestyle).

Using cancer registry data

All registries produce routine reports, usually on incidence and survival, so if your enquiry is simple just take the report off the shelf. If the enquiry is more complex, or if you are not quite sure what you need, the registry will advise you. However, there are some questions you will always be asked, so you must know:

- *Which cancers you are interested in:* cancers are classified by site (lung, brain, rectum, etc.) and type (adenocarcinoma, teratoma, etc.).
- *Which people you are interested in:* by age, or date of birth, year or age band, e.g. 35–40, or born between 1920 and 1930, sex, area of residence (in the UK usually health district, but any combination of postcodes can be used, but must be in the region covered by the registry).
- The year of diagnosis.

Most registries are willing to provide data from which individuals cannot be identified although there are issues around even anonymous data which may be 'disclosive' if the population is small or the tumour relatively rare in the age group. If individuals need to be identified or the data are potentially disclosive then release will depend on other factors, mainly related to ethical and confidentiality issues. These are spelt out in the UK Association of Cancer Registries Policy Document[4] whose procedures are similar to those established by the International Association of Cancer Registries. To summarize, you can have named data if you are the patient or the patient's doctor, or you want the data for the benefit of the patient or the direct benefit of others or for audit. For genetic counselling you need the consent of living relations, and for research you need research ethics committee permission.

Analysing the data

Before you obtain the data, you must have a reasonably detailed idea of what you intend to do with them. Essentially, as with any investigation of this kind, the analytical skills you need are epidemiological and statistical, but it pays to be quite clear which problems you are trying to solve, and whether the questions you ask will do it. All registries employ statisticians or epidemiologists, and part of their job is to advise on the use and the limitations of the data.

The limitations of the data

Cancer registries are the main source of epidemiological information on cancer, although there are limits to the information they can provide. They will *not* tell you:

- *About cancer more than 35 years ago (at least for the whole of the UK)*: before that, you have to rely on mortality information; other countries are similar though many have been started more recently.
- *About hospital activity*; they will tell you about patients resident in that region, but patients from outside the registry region will be entered on their home registry, and patients from outside the UK probably will fall through the net.
- *About patients diagnosed within the last year*: registries cannot provide survival data for a period longer than the time since diagnosis, e.g. 5-year survival in patients diagnosed the previous year. Actually, approximations and projections can be made, but they are not particularly accurate.
- *What has happened between 6 months after diagnosis and death*: unless there is active follow-up, some deaths may be missed—this also applies to local recurrence and prolonged treatment.

Myths and shortcomings

Data collection takes time, especially when it is manual, and therefore registers are unlikely to have a complete up-to-date collection of data. Cancer registries usually have complete data that are about six months to a year old, while the UK Office of National Statistics publish the data after 18 months. With the increase in electronic data feeds to registries data are being collected more rapidly and statistics are being released on-line more quickly. The data are never entirely complete because occasional data may appear many years after diagnosis.

A register is only as good as the data that are available to it. Remember, electronic data are no more accurate than paper data—but they may be easier to obtain and simpler to import into the register and therefore avoid some of the human errors that occur during data entry. If the diagnosis or the death certificate is wrong then even a complete data set will be flawed. Be skeptical and question all your data sources—even registers!

Further resources

International Association on Research on Cancer. *Epidemiology database* ℘ http://www-dep.iarc. fr/ (accessed 25 January 2010).

Cancer Research UK. *Statistics. Cancer facts and figures.* Available at: ℘ http: info.cancerresearchuk. org/cancerstats/ (accessed 25 January 2010).

National Statistics, UK. *Cancer.* Available at: ℘ http:www.statistics.gov.uk/CCI/nscl.asp?id=6279 (accessed 25 January 2010).

National Cancer Institute (USA). *SEER (surveillance, epidemiology and end results).* ℘ http://seer. cancer.gov (accessed 25 January 2010).

References

1 Newton J, Garner S. (2002). *Disease registers in England. Report for the Department of Health policy research programme.* Available at: ℘ www.erpho.org.uk/viewResource.aspx?id=12531 (accessed 21 January 2006).

2 Black N, Barker M, Payne M. (2004). Cross sectional survey of multi-centre clinical database in the United Kingdom. *British Medical Journal,* **328,** 1478–81.

3 Parkin DM, Whelan SL, Ferlay J, Teppo L, Thomas DB. (2003). *Cancer incidence in five continents,* Vol. VIII. IARC, Lyon.

4 UK Association of Cancer Registries. *Guidelines on the release of confidential data.* Available at: http://www.ukacr.org/confidentiality/ (accessed 3 September 2012).

Part 3

Direct action

3.1 Communicable disease epidemics

Sarah O'Brien

Objectives

After reading this chapter you should be able to:
- define the terms 'communicable disease', 'epidemic', and 'outbreak'
- explain the principles of preventing communicable disease
- explain the key features of different types of outbreaks or epidemics
- understand the key steps in investigating an outbreak or epidemic.

Definitions

A *communicable (or infectious) disease* is an illness due to the transmission of a specific infectious agent (or its toxic products) from an infected person, animal or inanimate source to a susceptible host, either directly or indirectly.[1]

A commonly used definition of an *epidemic* is that of Abram Benenson, who defined it as 'the occurrence in a community or region of cases of illness (or an outbreak) with a frequency clearly in excess of normal expectancy'. The meaning of the term epidemic is broad. It encompasses both communicable diseases, e.g. meningitis, and non-communicable diseases, e.g. obesity. In this chapter, however, we will concentrate on communicable diseases. The numbers of cases, geographic extent, and time period need to be specified to be able to describe an epidemic.

The term *outbreak* is often used to describe any of the following:
- *Two or more related (i.e. epidemiologically-linked) cases of a similar disease:* acute food poisoning after a wedding breakfast may present like this.
- *An increase in the observed incidence of cases over the expected incidence within a given time period:* this way of detecting outbreaks, through routine surveillance, implies a less acute onset but, paradoxically, may be more serious than the previous example. This is because the problem was detected later, there is no immediate indication as to source and many more cases may be pending.
- *A single case of a serious disease:* a single case of botulism or smallpox constitutes a public health emergency and should trigger a very detailed investigation.

Why does preventing epidemics matter?

Severe acute respiratory syndrome (SARS), the first new severe disease of the 21st century, reminded us that new diseases emerge in human/micro-organism interactions. Similarly, old diseases, like tuberculosis, re-emerge, this time with antimicrobial resistance. People's susceptibility and/or exposure to micro-organisms also changes so that communicable diseases pose a constant threat to global security either naturally or, potentially, through bioterrorism.

Communicable diseases lead to around 14.7 million deaths worldwide (26% of global mortality) (Table 3.1.1). Furthermore, they cause approximately 26% of cancers in the developing world and 8% of cancers in the industrialized world (Table 3.1.2).[2] So reducing mortality and morbidity means tackling these preventable infections.

Table 3.1.1 WHO estimates of global mortality from infectious diseases, 2001

Infectious disease	Deaths (millions)
Respiratory infections	3.9
Acquired immunodeficiency syndrome	2.9
Diarrhoeal disease	1.9
Malaria	1.1

Adapted from Kindhauser.[2]

Table 3.1.2 Selected infection/cancer combinations

Infectious agent	Cancer	% of cancers due to infection	No. of cases globally/yr
Helicobacter pylori	Gastric cancer	30	603,000
	MALT lymphoma	100	
Human papilloma virus	Cervix	100	490,000
Hepatitis B virus	Liver	50	340,000
Hepatitis C virus	Liver	25	195,000

Source: Infections and Cancer—an overview. Cancer Research UK, London. Available at: ℘ http://info.cancerresearchuk.org/cancerstats/causes/infectiousagents/virusesandcancer/#burden (accessed 31 August 2010).

How can we prevent epidemics?

Classically, prevention is described as primary, secondary, or tertiary.

Primary prevention: preventing disease onset

In the context of communicable diseases various options include:

- *Eliminating the organism:*
  - controlling organisms in their natural reservoir, e.g. maintaining
  - *Brucella*-free cattle herds to prevent human brucellosis.
- *Environmental protection:*
  - ensuring a safe drinking water supply, with proper separation of sewage from drinking water (taken for granted in high and some middle income countries!)
  - safeguarding the food supply.
- *Interrupting the chain of transmission:*
  - controlling the insect vector for arthropod-borne diseases, e.g. West Nile Virus—emerging cause of encephalitis in North America
  - controlling the rodent vector for diseases like leptospirosis
  - modifying behaviour, e.g. practicing safe sex or avoiding injecting drug use, to prevent the spread of STDs and blood-borne viruses like hepatitis B, hepatitis C, and HIV
  - personal hygiene—a simple yet effective means of control.
- *Reducing susceptibility in the host:*
  - reversing malnutrition and micronutrient deficiency to boost people's immunity in low-income countries helps to prevent the spread of, for example, tuberculosis
  - vaccination—perhaps the most successful example of primary prevention, leading to global eradication of smallpox and to a sustained reduction in the incidence and consequences of childhood diseases. Childhood vaccination schedules vary by country, but an up-to-date list is posted on the WHO website at: ℅ http://www.who.int/vaccines/GlobalSummary/Immunization/ScheduleSelect.cfm (accessed 31 August 2010). This is very useful for assessing if children moving into the community from overseas are likely to have completed their courses of vaccinations.
- *Health education and community participation:*
  - promoting vector control programmes, in particular the use of personal protection like insect repellents and mosquito nets
  - supporting personal hygiene and food hygiene measures in preventing gastroenteritis
  - endorsing vaccination campaigns.

Secondary prevention: arresting the progression of established disease

The options here include:

- *Screening:* where there is an asymptomatic or pre-symptomatic period in the infection process screening programmes are useful.
- Outbreak/epidemic investigation.

The main aims of epidemic/outbreak investigation are to:
- identify the causative agent, route of transmission, and risk factors for the outbreak
- develop and implement control and prevention strategies and provide advice to prevent a similar event in the future.

Tertiary prevention: limiting the consequences of established disease

One example of this is providing artificial limbs for a child who has needed amputations following severe meningococcal septicaemia.

What are the key tasks?

Epidemic/outbreak investigation needs to be systematic, thorough, and rapid.

Conventionally, investigating and managing outbreaks/epidemics is divided into stages, although in practice these often run in parallel. The technical stages (Box 3.1.1) are as follows.

Box 3.1.1 Key elements of outbreak/epidemic investigation and management

- Establish that there really is an outbreak
- Confirm the diagnosis
- Create a case definition
- Find and count cases
- Draw an epidemic curve
- Determine who is at risk
- Generate and test hypotheses for exposure
- Consider what additional evidence is needed
- Implement control measures
- Write up your findings.

Establish that there really is an outbreak

Look at your local surveillance data and combine this with your local knowledge to help you determine whether or not an epidemic/outbreak is occurring. Consider artefactual reasons why an epidemic/outbreak might appear to have occurred, including:
- changes in reporting practice
- introduction of new microbiological methods
- increasing awareness of an infection in the community leading to increased reports
- a laboratory contamination incident.

Confirm the diagnosis

Arrange for appropriate specimens to be obtained and examined. The types of specimens needed depend upon the precise circumstances so seek the advice of an expert in microbiology. If nothing else, warn laboratory staff of an impending influx of specimens so that they can organize their work, prioritizing outbreak samples. Agree with laboratory staff how to identify outbreak-related samples. Since laboratory diagnosis takes time and must not delay investigations, look for a degree of commonality of symptoms to form a case definition.

Create a case definition

Construct a case definition comprising clinical criteria, which should be simple and objective, with limitations on time, place, and person. Sometimes you will need different levels of case definition—probable (patients with similar symptoms) and confirmed (where a laboratory diagnosis is added to the definition for a probable case).

Count cases (case finding)

Where an outbreak is focused on an event or discrete location (e.g. a hotel or hall of residence) contacting everyone who might have been exposed and finding out if they have symptoms is relatively easy. Where the extent of the outbreak is less well defined, trawl through laboratory returns or approach primary care physicians to find additional cases. Whatever method you choose, the case definition should be applied without bias. Typically, information is recorded in a questionnaire.

- *Personal demographic data:* name, address, date of birth, gender, and occupation.
- *Clinical details:* date of illness onset, a listing of symptoms so that the case can select those affecting them, duration of illness, days off work, and need for admission to hospital, outcome of illness.
- *Data items determined by the nature of the outbreak:* for example, travel history, immunization history, exposure to possible causal sources, such as food, water, recreational, environmental, places visited, shopping habits, contacts with ill people or animals all depending on circumstances.

Draw an epidemic curve

Plot the number of cases over time on a graph. By convention cases are represented as square boxes. The shape of the epidemic curve provides clues to the nature of the outbreak. A point-source epidemic curve, where exposure has been limited in time, usually shows a sharp upswing and a fairly rapid tail-off (Figure 3.1.1). A propagated, or continuing source, epidemic curve tends to be flatter in shape and continues over a much longer time (Figure 3.1.2). In an outbreak transmitted from person to person, epidemic waves can be seen. The epidemic curve should be updated on a daily basis. In an outbreak of Legionnaires' disease, plotting cases on a map can also yield helpful clues to potential sources of contamination.

Determine who is at risk

Sometimes this is obvious, e.g. a food poisoning outbreak at a wedding breakfast where those at risk are the guests. Also consider other people who might have dined at the same place, but not been part of the wedding party.

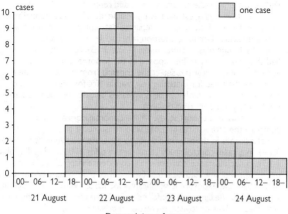

Figure 3.1.1 An example of a point source epidemic curve.

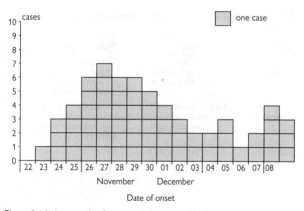

Figure 3.1.2 An example of a propagated source epidemic curve.

Generate and test hypotheses for exposure

Collate information about symptoms, circumstances, and diagnosis to form hypotheses about the cause of the outbreak, which can be tested using analytical epidemiology. Do not re-use the cases who were interviewed as part of the hypothesis-generation exercise. Decide on the appropriate study design. If the event is so well delineated that all those at risk, both ill and well, can be identified, then a cohort study is appropriate. If all those at risk cannot be delineated, e.g. where a general excess of disease is apparent in the community, but its origin is not, a case-control study is appropriate:

- *Data capture from the cohort, or cases and controls is usually using a standard structured questionnaire:* If possible, develop questionnaires on the Web to avoid the need for separate data entry, but ensure that data are secure. E-mailing questionnaires achieves rapid responses.
- *Control selection (case–control study) (Table 3.1.3):* controls must have had the opportunity to be exposed to the hypothesized source and, in a community outbreak, select the controls from that community. Consider the need for matching (e.g. within 10% for age), but avoid over-matching. Controls can be nominated by cases or recruited at random (e.g. random digit dialling).
- *Data analysis:* in a cohort study, where denominators are known, compare the attack rates in those who consumed a given food with the attack rate in those who did not to generate relative risks (Table 3.1.4). In a case–control study calculate the odds of becoming ill (Table 3.1.5). In each instance compute 95% confidence intervals (CIs) and use an appropriate statistical test (seek advice from a statistician). If more than one exposure is significantly associated with illness, look at strategies for dealing with confounding and potential interactions, e.g. stratified analysis or logistic regression modelling.

Alternative methods for analysis include case–case studies[3] and case cross-over studies.[4]

Table 3.1.3 Pros and cons of control selection in epidemic/outbreak investigations

Control type	Advantages	Disadvantages
Hospital or laboratory	Easy to access. Cases and controls comparable in terms of medical care	Patients may have other conditions that are associated with the disease of interest
Case-nominated	Easy to access. Useful for rare conditions. Participation rate usually good	Risk of over-matching—friends, relatives, or neighbours may share exposures with the cases
Community	Avoids bias inherent in using case-nominated controls	Method of recruitment may introduce new biases. Participation rate likely to be lower than with case-nominated controls

Consider what additional evidence is needed

Do you need additional laboratory tests, e.g. food, water, or environmental samples? What have investigations by your professional colleagues shown? For example, in a food poisoning outbreak, environmental health officers will collect important details, such as food preparation and storage practices, and carry out an inspection of the implicated premises. In an outbreak of Legionnaires' disease a specialist inspection by an environmental engineer may be needed. Combining information from epidemiological, environmental, and microbiological investigations means that you can develop a picture of what went wrong and why, and this will help you formulate both immediate control measures and measures to prevent a recurrence in the longer term.

Table 3.1.4 An example of how to present results from a single risk variable analysis in a retrospective cohort study

Variable	Category definitions	Ill	Not ill	Attack rate	Relative risk	95% CI for the relative risk	P value
Coleslaw	Yes	21	23	48	1.13	(0.62, 2.09)	0.89
	No	8	11	42			
	Missing	1	3				
Pasta salad	Yes	26	24	52	2.43	(0.86, 6.85)	0.08
	No	3	11	21			
	Missing	1	2				
Italian ciabatta and butter	Yes	16	14	53	1.39	(0.81, 2.40)	0.34
	No	13	21	38			
	Missing	1	2				
Lemon cheese-cake	Yes	9	11	45	0.92	(0.52, 1.64)	1.00
	No	20	21	49			
	Missing	1					
Strawberry gateau	Yes	13	17	43	0.92	(0.54, 1.58)	0.96
	No	16	18	47			
	Missing	1	2				
Orange juice	Yes	28	22	56	3.92	(1.06, 14.48)	0.01
	No	2	12	14			
	Missing	0	3				

Implement control measures

These can be initiated at any stage of the investigation, as soon as there is sufficient evidence to act upon. Seek specialist advice if necessary. The aims are to prevent new primary cases and secondary spread.

Table 3.1.5 An example of how to present results from a single risk variable analysis in a case–control study (in this instance the analysis was matched)

Variable	Exposed (%)		MOR*	95% CI		P Value
	Cases	Controls		Lower	Upper	
Cold food from take-away cafes	46 (58)	34 (26)	3.46	1.84	6.50	<0.001
Eat any eggs	56 (71)	67 (51)	2.41	1.26	4.61	0.006
Egg prepared away from home	35 (60)	14 (18)	25.74	3.24	204.55	<0.001
Any cold cows milk drunk	56 (71)	107 (81)	0.48	0.24	0.99	0.04
Sandwiches, rolls, etc., bought in plastic packs	47 (59)	26 (20)	4.34	2.33	8.07	<0.001
Ham sandwiches, etc.	10 (13)	5 (4)	3.68	1.12	12.07	0.02
Prawn/other seafood sandwiches, etc.	6 (8)	3 (2)	4.52	1.05	19.46	0.03
Egg mayonnaise sandwiches, etc.	13 (16)	1 (1)	18.11	2.33	140.51	0.0001

Note: the percentage of cases and controls exposed ignoring matching.
*Matched odds ratio.

Write up your findings
Keep contemporaneous (preferably hand-written) notes as you go along—this saves a lot of heartache in court later! At the end of the outbreak, write up your findings in an outbreak control team report. As well as being a record of what you did and what was found, lessons learned should be highlighted so that others may learn from what happened.

What skills and competencies are needed?

Public health professionals investigating outbreaks need expertise in the following areas:
• surveillance
• epidemiological study design
• statistics
• leadership
• management of programmes
• evaluation
• communication.

A sense of humour also helps! Remember that skills such as microbiology and environmental health are vested in other team members.

What is involved in getting something done?

Have an outbreak plan beforehand, exercise it regularly, and update it annually. It helps to know your colleagues before you come together in a crisis. Make sure that you can mobilize people to help 24 hr/day, set up an incident room, and access specialist advice.

Who else might need to be involved?

This depends to a certain extent on the nature of the outbreak/epidemic. For example, in an outbreak of food-borne disease the core team often comprises a public health practitioner with specialized training, an environmental health officer or sanitarian, a microbiologist, and a statistician. It might be appropriate to include a specialist food microbiologist, a clinician, and a veterinarian, depending on the exact circumstances. Assistance from a press officer usually proves invaluable.

Potential pitfalls

Probably the biggest potential pitfall is trying to run an investigation single-handed. Outbreak/epidemic investigation is genuinely a team effort. Do not rely on being able to conduct an investigation solely during office hours. By the time an outbreak comes to light, many of the cases may have recovered. This means that they are back at work during the daytime, just like you are! The best times to conduct interviews tend to be during the evening, up to 9.00 p.m., and at weekends, although make sure that you are aware of the major sporting fixtures—ringing people during a major cup final is unlikely to increase the response rate! Do not have more than one person speaking to the press. Agree at the outset who will do it, and stick to it. Finally, use your commonsense—a good descriptive study can provide better evidence than a poor analytic one!

Dogma, myths, and fallacies

It is sometimes said that there is no point in investigating point-source outbreaks because they are, by definition, over. However, you cannot know that an outbreak is over unless you have at least conducted a preliminary investigation. Requests for standard questionnaires are often made. Whilst it is true that certain elements, e.g. demographic and clinical details, rarely change—in reality there is no such thing as a standard outbreak. The danger is of being blinded by biological plausibility and, if taken to its logical conclusion, outbreaks of salmonellosis associated with contaminated lettuce or melons would never have been identified and controlled. Similarly, we would still be chasing contaminated hamburgers as the cause of outbreaks of *Escherichia coli* O157, ignoring transmission from the environment and animals. Standard questionnaires are not a substitute for thinking.

What are the key determinants of success?

These are skill, speed (including the ability to mobilize sufficient resources at very short notice), a pre-determined, tested plan, flexibility, and political clout.

How will you gauge success?

Continue to monitor the epidemic curve and routine surveillance data, which should show no new cases or a reduction in incidence.

Further resources

Connolly MA (ed.) (2005). *Communicable disease control in emergencies. A field manual*. World Health Organization, Geneva.

Giesecke J (2002). *Modern infectious disease epidemiology*, 2nd edn. Arnold, London.

Gregg MB (ed.) (2008). *Field epidemiology*, 3rd edn. Oxford University Press, Oxford.

Heymann DL (ed.) (2008). *Control of communicable diseases manual*, 19th edn. American Public Health Association, Washington DC.

Nelson KE, Williams CFM. (2006). *Infectious disease epidemiology: theory and practice*, 2nd edn. Jones and Bartlett Publishers, Sudbury.

References

1 Porta ℜ (ed.) (2008). *A dictionary of epidemiology*, 5th edn. Oxford University Press, Oxford.

2 Kindshauer MK (ed.) (2003). *Communicable diseases 2002—global defense against the infectious disease threat*, WHO/CDS/2003.15. World Health Organization, Geneva. Available at: ℜ http://www.who.int/infectious-disease-news/cds2002/intro.pdf (accessed 31 August 2010).

3 McCarthy N, Giesecke J. (1999). Case-case comparisons to study causation of common infectious diseases. *Int J Epidemiol*, **28:** 764–8.

4 Haegebaert S, Duche L, Desenclos JC. (2003). The use of the case-crossover design in a continuous common source food-borne outbreak. *Epidemiol Infect*, **131:** 809–13.

3.2 Environmental health risks

Roscoe Taylor and Charles Guest

Objectives

This chapter will help you to understand:
- environmental health in the rapidly changing context of health protection
- the usefulness of having a framework for environmental health risk assessment
- the process of identifying, evaluating, and planning a response to an environmental health threat.

Definitions

- *Environmental health* is concerned with all aspects of the natural and built environment that may affect human health, including physical, chemical, and biological factors. It encompasses the assessment and control of those factors, and is focused on preventing disease and creating health-supportive and sustainable environments. The occupational environment is generally excluded from consideration, but practitioners in both domains often share similar approaches.
- *Environmental health practitioners* may work in private, not-for-profit, government or academic sectors and operate at local (municipal), regional, or national and international levels, and be involved in a wide range of issues across many sectors.
- *Health protection* is the avoidance or reduction of potential harm from exposures through organized efforts, including direct action with individuals or communities, regulation, legislation, or other measures. Health protection may include environmental health services, food and water safety, communicable disease control, tobacco control, injury prevention, emergency planning and response, and other activities that aim to minimize preventable health risks. Health departments often organize public health governance along the lines of health protection, health promotion, and (depending on the jurisdiction) quality of care assurance.
- *Hazard* is the intrinsic capacity of an agent or mixture of agents that make it capable of causing adverse effects to organisms or the environment following exposure to that agent.
- *Exposure assessment* is the process of finding out how people come into contact with a hazardous agent, how often and for how long and

the amount with which they are in contact. Exposure pathways include inhalation, ingestion, or contact with the skin or eyes.

- *Dose* is the total amount of a substance or agent taken up by, or absorbed by an organism. Many processes including absorption, metabolism, storage, and excretion may affect the dose that ultimately reaches a target organ.
- *Dose–response* is the relationship between the dose of a substance and the resulting changes in body function or health (response).
- *Risk assessment* is the process of estimating the risk to individuals or populations resulting from a specific occurrence or use of an agent, including the identification of attendant uncertainties, and taking into account possible routes and duration of exposure. Where good information is available, risks may be quantifiable, but risk assessment is not an exact science. To be effective, qualitative information influencing the nature of health effects and concerns in the context of particular communities must also be taken into account.
- *Health impact assessment* utilizes risk assessment techniques in relation to development or policy proposals that may have consequences for environmental health. Increasingly, consideration of equity is being introduced into health impact assessment (see 📖 Chapter 1.5).

Why is this an important public health issue?

Risks to public health from environmental hazards are continually emerging, with impacts ranging from small-scale or local, to widespread exposures affecting whole populations.

Public health has its developmental roots in the identification and control of environmental health risks. 'Old' health protection issues, such as failures in sanitation, contamination of food or water supplies, and air pollution episodes continue to re-emerge, and new threats are evolving from our changing environments and patterns of human usage.

Environmental health practitioners must identify environmental hazards and understand how to predict, prevent, monitor, and respond to the threats that they present. Enforcement of statutory provisions (often through environment agencies) remains an important tool, but the emphasis now on prevention requires a broad range of strategies, including advocacy, intersectoral collaboration, and community development models in addition to development of policy, standards, and guidelines.

Environmental health practice at the grassroots level—such as the work carried out by local governments to ensure the safety of food and water—forms part of the bedrock of public health protection.

Public health practitioners understand that healthy environments, including healthy social and economic conditions, are needed to improve the health of the population. Effectively implementing systemic changes to reduce hazards at a broader population level usually requires a strong understanding of environmental health research, knowledge and skills as well as policy making, community action and regulation (see 📖 Chapters 3.4, 4.1, and 4.8).

It is also abundantly clear that environmental and ecosystem degradation threatens health at the global level, on a massive scale, in ways that are likely to affect disadvantaged people and developing nations most severely, and which will require environmental health practitioners to work collaboratively across a wide range of sectors and disciplines (see 📖 Chapter 7.6).

Dividing this work into defined tasks

In order to assess and then protect against a potential environmental health threat, it is useful to adopt a consistent framework for assessing and managing a health risk. The steps involved are:[1]
- issues identification
- hazard assessment, comprising hazard identification and dose–response assessment
- exposure assessment
- risk characterization
- risk management.

In practice, this is often an iterative, rather than linear process. Risk management strategies must sometimes be developed before all the information is available.

Issues identification

Before embarking on a formal risk assessment the specific issues should be identified with key stakeholders. Explore the underlying concerns and their context—including any existing health complaints that are being related to current exposures. Find out what interventions have been used and what may be available. Discuss whether the issue is amenable to risk assessment. Successful management of the issues (as distinct from producing a technically competent risk assessment) requires transparency and a strong involvement of affected communities as far as possible in the process.

Hazard identification

Hazard identification generally relies on prior knowledge and published scientific evidence of adverse effects associated with exposure to a substance or agent.

Dose–response assessment

Dose–response information involves detailed study of available data (including animal toxicology, epidemiology), although there are often gaps in such data. This can be due to difficulties in measuring exposure and dose in human studies (which tend to be opportunistic and retrospective), but methodological weaknesses are also common. Even when human data are available, it may be difficult to extrapolate dose–response relationships from high-exposure studies to situations involving low exposures.

Exposure assessment

Commonly, in developed nations, environmental exposures (e.g. via soil, water, or ambient air) present lower dose rates and total doses than those experienced through personal behaviours or occupational sources. Such exposures may incur relatively small increases in risk. However, because they are perceived as being outside the control of individuals, there is often a large outrage factor. It is important to understand and accept that such issues may require attention that seems out of proportion to their physical health impact if the exposure was involuntary (see 📖 Chapter 6.5). Knowing the source of emissions and environmental concentrations of contaminants is essential to environmental health protection, but does not indicate how much harmful agent or toxin is actually absorbed by an individual. An agent may be hazardous but not result in a risk until exposure occurs *and* a sufficient dose is delivered to target organs.

Risk characterization

Environmental factors with only a small, perhaps unmeasureable, additional risk at the individual level can still have a major impact on populations if many people are exposed, for example low-level childhood lead exposure, or particulate pollution of airsheds and cardiovascular disease. Rose's 'prevention paradox' is very relevant to environmental health and can be used to illustrate how small reductions of exposure across a population may reap significant health benefits overall, whilst offering little to the individual.[2]

Risk management

The above steps provide a sound basis for effective risk management, which is the process of evaluating alternative actions, selecting options, and implementing them. The goal is defensible, cost-effective, integrated actions that reduce or prevent risks while taking into account social, cultural, ethical, political and legal considerations. The decision-making process requires value judgements, and the more transparent these are the better it is for communication of health risk (see 📖 Chapters 3.8 and 6.5). The influences of risk perception and community outrage must also be addressed.

Competencies needed to achieve these tasks

Necessary competencies include communication, media, and 'people skills', interdisciplinary teamwork, advocacy, policy, and planning together with an understanding of epidemiology, toxicology, microbiology, and a range of other biological, physical, and social sciences. A low threshold for recognizing when additional specialist input is needed is desirable.

Systematic performance to make action more effective

Maintenance of a healthy environment requires a systematic approach that may include a range of strategies such as:
- healthy public policy
- legislation and other regulation, with enforcement
- appropriate guidelines and standards
- economic incentives
- demonstration projects
- interventions to bring about attitudinal change
- community involvement
- accurate information
- intersectoral action.

Although legislative controls and regulatory mechanisms may be available to deal with an environmental health threat (and are sometimes essential as a back-up measure), this is not usually the first course of action. It is preferable to establish collaborative approaches and to work with stakeholders, including affected communities, from an early stage in developing risk management strategies.

A capacity for monitoring and surveillance is necessary for verifying that control measures are working (e.g. drinking water supplies and catchment management).

Some environmental hazards are amenable to control more readily than lifestyle exposure factors and therefore present opportunities for efficient and effective public health interventions. This is analogous to 'engineered' injury prevention measures that separate the person from the hazard.

In establishing priorities when there are multiple environmental health problems to contend with, consider:
- the urgency of the threat (see 📖 Chapter 3.5)
- the number of people affected, and their experience of the impacts
- whether the exposure is increasing
- the consequences of 'doing nothing'
- the vulnerability and identifiability of population subgroups
- the amenability of issues to investigation
- the availability of interventions or remedies.

Periodic, systematic review is important to ensure that priorities are not only reactive. For example, there remains an urgent need to consider the long-term health perspective and address global environmental issues (including the abatement of greenhouse gas emissions), as well as respond to the immediate impacts of problems related to the environment.

Effective action for systemic changes to reduce a hazard (e.g. environmental tobacco smoke) can require careful building of a mandate, and political engagement via multiple pathways, to ultimately succeed.

Risk management options can be systematically considered as follows.

Reducing the hazard at its source

- Alteration of systems and human behaviours that underlie the production of a hazard, e.g. transport systems, housing and overcrowding, land use practices, food production methods, water catchment management.
- Alternative source materials, e.g. unleaded paint and petrol
- Cleaner processing systems and improved emission controls.
- Enforced shutdown of activity.

Protection at the community level

- *Removal of contaminant from a medium:* e.g. drinking water treatment.
- *Physical separation from the source:* e.g. relocation of activity; buffer zones; barriers (such as motorway noise barriers, creation of shade).
- *Altering behaviours to reduce exposure:* e.g. education to reduce intake of mercury-contaminated fish in pregnancy; boil water alerts; signage and access controls to prevent recreational water contact during blue-green algal blooms; regulation of environmental tobacco smoke.

Protection at the individual level

- Lead abatement of a household to protect a toddler
- Wearing personal protective equipment
- *Biological measures:* e.g. vaccination against hepatitis A to reduce the risk of the disease from unsafe food or water.

Options that reduce hazards at their source are generally preferable as they address root causes and tend to be more equitable and sustainable.

Who else should be involved?

Given the breadth of inputs and strategies mentioned above, efforts to protect public health from environmental threats typically require more engagement with stakeholders outside the health care system than within it (and this may in part explain why environmental health has been described as the 'Cinderella' of the health system, in terms of resourcing).

In controversial environmental health issues it can help to involve independent third parties who can objectively question an investigative or risk assessment process, or comment on the evidence available.

Potential pitfalls

Epidemiological approaches

Community members not uncommonly call for a study of the health status of local area when concerned about impacts from an existing or perceived exposure. However, epidemiological investigations in relation to environmental exposures should not be undertaken lightly and many factors need to be considered in examining their feasibility. Such studies can be resource-intensive, but inconclusive (particularly in small populations) and may actually cause delay in implementation of reasonable precautionary measures to reduce exposure. Cancer cluster investigations often suffer from these pitfalls and various agencies are refining their approach to deal with increases in demand (see ▢ Chapter 2.9).

It is often more appropriate and efficient to carry out thorough exposure assessment, which may include environmental sampling and sometimes biomonitoring, and rely on pre-existing information (e.g. dose–response data of a known toxicant, or application of environmental standards or guidelines) to help interpret the exposure data.

Well-conducted epidemiological studies of adverse health outcomes from environmental exposures provide critical evidence. However, health studies also have limitations and can be a weak link in health risk assessments.

Inadequate measurement of exposure is a particularly common failing when attempting to assess whether current health outcomes are attributable to past environmental exposures. Other problems may include lag times between exposures and potential health effects, health effects may be poorly defined, and low-level effects may be very difficult to distinguish from 'background' incidences of common health problems.

There may be groups within a population who are more susceptible to certain hazards, or more highly exposed, or both (e.g. children), and to whom standard risk assessment assumptions do not apply. Compounding of risk by other exposures or possible synergism between co-pollutants may also lead to underestimates of risk, or alternatively the significance of such risks may be over-played.

Uncertainty and the precautionary principle

Whilst an evidence-based approach should underpin environmental health action there are many instances where adequate information is lacking. In such circumstances, a precautionary approach should apply, recognizing the existence of uncertainty and ignorance and accepting that lack of full scientific certainty should not be used as a reason to postpone preventative measures (see Box 3.2.1).

Box 3.2.1 The precautionary principle

One of the outcomes of the United Nations Conference on Environment and Development (also known as the Earth Summit) held in Rio de Janeiro, Brazil, in June 1992 was the adoption of the Rio Declaration on Environment and Development, which contains 27 principles to underpin sustainable development.

One of these principles is Principle 15, which states:

> In order to protect the environment, the precautionary approach shall be widely applied by States according to their capabilities. Where there are threats of serious or irreversible damage, lack of full scientific certainty shall not be used as a reason for postponing cost-effective measures to prevent environmental degradation.

The 'cost-effective' component of this principle can be overlooked by protagonists, leading to conflict between stakeholders about the appropriate response to an issue. Nevertheless, proponents of environmental modification need to be able to demonstrate that, to a very high degree of probability, a project will not cause significant harm, either to the environment or to health.

In the development of standards and guidelines, it is common for government policy to be defined not in terms of the precautionary principle but on a science-based conservative approach, which underpins risk assessment and risk management regimes.

Health risk assessments need to be explicit about uncertainties. Looking for bias and identifying what further information could reduce the uncertainty also assists in setting priorities in research and monitoring.

Lessons from success and failure

Successful environmental health practice is usually invisible to the public, while failures often attract attention.

Disasters such as earthquakes and tsunamis powerfully illustrate the essential nature of local environmental health measures in reducing morbidity and mortality during recovery phases.

The international trend towards adoption of risk management frameworks in guidelines for drinking water quality, incorporating a multiple-barriers approach to hazards from catchment to tap, provides an excellent example of a systems approach to a profoundly important environmental health issue.[3,4]

There are many local examples of success from environmental health activities, with the Belfast Healthy Cities partnership being one such case from the WHO European Healthy Cities Network.[5]

Failures unfortunately are all too evident at the macro-level, if continued global ecosystems harms are a guide. With many contemporary environmental issues a technical approach alone is insufficient to achieve a satisfactory outcome, especially in terms of community ownership. Careful and transparent attention to the process of scoping out the range of concerns (and dialogue with relevant parties about what can and what cannot realistically be explored) is usually well worth the investment.

Key determinants of success

In acute situations where environmental exposures clearly threaten health, adequate legislation and emergency powers to support public health interventions may be essential to ensure that exposures are abated as soon as possible.

Risk assessment and management practices need to be sound and accountable. Knowing where and when to seek advice on technically complex matters is vital. Cultivate contacts who can rapidly steer you in the right direction if they do not know themselves.

Empowerment and support of local authorities and communities to integrate environment, health, and sustainable development in local strategies is fundamental to the creation of healthy environments.[5]

Developing a shared understanding with all partners is a key strategy, for example, in promoting active transport and reducing air pollution, and carbon emissions through town planning, road design, and transport measures.

Being prepared for and offering briefings to senior managers, politicians, and community meetings is often more productive in securing understanding and engagement, than reaction through the media dialogue (see 📖 Chapter 4.5)

How will you know if you have been successful?

Positive indicators include:
- reduced population exposures to a hazard (usually easier and quicker to measure than health outcomes, although there are exceptions e.g. food safety improvements)
- 'process' measures such as improvements in policy or community satisfaction with the process of risk assessment and management
- other sectors own and maintain the environmental control measures that you initiated
- reduced morbidity or mortality associated with the exposure, when health surveillance/epidemiological methods and time frames allow.

Emerging issues

Environmental health inequities may be widening, with major risks persisting or emerging in developing countries, while developed nations generally still focus inwardly on issues that are relatively minor in global terms.

The proliferation of chemical synthesis and usage in novel ways and the advent of new technologies (e.g. nanoparticles) present challenges for established methods of toxicological assessment. In the 21st century there is a need for better and more rapid toxicological assessment tools.

Improved epidemiological evidence is providing dose-response data that commonly shows there is no threshold or 'safe' level of exposure to a widely-distributed hazard (e.g. air pollution from fine particulate matter). In such cases, the policy and regulatory response is shifting from a standards compliance basis towards ongoing measures to further reduce population exposure.

The interrelationship between environment and chronic disease has long been recognized, but the momentum to achieve real change is still patchy outside of the public and environmental health sector. However, the profoundly urgent and complex issue of climate change is driving strategic recognition of the co-benefits of environmental action for sustainability with simultaneous improvements in more immediate population health problems such as obesity.[6,7]

Further resources

World Health Organization (Public Health & Environment) (2012). *Preliminary dose estimation from the nuclear accident after the 2011 Great East Japan earthquake and tsunami*. Available at: http://www.who.int/phe/en/

Health Protection Agency, United Kingdom. Available at: ℘ http://www.hpa.org.uk/

Agency for Toxic Substances and Disease Registry. Public Health Assessment Guidance Manual (2005). US Department of Health and Human Services. Available at: ℘ http://www.atsdr.cdc. gov/.

References

1 Australian Government. (2004). *Environmental health risk assessment—guidelines for assessing human health risk from environmental hazards*. Available at: ℘ http://www.health.gov.au/internet/publications/publishing.nsf/Content/CA25774C001857CACA2571E0000C8CF1/$File/EHRA%20 2004.pdf (accessed May 31, 2012)

2 Rose G. (1992). *The strategy of preventive medicine*. Oxford University Press, Oxford.

3 Australian Government NHMRC/NRMMC (2004). *Australian drinking water guidelines*. http://www. nhmrc.gov.au/publications/synopses/eh19syn.htm (accessed 3 August 2010).

4 World Health Organization (2006). Guidelines for drinking water quality, 3rd ed. Available at: ℘ http://www.who.int/water_sanitation_health/dwq/en/ (cited 3 August 2010).

5 Healthy Cities Belfast. Available at: ℘ http://www.belfasthealthycities.com/ (cited 1 August 2010).

6 *The Lancet*. (2009). *Health and Climate Change series*. Available at: ℘ www.thelancet.com (cited 29 August 2010).

7 Heart Foundation. (2010). Healthy by Design: a guide to planning and designing environments for active living in Tasmania. Available at: ℘ http://www.heartfoundation.org.au/Professional_Information/Lifestyle_risk/Physical_Activity/Active_by_Design/Pages/default.aspx (cited 3 August 2010).

3.3 Protecting and promoting health in the workplace

Tar-Ching Aw, Stuart Whitaker, and Malcolm Harrington

Objectives

After reading this chapter you will be able to understand:
- the nature and scope of occupational health practice
- how efforts to protect and promote health in the workplace will contribute to general public health.

Definition

Occupational health deals with the two-way interaction between health and work. It encompasses:
- prevention of occupationally related illness or injury resulting from exposure to workplace hazards
- ensuring that workers with pre-existing illnesses or disability are able to continue working without undue risk to their own health or those of third parties
- promoting general health and safe working practices in the workplace. The workplace setting can be a useful environment for health promotion for the working age population.

Why is this an important public health issue?

For many people, lack of work and unemployment, are recognized causes of ill-health, but the workplace itself poses many preventable health hazards. These include exposure to physical, chemical, biological, ergonomic, and psycho-social hazards.

Individuals at work constitute a significant proportion of the general population. Maintenance of their state of health is key to ensuring the well-being of their co-workers, their families, the employer, and the nation. Most people spend around a third of their life at work. Hence, the work that they do, the environments in which they work, and how they are treated in those workplaces, can all contribute to their physical, mental and social well-being.

Approaches to occupational health

Preventing occupationally-related illness or injury

- Identifying hazards in the work setting
- Determining the population exposed to such hazards
- Assessing the risks from exposure to the hazards (risk assessment)
- Taking appropriate preventive action by one or more of the following actions to reduce those risks:
  - elimination, substitution, or containment of the hazards; limiting the numbers of workers exposed
  - reducing the time each person is required to spend at specific work areas where hazards are not easily eliminated
  - providing personal protective equipment, as a last resort
- Auditing and reassessing the efficacy of the preventive measures
- Considering the need for a suitable health surveillance programme or periodic monitoring system for the workforce.

Workers with pre-existing illnesses or disability

- Identifying relevant risk factors, e.g. atopy, previous asthma, or previous history of several episodes of low back pain, so that suitable advice, job placement, and work modification can be considered
- Assessment of job duties, and providing advice on the reasonable adjustments or job modifications that would allow the worker to be employed safely
- Pre-placement assessment and advice
- Health surveillance, including periodic review of health status and sickness absence record.

For some occupational groups, e.g. health care workers, specific tasks include checking the immune status and providing immunization as required. An example is determination of the hepatitis B immune status for health-care workers.

Promoting general health in the workplace

The main tasks involved in health promotion at the workplace are:

- *General:* the workplace can be used as a setting to address non-occupational, lifestyle factors that affect general public health. Examples are advice and information on alcohol intake, smoking, diet, exercise, safe driving, safe sex, and precautions in the course of travelling or working abroad. The workplace, along with other venues such as the school, the home, and the local community, is an important setting for the delivery of health education and health promotion. Health promotion initiatives in the workplace can include measures, such as improving the quality of food provided in the works canteen, establishing a no-smoking policy, encouraging exercise at and away from the workplace and/or providing subsidized membership to sports and exercise facilities.
- *Specific:* suitable and sufficient information, instruction, and training in working safely should be provided where there are recognized hazards in the workplace.

The potential disadvantage of focusing on workplace health promotion alone is the diversion of attention and resources away from measures to assess and control the more serious occupational health and safety risks. These form part of the employer's legal responsibilities.

Conducting a HNA at the workplace, in conjunction with the workforce, can help identify priorities for action, and determining how these needs may be best met. Participatory approaches to workplace health promotion are likely to be effective, especially if it empowers workers to address their own health needs.

What are the tasks needed to achieve effective change?

- Proper assessment of risks by a competent person
- Commitment at the highest level to rectify the problem
- Clear strategy for implementing preventive measures
- Good communication between preventive medicine professionals and management and the workforce. Publicity through in-house newsletters, seminars, and effective use of the media are crucial elements for creating effective change
- Timely implementation of measures
- Review and evaluation of success or failure.

It is essential that the workforce is not only informed, but is actively engaged in the whole process of change where appropriate.

Competences required

- Occupational health training to assess hazards and risks at the workplace
- Clinical skills to determine the health status of the workforce
- Technical expertise to modify workplaces and recommend safer systems of work
- Communication skills to persuade workers to participate in behavioural change to improve health.

Who are the other people that might need to be involved?

- Management at all levels, as they ultimately have the responsibility for managing occupational health issues and controlling the access to resources
- The workforce and their representatives, as the measures proposed will affect them. Worker co-operation and participation is essential for the measures to succeed

- Occupational health and safety and public health professionals:
  - occupational physicians and nurses
  - public health practitioners
  - safety practitioners
  - occupational hygienists
  - occupational psychologists
  - ergonomists
  - health promotion personnel
  - toxicologists
  - epidemiologists
  - other health practitioners and specialists.

In order to engage the workforce with the actions being taken to protect and promote their health, it is important to understand that genuine teamwork is crucial.

The general practitioner (family physician) will also have a key role in providing advice to their patients on the importance of work to health and well-being, and in supporting a timely return to work after a period of sickness absence.

Ethical dilemmas

- A worker with occupational asthma wants to continue in his job where workplace exposure to the asthmagen cannot be eliminated. The medical advice is to avoid exposure. The worker has no other available job alternatives:
  - Should the worker be given all the necessary medical information, and then he/she chooses whether to continue being employed or to leave the job?
  - Is the physician avoiding responsibility by asking the patient to make a decision?
- A safety practitioner is informed by a worker about poor control of exposures at his workplace, and poor compliance with safe systems of work. However, he is asked to keep this information confidential and that no representations on this are made to management, since he might be identified as the source of this information with implications for his job security:
  - Should the safety practitioner approach management and ignore the request of the worker?
  - Or should the wishes of the worker be respected, and the unsafe work practices be allowed to continue?
- A nurse advises that a worker with prolonged 'absenteeism' from low back pain should be able to return to his work duties, and not wait until he is completely free of symptoms. The worker is prepared to do so, but has been advised by his colleagues that some people have remained at work despite not being in the best of health, thereby posing a risk to their health and that of their co-workers ('presenteeism'). Should the worker be advised to return to work, or to stay at home?

Consider these dilemmas, and see what advice is given by the professional bodies, e.g. The London and Irish Faculty of occupational medicine's publications on guidance on ethics,[1,2] and other publications on ethics (e.g. International Commission on Occupational Health (ICOH) code of ethics for occupational health professionals).

What are the potential pitfalls in occupational health?

- Misinterpretation of motives for action by either management or the workforce
- Misguided and ill-informed media coverage
- Inappropriate risk perception
- Inappropriate or inaccurate health belief models
- Lack of attention to social and cultural values.

Fallacies in occupational health

Fallacy 1: the data are abundant

For many occupational hazards there is often a lack of good data on the effects of exposure on human health. This is either because a good system for gathering information on health effects is non-existent, that compliance with current reporting requirements for occupational ill-health is poor, or that there are conflicting animal data, and human epidemiological data are limited. The explanation that is sometimes offered that 'We have never had a case of ill-health in our workplace resulting from the use of our chemicals or due to our work processes' may reflect an absence of a system for collecting data on occupational ill-health, instead of an absence of ill-health.

Fallacy 2: if there are no data, exhortation will be sufficient

Until accurate data on the incidence and prevalence of work-related conditions become available, it may be difficult to impress upon the public, employers, and government the extent of any problem. The absence of data will also limit the likelihood of obtaining resources for prevention. The classic case of John Snow removing the Broad street pump handle to stop the outbreak of cholera in London demonstrates that effective preventive measures can be taken even before full data or information is available about the causative agent. The *Vibrio cholerae* bacterium was not yet discovered at the time of the outbreak.

Fallacy 3: most clinicians are well trained in occupational health

Training in occupational medicine and occupational health in medical and nursing schools is limited. Consequently, medical and nursing professionals often have only a very general understanding of what can be done to prevent ill-health and injury at the workplace.

Fallacy 4: if we examine every potential worker, and exclude those that are not 100% fit, that will help reduce future ill-health and sickness absence

Pre-employment examinations are used in many parts of the world to exclude individuals who have a health problem, even if there is no obvious mismatch between the ill-health or disability detected and the job tasks involved. Over 98% of pre-employment assessments do not detect any clinical abnormalities. If at all warranted, such examinations should be restricted to specific jobs where there is residual exposure to significant risk despite the best measures to reduce the risk. The focus on prevention in the workplace should be on improving the workplace instead of excluding the worker. The new Equality Bill in the UK will outlaw many processes used for pre-employment screening. Clinical assessments, if indicated, will need to be performed at a pre-placement stage, and not as a condition for employment.

Case studies: occupational health incidents

- *The Bhopal disaster:*[3] an explosion in the workplace led to acute and chronic health effects among the workforce and surrounding community. The chemical agent involved was methyl isocyanate.
- *The Chernobyl incident:*[4] effects from an out-of-control 'industrial process', partly related to operator fatigue, became a major public health problem (occupational and environmental). The agents involved were radioactive materials.
- *The dibromochloropropane (DBCP) problem:*[5] questions on male infertility and the inability to start a family amongst a US workforce led to a factory and industry-wide epidemiological investigations that then identified DBCP as the cause. This resulted in cessation of manufacture of DBCP for use as a pesticide.
- *Gynecomastia in a pharmaceutical company in Puerto Rico:*[6] enlargement of male breasts in workers led to investigations confirming exposure to oestrogenic compounds. The main recommendations included ensuring an improved level of containment to prevent health effects.
- *Asbestos exposure:* pulmonary fibrosis, bronchogenic carcinoma, and pleural and peritoneal mesothelioma occurred in workers exposed to asbestos fibres. The risk of lung cancer for asbestos exposure was noted to be multiplied where there was concomitant cigarette smoking. Similar health effects occurred from secondary exposure of wives who had to clean the asbestos-contaminated overalls of these workers. Mesotheliomas have also been associated with non-occupational environmental exposure to asbestiform fibres.[7]
- *Vinyl chloride monomer:* a cluster of four cases of a very rare malignancy—angiosarcoma of the liver—occurred amongst workers responsible for cleaning polymerization chambers for manufacture of polyvinyl chloride (PVC). Prompt preventive action led to rapid reduction in worker exposure to the chemical agent—vinyl chloride

monomer.[8] This is a gas that is polymerized to form the relatively inert and non-toxic PVC. Corroborative animal evidence of similar tumors in rodents came to light at about the same time.

Four important lessons

- Prompt public health action may be needed even if not all of the desired information is available. Do not let the desire for perfection hinder the need for pragmatism
- Clusters of a rare disease (mesothelioma, angiosarcoma) are often easier to identify as resulting from an occupational exposure than more common pathology such as lung cancer or spontaneous abortions
- Effects on the workforce, the wider community, and the environment can result from workplace hazards
- Public health vigilance and clinical case reports can both lead to identification of health hazards in the workplace.

Predictors of success and failure

Success

- A good team of occupational and public health professionals can identify problems early in order to initiate effective preventive action
- Sympathetic and supportive management and workforce aid this process
- Engagement of primary and secondary care providers can assist in protecting and promoting workers' health.

Failure

- Health promotion in the workplace should not be done at the expense of control of workplace hazards
- A multidisciplinary approach will not work if co-ordination is poor and there is a lack of understanding of the roles of each team member
- An over-reliance on the medical model may prove to be ineffective in addressing the problems encountered in the workplace. Identification of cases, correct diagnosis, treatment, and reporting procedures, important though those activities are, will do little to prevent further cases from occurring unless risks to health can be communicated effectively to the public, politicians, decision-makers, employers, and employees. All of these groups have a part to play in ensuring that effective action is taken to prevent exposure to hazardous working conditions.

How will you know if you have been successful?

Criteria for success

These include:

- reduction in the incidence and prevalence of occupational ill-health and injury
- improvement in morale (and productivity) of the workforce
- reduction of risk or frequency of hazardous exposures
- improvement in knowledge of risks and awareness by the working population
- positive changes in behavior and attitudes towards occupational risks by the working population
- absence of inappropriate adverse media publicity.
- commitment and participation by managers and workers in initiatives to improve health at the workplace.

Emerging issues

- *The ageing worker:* longevity of the population and fewer offspring per family have contributed to a higher proportion of older workers in the workforce. Many countries have also proposed increasing the retirement age (mainly for fiscal reasons). Workplaces have to adapt to accommodate the physical capabilities of ageing workers. Degenerative disorders will be expected to increase amongst the causes of ill-health in the ageing workforce of the future.
- *Stress and mental health:* the main cause of sickness absence in many countries has shifted from infections and respiratory, gastrointestinal and skin problems to musculo-skeletal and mental health issues. The trend towards an increase in stress, anxiety and depression is seen in developed and rapidly developing countries, and especially when physical and chemical risks start to decrease with good control of exposures.
- *The 'fit note':* Dame Carol Black reviewed the health of workers in the UK and made a number of recommendations.[9] The most progressive reform proposed was a replacement of the traditional 'sick note' signed by general practitioners by an electronic 'fit note'. The aim is to encourage individuals back to work instead of indicating just the number of days the person should take as certified sickness absence. This was implemented on 6th April 2010.
- *New technology:* concerns have been raised about the possible impact of new technology on health. One example is the increasing applications that have been developed for nanotechnology. Nano particles have considerable potential for use in a wide range of

applications including clothing, computing, industrial coatings, and medicines, Studies on laboratory animals have demonstrated a potential for these minute particles to cause toxic effects, and there is a worry that nanoparticles may become the new 'asbestos' in regards to health effects.[10]

- *Mental health and well-being:* a UK government report on building mental capital and well-being has identified workplace factors that may help or hinder the promotion of mental health.

Further resources

Books

Aw TC, Harrington JM, Gardiner K. (2007). *Pocket consultant: occupational health*, 5th edn. Blackwell Publishing, Oxford.

Baxter PA, Aw TC, Cockcroft A, Durrington, P, Harrington JM. (eds.) (2010). *Hunter's diseases of occupations*, 10th edn. Hachette, London.

Palmer K, Cox RAF, Brown I. (eds) (2007). *Fitness for work: the medical aspects*, 4th edn. Oxford University Press, Oxford.

Gardiner K, Harrington JM. (eds) (2005). *Occupational Hygiene*, 3rd edn. Blackwell Publishing, Oxford.

Westerholm P, Nilstun T, Ovretveit, J. (eds) (2004). *Practical ethics in occupational health*. Radcliffe Medical Press, Oxford.

Occupational health journals

Occupational and Environmental Medicine
Scandinavian Journal of Work, Environment and Health
American Journal of Industrial Medicine
Journal of Occupational & Environmental Medicine
Occupational Medicine

Journal papers

Gochfeld M. (2005). Chronologic history of occupational medicine. *Journal of Occupational and Environmental Medicine*, **47,** 96–114.

Greenberg M. (2004). The British approach to asbestos standard setting: 1928–2000. *American Journal of Indian Medicine*, **46**, 534–41.

Norashikin M, Schonstein E, Schaafsma F, *et al.* (2010). *Pre-employment examinations for preventing occupational injury and disease in workers.* Cochrane Library (Wiley Online Library). Published online 8 Dec 2010. Available at: ℘ http://www.update-software.com/BCP/WileyPDF/EN/CD008881.pdf (accessed 31 May 2012).

Whitaker S, Aw TC (1995) Audit of pre-employment assessments by occupational health departments in the National Health Service. *Occupational Medicine* **45,** 75–80

Databases

Available on CD-ROM: (contact info@mdx.com and ℘ http://www.ovid.com)
TOMES (Toxicology, Occupational Medicine and Environmental Series).
HSELINE (Health and Safety Executive, UK).
NIOSHTIC and NIOSHTIC-2 (National Institute for Occupational Safety and Health, USA).
CISDOC (International Labour Office, Geneva).

Websites

American Conference of Governmental Industrial Hygienists, Inc. Available at: ℘ http://www.acgih.org/home.htm

Faculty of Occupational Medicine, UK. ℘ http://www.facoccmed.ac.uk/

Finnish Institute of Occupational Health. ℘ http://www.ttl.fi/en/Pages/default.aspx (accessed 31 May 2012)

Health and Safety Executive, UK. ℘ http://www.hse.gov.uk/

International commission on Occupational health (ICOH) ℘ http://www.icohweb.org

The Government Office for Science, London. Foresight Mental Capital and Wellbeing Project: http://www.bis.gov.uk/assets/biscore/corporate/migratedD/ec_group/116-08-FO_b (accessed 31 May 2012)

References

1 Faculty of Occupational Medicine (2006). *Guidance on ethics for occupational physicians*. Faculty of Occupational Medicine, Royal College of Physicians, London.
2 Faculty of Occupational Medicine, Ireland (2007). *Guidance on ethical practice for occupational physicians*. Faculty of Occupational Medicine, Dublin.
3 Dhara VR, Dhara R. (2002). The Union Carbide disaster in Bhopal: a review of health effects. *Archives of Environmental Health*, **57**, 391–404.
4 Tuttle RM, Becker DV (2006). The Chernobyl accident and its consequences: update at the millennium. *Seminars in Nuclear Medicine*, **30**, 133–40.
5 Whorton D, Krauss RM, Marshall S, Milby TH. (1977). Infertility in male pesticide workers. *Lancet*, **2**, 1259–61.
6 Harrington JM, Stein GF, Rivera RO, de Morales AV. (1978). Occupational hazards of formulating oral contraceptives—a survey of plant employees. *Archives of Environmental Health*, **33**, 12–15.
7 Pasetto R, Comba P, Marconi A (2005). Mesothelioma associated with environmental exposures. *La Medicina del Lavora*, **96**, 330–7.
8 Makk L, Delmore F, Creech Jr JL, *et al.* (2006). Clinical and morphologic features of hepatic angiosarcoma in vinyl chloride workers. *Cancer*, **37**, 148–63.
9 Black C. (2008). *Working for a healthier tomorrow*. TSO, London.
10 Seaton A, Donaldson K. (2005) Nanoscience, nanotechnology, and the need to think small. *Lancet*, **365**, 923–4.

3.4 Engaging communities in participatory research and action

Meredith Minkler and Charlotte Chang

Objectives

After reading this chapter you will be able to:
- define participatory research and its core principles
- describe how engaging communities in participatory research and action can add value to research, while building community capacity and helping achieve action to promote community health
- identify some of the challenges that arise in such work and how they may be addressed
- describe a case study that started with an important issue in the community and demonstrates core principles of CBPR, challenges faced in such work, and subsequent community action for change.

Definition and core principles

Participatory research is a generic term for a wide range of approaches that go by many names (e.g. community-based participatory research (CBPR), mutual inquiry, participatory action research and community-partnered research), but have as their centerpiece three interrelated elements: participation and education, research, and action.[1,2] Building on earlier work,[3] the Kellogg Community Health Scholars Program[4] defined community-based participatory research in the health field as: 'a collaborative approach to research that equitably involves all partners in the research process and recognizes the unique strengths that each brings. CBPR begins with a research topic of importance to the community with the aim of combining knowledge and action for social change to improve community health and eliminate health disparities.' The core principles of community-based participatory research are listed in Box 3.4.1.

Box 3.4.1 Core principles of participatory research

- Recognizes community as a unit of identity[5]
- Builds on strengths and resources within the community
- Facilitates a collaborative, equitable partnership in all phases of research, involving an empowering and power-sharing process that attends to social inequalities
- Fosters co-learning and capacity building among all partners
- Integrates and achieves a balance between knowledge generation and intervention for the mutual benefit of all partners.
- Focuses on the local relevance of public health problems and on ecological perspectives that attend to the multiple determinants of health
- Involves systems development using a cyclical and iterative process
- Disseminates results to all partners and involves them in the wider dissemination of results
- Involves a long term process and commitment to sustainability
- Openly addresses issues of race, ethnicity, racism and social class, and embodies 'cultural humility',[6] (acknowledging personal biases and the limitations of one's own knowledge about others' cultures, being open to learning, and committing to genuine and respectful partnership)[2]
- Works to assure research rigor and validity, but also 'broadens the bandwidth of validity'[7] by making sure that the issue comes from, or has real relevance to the community, and that different ways of knowing, including the community's lay knowledge, are called upon and respected.

Sources for principles: 1–9 (refs 3 & 5) and 10–11 (refs 2, 6, 7).

Why is this an important issue?

Recent decades have seen growing appreciation of the importance of working 'with', rather than 'on' communities to understand and address complex health problems. Participatory, community-partnered and action-orientated approaches, including CBPR, to problems ranging from asthma and HIV/AIDS to obesity, depression, and violence, are important parts of a health professional's tool kit.

Many of today's complex health problems have proven poorly suited to 'outside expert'-driven research and the often disappointing interventions to which it has given rise.[2] Too often, communities feel 'studied to death' by researchers, while seeing no real local benefit. With its accent on engaging community members throughout the research process and using study findings to help promote new or improved programmes, practices, and policies, community engagement both strengthens the research itself, and builds local capacity or problem-solving ability, while addressing concerns of genuine interest to the community and other stakeholders.

Approaches to participatory action and research

Following the principles of engagement of communities in participatory research and action requires:

- Ensuring that the problem under study comes from, or is of genuine interest to, the community
- Identifying and building on community strengths and assets
- Building genuine collegial relationships characterized by mutual respect and co-learning between the partners
- Engaging communities throughout the research process, including:
  - deciding on the research question
  - study design and methods, including the design of culturally appropriate instruments
  - data collection and interpretation
  - dissemination and use of findings to help bring about change
  - ongoing evaluation of the project's processes and outcomes.[2,3,5,8–12]

Who is the community and how do we begin?

- *Identification of the community is a critical starting point for participatory research and action:* although commonly identified in geographic terms, communities can also be based on identity, and a 'shared sense of personhood' resulting from common cultural beliefs, values and traditions. A local neighbourhood, a community of people with disabilities or people who identify as gay or lesbian, also may be an important starting point for participatory and action-orientated research.
- *Find out who the key opinion leaders are in that community:* who do people go to for advice or help? Who are the 'movers and shakers' who have helped in the past when the community has come together around a problem? Is there a strong, autonomous organization (e.g. a faith- or community-based organization (CBO), or community centre) that is widely respected and that might serve as a partner on an action-orientated participatory research effort?
- If an outside researcher or health department is interested in mobilizing the community to study and address a particular health issue, it is also important to find out whether that issue is, in fact, of genuine concern to the community. Key opinion leaders and respected local organizations can help us do this, or we may hold focus groups or interviews with community members to assess their views.

The spectrum of community engagement

Participatory research and action can be seen as taking place along a spectrum, depending on the level of community engagement involved:[13]

- *Informing communities about a project or study and inviting members to take part as subjects or participants:* although commonly listed as a form of participatory research, such an approach tends to be *community placed*, but not genuinely *community based*. While important for achieving informed consent, it is not truly participatory in nature and typically does not promote improved community health.

- *Inviting community members to have input on some aspects of the study:* e.g. the design of survey questions or dissemination of findings. This approach is important, and helpful in increasing response rate. However, it does not take full advantage of community engagement—or give back optimally to the community.
- *Engaging community members as collaborators on a research project or intervention that is designed by outside researchers:* even when outside researchers have already designed a study or intervention, significant mutual value can be added when community partners then are invited to participate collegially in providing input on each stage of the study project.
- *Collegial research for action, in which community members are involved as equal partners throughout the process:* here, the research comes from or is of real importance to the community partners who participate as colleagues from the study's inception through the dissemination and action phases of the work. Community partners control or share control of the entire project.

Competences required

- Ability to identify appropriate community members and other collaborators and respectfully engage with them as equal partners
- Familiarity with/commitment to the principles of participatory research
- Technical expertise in research methods, along with an openness to alternative ways of knowing (e.g. community's lay knowledge) and an ability to engage in research that draws upon both
- Communication skills, including skills in communicating cross-culturally and/or with low-literacy populations
- Comfort in and willingness to share power and engage in respectful conflict resolution as challenging issues arise
- Ability to commit to a participatory research project 'over the long haul' to ensure getting to the action phases of the work, which may extend well after formal funding for the project has ended.

Who are the other people that might need to be involved?

- Community-based organizations and groups, including neighborhood agencies and faith-based organizations
- Community organizers, CBO staff, or other 'bridge people' who have strong relationships with and cultural knowledge of both community members and academic researchers and can facilitate the development of trust and relationships between diverse partners
- Policy makers, funders, or other decision-makers with the power to help the partnership use its findings to foster health-promoting change

- Local health departments, hospitals, or academics knowledgeable about the topic and interested in engagement as equal partners.

What's the value added in using a participatory approach?

- Helps ensure that the topic under investigation comes from or is of genuine interest to the community
- Increases community buy-in and trust, which in turn can increase response rate
- Enhances our ability to develop meaningful informed consent procedures and materials, and to consider potential community as well as individual risks and benefits.[10]
- Improves cultural sensitivity and acceptability of surveys, and other research instruments and may improve their validity
- Enables the design of more locally appropriate interventions, increasing in the process the likelihood of success
- Improves interpretation of research findings
- Identifies new dissemination channels and approaches that can increase the value of study findings and recommendations for end-users
- Helps ensure that study findings are translated into action that can in turn result in programmes, policies or practices that can benefit the community and other stakeholders
- Empowers and increases capacity of communities to understand and take action on local health issues.[2,3,5,8–12]

Challenges in participatory research and action

Time and labour intensive nature of the work
Community-engaged participatory research requires more 'front-end time' than traditional research for building relationships, co-learning processes, and engaging community partners in each step of the process. As noted above, the action phase of the process, and the commitment of researchers to the community over the long term, also means that this work may engage well beyond a funded project period.

Conflict and power dynamics are part of the process
Health professionals who take part in a CBPR or related project should be comfortable dealing with conflict and should recognize that power sharing—and therefore likely struggles over power, resource allocation, etc.—are part of the process. Practitioners should be honest and upfront with community partners about institutional challenges to sharing power, for example, parameters required by human subjects review processes.[10] Developing 'ground rules' and memorandums of understanding (MOU's), using guidelines for assessing partnership processes[11,12] and building in

ongoing participatory evaluation can help address some of these concerns, but cannot be expected to fully prevent them.

Community engagement may involve trade-offs between scientific rigor, and community responsive interventions and measurement tools

One of the greatest strengths of participatory research and action—its ability to contribute to culturally sensitive and acceptable research instruments and interventions—may also be problematic when community concerns challenge study designs, or preclude the use of validated instruments in data collection. For example, community members facing urgent health problems may not believe that randomized studies with control groups are fair to those who don't receive the intervention, and may argue strongly for a less rigorous study design. Genuine dialogue about the meanings attached to terms like 'rigor' and 'validity,' the advantages of having stronger 'scientific' findings and the equally important need for community trust and acceptance, as well as openness to compromise and different ways of knowing, will help address these knotty issues.

Conflicts over the dissemination and use of findings to promote change

Price and Behrens[14] write about the mismatch that frequently occurs between the 'necessary skepticism of science' and the 'action imperative of the community.' Community partners thus may wish to move quickly from preliminary findings to advocating for a change in practice or policy, while health professionals feel a responsibility to ensure that the findings are accurate—and sometimes, that they have first gone through peer review! Sometimes, too, findings may emerge that could cast the community in a bad light if made public.[10] In these cases, ongoing dialogue and memoranda of understanding (MOUs) may be helpful, but cannot fully prevent tough issues from emerging that need to be addressed in ways that satisfy all concerned partners.

Case study: a participatory approach to studying and addressing occupational health and safety among immigrant workers in San Francisco's Chinatown restaurants

One-third of all residents in San Francisco's Chinatown district are employed in the restaurant industry. Health and safety problems abound in these workplaces, and include traditional occupational health concerns, such as cuts, burns, falls, and on-the-job stress. Health problems also encompass serious economic and other social vulnerabilities when employers do not pay the legal minimum wage and delay, or evade payment of wages earned, sometimes for periods as long as several months.

The Chinese Progressive Association (CPA) had been organizing campaigns around such worker issues in Chinatown restaurants for over 30 years when it formed a partnership with the University of California, Berkeley School of Public Health and its Labor Occupational Health Program, the San Francisco Department of Public Health, and the University of California San Francisco Division of Occupational and Environmental Medicine in 2007. The partnership used a participatory research approach to document working conditions and the health status of Chinatown restaurant workers, evaluate their process throughout, and use the study findings to take action. Research activities included initial focus groups, a community survey of 433 Chinatown restaurant workers, development and use of an observational checklist on the physical working environments of 106 of the 108 restaurants in Chinatown, and interviews and surveys of participating partners.[15]

The structure and dynamics of the partnership evolved over time and were adapted to changing circumstances. Many layers of complexity were involved in obtaining equitable participation on the project across the different partners who included Chinese restaurant workers, community organizers, university-based researchers, and health department professionals. These factors included the use of three languages, different educational and professional backgrounds, and differences in organizational as well as ethnic cultures. Mutual trust and respect, including 'leaps of faith' in other partners, the use of translation services, and much 'bridging' by key facilitating partners were keys to success in working across diversity and within the constraints of a tight budget and timeline. In the end, partners successfully collaborated to develop research instruments and questions, recruit participants, collect, analyze, and interpret data, and lay the foundation for policy action.

Findings from the research showed that of all Chinatown restaurant workers surveyed:

- 48% had been burned, 40% had been cut, and 17% had slipped or fallen at work in the last 12 months
- 50% did not receive the City's minimum wage
- 40% did not receive any breaks during the day

- 64% did not receive any training on how to perform their jobs
- 54% paid for healthcare out of pocket; just 3% had employer-covered insurance.[16]

From the observational check list component of the study, it was learned that:

- 65% of the 106 restaurants did not have any of the required labour law postings displayed
- 62% had wet and greasy floors
- under half (48%) had non-slip mats
- 82% did not have fully stocked first aid kits.

Outcomes from the project included:

- Major contributions to the development by worker partners and allies of a Worker Bill of Rights policy advocacy tool and its use in subsequent organizing.
- Development of leadership potential and 'courage to confront problems in their community' among worker partners
- Posting of the observational check list on the health department's web site (🖱 http://www.sfphes.org/elements/work/22-elements/work/80-chinatown-restaurant-health-and-safety) and subsequent interest among other agencies in partnering with health department food inspectors to address worker health and safety.
- The formal 'launch' of the study's report and recommendations for action at a community event attended by over 80 community members, media representatives, and agencies as a prelude to subsequent community action.
- Development by the community partner and a design co-operative of a glossy, professional quality brochure on key findings and action steps for use in subsequent education of employers, employees, and community members, and with the lay and ethnic media.
- Development of strong relationships among partners and their continued collaboration on the action phase of the work over a year past the end of funding.

Some important lessons

- Community participation in research, and inclusion of an action component, will likely slow down the process. However, the extra time and effort may be well counter-balanced by the added richness of the study, and its capacity for studying a problem of genuine local concern, doing so in ways that respect and honour local community beliefs and wisdom, and increase the likelihood of intervention success and follow-up action to promote improved community health
- Although there is no one set of principles for engaging communities in research and action, attending to the basic principles described,[2,3,5] and tailoring them to meet the specific needs of your own partnership, can be an important way to monitor and assess your progress, and facilitate the discussion of difficult issues before, or as, they occur

- Balancing research with action in participatory work with communities is a must, and all partners should commit 'to the long haul,' including staying engaged in the action phase of the work even if the money has run out.

Predictors of success and failure

Success

- A strong initial partnership, with plenty of front end attention to building trusting and collaborative relationships
- Shared goals, including assurance that the research topic matters to the local community and that the methods selected and interventions developed similarly reflect local knowledge and priorities
- Respect among all partners for the importance of community needs and priorities, as well as 'good science' as a prerequisite to effective action, particularly when the desired change requires action on the part of policy makers or other key decision-makers
- Engagement of multiple key stakeholders in the process, and the building of alliances well beyond the original partnership to instigate action
- Mutual respect, trust, and flexibility in working with partners from different perspectives and backgrounds.[1–5,8–12]

Failure

- 'Name only' participatory research and action, in which community members are rarely consulted and simply used to help bring in a grant or help increase response rates, often incur resentment and do not lead to authentic and effective partnerships
- Lack of community commitment to the research question under consideration misses both the spirit and the process of participatory research and action—often with disappointing results.
- Particularly when there are multiple partners or major differences in culture and educational level among partners, lack of sufficient attention to process and communication, and failure to use mechanisms that help ensure equal participation can doom an otherwise promising partnership.
- Failure to plan ahead for the dissemination and action phases of the study—including deciding on a dissemination strategy and commitment by all partners to the action phase of the work—can be disillusioning for the community while precluding a central tenet of participatory research and action.[1–5,8–12]

How will you know if you have been successful?

Criteria for success
- Partners have shown mutual respect and engaged in co-learning throughout the process
- Many clear examples exist of the ways in which community participation improved research quality, and built individual and community capacity in the process
- The final study shows evidence of the partners' commitment to academically strong research enriched by community members' deep knowledge of their community. Different ways of knowing have been valued and incorporated
- Study findings have been used by the partners to work for changes in programmes, practices, and policies promoting improved community health and well-being
- There is clear evidence of both community and individual capacity building as a result of community participation throughout the process
- The partners respond in the affirmative to the question, 'would you engage together again if you had the chance?'
- Partners agree that the group has successfully reached mutually determined goals for research and action.[2–5,8–12]

Emerging issues

- Participatory research has become a 'buzz word' in the USA, the UK, and elsewhere. With funders now mandating CBPR and related approaches in calls for proposals, it is essential that new mechanisms be developed to help foster authentic community engagement in the work.[2] From ethics review procedures (IRB's) that respect the different processes involved in CBPR[10] to easily accessible sample MOU's and other tools for monitoring process,[11–12] institutional help for partnerships interested in exploring this approach is needed
- The substantially longer time table involved in participatory research and action suggests the need for realistic, multi-year funding that includes ample support for partnership building processes and subsequent action aspects of the work, as well as the more traditional research components
- Appropriate institutional support for health practitioner and academic partners, and recognition and adequate compensation of community partners should be provided in recognition of the time and labour intensive nature of this work
- The Institute of Medicine[17] has named CBPR one of eight new content areas in which schools of public health should be offering training. How can such training be developed that builds in on-the-ground experience with participatory research and action processes, while also respecting the limitations of the typical academic

timetable and the long-term commitment required in improving community health
- There is increasing interest in using a CBPR orientation with such traditional approaches as randomized controlled trials (RCTs). How can these diverse approaches be brought together effectively? And is this even appropriate?[18]
- Due to the increasingly popular use of community-engaged and participatory research approaches to public health issues, there is a need to develop clearer ways to evaluate such efforts and strong criteria for what qualifies as an 'authentic' effort.

Further resources

Books and monographs

Corburn J. (2005). *Street science: community knowledge and environmental health justice.* MIT Press, Cambridge.

Green LW, George MA, Daniel M, *et al.* (1995). *Study of participatory research in health promotion: Review and recommendations for the development of participatory research in health promotion in Canada.* Royal Society of Canada, Vancouver.

Israel BA, Eng E, Schulz AJ, Parker EA. (eds) (2005). *Methods in community-based participatory research for health.* Jossey-Bass, San Francisco.

Minkler M, Wallerstein N. (eds) (2008). *Community-based participatory research for health: from process to outcomes,* 2nd edn.: Jossey-Bass, San Francisco.

Reason P, Bradbury H. (2006). *Handbook of action research: participatory inquiry and practice,* concise edn.: Sage Publications, London.

Journals featuring articles on participatory research and action (selected)

Health Education and Behavior
American Journal of Public Health
Action Research
Progress in Community Health Partnerships
Journal of Health Promotion Practice
Ethnicity and Disease
Journal of Urban Health
Health Promotion International
American Journal of Community Psychology

Journal papers

Cargo M, Mercer SL. (2008). The value and challenges of participatory research: strengthening its practice. *Annual Review of Public Health,* **29**.

Green LW, Mercer SL. (2001). Can public health researchers and agencies reconcile the push from funding bodies and the pull from communities? *American Journal of Public Health,* **91**, 1926–9.

Israel BA, Schulz AJ, Parker EA, Becker AB. (1998). Review of community-based research: assessing partnership approaches to improve public health. *Annual Review of Public Health,* **19**, 173–202.

Minkler M. (2005). Community-based research partnerships: challenges and opportunities. *Journal of Urban Health,* **82(Suppl. 2)**, ii3–12.

O'Fallon LR, Dearry A. (2002). Community-based participatory research as a tool to advance environmental health sciences. *Environmental Health Perspectives,* **110(Suppl. 2)**, 155–9.

Seifer SD. (2006). Building and sustaining community-institutional partnerships for prevention research: Findings from a national collaborative. *Journal of Urban Health-Bulletin of the New York Academy of Medicine,* **83**, 989–1003.

Websites

Community campus partnerships for health. Available at: ⌕ http://www.ccph.info

Developing and sustaining CBPR partnerships. CBPR resources for community partners. Available at: ⌕ http://depts.washington.edu/ccph/cbpr/u1/u11.php

The Community Tool Kit. Available at: ⌕ http://ctb.ku.edu

PolicyLink Inc. Available at: ⌕ www.policylink.org

References

1 Hall BL. (1992). From margins to center: The development and purpose of participatory action research. *American Sociologist*, **23**: 15–28.

2 Minkler M, Wallerstein N. (2008). Introduction to CBPR: New issues and emphases. In: Minkler M, Wallerstein N (eds) *Community-based participatory research for health*, pp. 5–24. Jossey-Bass, San Francisco.

3 Israel BA, Schulz AJ, Parker EA, Becker AB. (1998). Review of community-based research: assessing partnership approaches to improve public health. *Annual Review of Public Health*, **19**, 173–202.

4 W.K. Kellogg Community Health Scholars Program. (2001). *Stories of impact*. University of Michigan, School of Public Health, CHSP, National Program Office, Ann Arbor.

5 Israel BA, Eng E, Schulz AJ, Parker EA (eds) (2005). *Methods in community-based participatory research for health*. Jossey-Bass, San Francisco.

6 Tervalon M, Murray-Garcia J. (1998). Cultural humility versus cultural competence: a critical distinction in defining physician training outcomes in multicultural education. *Journal of Health Care for the Poor and Underserved*, **9**, 117–25.

7 Reason P, Bradbury H. (2006). *Handbook of action research: participatory inquiry and practice*, concise edn. Sage Publications, London.

8 Cargo M, Mercer SL. (2008). The value and challenges of participatory research: strengthening its practice. *Annual Review of Public Health*, **29**.

9 O'Fallon LR, Dearry A. (1992). Community-based participatory research as a tool to advance environmental health sciences. *Environmental Health Perspectives*, **110(Suppl. 2)**, 155–9.

10 Flicker S, Travers R, Guta A, McDonald S, Meagher A. (2007). Ethical dilemmas in community-based participatory research: recommendations for institutional review boards. *Journal of Urban Health*, **84**, 478–93.

11 Mercer SL, Green LW, Cargo M, *et al.* (2008). Reliability-tested guidelines for assessing participatory research projects. In: Minkler M, Wallerstein N, (eds) *Community-based participatory research for health: from process and outcomes*, 2nd edn. Jossey-Bass, San Francisco.

12 Israel BA, Lantz PM, McGranaghan RJ, *et al.* (2005). Detroit Community-Academic Urban Research Center: in-depth semistructured interview protocol for board evaluation, 1996–2002. In: Israel BA, Eng E, Schulz AJ, Parker EA (eds) *Methods in community-based participatory research for health*, pp. 425–9. Jossey-Bass, San Francisco.

13 Biggs SD. (1989). *Resource-poor farmer participation in research: a synthesis of experiences from nine national agricultural research systems*. The Hague, Netherlands.

14 Price RH, Behrens T. (2003). Working Pasteur's quadrant: harnessing science and action for community change. *American Journal of Community Psychology*, **31**, 219–23.

15 Minkler M, Lee PT, Tom A, *et al.* (2010). Using community-based participatory research to design and initiate a study on immigrant worker health and safety in San Francisco's Chinatown restaurants. *American Journal of Industrial Medicine*, **53**, 361–71.

16 Salvatore AL, Krause N. (2010). Health and working conditions of restaurant workers in San Francisco's Chinatown: report of preliminary findings. *Public Health Reports*, **126(Suppl. 3)**, 62–9.

17 Gebbie K, Rosenstock L, Hernandez LM (eds) (2003). *Who will keep the public healthy? Educating public health professionals for the 21st century*. National Academies Press, Washington DC.

18 Buchanan DR, Miller FG, Wallerstein N. (2007). Ethical issues in community-based participatory research: balancing rigorous research with community participation in community intervention studies. *Progress in Community Health Partnerships*, **1,**153–60.

3.5 Emergency response

Paul Bolton and Frederick M. Burkle, Jr

Objective

After reading this chapter you will be familiar with a basic public health approach to disasters and other crises.

Classification and definition

The term 'disaster' is used in many different ways. To get an overview of all the ways in which the word is used see Box 3.5.1.

A public health crisis is an event(s) that overwhelms the capacity of local systems to maintain a community's health. Therefore, outside resources are temporarily required. Crises can range from specific health issues, such as a disease outbreak in an otherwise unaffected community, to a full-scale disaster with property destruction and/or population displacement

---

Box 3.5.1 Natural and human disasters

Disasters of natural origin
- Sudden onset (earthquakes, landslides, floods, etc.)
- Slower onset (drought, famine, etc.).

Disasters of human origin
- Industrial (e.g. Chernobyl)
- Transportation (e.g. train crash)
- Complex emergencies (e.g. wars, civil strife, and other disasters causing displaced persons and refugees).

Adapted from Noji.[1]

---

and multiple public health issues. This chapter focuses on the more complex disasters and crises (with the understanding that any of the issues and approaches described applies equally to other types of disasters and lesser crises). During disasters mortality and morbidity classically result from the loss of public health social and physical protections (i.e. water, sanitation, health, food, shelter, and fuel). However, for example, loss of transportation, communications, and public safety, among others, can limit or prevent access to and availability of health services resulting in indirect, preventable, or excess mortality and morbidity in a public health crisis. The tsunami in December 2004 that impacted the public health protections in 20 countries, or the Haiti earthquake of 2010 exemplify how big the challenge can be, but smaller disasters can pose equally severe threats to public health.

A decade ago, refugees (those who cross their country's border) out-numbered internally-displaced populations. Currently, the world enjoys the fewest number of declared wars and refugees reported since 1994. However, increasing numbers of internally displaced populations live in tenuous post-conflict environments suffering various low levels of inten-sity of violence, poor governance, limited public health protections, and wide proliferation of weaponry. Despite some notable exceptions such as Rwanda, East Timor and Liberia, 47% of post-conflict countries risk returning to war within a decade. The numbers of internally displaced populations fleeing post-conflict despair or climate change consequences has risen dramatically. Many have fled to cities where dense urban popula-tions have marginal shelter and other essentials resulting in some of the highest infant mortality and under age five mortality rates.

Principles of response

The public health response to any disaster or crises is based on these principles:

1 Securing the basics that all humans require to maintain health.
2 Determining the current and likely health threats to the affected com-munity, given the local environment and the community's resources, knowledge, and behaviour.
3 Finding and providing the resources required to address points 1 and 2.

The first action is a rapid assessment of points 1 and 2 in order to initi-ate step 3 as soon as possible. Too often assessment is delayed due to a misguided fear of delaying assistance. Instead organizations may rush to supply materials and personnel without checking what is actually needed. After a major disaster, these supplies can choke the transport system with unneeded goods while goods that are needed cannot get through. Even in a limited crisis, time and money may be wasted sorting through, stor-ing, and/or destroying useless donated supplies. WHO has issued guide-lines on drug and equipment donations during disasters that have helped improve this situation. These guidelines are available from WHO at: ꙮ http://www.who.int/topics/disasters/en/ (accessed 07 June 2010).

Remember to quickly assess first, by the aphorism 'don't just do some-thing, stand there (and assess)'. If conducting an assessment for a particular agency, then any assessments should include coordination with local gov-ernment, community leaders, and other assisting and coordinating orga-nizations, such as the UN or 'non-governmental organizations' (NGOs). This is necessary to determine their capacities and intentions, to avoid duplication of efforts, and to gain their co-operation in future programmes to address the issues that emerge.

This chapter concentrates on the initial rapid assessment as the basis for response. More detailed assessments and response should be done after the practitioner has been joined by persons skilled in the necessary techniques.

The initial rapid assessment

Assessment involves determining what is needed, and how much. What is needed is decided by considering the principles mentioned above. The initial rapid assessment (IRA) provides an assessment of both direct and indirect (public health preventable) consequences of a disaster

Consider the basics required for health

Clean water and sanitation

Each person requires a minimum of 14 L/day—3 L for drinking (more in hot weather or with exertion), 2 L for food preparation, 5 L for personal hygiene, and 4 L for cleaning clothes and food utensils. Drinking water need not be pure, as long as it is reasonably clear, free of toxic substances and faecal contamination, and has acceptable taste. Simple kits for testing water quality are widely available. Where water is compromised, you should consult with a water and sanitation engineer as soon as possible to reconstruct damaged systems or set up temporary new ones.

Food

Food aid is most often required after disasters of human origin and when people have been displaced from their usual food sources. After natural disasters, crops usually remain intact and people usually do not leave the area, so that large supplies of food are not required. An exception to this can be in cases of flooding.

When outside supplies of food are required the major considerations are adequate calories, adequate micronutrients, acceptability to the local population, and ease of preparation. To survive, a population requires an average of at least 2100 kcal/person/day. If a population is already malnourished, or the emergency lasts months, they will require more. Acceptability to the population refers to supplying foods that people are familiar with and will eat. Ease of preparation is an important factor: if foods require cooking then supplies of fuel (such as piped gas or firewood) must be available. Alternatively, cooked meals may be provided directly in the short term.

When food must be supplied, a nutritional survey conducted by nutritional experts should be done as soon as possible to determine the correct food needs. Securing and transporting adequate supplies of food will require the expertise of a food logistician.

Shelter and clothing

People are best housed in their own homes, except if a disaster has rendered these structures unsafe. They should never be moved from their homes just to ease provision of assistance. If shelter must be provided, people should be housed in small groups, i.e. families or groups of families, to reduce general crowding and exposure to disease. In cold weather, attention to insulation and heating is necessary.

Additional clothing is rarely required as people already have clothes appropriate to their environment and usually manage to retain sufficient supplies. Exceptions may occur where a population is displaced from a hot to a cold area. However, facilities for washing clothes are more frequently required. Estimating and supplying shelter and clothing material needs fall under general logistics.

Health services

Adequate health care provides treatment for illness, reassurance to the population who will feel unsafe without it, and forms the basis of the health information system (see 📖 Information). 'Adequate' means reasonable access to drugs, equipment, and the infrastructure necessary to treat possible problems, as well as trained staff skilled in treating those problems with those facilities.

This is important in considering which, if any, outside medical staff are required. For example, an internist accustomed to Western illnesses and advanced diagnostic facilities is not considered appropriate for a crisis in a tropical area with limited resources; a skilled local nurse would probably be more useful. Good 'access' means that people know about the services, that they are eligible to use them, and they do not have to travel so far, wait so long, or pay so much as to discourage their usage. Setting up these services requires clinical, pharmaceutical, and medical supply personnel with emergency experience.

Medical personnel will also need to assess the potential for epidemics, and assess the need for vaccination. Keep in mind that epidemics cannot occur unless the causative organism is present. For example, cholera cannot occur in a community, no matter how crowded or how poor the sanitation, without the presence of *Vibrio cholerae*. Therefore, epidemic risk assessment includes finding out about the previous disease patterns of both the area of the disaster and the affected population.

Among disaster-affected populations exposed to exhaustion, malnutrition, and crowding, vaccination for preventable diseases, such as measles, assumes prime importance due to increased susceptibility, morbidity, and mortality under these conditions. Measles vaccination is recommended for children aged from 6 months to 12 years. This is particularly important among populations for which measles vaccine coverage prior to the disaster was low. Coverage of other routine child vaccinations should be maintained,

For large-scale emergencies WHO provides a recommended list of drugs and materials, including quantities, to serve 10,000 people for 3 months. These materials are available in kit forms.[2]

Information

This is often neglected, but is nevertheless a fundamental requirement of the disaster response. In unaccustomed circumstances, people require new information on how to maintain their health. They also require information on what is happening and what is likely to happen. In the absence of information rumour will take over, causing insecurity and mistrust of those handling the emergency. Rumours may even force inappropriate diversion of resources to minor or non-existent problems, to appease the population. Therefore, a system of good communication between those assessing the situation and in charge, and the affected population, is vital. Any accessible means of transmitting information is appropriate, as long as it communicates directly with the population and not through a third party, to avoid distortion. Collaboration with local persons in designing the messages is important to ensure a style and approach which is understandable to the population. Methods can include radio and TV, pamphlets, posters, advice by health workers in the clinics, and even megaphones.

Consider the current and likely health threats, given local conditions

Current health problems

Describing population health should include measurement of crude mortality rates, causes of mortality, and the nature of health problems—their current incidence and severity (including case fatality rates) and potential for change. Rates are important to determining disease trends in the face of varying population size. Measuring rates requires both numerators (the frequency of events, such as illness or death) and denominators (an estimate of population size).

For the initial assessment, numerator information can be gathered by visiting the available treatment centres, talking with staff, and reviewing daily records of diagnoses and treatment. These records form the basis of the HIS, which should be established as part of the initial assessment. In most cases setting up the Health Information System (HIS) requires developing case definitions for the important health problems and establishing treatment protocols to ensure sufficient medical supplies for treatment and prevention. Case definitions are required because laboratory facilities are usually not adequate to test all suspected cases of illness. Rather, the (usually limited) testing facilities are used to confirm the presence of specific illnesses among the population (particularly those with epidemic potential, such as meningitis) by testing the first suspect cases, and to develop case definitions for these diseases once confirmed. These case definitions are then used to diagnose subsequent suspected cases.

If the affected population is spread over a wide are and transport is poor, an effort should also be made to visit areas far from the treatment centres to ask people about the problems affecting them. In these situations, rates calculated on the basis of the HIS are likely to be underestimates, since many people will not attend the health centres. However, by visiting outlying areas you should still be able to form a general idea of the main problems and trends.

Denominators can be difficult to calculate. Although much less useful, proportional mortality ratios can be used if the denominator cannot be determined with any confidence. As soon as possible, resources need to be used to disaggregate the crude mortality rates to determine infant, under aged five, and maternal mortality rates. Disaggregating crude mortality rates defines vulnerable populations and the severity of involvement (i.e. children, women, elderly, and disabled).

All efforts should be made to identify the leaders among the population, to meet them early on, get their impressions of the main problems, and enlist their support for your efforts.

Another important aspect of current health and disease threat is the health knowledge and behaviour of the population. Failure to take precautions, such as washing hands, can render populations more susceptible to illness. Such behaviours are relatively more important when one is dealing with overcrowding, or with a specific health crisis like a single transmissible disease. Local knowledge and behaviour can be assessed by direct observation, and by interviews in which local people are asked how they prevent particular illnesses of concern, such as diarrhoea. Gaps in knowledge and behaviour form part of the information needs discussed previously.

General condition of the population

Talk with health workers and walk through the community. Observe and talk with people. The aim is to form an overall impression of the state of nutrition and available supplies, including clean water and food, cooking supplies and fuel, shelter and clothing, particularly in a cold environment:

- assess whether people appear to be getting enough supplies
- observe how people get water, to estimate the risk and potential for contamination
- ask how people are disposing of their faeces
- estimate the adequacy of access to medical treatment, given the distance, available transport, cost, and degree of crowding of the clinics.

Condition of the environment

Assess the need for shelter in terms of the weather. Get a weather report. Observe the water sources and whether the water from these sources looks clean or turbid. Observe where people are defaecating, the adequacy of available latrines, water drainage, and the likelihood that the water supply and faeces will come in contact. If there is a sewerage system, investigate whether the system has been damaged, whether it is being attended to, and whether water treatment supplies are adequate.

If the area is known to harbour transmissible disease, then monitor for those diseases as part of the disease surveillance system. Supplies needed to address these illnesses must be investigated, and prepared by the health team and logisticians. As previously noted, remember that transmissible agents can only occur if the agent is present in the environment. Information on disease endemicity is usually available from local authorities, and from regional health organizations like the Pan-American Health Organization (PAHO).

Injuries and diseases augmented by crowding—such as any respiratory or gastrointestinal infections—will be more likely where populations have left their homes and are crowded into an unfamiliar environment.

Security issues

These may be both health problems in their own right, such as violence, or threats that preclude access to resources and affect behaviour. For example, people may be unable to go to a clinic or collect supplies if this exposes them to danger. Similarly, health personnel may be unwilling to work or unable to do their jobs. Even limited health emergencies may engender violence, often through ill-feeling and rumour due to lack of information. Security can be assessed by talking with local people; addressing these issues requires close co-operation with the police or even the military. Having assessed what is needed, assess how much must be provided. This depends on how much is required less how much is available, which comes down to the size of the population and local capacity.

Size of the affected or vulnerable population

This is one of the most important pieces of information about the population. Without this 'denominator' the amounts of resources required cannot be assessed. Moreover, rates cannot be calculated, making it impossible, in public health terms, to determine the size of a problem or trends by prevalence or incidence.

Early in an emergency rough estimates are acceptable, and can be based on pre-existing information, estimates of knowledgeable persons, or even, in the case of a mass displacement of people to an open area, 'eyeballing' from a high piece of ground. Later more sophisticated sampling and survey methods should be used by a demographer or epidemiologist, or even a count if possible.

Demography of the affected population

Usually, some groups are more vulnerable to problems than others. In a limited crisis, such as a disease outbreak, this may be because of variations in disease susceptibility—children are more susceptible to vaccine-preventable diseases (i.e. polio, measles, H1N1). In a full-scale disaster with crowding and limited resources, some groups are at a disadvantage in securing their needs. This is particularly true in developing countries and can include women, particularly if pregnant or lactating, children, especially those without adult protectors, elderly people, and those with disabilities. The size and location of these groups should be determined and particular attention given to meeting their needs.

Assessing capacity

In meeting needs, the emphasis should be on reconstructing or supporting the system that met those needs before the emergency, rather than on creating a parallel system. Determine what that system was or is, and who is in charge. Work with that person to identify what they need to meet the current crisis, and try to provide it. This is particularly true after a disaster, yet this simple principle is often ignored. Where a system has been damaged, rather than simply overwhelmed, this does not mean reconstituting it the way it was, but rather providing those elements required to meet demand. For example, in an emergency it is not be possible to rebuild a hospital, but tents, supplies, etc. can be provided

Compared with the creation of a new system, reconstruction:
- requires fewer outside resources
- uses locally appropriate resources and so will be sustainable
- builds local capacity to address this emergency, other problems, and future emergencies
- provides employment
- uses people who know the local population best
- restores a sense of self-reliance.

Assessing local systems in detail requires persons skilled in that field, for example, a sanitation engineer to assess sewerage, a health information specialist or epidemiologist to assess a health information system. Suitable local people with these skills are preferable to outsiders because these will be the people who will maintain these systems in the long term.

Surveillance

After the initial assessment, a surveillance system must be created to monitor health trends and detect incipient epidemics. In any displaced and crowded population, surveillance should include measles and the common serious diseases known to occur among the population and in the geographic area. These may include important epidemic diseases like cholera and other diarrhoeal diseases, dysentery, malaria, dengue fever, meningitis, hepatitis, typhoid and paratyphoid, typhus, and viral encephalitis. Although measles and other vaccine preventable diseases are on the wane in many parts of Africa and the developing world, most countries, especially the least developed, remain at risk for reversals when politico-military situations worsen.

Surveillance information must be provided to all involved, including the affected population and those in charge politically. It will provide the information to determine whether the response to the crisis is effective. The surveillance system must be capable of rapidly investigating and either confirming or debunking rumours.

Setting up surveillance will require consultation with the other organizations providing health assistance to agree on standard case definitions and reporting formats. Access to a laboratory will be required to confirm diagnoses, particularly in the early phases of an epidemic. The system should be under the direction of an epidemiologist.

The International Health Regulations (IHR) treaty was put into effect in 2007 following the SARS pandemic, and provides for improved surveillance capacity and response assistance from neighbouring countries in those nations with limited resources. Although much needs to be accomplished to improve surveillance in many regions of the world, clearly the IHR has improved capacity to monitor and manage outbreaks.

Logistics

For all external supplies, consider:
- where to get them in sufficient quality and quantity
- how to pay for them
- how quickly they are needed
- available transportation methods for these requirements
- how the situation is likely to change.

All these considerations will require co-operation between an experienced logistician and local people familiar with local suppliers and markets.

Skills and knowledge

After a disaster, the following skills and knowledge are required:
- rapid assessment and survey skills
- clinical skills
- water and sanitation
- food and nutrition
- logistics knowledge
- familiarity with the local language, culture, environment, and affected population
- relationships with important local persons whose assistance and support will be needed
- sensitivity in dealing with the affected population
- the ability to communicate ideas and problems well, and to write coherent and clear reports
- the ability to deal with the media.

Personnel

The following personnel are required:
- project director
- epidemiologist
- logistician
- local people familiar with local culture and language
- water and sanitation expert
- nutritionist
- clinical staff familiar with likely problems and resources.

Fallacies

In his book *The public health consequences of disasters*,[1] Eric Noji describes some of the important myths and realities about disasters collected by the PAHO. Awareness of these myths is useful in approaching emergency response:

1 Foreign medical volunteers are always needed
2 Any kind of international assistance is urgently required
3 Epidemics are inevitable after disasters
4 Disasters bring out the worst in people
5 Affected populations are too shocked and helpless to help themselves
6 Disasters kill randomly
7 Locating disaster victims in temporary settlements is the best shelter solution
8 Food aid is always required after natural disasters
9 Clothing is always needed
10 Conditions return to normal after a few weeks.

All of these myths, except 4 and 10, have been dealt with previously in this chapter. Most workers would agree that disasters overwhelmingly bring out the positive side of human nature, and that community spirit is usually enhanced. Far from resolving quickly, the effects of most disasters last for years or even decades. This is true even in developed countries, where increased debt and interruption in economic activity can create long-term financial burdens.

Future humanitarian crises

2008 country-specific surveillance estimates of the major causes of child mortality reveal that 49% of deaths under age five occur in five countries: India, Nigeria, Democratic Republic of the Congo, Pakistan, and China. Infectious diseases caused 68% of deaths; with the largest percentage from pneumonia, diarrhoea, and malaria.[3] Yet, there is encouraging evidence of an accelerating decline in childhood mortality in 13 regions of the world, including sub-Saharan Africa.[4]

Meanwhile, the risk of asymmetrical or unconventional wars and conflicts, such as those seen in Iraq and Afghanistan, remains high. They characteristically result in pervasive insecurity, especially for civilians and aid workers, and in prolonged and catastrophic loss of public health protections, infrastructure and services.

More people now live in urban than in rural settings. Rapid urbanization in many African and Asian countries has proved unsustainable. Sanitation is being ignored and the prevalence of infectious diseases has increased, contributing to severe health indices and large gaps between the 'have' and 'have-not' populations. Many urbanites are relegated to living in dense disaster-prone areas (e.g. Mumbai, India, or Port au Prince, Haiti), devoid of public health protections.

Climate change migration from rising oceans has already taken place in Kiribati and other Polynesian islands where public health emphasis is on educating populations in adaptation, resilience, and the inevitable migration planning. It is estimated that up to 75 million island refugees will require placement and aid by 2050.

'Emergencies of scarcity' the term used to describe increasing areas of the world suffering from scarcity of water, food, and energy have resulted in unaffordable food prices and stunted growth in children in developing countries like Guatemala and in 'land grabbing' of arable lands in fragile poverty-stricken countries (i.e. Madagascar) by rich food import-dependent countries. Eighty per cent of the wars during the last 3 decades occurred in 23 of the 34 most biodiverse areas of the world, where many highly sensitive sustainable vascular plants and vertebrae are being threatened. Many biodiverse areas have not recovered.

These and other public health crises threaten to dominate humanitarian requirements in the coming decades.[5] The aforementioned principles of assessment and response are critical as well, although ensuring population-based public health protections will be more challenging to humanitarian practice.

Conclusion

As a public health professional or team there is much you can do to help in a disaster. Effective disaster and crisis response is predicated on rapid assessment of the situation prior to initiating a response and on focusing on the public health principles outlined in this chapter.

Further resources

Hanquet G. (ed.) (1997) *Refugee health: an approach to emergency situations*. Macmillan/Medecins Sans Frontieres, London.

Heymann DL. (ed.) (2005). *Control of communicable diseases manual*. American Public Health Association, Washington, DC.

Office for Foreign Disaster Assistance. (2006). *Field operations guide*. Available at: ✍ http://www. usaid.gov/our_work/humanitarian_assistance/disaster_assistance/resources/pdf/fog_v4.pdf (accessed 30 January 2006).

Perrin P. (1966). *War and public health*. International Committee of the Red Cross, Geneva.

References

1 Noji E (ed.) (1997). *The public health consequences of disasters*. Oxford University Press, New York.

2 World Health Organization (1998). *The new emergency health kit*, WHO document WHO/ DAP/98.10. World Health Organization, Geneva.

3 Black RE, Cousens S, Johnson HL, *et al.* (2010). Global, regional, and national causes of child mortality in 2008: a systematic analysis. *Lancet*, **375**, 1967–87.

4 Rajaratnam JK, Marcus JR, Flaxman AD, *et al.* (2010). Neonatal, postnatal, childhood, and under-5 mortality for 187 countries, 1970–2010: a systematic analysis of progress towards Millennium Development Goal 4. *Lancet*, **375**, 1988–2008.

5 Burkle FM Jr. (2010). Future humanitarian crises: challenges to practice, policy, and public health. *Prehospital and Disaster Medicine*, **25**, 194–9.

3.6 Assuring screening programmes

Angela Raffle, Alex Barratt, and
J. A. Muir Gray

All screening programmes do harm, some do good as well.
UK National Screening Committee

Objectives

After reading this chapter, you will:
- understand why screening needs a programme not just a test
- recognize the biases that limit the validity of observational evidence
- be clearer about the public health tasks in screening
- understand that values and beliefs shape screening policy as much as evidence.

What screening is and is not: definitions

Screening is testing people who do not suspect they have a problem. It is done:
- to reduce risk of future ill health (e.g. screen for raised blood pressure, intervene with drugs, reduce risk of stroke)
- to give information (e.g. screen pregnant woman, identify unborn baby has Down's syndrome, couple keeps baby, but is forewarned).

Tests or inquiries once disease is symptomatic are not screening. They are for prompt recognition or for clinical management.

Screening involves a system not just a test

There are two ways of looking at a screening system. You can:
- Consider everything that must be in place to deliver a service. This helps you ensure that high quality programmes are delivered to your population. The elements include:
  - a register for issuing invitations and reminders
  - a system for checking that follow-up steps happen
  - screening tests
  - investigations
  - interventions
  - information and support for participants
  - staff training
  - policy making

- co-ordination locally and nationally
- setting standards and ensuring they are met
- commissioning research to improve screening
- Consider the basics steps that a participant goes through. This looks like a flow diagram (see Figure 3.6.1); it helps with understanding what screening does.

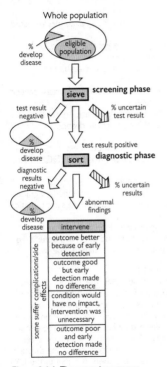

Figure 3.6.1 The screening process.

What screening does

You need to know the range, and likelihood, of different consequences in order to make decisions about policy. Individuals need this information so they can decide whether to participate. Whether a consequence is judged 'good' or 'bad' varies from person to person. Figure 3.6.1 can help you map the consequences.

The screening test is not a diagnostic test. It is only like a sieve. It sorts large numbers of low risk people, into a group at higher risk who then go on to a diagnostic phase, and those at lower risk (but not no risk).

The main consequences, using breast screening as an example, are listed below. The individual may:
- be reassured at the time of screening and not get the disease, i.e. have a negative result and not develop breast cancer
- be reassured, but get the disease, i.e. have a negative result but subsequently be diagnosed with breast cancer
- have a life-impacting disease averted, i.e. screen-detected breast cancer whose treatment prevents breast cancer death
- have an intervention but develop life-impacting disease, i.e. screen-detected breast cancer, but still die of breast cancer despite intervention
- have a potentially harmful intervention for a symptomless phenomenon i.e. screen-detected ductal carcinoma *in situ* (DCIS) that would have caused no problem
- have an intervention, but with no extra benefit, with an equally good prognosis if diagnosed symptomatically, i.e. screen-detected low grade breast cancer, or DCIS, that would have been curable on symptomatic presentation
- have an abnormality of uncertain significance detected, leading to follow-up, surveillance, possible intervention, and uncertain benefit, i.e. mammographic changes leading to annual repeat mammography.

Who is helped and who is harmed?

As a public health practitioner you will see that the people genuinely helped are those who, as a direct result of screen-detection, avoid death or serious disease. The perception of most participants and clinicians can be very different. Almost everyone with a screen-detected abnormality feels thankful, and some clinicians believe they have cured all the people detected. This is the *popularity paradox*. *Over-detection* is a major screening-related harm, yet it contributes to the popularity of screening through the illusion that large numbers of people are helped. A nurse in the UK cervical screening programme will see over 150 women with screen-detected abnormality, for each one who has serious disease prevented.[1] For 10,000 men age 50, the number who would die of prostate cancer is 30, yet 4200 of them will have histologically-confirmed prostate cancer if screened,[2] which leads to substantial harm from treatment-related deaths and side-effects, such as incontinence and impotence.

Balancing harm, benefit, and affordability

There is always a trade-off between benefit, harm, and affordability. The numbers flowing into different parts of the system are influenced by:
* the acceptability and accessibility of screening, e.g. convenience, publicity, information, frequency of testing
* the definition of the eligible group, e.g. age range
* changing the numbers of people with positive screening results, e.g. by more tests, by double or treble reading, or by changing the cut-off between positive and negative
* changing the number of people diagnosed with the disease, e.g. multiple investigations or changing the cut-off used to distinguish people with the disease from those without it.

Measuring the impact of screening

Observational evidence can be highly misleading because of biases that make outcome in screened people look good even if screening makes no difference.

Three key biases in screening
* *The healthy screening effect:* people who come for screening tend to be healthier than those who do not.
* *Length time bias:* screening is best at picking up long-lasting, slow-growing disease. This pulls good-prognosis cases into the observed group, whereas rapidly progressive, and therefore poor-prognosis cases, are less likely to be picked up.
* *Lead time bias:* the apparent survival time for people with screen-detected disease is longer simply because they are detected at an earlier point in the course of the disease.

Three sources of evidence for evaluating screening in the population
Measures of test performance tell you little about the impact on health of the whole programme so do not count as evidence.
* *Randomized controlled trials (RCTs):* people are recruited, then randomly assigned to receive screening or usual care. RCTs need to be large and last a long time, but are less expensive than allowing unevaluated screening to develop haphazardly. They are the only reliable source of evidence of benefit and harm.
* *Time trend studies:* these involve observation of trends in incidence and deaths once screening is in place. They are useful if properly conducted, and comparison with countries or regions without screening can help.
* *Case control studies:* these compare past screening in people with the disease, or who have died from the disease, and controls. Even with matching and validation of screening history they still consistently overestimate the effect of screening[3] because of confounding .

If more than one study of a particular method has been done, a systematic review of all the evidence should be prepared.

Two additional sources of information about screening
in the population

Modelling studies

These make theoretical predictions about screening outcomes and examine the effect of varying frequency, age range, intervention threshold, etc.
They are strongest if based on RCT evidence.

Pilot or demonstration projects

These can solve practical issues. They are not reliable for assessing benefit
and harm.

Presenting information about benefits and harms

Concern about uptake rates has meant that benefits of screening have
been emphasized more than harms. This slanted approach disregards the
rights of autonomous adults to reach informed decisions and is no longer considered appropriate or ethical. Policy in the UK and elsewhere
now requires that balanced information be available to people considering
screening. Decision aids for presenting such information are starting to
be developed.[4]

Practical tasks: implementing screening programmes

Starting a programme from scratch

It helps if you have:
- an agreed national policy and roll-out plan
- ring-fenced resources which can be spent only on screening
- training centres and demonstration sites
- consumer involvement
- reliable information technology.

Some of your challenges locally are:
- *Agreeing the boundary of the local programme:* administrative and
  provider catchments seldom match
- Getting co-operation from all organizations with a part to play.
- *Communicating understanding of the programme:* to staff, participants
  and public.

Sorting out a mess

Haphazard testing often starts ahead of national policy. Converting this
to a quality assured equitable screening programme is difficult, but can be
done. Major problems are:
- there is inconsistent training and practice but everyone thinks their
  way is right
- commercial, private practice, and research vested interests abound
- meeting resistance when you change from intense screening for a few,
  to less intense for all.

Carrying on screening

Once a programme is up and running, things will go wrong unless you keep an eye on it. Make sure there is:

- a nominated public health lead who knows the key players and understands the performance data
- a co-ordinating group meeting 1–3 times a year
- an annual report including a forward plan
- regular training/updating for all staff.

Quality assurance

Achieving quality depends on:

- system design and resources, e.g. staff training
- monitoring and readjustment, e.g. region-wide collation of annual performance data.

Box 3.6.1 illustrates an example of a quality assurance standard, taken from the programme to reduce risk of sight-threatening retinopathy in people with insulin dependent diabetes:[5]

Box 3.6.1 Example of a quality standard

- *Objective:* to take retinal photographs that are of adequate quality
- *Criteria:* percentage of patients whose photographs are ungradeable for at least one eye, excluding eyes with cataracts
- *Minimum standard (all programmes must meet):* less than or equal to 5%
- *Achievable standard (current top quartile):* less than or equal to 3%.

Quality is not solely about effectiveness. The seven components in Donabedian's definition of quality[6] include optimality and equity. Exclusive pursuit of effectiveness increases resource use irrespective of opportunity cost.

Practical tasks: controlling unwanted screening

You need to be able to stop unwanted screening in order to protect your public from diversion of resources and direct harm.

Unwanted screening arises because:

- *New screening self-starts irrespective of evidence:* drivers include market forces, consumer pressure, clinician enthusiasm, and media pressure, including celebrity endorsement, with usually a complex and manipulative inter-relationship between them
- Within existing programmes there is pressure to intensify irrespective of marginal cost-benefit. This is a response to inherent limitations (undetectable cases, cases outside the eligible group).

Key steps in controlling unwanted screening are:
- *Understand why people want the screening:* go and meet with and listen to clinicians, pressure groups, campaigning journalists.
- *Explicitly acknowledge the reasons why people want it:* don't dismiss concerns or belittle their interpretation of evidence.
- Assemble and communicate evidence and information about the consequences the screening would really have, and about alternative ways of addressing the problem.
- *Carefully introduce specific enforcement measures:* for publicly-funded programmes this could include declining requests for unscheduled tests.
- Regulate the advertising of tests so that consumers are guaranteed to receive balanced, accurate, and evidence-based information about benefits, harms, quality and price for the tests they are being offered.[7]

Screening and the law

Out of court settlements are commonplace. In rare cases that have been defended, some judgements have related to standards you would expect from diagnosis, not screening. Judges are influenced by the fact that an expert witness finds abnormality in the test the screener judged normal. This ignores:
- *Outcome bias:* the witness knows the outcome for the subject, the screener does not
- *Context bias:* the witness is an experienced doctor and has days to look at the sample, the screener is competent only at screening and has a few minutes.

Equipped with careful preparation and an expert lawyer who understands screening it is possible to successfully defend a service that meets recognized standards. We think it vital that Health Departments enable this to happen more.

Making screening policy

Who makes policy decisions about screening
Generally decisions are regional or national. They may relate to:
- state-funded provision of quality assured national programmes (as in the UK)
- state reimbursement for approved screening, with provision by both public and private providers (as in Australia)
- recommendations to consumers, who decide if they can afford a health policy that includes the screening (as in the USA).

What factors influence screening policy

In theory you base your policy on evidence and resources. In practice, values and beliefs have a profound influence. Box 3.6.2 illustrates the case of mammography recommendations in the USA.

Box 3.6.2 Case study: mammography recommendations in USA

When the USA National Institutes of Health recommended in January 1997 that evidence was insufficient to recommend screening mammography for all women in their forties, the response was dramatic.

- At the news conference the Panel was accused of condemning American women to death.
- The Panel's chairman was summoned to a Senate Sub-Committee.
- The Senate voted 98 to 0 in favour of supporting mammography for this age group.
- The head of the NIH said he was shocked by the report and asked for the evidence to be looked at again.

By March 1997 the Panel had changed its recommendation and advised that women in their forties should get a screening mammogram every 1–2 years.

The *New England Journal of Medicine* published a review article[8] lamenting the lack of logic. However, what the Senate was articulating were the values of American society. If mammography offers any potential for health gain how dare anyone recommend that the individual should not have it?

Many other societies take a collectivist approach and 'take it as read' that the rights of an individual to have any intervention that could be beneficial has to be balanced with the needs of others who require a share of the health care resource.

The public health role is to present information for decision-making as clearly as we can, but the wise politician, who needs to survive the next election, may take a decision that matches public values and beliefs. In the UK, for example, we have an evidence-based national decision against introducing a prostate cancer screening programme, but the NHS provides prostate-specific antigen (PSA) testing for individual men. The strong belief in PSA testing among public and politicians made it politically unacceptable to have an outright embargo.

The last word

Screening, like most other public health services, is at best a zero gratitude business.

Further resources

Barratt A, Irwig I, Glasziou P, *et al*. (1999). Users' Guides to the Medical Literature XVII: how to use guidelines and recommendations about screening. *Journal of the American Medical Association* **281**, 2029–34.

NHS Evidence—Screening (formerly a Specialist Library of the National Electronic Library for Health). Available at: ℘ http://www.phgen-meeting.eu/programme/graph-int (accessed 31 May 2012)

Russell LB. (1994). *Educated guesses, making policy decisions about screening tests*. University of California Press, Ewing.

Raffle A. (2009). Screening. Interactive learning. Health knowledge. Available at: ℘ http://www.healthknowledge.org.uk/interactive-learning/screening (accessed August 2010).

Raffle A, Gray JAM. (2007). *Screening; evidence and practice*. Oxford University Press, Oxford.

Tritter J. (ed.) (2001). *Health Expectations*, Vol. 4. Blackwell Science Ltd, Oxford.

References

1 Raffle AE, Alden B, Quinn M, Babb PJ, Brett MT. (2003). Outcomes of screening to prevent cancer: analysis of cumulative incidence of cervical abnormality and modelling of cases and deaths prevented. *British Medical Journal* **326**, 901–4.

2 Frankel S, Davey Smith G, Donovan J, Neal D. (2003). Screening for prostate cancer. *Lancet* **361**, 1122–8.

3. Moss SM. (1991). Case-control studies of screening. *International Journal of Epidemiology* **20**, 1–6.

4. Barratt A, Trevena L, Davey HM, McCaffery K. (2004). Use of decision aids to support informed choices about screening. *British Medical Journal*, **329**, 507–10.

5 NHS Diabetic Eye Screening Programme. National screening programme for sight-threatening retinopathy website. Available at: ℘ www.nscretinopathy.org.uk (accessed (30 November 2004).

6 Donabedian A. (2003). *An introduction to quality assurance in health care*. Oxford University Press, Oxford.

7 Raffle, A. (2010). Guest editorial: advertising private tests for well people. *Clinical Evidence*, **2**.

8 Fletcher SW. (1997). Whither scientific deliberation in health policy recommendation? Alice in the Wonderland of breast-cancer screening. *New England Journal of Medicine*, **336**, 1180–3.

3.7 Genetics

Alison Stewart and Hilary Burton

Objectives

After studying this chapter you should:
- appreciate that genes are important determinants of health and that almost all disease results from the combined effects of genetic and environmental factors
- be aware that new knowledge about the relationships between genetic variants and disease is changing aspects of disease management and prevention
- understand the use of genetics in screening programmes and other disease prevention strategies
- be able to use a knowledge of genetics within routine public health practice, for example in health needs assessment, health technology assessment, service review and evaluation
- be aware of the debate on the ethical, legal and social issues surrounding the use of genetic information in public health and healthcare
- be aware of the potential impact of new technologies that enable rapid and inexpensive sequencing of whole genomes and of the need for critical, evidence-based assessment of new genomic tests and interventions

Introduction

Almost all human variation and disease processes are determined both by environmental and by genetic factors. Traditionally, public health has focused on the environmental determinants of health. Although this focus remains valid, new knowledge about the relationships between genetic variation and disease is leading to opportunities for both disease management and prevention. Public health practitioners need a basic understanding of developments in genetic and genomic science, and to be aware of the implications for their practice.

Genetics: the basics

Genetic variation exists in all populations. This variation arises from changes in the DNA sequences of genes. Rare genetic variants are usually known as mutations and are generally harmful. More common variants, known as polymorphisms, tend to have more subtle effects on function. Each individual has two copies of every gene; one copy is inherited from each parent. The two copies, known as alleles, may be identical in sequence or may differ from each other.

Many genetic variants relevant for clinical disease have been identified in almost every sphere of medicine and the pace of discovery is accelerating. Genetic variation also affects responses to pharmaceutical agents, diet, and environmental exposures such as smoking.

The frequencies of specific genetic mutations and polymorphisms vary in different populations. For example, genetic mutations causing sickle cell disease are much more frequent in Afro-Caribbean populations than in northern European populations.

Although the nature of the interaction between genes and environment ranges over a wide spectrum, three main categories can be distinguished, as follows (for examples, see Box 3.7.1).

Box 3.7.1 Relationships between genes and disease

Examples of genetic diseases
- Duchenne muscular dystrophy
- Cystic fibrosis
- Adult polycystic kidney disease
- Phenylketonuria
- Sickle cell disease
- Neurofibromatosis

Examples of rare genetic subtypes of common complex diseases
- Familial hypercholesterolaemia (atherosclerosis)
- BRCA1 and BRCA2 in breast cancer
- Hereditary non-polyposis colorectal cancer (HNPCC)
- PSEN1 and PSEN2 in Alzheimer disease
- Maturity onset diabetes of the young

Examples of polymorphisms associated with common complex disorders
- ACE gene, DD polymorphism (myocardial infarction)
- Factor 5 Leiden (preeclampsia)
- TCF7L2 gene, IVS3C>T polymorphism (Type 2 diabetes).

Conditions where a mutation(s) in a single gene diagnoses or strongly predicts disease development

Dominant conditions (for example, neurofibromatosis type 1) occur if one allele is mutated, whereas recessive conditions (for example cystic fibrosis) arise only if both alleles are mutant. These diseases, conventionally referred to as genetic diseases, can be transmitted from generation to generation according to recognizable patterns of inheritance or may arise sporadically as a result of a mutation in one of the gametes (sperm or egg) that gave rise to the affected individual.

Genetic diseases are often characterized by high penetrance: that is, there is a high probability that an individual who carries a mutation will develop the disease, though symptoms and severity may vary. Genetic diseases are usually rare, but collectively contribute significantly to mortality and morbidity within the population. Many thousands of mutations causing genetic disease have now been identified. Note also that some genetic diseases are caused not by mutations in single genes but by deletions, duplications or rearrangements of whole chromosomes or large sections of chromosomes. An example is Down syndrome, caused by an extra copy of chromosome 21.

Rare, highly penetrant genetic subsets of common complex diseases

For example, coronary heart disease, cancers, and diabetes. Such single-gene subsets of common disease typically account for up to 5% of the total burden of the disease in a population.

The bulk of common complex disorders

This is where the presence of a polymorphism in a particular gene may increase the risk of the condition, but is not strongly predictive. Whether the disease actually develops or not depends on the consequence of interactions with other genes and with environmental factors. Polymorphisms associated with common diseases are being identified by large case-control studies known as genome-wide association studies.

At present most public health applications of genetics are concerned with the management or prevention of genetic diseases or the rare genetic subtypes of common disease.

What is a genetic test?

Most clinical applications of genetics involve the use of genetic tests. There is much confusion about what the term means. There are two main usages:

- A test for a *genetic disease:* when used in this way, a 'genetic test' may mean any type of test—DNA-based, biochemical, radiological, etc.—that can be used to diagnose or predict the disease. For example, sickle cell disease is typically diagnosed by biochemical analysis of haemoglobin variants.
- A test of the *genetic material* (usually DNA).

It is important to understand that the implications of a test result depend on its diagnostic or predictive power, not on what material is being tested. Any sort of test for a genetic disease is usually strongly predictive or diagnostic for the disease. However, the predictive power of DNA tests varies widely: a test for the mutation that causes Huntington disease has a very high predictive power, but the predictive power of a test for a common DNA polymorphism associated with coronary heart disease is likely to be no higher—and may be lower—than a test for, say, blood lipid levels. Weakly predictive DNA tests are sometimes called susceptibility or predisposition tests, to indicate their lower predictive power.

At present, most DNA tests that are used in a clinical context are tests for genetic diseases (that is, single-gene or chromosomal disorders). They are typically carried out by specialized clinical laboratories. Test interpretation can be very complex, requiring the skills and experience of both laboratory scientists and clinical geneticists.

You should be aware of the importance of thorough evaluation of any genetic tests (DNA based or otherwise) that are used in clinical practice.[1] A framework for evaluation of genetic tests has been developed: the ACCE framework (Box 3.7.2). Increasingly, public health skills are required both for test evaluation and in the assessment of new genetic technologies (for a case study, see Box 3.7.3).

Box 3.7.2 The ACCE framework for evaluation of genetic tests

The ACCE framework[2] comprises assessment of a test's:

- *Analytical validity*: the accuracy with which it measures or detects the analyte (for example, a specific DNA variant(s)).
- *Clinical validity*: its ability to diagnose or predict a specific disease
- *Clinical utility*: the likelihood that its use will lead to an improved health outcome
- *Ethical, legal and social implications*: its impact on, for example, psychosocial well-being or the potential for stigmatization or discrimination. (Some commentators suggest that ethical, legal and social implications should be thought of as an aspect of clinical utility).

Box 3.7.3 Cell-free foetal DNA

Cell-free nucleic acids (both DNA and RNA) originating from the foetus are present in the maternal blood from early pregnancy and are a potential source of genetic information about the unborn baby. Analysis of cell-free foetal DNA can be used for foetal sex determination (important for sex-linked conditions), assessment of foetal Rh blood group status, antenatal diagnosis of certain genetic diseases and, potentially in the future, identification of chromosomal abnormalities such as Down syndrome. It is vital that the use of this technology is meticulously evaluated against current testing that involves more invasive methods (amniocentesis or chorionic villus sampling of fetal tissue), particularly with regard to test performance, clinical utility and wider ethical issues such as the possible use of sex determination for non-medical reasons.

Genetics and disease prevention

There are applications of genetics in disease prevention at all stages of life. The ethical implications of each type of preventive strategy must be carefully considered.

Antenatal and preconception genetic screening

You should be aware of the distinction between genetic *testing* and genetic *screening*. If a couple know they are at risk of conceiving a child affected by a specific genetic disease (usually because of a family history of the disease, or the previous birth of an affected child) they may choose to undertake *antenatal genetic testing* within the context of specialist genetic services. If the foetus is affected the couple may, if they wish, decide to terminate the pregnancy. For some conditions the option of pre-implantation genetic diagnosis may be available. This procedure involves the use of *in vitro* fertilization to create embryos. One or two cells from each embryo are tested to see if the embryo is affected by the disease; only unaffected embryos are used to establish a pregnancy. Here, there will generally be no public health involvement unless there are issues of prioritization or resource allocation.

In contrast, programmes of *antenatal genetic screening* operate at the population level; those who are offered screening have no individual increased risk. An antenatal genetic screening programme may be considered if a serious genetic disease occurs at an appreciable frequency in a particular population or subpopulation. The aim is to make it possible for couples to avoid the birth of an affected child, should they wish to do so. Examples include sickle cell disease in populations of Afro-Caribbean origin, and beta-thalassaemia in Asian and some Mediterranean populations. Most programmes involve an initial screening test to identify individuals or couples at increased risk.[3] At-risk couples are then offered definitive diagnostic testing of the foetus. It is essential that couples taking up an offer of screening do so voluntarily and without coercion.

In some communities screening may be offered before conception to identify carriers of recessive disorders and provide advice on how to avoid the subsequent birth of an affected child. One example of such *preconception screening* is carrier testing for Tay Sachs disease and a small panel of other conditions in communities of Ashkenazi Jewish origin, where carrier frequencies for these conditions are elevated. There are examples of such programmes in Canada, the US and Australia.

The basic public health principles that apply to all screening programmes (for example, definition of the target population group; evaluation of the screening and diagnostic tests; ensuring autonomous informed choice) also apply to antenatal genetic screening. As a public health practitioner involved in setting up, supervising or auditing a genetic screening programme you should be aware of additional criteria that are relevant to screening for genetic conditions (Box 3.7.4).

Box 3.7.4 **Extra issues in screening for genetic conditions**

• Where a specific ethnic group is targeted, the programme must be sensitive to the cultural and ethical norms of the population and to the dangers of stigmatization.
• For those undergoing diagnostic testing, professional genetic counseling is generally required.
• If antenatal screening for a recessive condition also identifies unaffected carriers of the condition, policies must be in place for deciding whether and when the child should be informed of their carrier status.
• The implications for other family members (including future siblings) must be considered.
• Staff involved in implementing the programme must be adequately trained and supported and must be aware of the ethical implications of handling genetic information.

Newborn screening

Morbidity from some genetic conditions can be prevented, or the condition more effectively treated, if diagnosed very early in life. Examples include cystic fibrosis, sickle cell disease, and genetic metabolic disorders such as phenylketonuria (PKU) and medium chain acylCoA dehydrogenase deficiency (MCADD). Many countries in the developed world have set up newborn screening programmes to identify affected infants and institute preventive management strategies (Box 3.7.5).[4]

Box 3.7.5 **Newborn screening**

Tandem mass spectrometry has been introduced in many countries to screen for inherited metabolic conditions. PKU and MCADD have commonly been the initial targets for screening, but the technology potentially allows a further 50 or so conditions to be added to the panel at marginal cost. Public health specialists involved in decision making face particular difficulties related to the rarity and genetic heterogeneity (variability) of these conditions.

• What public health priority should be given to screening for extremely rare conditions (birth prevalence commonly between 1 in 100,000 and 1 in 400,000), which collectively cause appreciable infant and child mortality and disability, and which can be ameliorated by early diagnosis and treatment?
• How can robust evidence on effectiveness be obtained? For example, without screening, diagnosis is difficult. Milder cases or cases that present as catastrophic metabolic crisis (and commonly death) are likely to be missed. This causes biases in research that attempts to compare outcome in screen-detected versus clinically diagnosed cases.
• How should test cut-offs be set to optimize the balance between sensitivity (not missing cases) and specificity (not raising anxiety for parents and creating extra laboratory and clinical work by identifying many false positives)?

Predictive testing

Although many genetic conditions are manifest at birth or in early childhood, some have a later age of onset, during adolescence, early adulthood or middle age. In some cases, a predictive or presymptomatic genetic test may indicate whether an at-risk individual has inherited a disease-causing mutation, and prophylactic interventions may be offered. Predictive testing can make an important contribution to disease prevention in the case of single-gene subtypes of common disease. This is area in which genetics is beginning to be incorporated into mainstream medical practice (Table 3.7.1). The involvement of the extended family is crucial in the investigation, diagnosis and management of these conditions.

As a public health practitioner you may be involved in aspects such as:

- *Needs assessment:* including epidemiological work to define the incidence and prevalence of the genetic condition, estimates of its penetrance, and expected and actual numbers of cases presenting to health services (for a case study, see Box 3.7.6).
- *Quantification of risk:* including both relative risk and absolute risk over a defined time period.
- *Advising on measures to identify affected individuals and families:* possibilities include systematic population-level screening programmes or, more often, targeted family-based approaches based on known individuals with disease. This method is known as cascade testing.
- *Evaluation and critical comparison* of DNA-based and phenotypic diagnostic tests
- *Assessment of the role of specialist genetic services:* which work alongside other clinicians in diagnosis and management of the condition. Here, it is important that you appreciate that the geneticist will focus on the family as the unit of care, rather than the individual.
- *Assessment of the risks and benefits* of the available interventions and the way management might vary if, as is usually the case, many different mutations can cause the same or a similar clinical condition.
- Where public health has a role in the commissioning and organization of services, advising on optimal service size, configuration, staffing, professional competences and training, quality criteria and audit.

Table 3.7.1 Examples of intervention strategies for prevention or reducing mortality in some genetic subtypes of common disease

Condition	Preventive strategy
Highly penetrant subsets of breast cancer (BRCA1 and BRCA2), and colorectal cancer (HNPCC)	Mammography or MRI, chemo-prophylaxis or mastectomy for breast cancer; colonoscopy for colorectal cancer
Sudden cardiac death in arrhythmia syndromes such as long QT syndrome	Beta blockers, calcium channel blockers or implantable cardioverter defibrillators
Coronary heart disease in familial hypercholesterolaemia	Statin drugs

Susceptibility testing

Much current research in genetics and genomics is aimed at identifying polymorphisms associated with common, complex disease. It has been suggested that genetic susceptibility tests may help refine disease risk estimates and enable preventive interventions to be targeted more effectively. Although some validated gene-disease associations are known, you should be aware that susceptibility tests based on these associations have not so far led to clinical applications.[5]

Factors relevant to the debate on susceptibility testing include:

- Tests based on single common polymorphisms will generally have very low predictive value
- The penetrance and population prevalence of polymorphisms affecting risk will together determine their population attributable fraction, an indicator of their contribution to the burden of disease
- Interactions between genetic polymorphisms and environmental factors (meaning that some genetic variants may only increase or decrease disease risk in the presence of specific environmental factors) are difficult to study and far from being understood
- Rather than providing precise estimates of individual risk, DNA-based susceptibility tests may prove useful to stratify a population into broad risk groups for whom appropriate surveillance or preventive interventions may be devised. For example, it has been suggested that in the future breast screening may be targeted to women identified as at greater risk on the basis of genetic susceptibility[6]
- Ongoing research may lead to improved clinical utility for genetic susceptibility tests; public health practitioners should maintain a watching brief on developments in the science.

In the meantime, it has been suggested that family history, which reflects both shared genetic factors and shared environmental and behavioural factors, might be useful as a public health tool in disease prevention and health promotion. Its utility for this purpose requires careful evaluation.[7]

Box 3.7.6 Needs-based services for people with inherited cardiovascular conditions: a case study

- *Background:* advances in scientific and clinical understanding of inherited cardiovascular conditions (ICCs) and the development of genetic tests mean that individuals with these conditions can now be identified and treatments provided to prevent morbidity and sudden cardiac death. Conditions include long QT syndrome, hypertrophic cardiomyopathy, and Marfan syndrome. The aim of the study was to assess needs for specialist ICC services across the UK, define the current service provision and make recommendations for development.[8]
- *Method:* the needs assessment was undertaken by a multi-disciplinary working group that included cardiological and genetic expertise, patient groups, commissioners and others. Work included a review of epidemiological literature, clinical management and evidence.

of effectiveness, focus groups to obtain the patients' perspective and use of case histories to develop expert consensus on the components of a specialist service. A questionnaire survey of all 19 services in the UK was used to obtain information on structure and activities of these services.

• *Results:* key findings were:
  • the prevalence of these conditions in the UK may be around 200,000 (based on UK population of 61 million);
  • services lack capacity to meet current or likely future needs and are uneven in quality and quantity;
  • the estimated current unmet need is at least 7,000 new patients per year;
  • systems to identify at-risk individuals and families are not optimal;
  • the availability and use of genetic testing (both for diagnosis and to guide management) is highly unequal across the country.
• *Outcome:* the needs assessment led to national recommendations that ICC services should be developed through specialized commissioning and the development of a commissioning framework setting out service components and indicative capacity required. A professional group was set up to lead on supporting issues such as development of protocols and guidelines and professional education.

Ethical, legal, and social considerations

Like all aspects of medical and public health practice, the use of genetics in disease management and prevention has ethical implications. You should, however, beware of genetic exceptionalism—the belief that genetic information *necessarily* entails problems that are unique and more serious than those associated with other types of medical information.

You should bear in mind that:
• genetic information, like all medical information, must be kept confidential
• the most important criterion for assessing the personal sensitivity of genetic information is its predictive value
• generally, genetic information is only strongly predictive when it relates to highly penetrant genetic diseases
• information relating to genetic diseases has implications for other family members, who may also carry the disease-causing mutation
• information about polymorphisms associated with common disease does *not* generally have significant implications for family members.

It is important also to be aware that the relationship between genetics and public health is a highly sensitive one. In the past, there have been attempts to use coercive programmes to attempt to 'improve' the genetic fitness of populations. These eugenics programmes were both morally repugnant and scientifically flawed. Their legacy has been a widespread fear of genetics throughout society that can only be counteracted by careful safe-guards and education to promote public knowledge and confidence.

The future

Genetics will make an increasing impact on all areas of medicine. New technologies that enable rapid and inexpensive sequencing of whole genomes promise to improve the ability to identify the genetic mutations responsible for single gene diseases and may have applications in areas such as carrier screening, oncology, and pharmacogenetics. Some commentators predict that whole-genome sequencing will make susceptibility testing (based on a range of both genetic and environmental factors) a clinical reality. You should be wary of unjustified 'hype', but alert to developments that offer clear, evidence-based benefits. An important element of such evidence will be a better understanding of the relationship between genetic risk information and health-related behaviour.

As gene–environment interactions become better understood, there may be implications for nutrition, infectious disease control, and dealing with the effects of exposure to environmental toxins and pollutants.

Advances in understanding the genetics of non-human organisms also offer opportunities for improved health. For example, rapid genetic characterization of new pathogenic viruses, such as avian or swine flu, provides information that can be used for timely development of diagnostics and vaccines.[9]

Public health practitioners have a responsibility to ensure that genome-based tests and interventions are evidence-based and ethically applied to benefit the health of individuals and populations. The discipline of public health genomics promotes this aim.[10]

Further resources

Foundation for Genomics and Population Health, Cambridge UK. Available at: ℘ www.phgfoundation. org

GraPH-Int, International Network for Public Health Genomics. Available at: ℘ http://www. phgen-meeting.eu/programme/graph-int (accessed 31 May 2012)

HuGENet, the human genome epidemiology network, established by the US National Office of Public Health Genomics to help translate genetic research findings into opportunities for preventive medicine and public health by advancing the synthesis, interpretation, and dissemination of population-based data on human genetic variation in health and disease. Available at: ℘ www.cdc.gov/genomics/hugenet/default.htm

HumGen resource on ethical, legal and social implications of genetics. Available at: ℘ www. humgen.org/int/

National Office of Public Health Genomics at the US Centers for Disease Control and Prevention. Available at: ℘ www.cdc.gov/genomics/

References

1 Burke W, Zimmern R. (2004). Ensuring the appropriate use of genetic tests. *National Review of Genetics*, **5**, 955–9.

2 Haddow J, Palomaki G. (2004). ACCE: a model process for evaluating data on emerging genetic tests. In: Khoury M, Little J, Burke W, eds, *Human genome epidemiology*, pp. 217–33. Oxford University Press, Oxford.

3 Ram KT, Klugman SD. (2010). Best practices: antenatal screening for common genetic conditions other than aneuploidy. *Current Opinion in Obstetrics and Gynecology*, **22**, 139–45.

4 Khoury MJ, McCabe LL, McCabe ERB. (2004) Population screening in the age of genomic medicine. *New England Journal of Medicine*, **348**, 50–8.

5 Janssens AC, van Duijn C. (2009). Genome-based prediction of common diseases: methodological considerations for future research. *Genome Medicine*, **18**, 20.

6 Pharoah PDP, Antoniou AC, Easton DF, Ponder BAJ. (2008). Polygenes, risk prediction, and targeted prevention of breast cancer. *New England Journal of Medicine*, **358**, 2796–803.

7 Valdez R, Yoon PW, Qureshi N, Green RF, Khoury MJ. (2010). Family history in public health practice: a genomic tool for disease prevention and health promotion. *Annual Review of Public Health*, **31**, 69–87.

8 Burton H, Alberg C, Stewart A. (2010). Mainstreaming genetics: a comparative review of clinical services for inherited cardiovascular conditions in the UK. *Public Health Genomics*, **13**, 235–45.

9 Seib KL, Dougan G, Rappuoli R. (2009). The key role of genomics in modern vaccine and drug design for emerging infectious diseases. *PLoS Genetics* **5**, e1000612.

10 Stewart A, Burke W, Khoury MJ, Zimmern R. (2009). Genomics and public health. In: Detels R, Beaglehole R, Lansang MA, Gulliford M, eds, *Oxford Textbook of Public Health*, chapter 1.6. Oxford University Press, Oxford.

3.8 Health communication

Kasisomayajula Viswanath

Objectives

After reading this chapter you will be able to:
● understand why health communication is important in health promotion and disease prevention
● explain how communication messages are produced by different organizations
● identify different types of communication content and genres, such as entertainment, news and advertising
● understand the effects of exposure to communication messages on health outcomes.

Introduction

The twin revolutions in communication and biomedical sciences have made the role of communication critical for mitigating or exacerbating health problems.[1] The dizzying array of delivery platforms, from conventional channels, such as interpersonal networks and radio, to more recent developments, such as 'social media', magnified the interest in health communication among researchers, funders, and practitioners.

The primary focus of this chapter will be on 'mediated communications', rather than communication between patients and physicians.

Why is health communication important?

The interest in health communication stems partly from the sheer amount of time one spends interacting with mass media or communication technologies of one kind or other. For example, in the USA, almost 69% of people have access to the Internet at home and about 77% have someone in the household who has access at some place or other. Other indicators regarding media exposure, particularly, ownership of communication gadgets, are equally impressive. About 85% of Americans own cell phones and 42% own gaming devices.[2] Time spent with media even among children is yet another indicator of media dominance in our contemporary lives. According to one study:[3]

- 74 per cent of all infants and toddlers have watched TV before age[2]
- 99 per cent of all children aged 0–6 years live in a home with a TV set
- 97 per cent have products, like clothes and toys, based on characters from TV shows or movies
- children under 6 spend about 2 hours a day with screen media, about the same amount of time that they spend playing outside, and three times as much time as they spend reading or being read to
- total time spent with all media by those aged 8–18 years increased from 6.19 to 7.38 hours on a 'typical day.'

Thus, the sheer breadth and depth of penetration of various communication technologies has public health practitioners wonder about the value and efficacy of the platforms to communicate health information to diverse audiences. The value of health communications to promote health stems from several reasons:

- Recognition of importance of health communication by such organizations as the World Health Organization (WHO) to United States' Institute of Medicine (IOM)
- Research suggesting that communication is a significant factor in major public health problems such as obesity, tobacco use, unsafe sex, and violence.

Given these diverse opinions, fast-evolving technologies and platforms, characterizing the role of communication for public health practice is important although challenging.

Dimensions of communication and health

Given its vast scope, inter-disciplinary roots, cross-cutting appeal, and the fast-evolving technologies, from a public health point of view, it is critical to get a clear understanding of the scope of health communication and how it can be used in health promotion and disease prevention.

At the outset, health communication is pursued and understood at multiple levels: individual, organizational, and societal.[4,5] Literature at these different levels offer useful insights into how communication messages are produced, processed, and disseminated within organizational contexts and how they are consumed with different effects at individual, group, and

social levels. Within this framework, studies have focused on two broad areas as they affect health:
- research has offered insights on how use of media and exposure to messages during *routine* use of media may impact health
- another line of work has looked at how communications may be used strategically to promote health.

One way to map health communication is to look at it along three dimensions:
- *Production of communication messages:* a process of generating information as a result of interaction between those who generate information or act as sources of information and media personnel who gather, process and disseminate information across different platforms.
- *Communication content:* that includes genres of advertising, news and entertainment that could promote health such as latest scientific developments or content that could detract from health.
- *Communication effects* of messages on individual and population health.

This section will summarize what we know about health communication along these three dimensions to map the field and understand health communication from a population perspective. Such an understanding will help practitioners to more skillfully use media for public promotion.

How are communication messages produced?

Much of what we see in the health information environment is a product of interaction between the 'suppliers' or generators of health information and producers representing media organizations that amass, process the content per imperatives of organizations they are working in and disseminate the information. We will briefly elaborate on these points.

In general, there are three types of information that pertains to health directly or indirectly—news, entertainment, and advertising. Each of these types is a product of organizational cultures, structures, and process that are somewhat unique to each with varying impact on health. It must be noted that while most advertising is not focused on promoting health *per se*, it nonetheless affects health, often adversely.

Despite the creative nature of media products, such creativity generally occurs within the constraints of organizations with defined hierarchies, cultures, norms, rules and operating procedures. These bureaucratic structures drive how information is gathered, processed and distributed.

New coverage of health is a good example. Coverage of topics increases the salience for those issues in the minds of the audience, 'frame' the topic, and influence audiences' beliefs, attitudes, and behaviours. News media are also a critical channel that translates scientific developments in health and medicine for different audiences including consumers, but also often to health care providers and policy makers. Journalists who report on health rely on 'sources' such as media or public relations personnel, 'spokespersons', or news or video-releases from scientific organizations or from medical journals for their initial ideas on what issues to report on. Health journalists use certain 'newsworthiness criteria' or rules of thumb to develop their stories, including 'potential for public impact,' 'new information or development' and whether the story allows them 'to provide a human angle' among others.[6]

Journalists also work under constraints of shaping the story to the imperatives of their medium. These include:

- potential length of the story
- deadline pressures
- the literacy levels of their audience, and
- the need for visuals in case of television.

These imperatives and priorities often clash with the practices of scientists who emphasize specialized use of language, long lead times to conduct and report research, and careful and qualified expression of their results. This 'clash of cultures' could lead to potential misunderstandings and frustrations and mutual stereotyping. If one were to understand and work within the journalistic constraints, news media are a helpful ally in shaping public beliefs and behaviours on health.

While the genres may differ, entertainment and advertising are also influenced by their respective organizational cultures though the degree of control exercised by producers and sponsors may vary with sponsors exercising great deal of control in advertising and entertainment.

Understanding and using these organizational rules and cultures could be particularly helpful for public health practitioners.

Communication content: genres and public health

Three broad genres of messages are worth paying attention to in understanding health communication: advertising, news and entertainment.

Advertising has drawn considerable attention in health, primarily for promoting beliefs and behaviours that are generally considered harmful to health and in contributing to an increase in disease burden. The sources of material and funding for generating the information are manufacturers, such as the tobacco industry or the food industry who have worked closely with the advertising and marketing agencies to promote certain values, beliefs, and lifestyles. The influence of advertising on certain lifestyle factors has garnered quite a bit of attention among researchers and policy makers. For example, an exhaustive review by the United States' National Cancer Institute (NCI) concluded that advertising and promotion are 'causally' related to the promotion and increased use of tobacco.[4] Similarly, food marketing has been implicated as one of the principal contributors to the growing problem of obesity worldwide.

Entertainment media expose people to content that could be both harmful, as well as conducive to health. The reason entertainment media are particularly more effective is because the exposure to health messages is 'incidental' or unintentional. Audiences who are watching stories in entertainment media such as movies or television shows are 'transported' to the fictionalized world and often let their guard down.[7] The consequence is that they are less likely to engage in critical viewing and thus more susceptible to media messages. Exposure to tobacco use in movies leading to greater initiation among youth is one of the most well documented effects of entertainment on health in the literature. Some have used entertainment or narratives to promote family planning, cancer screening, life skills, and maternal and child health among others.

News is a major source of information on health to general, as well as specialized audience, such as physicians and policy makers. Exposure to news is generally intentional and, hence, the audience is more engaged. Considerable work shows that people' exposure to health news, such as coverage of harmful effects of tobacco, are likely to lead to anti-tobacco beliefs and even change behaviour.[4] More effective is news in 'setting' the agenda, shaping the social norms about health and creating public opinion that is conducive to change or deters change. Social norms around smoking, including second-hand smoking, has led to the enactment of stricter laws restricting smoking in public places. Cultivating and working with reporters to improve health news coverage is one effective way to promote health.

What are the 'effects' of communication?

Given the immense exposure to mediated information, it is reasonable to assume that such exposure may potentially lead to 'effects' shaping audiences' knowledge, attitudes, and normative beliefs, and their behaviours. Communication effects could result not only through direct exposure to media, but also indirectly through 'interpersonal' channels, such as family members, peers, and co-workers. In fact, reactions to exposure to communication content may be 'mediated,' or in other words, influenced by others in one's social networks. The body of research documenting communication effects on various health outcomes is extensive, and in some cases, incontrovertible. Despite the well-documented observations, the difficulty in drawing causal connections between exposure and outcomes has resulted in controversial interpretations of media effects. Given the large body of work, it may be more useful to discuss 'effects' of communication on some major public health problems.

Tobacco use

Tobacco use is the most preventable public health threat and is implicated in almost 5 million deaths a year according to WHO with the heavier burden being faced by low and middle income countries. In many ways, media had a significant role in normalizing and glamorizing cigarette use starting with advertising and then Hollywood movies. Prominent Hollywood actors and actresses, such as former president Ronald Reagan served as spokespersons promoting cigarettes.

Content analytic studies show that tobacco use is portrayed in prime time TV, music videos, and movies, even in those rated for children over

13 years. While the recent trends shows some decline in smoking incidence in the movies, almost half of the movies for children over 17 years still showed tobacco use.

With a global focus, span, and reach, the tobacco industry has effectively used advertising and marketing to both initiate and sustain tobacco use though several countries have begun to place restrictions on tobacco advertising. One of the most, if not the most extensively documented bodies of work in public health communication on health is in the areas of tobacco, summarized in, 'The role of the media in promoting and reducing tobacco use,'[4] published by the NCI in the USA. This review of hundreds of studies and evidence reviews came to some far-reaching conclusions about the influence of media in tobacco use:

- Movies glamorized tobacco use, particularly, cigarette use and smoking is quite prevalent in movies
- The total weight of evidence from multiple studies using a variety of research designs and from different countries shows a causal relationship between tobacco advertising and promotion and increased tobacco use
- In a similar vein, the total weight of evidence from cross-sectional, longitudinal, and experimental studies indicates a causal relationship between exposure to depictions of smoking in movies and youth smoking initiation
- On the other hand, both controlled field experiments and population studies demonstrate that mass media tobacco control campaigns could change beliefs, curb initiation and encourage cessation. Mass media campaigns are particularly effective when combined with other tobacco control programmes.

Obesity

That there is growing 'epidemic' of obesity in industrialized countries is widely accepted. It is a major risk factor for a variety of chronic diseases including cardiovascular disease, diabetes, and cancer among others. The WHO estimated that in 2005, there were approximately 1.6 billion adults (age 15+) who were overweight and more than 400 million adults who were obese. More critically, at least 20 million children under age 5 were considered overweight foreshadowing a looming public health crisis.[8]

Communications media, particularly TV and screen media, were implicated as contributing to the growing obesity crisis. To be more specific, communications may contribute to the overweight and obesity problem through two mechanisms:

- by reducing time spent on physical activity (PA)
- in encouraging consumption of unhealthy foods, primarily through advertising.

Advertising and promotion as a part of food marketing has been a focus of attention by those concerned with the growing obesity problem. The IOM in the United States reported that in 2004, the food, beverage and restaurant industry has spent more than $11 billion on advertising with more $5 billion going to television.[9] Children and young adults are a particular target with more than $10 billion per year being spent on marketing food and beverages to them.

These intense marketing and advertising efforts have likely led children and adults learn to become consumers in the marketplace. In fact, children as young as 2–3 years, according to IOM, recognize packages and spokespersons and, by pre-school, recall brand names from exposure to televised advertising. The effect is that children are likely to ask for branded products when making requests and are often loyal to brands among beverages and the fast food industry. Consumption of sugar-sweetened beverages is one of the largest contributors to the problem of obesity.

Some have argued that time spent using media such as television and computers—'screen time'—may eat into time spent being physically active, contributing to a sedentary lifestyle. Although there are a large number of studies documenting the relationship between screen time and lower PA, with some exceptions, most are cross-sectional studies and seldom control for all other variables, such as social context, which influence PA. On the other hand, reducing screen time among children has found to have had positive outcome on body mass index (BMI), thus making this relationship plausible.

It is little wonder that this double-dose of lowering PA and increasing food consumption that is unhealthy has led many to zero in on the role of communications media in obesity and how to address this relationship.

Alcohol

According to the American Academy of Pediatrics (AAP) (2010), excessive alcohol consumption is responsible for more than 100,000 lives every year including 5000 of who are younger than 21 years. Alcohol and cigarettes serve as gateway drugs to other more serious drug abuse, such as marijuana. Alcohol consumption is related to a variety of other social ills and problems including risky sex and abuse. As is the case with other risk factors, communications media are important environmental contributors to alcohol through advertising and entertainment.

Opportunities for exposure to pro-alcohol content are widely prevalent in the media. The AAP position statement (2010) reported that about $6 billion are spent annually on alcohol advertising and promotion and that youth are exposed to 1000–2000 alcohol commercials a year.[10] Most of the advertising is in sports programmes that attract young viewers. In entertainment programmes, on American television for example, alcohol use is widely prevalent including during prime time. The portrayal of alcohol use is usually positive and seldom shows the negative consequence of the use. Music videos and movies also contain high depictions of alcohol use.

The consequence of such broad and extensive portrayal of alcohol use and its promotion in the media is that the audience, especially, young viewers' knowledge, and beliefs are influenced by it. For example, exposure to heavy alcohol advertising has major consequences such as:

- brand recognition ('Budweiser frogs') among children as shown in one study
- more favorable beliefs towards drinking
- potentially 'normalizing' alcohol use among the viewers, especially teenagers
- *drinking itself*—watching alcohol use in music videos and television is associated with beginning of alcohol use and even higher consumption.

Media violence

The impact of exposure to violent programmes on television and movies, and, more recently, in computer games has drawn attention from researchers, policy makers, and activists. As George Gerbner and colleagues have argued, television is the 'storyteller' of our times providing a 'common symbolic environment' for all people irrespective of their personal and social backgrounds.[11]

With more than 98% of the US households owning at least one television set, and most households, an average of almost three television sets, TV so far is the primary socialization agent. Because of massive exposure and broad reach, and arguably high levels of violent content, considerable research has been done to assess the impact of exposure to violent programmes and games, particularly on children, considered as 'vulnerable audience.' Several congressional committees have held hearings and the Office of Surgeon General has released reports.

The evidence for the impact of violent programmes comes from studies using a variety of research designs, including longitudinal studies, cross-sectional studies, field and laboratory experiments. Research has concluded that:

- There is a 'causal connection between media violence and aggressive behavior in some children'[12]
- Exposure to violence in childhood could lead to aggression among adults thus suggesting a longitudinal impact. Several explanations have been offered for documented effects of violent programming including how the programmes can 'model' actions to children leading to social learning; provide 'cognitive shortcuts' for quick and unthinking action to resolve social problems and priming
- Heavy exposure to television, especially violent programmes on television could lead to a heightened sense of vulnerability and susceptibility to violence among the viewers.[11]
- TV and games can also promote pro-social behavior, such as sharing, co-learning, fair exchange, build relationships and engagement among children
- Similar effects of violent computer and videogames are now being documented with studies showing playing games is associated with a temporary decrease in pro-social behaviour, and engendering aggressive thoughts, feelings and arousal.

With a capacity for mass production and distribution, the influence of American entertainment programmes spans across the globe, thus enhancing the importance of studying the impact of such entertainment on violence and taking steps to mitigating the impact.

Media campaigns and health

Mass media campaigns have been used strategically in health promotion and disease prevention.[13–15] Research suggests that mass media campaigns are successful when done right and when they achieve sufficient exposure in:
• changing social norms
• promoting pro-healthy behaviours
• preventing unhealthy behaviours
• changing people's knowledge and attitudes towards health risks.

Communication campaigns are particularly effective when they are accompanied by environmental supports, such as creating structural opportunities in the community and appropriate policy changes.

Communication technologies and health

The explosion in new information delivery platforms such as the Internet, mobile communications, such as smart phones and other such telecommunication developments offer tremendous challenges and opportunities in public health communications. The widespread adoption of Internet in a number of countries is changing the way we conduct commerce, communicate, seek information and entertain ourselves.

Some broad figures of 'new media' reach demonstrate why this matters. A recent government report in the United States[16] showed that about 69% of American households access Internet from home, predominantly through broadband technology that allows faster downloads and uploads. Similar such numbers are reported by the International Telecommunication Union[17] with particularly impressive penetration of almost 80 mobile phone subscribers and 30 Internet users for every 100 inhabitants worldwide.

Equally compelling are the uses of new communication technologies for health. Data from Pew Internet and American Life,[18] a research agency in the United States show that about 57% of online users used the Internet to look for health information and more than half such queries are on behalf of someone else. The so-called 'social media' or social networking sites have become hugely popular. One such site, *facebook* claims it has more than 500 million active users worldwide with more than half of them logging on 'any given day' spending an estimated 700 billion minutes a month.

The opportunities to use these technologies to widen and deepen reach and overcome barriers of geography are tremendous. Nonetheless, they also pose some compelling challenges:
• One major challenge is that people are getting their information from a variety of sources and often from multiple sources leading to increasing fragmentation of audience. One advantage of such fragmentation and specialization is that health information can often by customized more narrowly to the interests and needs of the audience allowing for better reception, attention, and communication effects.

- More interesting is the fact that people are forming online communities and relying on experiences of others similar to them when engaging in online health information. This has the potential to increase engagement of the audience. For example, the Pew data[18] show that 4 out of 10 'e-patients' have followed someone else experience on a blog or another site and 2 out of 10 have consulted on rankings of reviews of providers or hospitals.
- On the other hand, the diversity of sources, 'gatekeepers,' makes it challenging to provide accurate information that has been vetted for accuracy and relevance. The millions of websites on health mean that there are multiple interpreters of health information that may or may not be accurate.
- It also could potentially confuse some people and overwhelm them with choices. For example, Pew reports that there are more almost 300,000 apps for mobile phone users on a variety of health topics including nutrition, physical activity, counting calories, estimating risk, assisting in smoking cessation and keeping personal health records. The value, utility, accuracy and reliability of such applications and websites and the consequences for population health remain to be investigated.

Communication inequalities and health disparities

One of the most significant, if not transformative movements in public health is the insights from research in social epidemiology on identifying social factors or 'social determinants' that affect population health.[19,20] leading to disparities in mortality and morbidity among social classes, races, geographies, and countries. A number of social determinants such as social class, race, ethnicity, urbanicity, access to medical care, neighbourhood, social capital, social and economic policies among others have been examined by researchers. The significance of this research has been a shift in focus from more medical and biological lens for disease causation to a focus on social, economic and cultural factors.

In parallel, in public health communication researchers are beginning to document 'communication inequalities' as one type of social determinants that could potentially explain disparities in health outcomes. Communication Inequality may be defined as differences among social classes in the generation, manipulation, and distribution of information at the group level and differences in access to and ability to take advantage of information at the individual level.[21] Several studies have documented significant differences among social classes, and racial and ethnic groups in preferences for, accessing, using, and understanding health information from a variety of media including newspapers, television, radio, and the Internet.

For example, the American government report on broadband Internet use cited earlier suggests that those with higher education and income, Whites and those living in urban areas are likely to access the Internet through Broadband technology. The reasons for not accessing through broadband include lack of affordability, perceived need and availability. Similarly, at global level, the ITU reports that there are more than 70 Internet users per 100 people in the 'developed world' compared with about 21 users per 100 people in the developing world. For example, Europe is estimated to have more than 60 users per 100 people compared with a little less than 10 per 100 people in Africa.

The consequences of communication inequalities are growing 'knowledge gaps' in health between the haves and have-nots, and the ensuing gaps in health behaviours and health outcomes. The inequities become even more pernicious at a time when more information on health is being made available for public consumption and greater responsibility in the guise of 'informed' and 'shared' decision-making is expected of patients and their families.

At the same time, communication inequalities are much more addressable than other social determinants through the development of appropriate interventions at group and policy levels. Also, under certain conditions technological developments have the potential to narrow the gap.

Conclusions

This brief essay cannot do justice to the rapidly changing field of health communications and the opportunities and challenges it offers to public health. In parallel to biomedical revolution at the molecular and clinical levels, revolutionary changes in communication technologies may radically transform how scientific developments in health and medicine are translated to influence public health. These radical developments are upending the conventional approach of controlled dissemination of health information to public and patients. While the advantage is that this democratizes health information to spread beyond specialists and those with advantages, the speed with which it is spread as well as multiple players, institutions and interpretations also overwhelm people leading to confusion and frustration. The greatest challenge of public health in the 21st century, one may contend, is the explosion in health information and taming the tide of this explosion is one of the most significant roles that public health practitioners may be able to play.

References

1 Viswanath K. (2005). Science and society: the communications revolution and cancer control. *Nature Reviews Cancer,* **5,** 828–35.

2 Smith A. (2010). *Americans and their Gadgets* [Report on the Internet]. Pew Research Center's Internet & American Life Project, Washington, DC Available at: ℗ http://www.pewinternet.org/Reports/2010/Gadgets.aspx

3 Rideout V, Foehr UG, Roberts DF. (2010). Generation M2: Media in the lives of 8- to 18-year-olds [Report on the Internet]. Henry J. Kaiser Family Foundation, Menlo Park. Available at: ℗ http://www.kff.org/entmedia/upload/8010.pdf

4 National Cancer Institute. (2008). *The role of the media in promoting and reducing tobacco use,* Tobacco Monograph Series 19. Department of Health and Human Services, National Cancer Institute, Washington DC.

5 Finnegan JR, Viswanath K. (2008). Communication theory and health behavior change: the media studies framework. In: Glanz K, Rimer B, Viswanath K, eds, *Health behavior and health education: theory, research, and practice,* 4th edn, pp. 363-87. Jossey-Bass, San Francisco.

6 Viswanath K, Blake KD, Meissner HI, *et al.* (2008). Occupational practices and the making of health news: a national survey of US health and medical science journalists. *Journal of Health Communication*, **13**, 759–77.

7 Green MC. (2006). Narratives and cancer communication. *Journal of Communication*, **56**, S163–83.

8 World Health Organization. (2010). *Obesity and overweight* [Report on Internet]. WHO, Geneva. Available at: ℘ http://www.who.int/mediacentre/factsheets/fs311/en/ / (accessed 31 May, 2012).

9 Institute of Medicine. (2006). *Food marketing to children and youth: threat or opportunity?* Institute of Medicine, Washington, DC.

10 Strasburger VC, The Council on Communications and Media, American Association of Pediatrics. (2006). Children, adolescents, substance abuse, and the media. *Pediatrics*, **126**, 791–9.

11 Gerbner G, Gross L, Morgan M, Signorielli N, Shanahan J. (2002). Growing up with television: Cultivation process (pp. 43-67). In: Bryant J, Zillmann D, eds, *Media effects: advances in theory and research*. Lawrence Erlbaum, Mahwah.

12 Anderson CA, Bushman BJ. (2001). Effects of violent video games on aggressive behavior, aggressive cognition, aggressive affect, physiological arousal, and pro-social behavior. A metanalytic review of the scientific literature. *Psychological Science*, **12**, 353–83.

13 Hornik RC. (2002). Public health communication: making sense of contradictory evidence. In: Hornik RC, ed., *Public health communication: evidence for behavior change*, pp. 1–19. Lawrence Erlbaum, New York.

14 Randolph, W., Viswanath K. (2004). Lessons Learned from public health mass media campaigns: marketing health in a crowded media world. *Annual Review of Public Health* **25**, 419–37.

15 Wakefield, MA, Loken B, Hornik RC. (2010). Use of mass media campaigns to change health behaviour. *Lancet* **376**, 1261–71.

16 National Telecommunication and Information Administration, United States Department of Commerce (2010). *Exploring the digital nation: home broadband Internet adoption in the United States*. [Report on the Internet]. Available at: ℘ http://www.esa.doc.gov/DN/

17 International Telecommunication Union (2010). *World Telecommunication/ICT Indicators Database* [Report on the Internet]. Available at: ℘ http://www.itu.int/ITU-D/ict/statistics/ (accessed 24 November, 2010).

18 Fox S, Jones S. (2009). *The social life of health information* [Report on the Internet]. Pew Research Center's Internet & American Life Project, Washington DC. Available at: ℘ http://www.pewinternet.org/Reports/2009/8-The-Social-Life-of-Health-Information.aspx

19 Berkman LF, Kawachi I. (2000). A historical framework for social epidemiology. In: Berkman LF, Kawachi I, eds, *Social epidemiology*, pp. 3–12. Oxford University Press, New York.

20 CSDH (2008). *Closing the gap in a generation: health equity through action on the social determinants of health*, Final Report of the Commission on Social Determinants of Health. WHO, Geneva.

21 Viswanath K. (2006). Public communications and its role in reducing and eliminating health disparities. In: Thomson GE, Mitchell F, Williams MB, eds, *Examining the health disparities research plan of the National Institutes of Health: unfinished business*, pp. 215–53. Institute of Medicine, Washington DC.

3.9 Public health practice in primary care

Steve Gillam

Objectives

Having read this chapter, you should:
- understand why effective systems of primary care are integral to delivering public health objectives
- know those public health interventions that primary care professionals provide
- be able to define those elements of primary care that need strengthening in order to deliver public health objectives.

Definitions

The central importance of primary care for public health has long been acknowledged. In 1978 at Alma Ata, primary health care was declared to be the key to delivering 'health for all' by the year 2000. Primary health care 'based on practical, scientifically sound and socially acceptable methods and technology made universally accessible through people's full participation and at a cost that the community and country can afford' was carefully distinguished from primary medical care.[1] The social and political goals of those epochal declarations—acknowledging as they did the social and economic determinants of health—were subsequently diluted. So called 'selective primary health care' and packages of low cost interventions such as GOBI-FFF (growth monitoring, oral rehydration, breast feeding, immunization; female education, family spacing, food supplements) in some respects distorted the spirit of Alma Ata.[2] Nevertheless, a central justification for universal primary care is ethical: the public health preoccupation with equity.

Primary care is often defined in terms of 'four Cs': it is continuous, comprehensive, the point of first contact, and co-ordinates other care. This co-ordinating function underlines a second set of arguments in support of primary care concerning efficiency and cost-effectiveness. International comparisons of the extent to which health systems are primary care oriented suggest that those countries with more generalist family doctors with registered lists acting as gatekeepers are more likely to deliver better health outcomes, lower costs and greater public satisfaction.[3] In 2008, the WHO reaffirmed the central place of primary care in delivering the Millennium Development Goals.[4]

Bridging the divide

General practitioners and public health specialists improve health by different means. General practitioners concentrate on personal, continuing health care while public health physicians focus on the population through changes in the environment, society and health service provision.[5] At the heart of the relationship between general practice and public health is an ethical conflict between individual and collective freedom.[6,7] The utilitarian values underpinning population-orientated care are at odds with the individualistic nature of the traditional doctor-patient relationship. The roles of carer, advocate and enabler may overlap and conflict with one another.[8]

The clinical generalist develops a unique understanding of the personal and social determinants of their patients' health.[9] However, traditional primary care based on the perspective of the clinician exposed exclusively to individual patients presenting for care has evident limitations. Knowledge about the distribution of health problems in the community cannot be derived from experience in the practice alone for most episodes of ill health do not lead to a medical consultation. An understanding of how disease presents is not obtainable without a population focus. Doctors over estimate their role in the provision of care. Primary health care is not, of course, synonymous with general practice and is provided by a range of other health personnel. Finally, professional knowledge about disease does not necessarily reflect people's illness experiences and needs to be supplemented with the insights of the community.

Several international trends in the delivery of health services are facilitating community-oriented approaches to primary care. Public health competencies, especially as they relate to the management of chronic disease, are of increasing importance to the 21st century primary care workforce.[10] More training is now taking place in community settings. An emphasis on more effective and more efficient health care will entrench community-oriented approaches if they prevent disease and encourage more discriminating use of medical technologies. In high income countries, a 'secondary to primary shift' is relocating specialist care closer to patients. Primary health care teams have always been pivotally placed to combine high risk and population approaches to disease prevention.[11] Meeting the challenge of non-communicable disease in low and middle income countries will require universal coverage of horizontally integrated programmes accessible through primary care.[12]

How does primary care deliver public health?

With the decline in infectious diseases and ageing of the population, an increasing proportion of the workload in general practice deals with the consequences of chronic disease. This has required the development of new services and changing systems of care. Many diseases, such as diabetes, which were once the exclusive preserve of hospital specialists are now managed by teams in the community.[13] If the 1970s saw the birth of a 'New Public Health', the first decade of the millennium has seen the emergence of a 'New Primary Care' at least in the UK (Box 3.9.1). How each of these five elements contributes to public health is considered below.

> **Box 3.9.1 Elements of today's primary care**
> * Self-care
> * First contact care
> * Chronic disease management
> * Health promotion in primary care
> * Primary care management.

Self-care

Less than one in ten ailments experienced is brought into contact with the formal system of health care. Most are self-managed using whatever knowledge and support is available to the sufferer. Increasingly, many patients are more knowledgeable than their doctors about the management of their chronic disease. Nevertheless, they sometimes need help in making sense of the surfeit of information available. The computer screen threatens the personal nature of the consultation, but new tools are changing clinicians from being repositories of facts to being managers of knowledge.[14] Some clinicians are nervous of giving patients better information and not all patients want it. However, most people want to be in charge of decisions about their health—for the default approach to be empowerment, rather than paternalism. Giving patients more knowledge or a consultation style that facilitates shared decision-making improves not only patient satisfaction, but also clinical outcomes. Indeed, as people gain access to information about risk, a higher proportion may choose not to accept the offer of screening or treatment.[15]

First contact care

If the bulk of first contact care is provided by friends and relatives, the next port of call has traditionally been general practice. However, there is an increasing plurality of routes through which primary care can be obtained (figure 3.9.1). These include the telephone helpline NHS Direct, Walk In Centres and community pharmacies. Experience in other countries has suggested that multiple access points with poorly co-ordinated record-keeping may result in fragmented care.[16] Questions over the cost efficiency of these services remain. Nevertheless, they have exposed the limitations of conventional general practice in providing basic care for populations who have not, for reasons of culture or convenience, gained satisfactory access to primary care in the past.

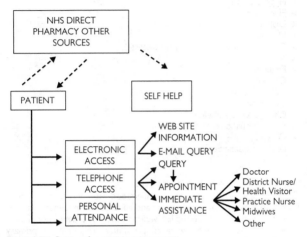

Figure 3.9.1 Routes of access into primary care.

Chronic disease management

Numerous studies attest to the variable quality of care provided to people with chronic diseases. The GP Contract in the UK provides financial incentives for practices to enhance the quality of their care in specific areas through the Quality and Outcomes Framework (QOF, Box 3.9.2). Much infrastructural investment is required to develop registers and call-recall systems, but the benefits in terms of public health are potentially significant. There is evidence that the QOF has led to better recorded care, improved intermediate outcomes, and reductions in health inequalities (although pay-for-performance schemes can yield perverse consequences for continuity, patient-centredness and professionalism).[17] Routine disease monitoring is increasingly undertaken by practice nurses with extended training. Disease management is becoming more complicated as pharmaceutical advances allow more care to be shifted from secondary to primary care. There is growing interest once more in North American techniques of managed care: risk stratification, targeting the heaviest consumers of care and utilization review—but little clear cut evidence to guide policy makers.[18]

Box 3.9.2 Chronic diseases targeted in the Quality and Outcomes Framework (QOF)

- Coronary heart disease
- Stroke and transient ischaemic attack (TIA)
- Hypertension
- Hypothyroidism
- Diabetes
- Mental health
- Chronic obstructive pulmonary disease
- Asthma
- Epilepsy
- Cancer
- Palliative care
- Dementia
- Chronic kidney disease
- Atrial fibrillation
- Obesity
- Learning disabilities.

Health promotion in primary care

General practitioners have always understood the importance of social factors such as housing, employment and education as influences on their patients' health. The registered list, which defines the practice population, provides the basis for effective health promotion programmes in primary care. Preventive activities within primary care can be divided into individual, organizational and community interventions.[19,20] *Individual* interventions take place between health professionals and patients, often classified into primary, secondary, and tertiary prevention (Box 3.9.3). The public health approach to screening focuses on maximizing participation in screening, rather than on informed participation. For example, current recommendations for the primary prevention of coronary heart disease in groups at high risk depend on screening through primary care and provision of risk-related advice or treatment. However, we lack evidence for the cost effectiveness of multiple risk factor interventions delivered through primary care.[21] Presenting the uncertainties associated with the assessment and reduction of cardiovascular risk has the potential to be more cost effective than screening conducted in a traditional, public health paradigm if it results in participants who are more motivated to reduce their risks.[22]

Organizational interventions are concerned with improving the management of care and access to services for disadvantaged groups. Such interventions may take place at the level of the practice or the whole health system. An example of the former might be changes to make cervical screening more accessible to certain ethnic groups by providing information in different languages and increasing the availability of female health professionals. More wide-ranging organizational changes could include allowing private sector providers to address previously unmet needs in deprived, under-doctored locations under the terms of the Alternative Personal Medical Services scheme.[23]

> **Box 3.9.3 Individual interventions between health professionals and patients**
>
> *Primary prevention*
> - *Health education and behavioural change:* e.g. dietary, smoking cessation, exercise.
> - *Immunization:* for an ever-increasing range of infections.
> - Welfare benefits advice
> - Community development
>
> *Secondary prevention*
> - Detection and management of ischaemic heart disease
> - *Screening:* e.g. for cervical, breast cancer and colon cancer
>
> *Tertiary prevention*
> *Chronic disease management:* e.g. diabetes mellitus.

The third category of interventions is **community**-wide. For example, in their roles as employers, users of resources, procurers, producers of waste, deployers, and vendors of land, primary care organizations have opportunities to enhance community health that have as yet been neglected by practitioners in the UK. They are just beginning to understand their role in promoting sustainable health care in a future low carbon health system.[24]

Community development has a stronger pedigree in developing countries. Every year over 500,000 women die from maternal causes, four million infants die in the neonatal period, and a similar number are stillborn. If the millennium development goals to reduce maternal and child mortality are to be achieved, public health programmes need to reach the poorest households. Most maternal and neonatal deaths take place at home, beyond the reach of health facilities. Evidence is growing that primary care strategies centred on community based interventions are effective in reducing maternal and neonatal deaths in countries with high mortality rates, even if institutional approaches are necessary to reduce them further.[25]

Primary care management

New public management with its emphasis on targets and objective-setting has permeated all parts of the health service. One important consequence of the growth of large practice-based teams has been the differentiation of administrative functions. Increasingly, primary care teams need to accept responsibility for auditing the health status of their patients, publicizing the results, monitoring and controlling environmentally determined disease, auditing the effectiveness of preventative programmes, and evaluating the effect of medical interventions. Their newly devolved role in commissioning health services gives general practitioners particular responsibilities for local strategy development and budgetary management.[26] Public health specialists remain crucial in supporting these functions.

Key challenges for public health practitioners

- *What kind of primary care?* The difficulty of transposing health systems across international boundaries is universally acknowledged. Care at the level of the community within any system reflects different histories and cultural contexts. No single model of primary health care will be universally applicable. For example, community-orientated primary care (COPC) seeks to integrate public health practice by delivering primary care to defined communities on the basis of its assessed health needs.[27] COPC remains a powerful, enduring concept, but its protagonists have made little mark beyond developing countries. In part, this reflects the lack of financial incentives within hospital-orientated health systems.

- *The politics of public and patient involvement:* There is a fundamental difference between health care that is multi-sectoral, preventive, participatory, and decentralized, and low cost (low quality), curative treatment aimed at the poorest and most marginalized segments of the population, particularly if that care is provided through programmes that are parallel to the rest of the health care system without active participation of the full population. Julian Tudor Hart, an eloquent exponent of COPC in the Welsh mining village where he practiced, has argued for the need to look in a new way at the relationship between doctors and patients as 'co-producers of health' and develop alliances between health workers and the public in defence of health.[28]

- *Information systems:* the creation of a single, longitudinal electronic patient record could create powerful new means of monitoring and improving care. An easily accessible, portable record ought to increase the involvement of users in their own management.

- *Evaluation:* assessing the health impact at the level of the organization or individual health worker is challenging. Even large UK general practices serve populations that are usually too small to compare health outcomes such as all-cause or disease specific mortality rates. The focus is on intermediate outcomes—changes in established markers of quality care. The QOF provides an example of an evidence-based approach to measuring (and rewarding) improvements in the management of common chronic diseases. Public health practitioners will be familiar with the measurement challenges listed in Box 3.9.4.

Box 3.9.4 Factors complicating the assessment of primary care

- Small denominators and the play of chance
- 'Street lamp effect': focusing on what is measured (paid for), ignoring the penumbra
- Measuring the easily measurable, but unimportant . . .
- . . . while ignoring the difficult to measure (e.g. communication skills, continuity of care).

- *Ensuring equity at practice level:* one well-attested form of differential access to care is the so-called 'inverse prevention' effect whereby communities most at risk of ill health tend to experience the least satisfactory access to the full range of preventive services.[29] Access may be affected in more material ways, e.g. through the provision of aids of wheel chair users or translated materials for people for whom English is not their first language. User charges for primary care have been repeatedly shown to deter those most likely to benefit from preventive activities.[30]
- *Continuing professional development and the workforce:* primary care like public health is a multi-disciplinary endeavour. In the UK presently, labour is being divided in new ways between many different health workers. A new cadre of primary care nurses is taking responsibility for minor illness management, triage, and routine care of common chronic diseases. The particular skills of others such as community pharmacists are being recognized. Beyond strengthening appraisal and revalidation mechanisms within different disciplines, there lies the challenge of ensuring that professional development activities are congruent and co-ordinated across teams.
- *Maximizing effectiveness:* the dearth of evidence in support of many preventive interventions highlights the need for further research. Reasons for the failure to implement best practice go beyond the quality of the research and accumulating further technical evidence may not be the most useful response. Barriers to implementation include a consistent failure to address the opportunity costs of new or different activities in primary care. For example, increasing primary care's public health role may mean doing less of something else. Related to this is a failure to address adequately and with all relevant stakeholders, the question of the role of primary care. This is not a technical agenda but one of achieving shared values as a starting point for any changes in professional roles.

Conclusions

Health systems are in constant flux. Everywhere the generalist seems to be under threat. What were once seen as strengths of general practice within the NHS are now regarded as liabilities—the registered list (restricting choice), personal (paternalistic care), gate-keeping (rationing). Public health practitioners should be mindful of the law of unintended consequences. For example, one result of increasing access points may be discontinuous, poorly co-ordinated services for those most in need. Paying practitioners by results may create disincentives to practice exactly where care is already weakest. Fragmented primary care will yield poorer public health. Public health practitioners who understand the complementary nature of these disciplines (Table 3.9.1) will mobilize the resources of primary care more effectively.

Table 3.9.1 Public health and primary care practitioners—core competencies contrasted

Public health practitioners	Primary care practitioners
Care for populations	Care for individuals on practice lists
Use of environmental, social, organizational, legislative interventions	Use of predominantly medical, technical interventions
Prevention through the organized efforts of society	Care of the sick as their prime function with the consultation as central
Application of public health sciences (e.g. epidemiology/medical statistics)	Application of broad clinical training and knowledge about local patterns of disease
Skills in health services research, report and policy writing	Skills in clinical management and communicating with individuals
Analysis of information on populations and their health in large areas	Analysis of detailed practice/disease registers and information on individuals
Use of networks that are administrative: health and social care authorities, voluntary organizations	Use of networks that are less bureaucratic: frontline health and social care providers, other primary care teams

References

1 World Health Organization. (1978). *Primary health care*, Report of the International Conference on Primary Health Care, Alma-Ata, USSR, 6–12 September. WHO, Geneva.

2 Gillam S. (2008). Is the declaration of Alma Ata still relevant to primary health care? *British Medical Journal*, **336**, 536–8.

3 Starfield B. (1994). Is primary care essential? *Lancet*, **344**, 1129–33.

4 World Health Organization. (2008). *Primary health care (now more than ever)*, World Health Report. WHO, Geneva.

5 Bhopal RJ. (1995). Public health medicine and primary health care: convergent, divergent or parallel paths? *Journal of Epidemiology and Community Health*, **49**, 113–16.

6 Pratt J. (1995). *Practitioners and practices. A conflict of values?* Radcliffe Medical Press, Oxford.

7 Fitzpatrick M. (2001). *The tyranny of health—doctors and the regulation of lifestyle.* Routledge, London.

8 Gillam S, Meads G. (2001). *Modernisation and the future of general practice.* King's Fund, London.

9 Heath I. (1995). *The mystery of general practice.* Nuffield Provincial Hospitals Trust, London.

10 World Health Organization. (2006). *Preparing a workforce for the 21st century: the challenge of chronic conditions.* WHO, Geneva.

11 Rose G. (1992). *The strategy of preventive medicine.* Oxford University Press, Oxford.

12 World Health Organization. (2011). *A prioritized research agenda for prevention and control of noncommunicable disease.* WHO, Geneva.

13 Moore G. (2000). *Managing to do better. General practice for the twenty-first century.* Office of Health Economics, London.

14 Muir Gray JA. (1999). Post-modern medicine. *Lancet*, **354**, 1550–2.

15 Coulter A, Ellins J. (2007). Effectiveness of strategies for informing, educating, and involving patients. *British Medical Journal*, **335**, 24–7.

16 Jones M. (2000). Walk-In primary care centres: lessons from Canada. *British Medical Journal*, **321**, 928–31.

17 Gillam S, Siriwardena N, eds (2010). *The Quality and Outcomes Framework: transforming general practice.* Radcliffe, Oxford.

18 Gillam S. (2004). What can we learn about quality of care from US health maintenance organisations? *Quality in Primary Care* **12**, 3–4.

19 Hulscher MEJL, Wensing M, van der Weijden T, Grol R. (2001). *Interventions to implement prevention in primary care*, Cochrane Review. The Cochrane Library, **Issue 1**, Update Software, Oxford.

20 Ashenden R, Silagy C, Weller D. (1997). A systematic review of the effectiveness of promoting lifestyle change in general practice. *Family Practice*, **14**, 160–75.

21 Rouse A, Adab P. (2001). Is population coronary heart disease risk screening justified? A discussion of the national service framework for coronary heart disease (standard 4). *British Journal of General Practice*, **51**, 834–7.

22 Kinmonth A-L, Marteau T. (2002). Screening for cardiovascular risk: public health imperative or matter for individual informed choice? *British Medical Journal*, **325**, 78–80.

23 NHS Confederation. (2005). *Alternative providers of medical services—a contracting guide for primary care trusts.* NHS Confederation, London.

24 Gillam S, Barna S. (2011). Sustainable general practice: another challenge for trainers. *Primary Care Education*, **22**, 7–10.

25 Costello A, Osrin D, Manandhar D. (2004). Reducing maternal and neonatal mortality in the poorest communities. *British Medical Journal*, **329**, 1166–8.

26 Secretary of State for Health. (2010). *Equity and excellence: liberating the NHS.* Department of Health, HMSO, London.

27 Mullan F, Epstein L. (2002). Community-oriented primary care: new relevance in a changing world. *American Journal of Public Health*, **92**, 1748–55.

28 Tudor Hart J. (1988). *A new kind of doctor.* Merlin Press, London.

29 Marmot M. (2011). *Fair Society, Healthy Lives—the Marmot Review.* Available at: ℘ www.ucl.ac.uk/marmotreview

30 NHS Centre for Reviews and Dissemination. Evidence from systematic reviews of the research relevant to implementing the 'wider public health' agenda. York: University of York, NHS Centre for Reviews and Dissemination, 2000.

4.1 Developing healthy public policy

Don Nutbeam

Objectives

Reading this chapter should help you better understand:
- the process of policy making and the role of public health information and evidence in shaping policy
- the role of public health practitioners in influencing the policy process through the provision of evidence and advocacy.

Definition of key terms

- Public policy: public policy is comprised of public issues identified for attention by the government and the courses of action that are taken to address them.
- Public policy making: policy is often enacted through legislation or other forms of rule-making that define regulations and incentives and enable the provision of resources, programmes and services to address public issues.
- Healthy public policy: healthy public policy is a concept promoted by the WHO to highlight the potential impact all government policies have on health. Healthy public policy is policy that makes explicit the impact it may have on health. The WHO's *Ottawa Charter* emphasizes that health should be a consideration in policy making in all sectors at all levels of government, and that governments should be held to account for the health consequences of their policies.[1]
- Health impact assessment: health impact assessment is a methodology for prospectively assessing the potential impact of policy proposals in order to improve their positive impact on the health of a population and to minimize inequalities in health (see 📖 Chapter 1.5).[2]

Evidence

Evidence may be simply defined as proof of an unknown or disputed fact and is generally derived from research. In public policy making, 'evidence' is derived from information gathered from a wide variety of sources including, though not exclusively, peer-reviewed research. A great deal of policy-relevant evidence can be gathered from programmes already in existence by observing the way they operate, identifying what has worked in the past and what has not, and learning from the experience of practitioners in delivering programmes. Evidence from more conventional research is often blended with this contextual, 'real world' knowledge.[3] (For more on evidence see 📖 Chapter 2.7)

Why is it important to be able to use evidence to inform/influence policy?

Public health practitioners are often frustrated that public health evidence and a population-based perspective on health do not adequately influence the development of public policy, particularly in sectors other than health. An improved understanding of the policy making process and how to influence it will enable public health practitioners and researchers to engage more effectively in the development of healthy public policy.

How is healthy public policy made?

Policy develops and changes on the basis of underlying beliefs about both the cause of a problem and the potential effect of proposed interventions. These beliefs contribute to the policy making process and final policy direction along with the social and political context in which the decision is made. The ability to interpret the causes of a problem and identify effective solutions are skills that enable public health practitioners to influence policy decisions. These basic skills will be enhanced by an understanding of the social and political context of a problem and its possible policy solutions.[4]

Policy making is rarely an 'event' or even an explicit set of decisions derived from an appraisal of evidence and following a pre-planned course. Policy tends to evolve through an iterative process and to be subject to continuous review and incremental change. Policy making is an inherently 'political' process and the timing of decisions is usually dictated as much by political considerations as the state of the evidence. As such, policy making requires a point-in-time appraisal of:

- What is scientifically plausible, based on an appraisal of the best available evidence at the time it is needed?
- What is politically acceptable, based on an appraisal of the political context in which policies are being made?
- What is practical for implementation, based on an appraisal of the experience of practitioners in delivering programmes?[5]

Models to help explain the relationship between public health evidence and the policy making process

Evidence can be used in a variety of ways to lead, justify or support policy development. A range of models explain the different ways in which evidence has been used to guide the policy making process[6] including:

- *The knowledge-driven model:* where the emergence of new knowledge from research will automatically create pressure for its application in policy. In public health, developments such as the development of new vaccines or screening tools may lead to public pressure for their immediate adoption, often regardless of their cost relative to benefit.
- *The problem-solving model:* where evidence derived from a variety of sources is gathered and applied as a starting point for the development of policy and used as part of a rational process with a clear beginning and end. For example, the government of the Netherlands introduced a limited range of interventions to tackle health inequalities for which there was good evidence and an established system for monitoring progress.[7]
- *The interactive model:* where research knowledge is only one input in the decision-making process, along with experience, social pressures, and political considerations. Recent approaches to tackling health inequalities in the UK reflect this complex process and mix of influences.[8]
- *The political model:* where evidence is selectively used to justify a pre-determined position. The exclusive use of mass-media campaigns and/or school-based interventions to address complex problems such as drug misuse and anti-social behaviour can be seen as examples of this model. Evaluation of the US drug-use-prevention programme D.A.R.E. provides an example of this type.[9]
- *The tactical model:* where the normal uncertainty of research findings is exploited to delay a decision or where weak evidence is used to justify an unpopular decision. The early responses of some governments to the rise of HIV/AIDS in the 1980s provide an example of this model.

In reality, policy decisions emerge from political ideology, judgement, and debate alongside analysis of research findings. It is likely evidence will be used in policy development in ways that correspond to the interactive, political and tactical models described above. In order to better influence public policy, public health practitioners need to understand the place of evidence in the political processes that occur during policy development.

Who is involved in developing healthy public policy, and what role can I play?

Four key players have been identified in the development of healthy public policy:[4]

- *Policy makers:* (usually politicians and bureaucracies) who have initiated or hold a mandate for a specific policy and move the policy at a pace that meets their interests. Public health practitioners can get to know this group and, where feasible, develop a working relationship with individual policy makers.
- *Policy influencers:* are groups (inside or outside government) with an interest in an issue and may try to influence the content of the policy and the speed and way in which it is implemented. Public health practitioners can contribute to such groups and actively engage in influencing policy content and the process of implementation.
- *The public:* (audiences, consumers, taxpayers, and voters) whose opinion will ultimately affect the adoption of the policy. Public health practitioners can play an important role as community leaders and opinion makers with the public, especially by making effective use of the media.
- *The media:* (print and electronic) who influence both the policy makers' and public's understanding of, and attitude towards, an issue. Public health practitioners can engage with the media to provide credible information and expert advice, as well as more active media advocacy (see Chapter 4.5 for more on media advocacy).

The ways in which evidence is used in the policy-making process will vary according to the beliefs of those who create and influence policy.[8] 'Evidence' can be used internally to monitor, analyze, and critique policy options, or externally to persuade or mobilize others into action. The media has an important role in creating public opinion not only in relation to what they report, but by choosing who is allowed to speak, how much prominence an issue is given, and how an issue is framed.[4]

What determines success in developing healthy public policy?

Public health practitioners and academics often complain their evidence is ignored by policy makers. However, our choice of research, methods of communication, and general dislocation from the policymaking process all exacerbate this situation.[10]

A 'hierarchy of evidence' is well established in the public health and broader scientific community. Systematic reviews and meta-analyses of randomized trials have become far more accessible and policy-makers have become more adept at using this type of evidence. There is little doubt that this high quality evidence has been influential in policymaking and countries like the UK (through its NICE) have established formal structures to systematize the use of evidence in health policy making.

(For more on the transfer of evidence into policy see 📖 Translating evidence to policy.)

However, not all randomized trials produce evidence that is policy relevant and not all policy-relevant evidence comes from randomized trials. Evaluations based on prospective experimental designs are simply not possible in many areas of public health policy. From a policy making perspective, a large amount of public health research appears to offer no practical way forward and provide no solutions to the problems examined.

In contrast, a great deal of policy-relevant evidence is gathered from case studies of practice, reflecting expert opinion or even anecdotal evidence. Such 'evidence' generally ranks at the bottom in established hierarchies of evidence but is frequently highly valued by policy makers, particularly as it is often available when needed, addresses issues of current concern, and offers solutions that are practical for implementation. Policy making is an inherently political process and the timing of decisions is usually dictated as much by political considerations as the state of the evidence.

Policy is most likely to reflect public health priorities and the evidence that informs them if:
- evidence is available and accessible when needed
- the evidence is presented in a way that fits with the political vision of the government (or can be made to fit)
- the evidence points to actions for which powers and resources are (or could be) available, and the systems, structures, and capacity for action exist
- there is successful public health advocacy within and outside of the political system, and
- policy makers have basic critical appraisal skills and are supported in using evidence in policy development.

While there are many obstacles to using public health evidence in developing healthy public policy there are real signs of progress in many countries, including:
- overt commitments by governments to use evidence in policy making
- the growth of active public health communities and a strengthened voice in public debate
- changes to research funding to better align research with policy needs, and
- investments in institutions to build the public health evidence base.

What are the potential pitfalls?

Public health researchers and practitioners often fail to understand the intensely political nature of policy making. We need to develop a better understanding of how policy is made and be more realistic and pragmatic about the possible contribution of their evidence to the policy process. We also need to be aware of rare 'windows of opportunity' for the uptake of evidence into policy, when policy makers' interests and the social climate coincide to support the use of public health evidence in policy making. Timing is everything.

What competencies are required for public policy making?

Public health practitioners need to develop advocacy skills. This may involve building relationships with civil servants and policy makers within government departments, establishing partnerships and alliances with organizations and individuals with similar objectives, and effectively engaging with the media (see 📖 Media advocacy for policy influence). Importantly, researchers need to develop closer working relationships with policy makers, from the earliest stages of research design through to programme implementation and beyond (see case study).

The transfer of evidence into policy is further hampered by a lack of knowledge and skill in handling research evidence among policy makers. The ability to critically appraise the quality of research, interpret results and draw wider conclusions from the research findings are skills that enable policy makers to competently and comfortably consider research evidence in their decisions. Public health practitioners who can make evidence accessible and comprehensible to policy makers will have an advantage when it comes to advocating and influencing.

Myths and misconceptions

The emergence of evidence-based medicine in the early 1990s put pressure on policy makers to become more evidence-based in their decision-making. In the scientific and medical communities, where evidence-based practice is highly regarded, there is a common misconception that policy making is and should be a purely evidence-based and rational process. As Nick Black points out, policy makers often have other valid and competing concerns when formulating policy.[10] Political survival, financial constraints, and public opinion are strong motivators in policy decisions and tapping into these motivators will greatly increase the chances of influencing policy.

Case study: successful healthy public policy and lessons learned: Physical Activity in Schools

Research and the policy process

The New South Wales (NSW) Schools Fitness and Physical Activity Survey was undertaken to provide reliable scientific evidence in response to growing professional and community concern around reduced physical activity and rising levels of obesity in Australian children.[11]

The study measured the body composition, health-related fitness, physical activity habits and fundamental motor skills of primary and high school students in NSW. It also investigated the school facilities, policies and practices relevant to students' participation in physical activity.

Fundamental movement skills include running, jumping, catching, throwing, kicking, and forehand strike, and are essential prerequisites for participation and enjoyment of sports and other forms of physical activity. The results from the study showed only about 30% of students had completely mastered running and jumping, with another 30% close to mastery. Girls in particular scored poorly on some skills, with less than 20% showing mastery or near mastery of kicking and forehand strike. Most of these skills should be mastered by the age of 10 and the results showed NSW school children had surprisingly poor physical skills.

Two relatively small and achievable recommendations were made to policy makers:

- that two hours per week be allocated to physical education in primary schools
- and that one hour of this be used for developing fundamental movement skills.

These recommendations were taken by contacts within the department to higher levels in the organization until they reached the Minister and were accepted.

The resulting skills development programme in primary schools was well supported. Resources developed to support the teachers in implementing the programme included videos, workbooks, phone support, and face-to-face training.

Subsequent research showed improvements in the fundamental movement skills of NSW primary school children and an association between skill proficiency and higher levels of physical activity. Long-term effects on obesity were mixed.

Lessons learned

Several conditions assisted this transfer of evidence into education policy:

- Public health researchers engaged in a sustained media advocacy campaign, using their evidence to portray the lack of physical skills in Australian children as an important problem for society. This created the social and political climate needed for the adoption of healthy policy change

- Public health researchers worked collaboratively with contacts in the Department of School Education throughout the process, from the design and implementation of the study through to the evaluation of the subsequent skills development programme
- The involvement of policy makers in the design phase of the survey meant factors amenable to policy change and implementation were measured. For example, school facilities, sports equipment, and time allocated to physical education were assessed
- Lastly, the policy changes were consistent with the Australian Department of School Education's broader goals and within their capability to implement.

References

1 World Health Organization. (1986). *Ottawa Charter for Health Promotion*. WHO, Geneva.
2 Mindell JS, Boltong A, Forde I. (2008). A review of health impact assessment frameworks. *Public Health*. **122,** 1177–87.
3 Brownson RC, Fielding JE, Maylahn CM. (2009). Evidence-based public health: a fundamental concept for public health practice. *Annual Review of Public Health*, **30,** 175–201.
4 Milio N. (1987.) Making healthy public policy: developing the science by learning the art. *Health Promotion International*, **2,** 263–74.
5 Head BW. (2008). Three lenses of evidence-based policy. *Australian Journal of Public Administration*. **67,** 1–11.
6 Weiss CH. (1979). The many meanings of research utilization. *Public Administration Review*, **39,** 426–31.
7 Mackenbach J, Stronks K. (2002). A strategy for tackling health inequalities in the Netherlands; *British Medical Journal*, **325,** 1029–32.
8 Nutbeam D, Boxhall AM. (2008). What influences the transfer of research into health policy? Observations from England and Australia. *Public Health*. **122(8),** 747–53.
9 West SL, O'Neal KK. (2004). Project DARE outcome effectiveness revisited. *American Journal of Public Health*, **94,** 1027–9.
10 Black N. (2001). Evidence-based policy: proceed with care; *British Medical Journal*, **323,** 275–9.
11 Hardy LL, Okely AD, Dobbins TA, Booth ML. (2008). Physical activity among adolescents in New South Wales (Australia): 1997–2004. *Journal of Science and Medicine and Science in Sports and Exercise,.* **40,** 835–41.

4.2   Translating evidence to policy

Lauren Smith, Jane An, and Ichiro Kawachi

Objectives

As a result of reading this chapter you will be more able to:
- identify the challenges that arise in translating research findings to public policy
- understand the frequently cited barriers to evidence-based public health policy making from the perspective of legislators
- take steps to bridge the gap between evidence and policy formation.

Introduction

The three critical ingredients to public health policy formation are: a) the development of the evidence base, b) the political will to act, and c) the identification of sustainable strategies.[1] Yet evidence-based public health policy remains limited because of the challenges that arise in bridging research and policy.

Considering the 'supply side' of evidence production, some researchers express reluctance to be involved in the policy process because they do not want short-term political interests to direct their research agendas, and there are few incentives for them to address the policy relevance of their work.[2] From the perspective of the potential users of evidence (i.e. the 'demand side' of the equation), legislators/regulators are often forced to make policy under budgetary and time constraints. For instance, if there is a pressing political agenda to tackle childhood obesity, laws will be formulated with or without scientific input. At the same time, supplying the most rigorous evidence does not guarantee that policy actions will follow. The goal of this chapter is start you thinking about overcoming the barriers to translating evidence into policy.

Barriers to translating evidence to policy

What are the barriers that impede an effective incorporation of public health knowledge into policy?
- Rapid pace of decision making, which can be uncomfortable for academics
- The unavoidable tension between the sufficiency of information available for decision making versus the need to act now

- Researchers and policy makers place different weights on evidence versus experience
- There is unquestionable appeal of policy making based on anecdotes.

What do researchers need to understand about the policy making process?

Evidence for action is produced by several sets of people—not just academic researchers, but also practitioners. From the perspective of decision-makers, the following is a list of things you need to understand about translating evidence to action.

Public health researchers are not well prepared to convey the impact of 'intersectoral effects'

As a public health researcher, you need to explicitly 'connect the dots' to inform policy makers of the 'upstream' social determinants that influence population health. Often, decision makers in the sectors controlling these determinants (e.g. community development, education, employment, zoning, etc.) do not view population health as belonging to their domain. The strategic use of health impact assessments can be a useful tool to educate key stakeholders and policy makers on the health impacts of these social determinants (see also 📖 Assessing health impacts).

Public health researchers often do not recognize the 'supply vs demand' dynamic of data

Public health researchers (including practitioners engaged in the production of evidence) are usually more accustomed to the passive diffusion of data through peer-reviewed journals or presentations at professional conferences. A more effective strategy is to position your work so that the decision makers (policy makers and legislators) can reach out to you for information and advice at the specific time when they need it. This requires the cultivation of relationships ahead of time, before the decision maker needs information immediately and wants to turn to a credible, experienced, and known source.

Public health researchers devote inadequate attention to the 'framing' of their arguments

You need to understand that the language you use to present your data matters and must be chosen carefully. You may need training and experience in how to frame your ideas and evidence effectively, particularly when presenting evidence that may be inconsistent with the cognitive frames of the audience. As a result, you need to learn and consistently apply the lessons supplied by the field of cognitive linguistics and strategic frame analysis.[3] If you do not, your hard-earned knowledge may be dismissed.

Existing public health research training does not adequately prepare or support public health professionals who seek to work at the intersection of evidence production and public health policy

From the perspective of professional training in public health, you need to be aware of the gaps between evidence production and policy translation that you will need to bridge during your training:
● the inconsistent emphasis within public health training curricula on the requisite skills required to operate at this intersection
● an unclear pathway of career advancement for those interested in this kind of work
● public health training curricular requirements do not consistently emphasize the specific skills necessary to bridge the gap between evidence and policy (see Box 4.2.1).

Unclear pathway for career advancement for those interested in working at the intersection of public health and public policy

Even if you successfully bridge the gap between the worlds of evidence production and policy translation, you need to be aware of the barriers to career advancement as a result of working at the intersection between the two worlds. Different things are valued in the worlds of evidence production and policy translation. In the research world, what counts for career advancement are publications, publications, and publications. However, in a world where policy translation is valued, you should get credit for doing things such as:
● providing testimony at legislative hearings
● providing expert guidance, in the form of policy briefs or reports to decision makers
● participating in developing legislation or regulations
● providing policy briefings based on sound interpretation of available evidence to legislators, agency staff, and elected officials.

Box 4.2.1 Public health professional competencies in US Schools of Public Health

In the USA, schools of public health fully accredited by the Council on Education of Public Health (CEPH) must identify required competencies that define the knowledge, skills, and abilities that a successful graduate should be able to demonstrate at the conclusion of their programme.[4] The Association of Schools of Public Health recommends core competencies in five core disciplines, specifically for the master of public health (MPH) degree.[5] Some of the core competencies touch upon the skills necessary to bridge the gap between public health and policy but none addresses it comprehensively (Table 4.2.1).

Table 4.2.1. Competencies addressing the intersection between research and policy in the core disciplines for the MPH degree

Core disciplines	Competencies addressing the intersection between research and policy
Biostatistics	• Develop written and oral presentations on the basis of statistical analyses for both public health professionals and educated lay audiences
Environmental Health Sciences	None identified
Epidemiology	• Explain the importance of epidemiology for informing scientific, ethical, economic, and political discussions of health issues • Communicate epidemiological information to lay and professional audiences
Health Policy and Management	• Discuss the policy process for improving the health status of populations • Communicate health policy and management issues using appropriate channels and technologies • Demonstrate leadership skills for building partnerships
Social and Behavioural Sciences	• Describe the merits of social and behavioural science interventions and policies • Identify critical stakeholders for the planning, implementation, and evaluation of public health programmes, policies, and interventions • Specify multiple targets and levels of intervention for social and behavioral science programmes or policies

Adapted from reference:[5] Calhoun JG, Ramiah K, Weist EM, Shortell SM. (2008). Development of a core competency model for the Master of Public Health Degree. *American Journal of Public Health*, **98**, 1598–607.

The disconnect between emphasis on social determinants of health and insufficient support for assessing and communicating public health effects of policies originating outside the public health domain

There is increasing consensus on the need to focus on the fundamental drivers of population health, which often lie outside the domains of public health and health care. As a public health professional, you need to develop a deeper understanding of how these sectors are organized and how to develop effective collaborations with colleagues in those sectors who may be better positioned to identify potential policy issues to be addressed and the kinds of questions that would be most useful to answer (see Box 4.2.2).

Box 4.2.2 Case study: a child health impact assessment of energy costs and the Low Income Energy Assistance Programme

The Department of Pediatrics at Boston Medical Center (Massachusetts, USA) convened an interdisciplinary, inter-institutional working group to develop a Child Health Impact Assessment strategy to make the relationship of public policy to child health more comprehensible to policy makers and the public in Massachusetts. Below is a case study of one of the health impact assessments they conducted in 2007.[6]

- Purpose:
  - to conduct a timely health impact assessment to determine the influence of home energy costs on children's health and well-being, particularly among children from low-income families
  - to identify and inform key stakeholders of the findings and recommendations

- Who participated:
  - representatives from Boston University School of Medicine, Boston University School of Public Health, Brandeis University, Children's Hospital, Boston, Harvard Medical School, Harvard School of Public Health, and University of Massachusetts
  - state and federal programme officers from the Low Income Home Energy Assistance Program (LIHEAP)
  - energy assistance programme directors at Massachusetts community action agencies
  - energy advocates and researchers at the local, state and federal levels.

- Findings:
  - Low-income families facing disproportionately high energy costs are forced to make household budget trade-offs that jeopardize child health.
  - Families facing high heating costs resort to alternative heat sources that jeopardize child health and safety.

- High energy costs combined with unaffordable housing creates important budget constraints that force low-income families to endure unhealthy housing conditions that threaten child health.
- The growing gap between rising energy prices and LIHEAP benefits means more Massachusetts families accumulate substantial unpaid utility bills, leading to arrearages and disconnections that adversely affect child and family well-being

- Resulting policy actions:
  - members of the Child Health Impact Assessment Working Group presented their findings to the state legislature in testimony before the joint committee on housing. State expenditures for LIHEAP were subsequently increased
  - members of the Child Health Impact Assessment Working Group presented the findings to the National Energy Assistance Directors Association stimulating what has become an ongoing interest in the connection between health and energy costs. Some energy assistance programmes developed outreach programmes located in community health centres.

Bridging the gap between evidence and policy

Evidence producers and policy makers differ in their priorities, their time horizons, and their information communication and presentation styles.[7,8] If your work involves evidence production, you can increase the impact of your findings by taking the following steps:

- getting more involved in the policy process to gain an understanding of political decision making[9]
- translating and communicating findings so they are accessible and understandable by policy makers[10]
- building formal partnerships and informal relationships with policy makers[11]
- preparing for windows of opportunity when evidence can have maximal impact[12]
- conducting systematic reviews and meta-analyses to synthesize findings from large bodies of research[13]
- conducting health impact assessments that can increase recognition of social determinants of health and of inter-sectoral responsibility for health[14] (see also Chapter 1.5)
- Employing cost-effectiveness studies to compare costs of a programme or policy with some measure of health impact or outcome[15] (see also Chapter 1.6).

Further resources

Braveman PA, Egerter SA, Woolf SH, Marks JS. (2011). When do we know enough to recommend action on the social determinants of health? *American Journal of Preventive Medicine*, **40(Suppl. 1)**, S58–66.

Brownson Royer C, Ewing R, McBride TD. (2006). Researchers and policymakers: travelers in parallel universes. *American Journal of Preventive Medicine*, **30**, 164–72.

Choi BC, Pang T, Lin V, Puska P, Sherman G, Goddard M, et al. (2005). Can scientists and policy makers work together? *Journal of Epidemiology and Community Health*, **59**, 632–7.

Dannenberg AL, Bhatia R, Cole BL, *et al.* (2008). Use of health impact assessment in the U.S.: 27 case studies, 1999–2007. *American Journal of Preventive Medicine*, **34**, 241–56.

Frenk J. (1992). Balancing relevance and excellence: organizational responses to link research with decision making. *Social Science & Medicine*, **35**, 1397–404.

Innvaer S, Vist G, Trommald M, Oxman A. (2002). Health policy-makers' perceptions of their use of evidence: a systematic review. *Journal of Health Services Research & Policy*, **7**, 239–44.

Kelly MP, Morgan A, Bonnefoy J, Butt J, and Bergman V. (2007). *The social determinants of health: developing an evidence base for political action: final report to World Health Organization Commission on the Social Determinants of Health.* WHO, Geneva.

Nelson DE, Brownson RC, Remington PL, Parvanta C, eds (2002). *Communicating public health information effectively: a guide for practitioners.*: American Public Health Association. Washington, DC.

References

1 Atwood K, Colditz GA, Kawachi I. (1997). From public health science to preventive policy. Placing science in its social and political contexts. *American Journal of Public Health*. **87**, 1603–6.

2 Rychetnik L, Wise M. (2004). Advocating evidence-based health promotion: reflections and a way forward. *Health Promotion International*, **19**, 247–57.

3 Dorfman L, Wallack L, Woodruff K. (2005). More than a message: framing public health advocacy to change corporate practices. *Health Education & Behavior*, **32**, 320–36;

4 Council on Education for Public Health. (2011). *Accreditation Criteria: Schools of Public Health.* CEPH, Washington, DC.

5 Calhoun JG, Ramiah K, Weist EM, Shortell SM. (2008). Development of a core competency model for the master of public health degree. *American Journal of Public Health*, **98**, 1598–607.

6 Child Health Impact Working Group. (2007). *Unhealthy consequences: energy costs and child health impact assessment of energy costs and the low income home energy assistance program.* CHIWG, Boston.

7 Brownson RC, Royer C, Ewing R, McBride TD. (2006). Researchers and policymakers: travelers in parallel universes. *American Journal of Preventive Medicine*, **30**, 164–72.

8 Whitehead M, Petticrew M, Graham H, et al. (2004). Evidence for public health policy on inequalities: 2: assembling the evidence jigsaw. *Journal of Epidemiology and Community Health*, **58(10)**, 817–21.

9 Black N. (2001). Evidence based policy: proceed with care. *British Medical Journal*, **323**, 275–9.

10 Sorian R, Baugh T. (2002). Power of information: closing the gap between research and policy. *Health Affairs*, **21**, 264–73.

11 Martens PJ, Roos NP. (2005). When health services researchers and policy makers interact: tales from the tectonic plates. *Healthcare Policy*, **1**, 72–84.

12 Brownson RC, Chriqui JF, Stamatakis KA. (2009). Understanding evidence-based public health policy. *American Journal of Public Health*, **99**, 1576–83.

13 Anderson LM, Brownson RC, Fullilove MT, *et al.* (2005). Evidence-based public health policy and practice: promises and limits. *American Journal of Preventive Medicine*, **28(Suppl. 5)**, 226–30.

14 Cole BL, Fielding JE. (2007). Health impact assessment: a tool to help policy makers understand health beyond health care. *Annual Review of Public Health*, **28**, 393–412.

15. Brownson RC, Gurney JG, Land GH. (1999). Evidence-based decision making in public health. *Journal of Public Health Management and Practice*, **5**, 86–97.

4.3 Translating policy into indicators and targets

John Battersby

Objectives

Indicators and targets have been used in industry for many years and are widely used to measure and manage health systems; like them or not, they are here to stay.. Reports to hospital boards routinely include indicators to show performance and many organizations now use sets of indicators or dashboards.

An understanding of what indicators are and how indicators and targets are constructed is essential for public health practitioners. You will be called upon to interpret indicators, the performance of your department or team may be monitored using indicators, and you will be expected to meet targets. You may well also have to construct indicators and set targets for others.

Reading this chapter should improve your understanding of:
- what targets and indicators are
- what they can be used for
- how to go about constructing a good indicator
- how to go about setting a target
- when to avoid using indicators and targets.

The focus of this chapter is on constructing indicators and setting targets. To learn about using existing goals, targets, and indicators to best advantage see 📖 Translating goals, indicators, and targets into public health action.

Definitions

There are a number of definitions of the terms indicator and target. For the purposes of this chapter the following definitions have been used:
- *Indicator:* a summary measure that describes the condition or performance of a system, implying a direction.
- *Target:* a specific, time bound, destination.

In other words, an indicator suggests what you are trying to achieve, whilst a target shows you how close you are to achieving it.

Why should you use indicators and targets?

Turkey farmers in Norfolk, UK know the old saying 'You can't fatten a turkey by weighing it'. What applies to turkeys also applies to health systems: measuring performance does not necessarily improve it. There are two reasons for measuring performance:

- So you know when things are going wrong. For example, if you do not measure infection rates following surgery you will not know when they are getting worse.
- So you know when things are going right. If you redesign a care pathway you need to measure its outcomes to know whether you have improved care or not.

Indicators can be used to measure various elements of health and health care. What a particular indicator measures will be determined by how that indicator is constructed but it will measure either health status (inequality), the provision of health services (equity), or the performance of the system itself.

Performance can be measured:

- at different places, either geographic or organizational
- at different stages in a pathway, for example in relation to structures, processes, outputs, or outcomes
- at different times (e.g. the same measure repeated annually).

Understanding variation

Have you ever considered why you measure things? If nothing ever varied we would not need to measure but just as physiological parameters like blood pressure or weight vary, so do aspects of health and health systems.

Indicators are typically used to make a comparison with an average or benchmark so the key to making effective use of indicators is understanding variation. There are three causes of variation:

- chance
- artifact
- real differences.

Variation due to chance, sometimes called *common cause variation*, occurs with all measurement. There are a variety of statistical techniques for distinguishing whether variation is due to chance or whether it reflects a real difference between measurements (special cause variation). These include tools such as funnel plots,[1] process control charts,[2] and, particularly for measuring individual performance, cumulative sum monitoring.[3] Figure 4.3.1 shows an example of a process control chart.

These techniques, which are all forms of *statistical process control (SPC)*, separate out common cause variation from special cause variation.[4] Such techniques have been used in industry for many years and are now often used to understand indicators and targets in health care. Common cause variation is normal and inevitable; in contrast, special cause variation requires further investigation to understand what is causing it and what action to take.

Variation due to artifact may often show itself as special cause variation and investigation of special cause variation needs to exclude artifacts as a possible cause. Common types of artifact are changes in the definition of an indicator, changes in the method of data collection, and errors in coding or classification of data.

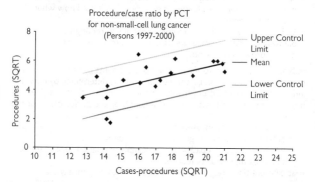

Figure 4.3.1 A process control chart plotting lung cancer cases not receiving surgical treatment (x-axis) against cases receiving surgical treatment (y-axis). Note that both axes are on a square-root scale. The plot shows health districts in the east of England, with control limits based on the regional mean of 9% of cases undergoing surgery—these limits are indicated by the upper and lower lines. Districts falling outside the control limits (i.e. falling above the top line or below the bottom line) have more than the expected degree of variation and should be investigated further.[5]

How is an indicator constructed?

An indicator is constructed from a numerator and a denominator. The resulting proportion or rate can then be compared with a standard (e.g. a regional average or benchmark). Box 4.3.1 gives an example of how data on the number of obese children in a school can be used to construct an indicator suitable for comparison. Statistical tests, such as the SPC techniques used for understanding variation, can be applied to show whether the difference between the measurement and the comparator is due to common cause or special cause variation.

Box 4.3.1 How data on the number of obese children in a school can be used to construct an indicator suitable for comparison

Measurement:	Comparator:
a (numerator), e.g. number of obese children aged 6 at a school	
―――――――――――	*c* (average or benchmark), e.g. mean proportion of obese children aged 6 at schools in the region
b (denominator), e.g. all children aged 6 at the school	

How do you choose and use indicators?

Choosing indicators is not always straightforward. Important issues to consider when choosing an indicator include:

● Is the issue you want to measure important?
● Does the indicator you want to use measure a relevant aspect of the issue?
● Is the indicator you plan to use valid, i.e. does it measure what it is supposed to measure?
● Can you obtain the data you need for the indicator and will they be timely?
● Is the indicator you plan to use sufficiently sensitive, i.e. will it detect changes in the system?
● Is the indicator meaningful? A useful test is whether you can explain it to somebody else.
● Do you know how to respond if the indicator is high or low? If not, do not use it!

Sometimes managers ask for an indicator that sums up a whole system but it is rarely possible to develop a single indicator and you might instead consider using a selection of indicators that measure different but important parts of the system. Such a selection is often referred to as a *balanced scorecard*.

You will often find someone else has already done the work for you. There are many examples of *baskets of indicators* which allow you to choose from a selection of validated indicators. In some countries there may be nationally developed sets of validated indicators which can be used. For example, the London Health Observatory has developed a basket of 70 indicators to assess health inequalities in England.[6]

The secret to using indicators successfully lies in communication. Indicators on their own are rarely sufficient to persuade people or organizations to change but if communicated effectively they can help to drive change. A useful tip when using indicators to change behavior is to involve stakeholders in the choice or development of the indicators that you will be using to monitor them.

Understanding targets

Targets are widely used in the management of healthcare systems and can be useful for clarifying priorities and setting expectations. Targets may also be linked to sanctions and this is often the case for performance management targets, or rewards, such as the use of stretch targets where success is linked to additional financial reward. Whatever their purpose targets should be SMART: Specific, Measurable, Achievable, Relevant/Realistic, Time bound.

Some measures can act as both targets and indicators depending on how they are used. For example, life expectancy is commonly used as an indicator of the health of a population and to compare the health of different populations. Life expectancy has many of the properties of an indicator, is objectively quantifiable, and is a proxy measure, as health itself cannot readily be measured. Life expectancy can also be used as a target.

How do you set and use targets?

The process of setting a target can be split into three stages:
- scoping
- gathering baseline data
- pitching.

Scoping

This involves deciding what the target should cover and what indicator (or indicators) you are going to use to monitor it. You need to be very clear about what outcome you are trying to achieve. For example, are you trying to motivate an effective team to deliver even better results or do you want to set a clear standard against which to judge performance? As targets are increasingly used to hold people or organizations to account it is important to include stakeholders in the scoping process.

Gathering baseline data

You will need to understand both current and historical patterns in the indicators you have chosen. For example, mortality rates from cardiovascular disease in most developed countries are falling. If the historical trend in mortality is not considered when setting a target it is easy to choose a target that can be reached with no additional action being taken.

Availability of data over the full time period may be a problem. It may be impossible to establish a trend accurately if the method of data collection has changed. Similarly, the quality of data coding needs to be considered as poor quality coding may prevent certain data from being used to measure progress towards a target.

Pitching

Pitching is the process of deciding how much change you are aiming for. This requires an understanding of how much change is possible and, given the likely effort and resource required to achieve change, how much change is realistic. Too often you see targets that have been chosen seemingly at random, e.g. a 10% reduction in emergency admissions over the next year, when proper pitching of the target would have shown clearly that it was either impossible to achieve or could only have been achieved by investing more resource than was available.

Deciding the way in which a target is expressed is also part of the pitching process:

- *Absolute:* reducing waiting times for potential cancer patients to two weeks.
- *Proportional:* reducing teenage pregnancy by 25%.
- *Relative to a benchmark or expected level:* reducing cardiovascular disease mortality to the level of the lowest in Europe.

When using targets you should:

- have a clear monitoring process
- provide regular feedback to those involved in delivery
- avoid blame—try to understand why a target is not being met
- periodically review the target.
- do not expect all targets to be met—if targets are always met they are probably not sufficiently challenging!

What are the potential pitfalls of indicators and targets?

There are several problems associated with the use of indicators and targets:

- Their appeal. Indicators and targets appeal to people who exercise authority (e.g. managers and politicians) but that appeal may not be matched by an understanding of how the indicator or target has been constructed.
- They can make people feel very threatened and a missed target or judgment of poor performance can be very demoralizing.
- Resources are required to construct and particularly to collect the necessary data to populate indicators or to assess the achievement of a target—those resources could be used elsewhere.
- They may encourage people to focus on the wrong issue. For example, in England targets associated with smoking cessation services have at times diverted attention away from the broader work of reducing smoking prevalence.
- They can create unintended outcomes. For example, a focus on shortening emergency waits may result in unnecessary hospital admissions.

- Targets may work against each other. For example, a target to increase the numbers of laboratory samples requested by clinicians may result in 'apparent' increases in certain infections because the laboratory is detecting infections that are not clinically important.
- The final pitfall is associated with not using them. Failure to use indicators and targets correctly can result in wasted resources and potentially can result in harm to patients.

The key to avoiding most of these pitfalls is for those who are measuring (often managers) and those who are being measured (often clinicians) to have a shared understanding of how the indicator or target has been developed and how it is going to be used.

Some myths about indicators and targets

- *You can develop a single indicator to measure a whole system:* unfortunately you cannot—no one measure can reflect the complexity of health systems.
- *You always need to develop an indicator from scratch:* much work has been done on developing validated indicators for use across health and social care; more often than not you will find one that exists already.
- *Indicators tell you what to do:* in fact, indicators generally give rise to questions. Their usefulness is in pinpointing what questions to ask.
- *Targets are bad:* although this view is often expressed the reality is that targets can be used badly or can be poorly constructed but are not in themselves bad.
- *Data need to be perfect:* data are never perfect and are often good enough. Part of the skill in constructing an indicator is in ensuring the data source is good enough and recognizing it is acceptable to improve the indicator rather than the system.

How will you know when you have identified a good indicator?

You will know you have got it about right when:
- those affected by the indicator feel motivated and encouraged
- nobody complains about it
- managers can use it to demonstrate service improvement
- politicians ask you to develop some more!

Emerging issues

Indicators have been used for many years to measure processes, outputs and outcomes. There is an increasing focus on using indicators to measure quality of care (see also 📖 Improving quality)—in England this has been reflected in the establishment of NHS Quality Observatories intended to enable local benchmarking, development of indicators and metrics, and identification of opportunities to help healthcare staff innovate and improve.

Quality has often been defined in terms of clinical outcomes but more and more often there is a requirement to include measures derived from users of services. This can be challenging as collecting data through surveys is time-consuming and expensive.

The other emerging issue is the increasing public availability of data. Both raw data and indicators will become more widely available through the Internet. There is a risk, that the increasing availability of data will not be matched by the increasing level of skill required to interpret and understand it.

Further resources

Audit Commission and I&DeA. (2005).*Target setting: a practical guide*. Available at: ℅ http://www.idea.gov.uk/idk/aio/985665.

Battersby J, Williams C. (2003). *Quantifying performance: using performance indicators*. Briefing papers on topical public health issues, 4. Eastern Region Public Health Observatory, INpho, Cambridge.

Dancox M. (2008). *Technical briefing 4: target setting in a multi-agency environment*. APHO, York. Available at: ℅ http://www.apho.org.uk/resource/item.aspx?RID=54328.

Pencheon D. (2008). *The Good Indicators Guide: Understanding how to use and choose indicators*. Association of Public Health Observatories and the NHS Institute for Innovation and Improvement, Coventry.

References

1 Spiegelhalter D. (2002). Funnel plots for institutional comparison [comment]. *Quality and Safety in Health Care,*. **11**, 390–1.

2 Mohammed MA, Cheng KK, Rouse A, Marshall T. (2001). Use of Shewhart's technique. *Lancet.*, **358**, 512.

3 Bolsin S, Colson M. (2000). The use of the Cusum technique in the assessment of trainee competence in new procedures. *International Journal of Quality Health Care*, **12**, 433–8.

4 Flowers J. (2007). *Technical Briefing 2: Statistical process control methods in public health intelligence*. APHO, York. Available at: http://www.apho.org.uk/resource/item.aspx?RID=39445

5 Battersby J, Flowers J, Harvey I. (2004). An alternative approach to quantifying and addressing inequity in healthcare provision: access to surgery for lung cancer in the east of England. *Journal of Epidemiology and Community Health*, **58**, 623–5.

6 London Health Observatory. (2011). *Basket of Indicators*. Available at: ℅ http://www.lho.org.uk/LHO_Topics/national_lead_areas/Basket_of_indicators/BasketOfIndicators.aspx

4.4 Translating goals, indicators, and targets into public health action

Rebekah A. Jenkin, Christine M. Jorm, and Michael S. Frommer

Objective

The objective of this chapter is to help you improve your use of goals, targets and indicators in guiding and informing the choice, implementation, and evaluation of public health action. For definitions and details of how to construct indicators and set targets see 📖 Translating policy into indicators and targets.

Why is this an important public health skill?

In public health practice the effort to base policy on evidence is crucial. Goals, indicators, and targets enable governments and health agencies to specify responsibilities for the health of populations and communities. They also help to galvanise public health action and the compilation of indicator data provides metrics for gauging the extent of progress. The depth of organizational and community commitment to the policies and programmes that goals promote and represent is important. Specific, challenging, well-defined, time-limited goals lead to higher levels of task performance than vague, easily-realized goals or a lack of goals.[1] Goals are only motivational if individuals and organizations are *committed* to them. Commitment is determined by such factors as the perceived value of specific goals, the perceived potential for goal attainment, the source and legitimacy of goals and the use of sanctions and incentives.[1]

Uses of goals, targets, and indicators

We can use goals, targets, and indicators:
- to guide the design and selection of interventions
- to help focus implementation efforts
- to provide a means of evaluating programmes and policies.

Using goals, targets, and indicators at different levels of public health practice

The international level

The eight ambitious United Nations' Millennium Development Goals (MDGs)[2] were adopted in 2000 to halve abject poverty by 2015 and address problems such as infectious disease, education, and gender equality. The MDGs were widely publicized and promoted and many international luminaries and bodies publically committed to pursuing them. It is now clear some of those goals will be met and others will not. For some regions (particularly sub-Saharan Africa and South Asia) the lack of prioritization of development needs coupled with a lack of ownership and complexity has stymied progress.[3] Self evidently, goals with such breadth may have limited utility at the local or even national level. Moreover, high-level global goals may overlook questions of local sustainability, local priorities, and capacity for implementation.[4] For instance, while maternal mortality remains an important problem internationally, the numbers of maternal deaths amenable to prevention in developed countries is very small. Programmes to prevent maternal deaths may therefore not constitute a public health priority in developed countries where reducing the 'burden of wealth-related disease' is likely to bring much greater benefit.[5]

The real value of international goals and targets in public health is perhaps in setting a worldwide policy agenda to which individual nations can subscribe, enabling them to use relevant goals to energize national agendas.

The national level

In most countries, mechanisms exist to ensure the priorities of regional or local health authorities reflect national priorities. In Australia, for example, regional health authorities are accountable to State and Territory governments that, in turn, have performance-based funding agreements with the Australian Government. These agreements require reporting on the implementation of specified health programmes and, where possible, health outcomes.[6,7] Analogous arrangements exist in other countries where funds flow from a central health policy agency to local health service agencies.

A recent example of national health goals promoted with the aim of directing regional and local public health activities in Australia is the Australian National Preventative Health Strategy (2009). The Strategy recommended a range of interventions aimed at reducing the chronic disease burden associated with three lifestyle risk factors—obesity, tobacco and alcohol—(see Box 4.4.1).

National level activity can be particularly effective in situations where a policy or legislative change is required to achieve a public health goal. For example, legislation is an effective tool in regulating the sale of cigarettes or alcohol by banning smoking from public places or the serving of alcohol to intoxicated persons. Enforcement of legislation such as the wearing of

> **Box 4.4.1 Examples of targets and associated projected national outcomes from the Australian National Preventative Health Strategy**
>
> **Aim:** halt and reverse the rise in overweight and obesity
> **Target:** prevention of half a million premature deaths if obesity is maintained at current levels between now and 2050
> **Aim:** reduce the prevalence of daily smoking to 10% or less
> **Target:** 1 million fewer people smoking in Australia by 2020, resulting in prevention of 300,000 premature deaths from four of the most common smoking-related diseases alone
> **Aim:** reduce the proportion of Australians who drink at short-term risky or high-risk levels from 20% to 14% and the proportion of Australians drinking at high-risk levels from 10% to 7%
> **Target:** prevention of (a) more than 7200 premature deaths; (b) the loss of 94,000 person-years of life; (c) 330,000 hospital admissions; (d) 1.5 million bed days. Savings of nearly $2 billion to the national health sector by 2020.[8]

seat belts, or correct labeling of foods so consumers can monitor their fat or salt intake, can also be effective.

The key in each case is to link the goal or target with an effective mechanism. At a national level such mechanisms tend to focus on the population, rather than the individual, although the message and effect may have an individual level outcome—for example, children cannot purchase cigarettes or alcohol under laws setting minimum consumer ages for sale of these products. Often, though, local mechanisms must be identified to translate higher-level goals into action.

The local level

The success of any large-scale effort to hit a target in public health typically relies heavily on local actions and success. Whilst national and regional level activities are important in establishing and maintaining policy and funding environments that enable change to occur, most of the activity occurs at a local level.

Local and regional health services have limited financial and human resources. Specialist expertise is often in short supply and community services often rely on a core of dedicated but overworked staff. Teams may be reluctant to take on new responsibilities and engage with new policies and programmes. Nationally proscribed activities such as action plans and related goals and targets may also seem irrelevant to those who face the day-to-day reality of dealing with disadvantaged communities that have heavy burdens of morbidity and complex social problems.

Conversely, once convinced of the value of a programme or the urgent need for a solution, local health services are often opportunistic and creative in identifying and using resources to support global, national and regional political commitment to goals and targets. These resources (funds or intellectual capacity) can be used for local priorities that mirror high-level priorities and may often provide incidental support for other (regional) priorities.

Ideally, a regional or local action plan will identify regional or local goals and targets. These set appropriate local expectations, taking account of baseline rates. Local targets may differ substantially from national or regional targets because of characteristics unique to the locality and translation of interventions and problems into a local context.

Even in taking local action it is important to recognize the heterogeneity of the population within defined geographic areas, not only because of variations in baseline occurrence of diseases or risk factors but also because of the varying responsiveness of particular groups to specific interventions. For some conditions, variations in baseline rates are enormous. For example, the prevalence of type 2 diabetes in many Australian Indigenous communities is up to seven times that of the rest of the population.[9] The setting of targets for diabetes control in these communities requires both knowledge of the medical interventions and an understanding of Indigenous social values, attitudes to illness, and community processes.[10–12]

Using targets to select interventions

There are likely to be a range of actions that could be taken to address a particular public health problem. Using established goals and targets, and being aware of the agreed indicators of performance, can help you select or set priorities among intervention options. Guidelines can assist in this process (e.g. *Deciding and specifying an intervention portfolio*[13]) as can schema for evaluating evidence to assess possible public health interventions.[14]

Criteria for selecting interventions include:

- *Assessment of feasibility*: of the interventions if they were applied locally, including estimates of necessary resources: financial, infrastructural, and human.
- *Assessment of the effectiveness of the interventions*: whether they will provide short-, medium-, or longer-term solutions to the health problem; the likely magnitude of their effect in a given time period; their sustainability; other effects on current services, positive or negative.
- *The ethics, acceptability and distribution of the interventions*: are the expected benefits likely to reach all groups? Are they evenly distributed? Do they particularly affect some groups to the detriment of others? Are the proposed interventions appropriate and acceptable, politically, socially, and culturally, to the target communities? Are the resources required to implement the interventions equitable given the burden of the problem for different population groups or subgroups? (For more on priorities and ethics see 📖 Chapter 1.2.)
- *Assessment of the costs associated with the potential interventions*: has an economic evaluation of the potential interventions been conducted?
- *Timing*: how soon can the potential interventions be introduced? How soon will the benefits be realized?
- *Risks*: relating to successful implementation of the interventions, which may include changes in the political and policy environment, shifts in priorities, escalation of costs, and unanticipated effects.
- *Availability of mechanisms to promote implementation*: which may include regulations, funding incentives, a requirement for public reporting, and individual performance agreements.[13-15]

- *Capacity to evaluate the intervention:* are the necessary data and expertise available to allow assessment of both baseline levels and the effect of the intervention?[14,15]

Taking into account these criteria, and the goals, targets, and indications, local action plans will include:
- New interventions, i.e. those to be initiated.
- Maintenance of existing interventions, either at their current level or with some enhancement or diminution.
- Cessation of existing interventions because they are inappropriate, ineffective, or too costly. (Cessation of interventions and disinvestment in them can be difficult and is often avoided but continuing ineffective interventions risks diluting the impact of new interventions and sending mixed and confusing messages to all stakeholders. Staged removal may be an acceptable compromise rather than immediate shut-down.)

Implementation

Implementation requires the translation of knowledge on interventions into specific local contexts, taking into account:
- local resources
- specific characteristics of the population
- incidence or prevalence of the health problem of interest
- the latency period before an effect of the intervention is observable
- local variations in the likely effectiveness of interventions.[16,17]

Once appropriate interventions have been identified you may find it useful to check that these interventions and the local goals and targets they are aimed at achieving:
- are consistent with higher-level (regional and national) goals and targets, if these are explicit
- reflect policies and principles such as equity of access and outcome, service quality, cost-effectiveness, and efficiency
- take account of particular areas of need, such as those of disadvantaged groups.

Implementation is likely to require the following steps:
- *Definition of terms* using existing datasets and dictionaries where available. It is essential the same definitions and measures of terms are used throughout the period of implementation and evaluation. For example, terms such as disadvantage, independence, and need may be interpreted in a range of ways and even contested, so ensuring they are clearly defined for the purposes of your programme—even if these definitions are not universally agreed upon—is important.
- *Analysis of regional expectations* and assessment of any significant differences between local intentions and the intentions expressed in higher-level (e.g. regional or national) goals and targets. This may include analysis of particular local problems or populations (and sub-populations at very high risk) not specifically addressed in the higher-level goals and targets.
- *Understanding context and local circumstances* that may influence the problem and understanding the acceptability of a programme at a local level. This will include setting priorities to mitigate the effects of the determinants, taking account of the risks and benefits.

- *Reviewing the existence, effectiveness, and cost* of current local objectives and programmes relevant to the new action plan.
- *Consulting* on the validity of the goals and targets and the action plan, their acceptability to local communities (both from a consumer and professional practice perspective), and their priorities for implementation. Consultation can inform the action plan (content) *and* is a central part of the action itself (agreement and implementation).[18]
- *Utilizing* existing partnerships and recruitment of community organizations to support the action plan. (see Chapter 7.4)
- *Quantifying* resources needed and resources available. The latter include existing programmes that might be relevant and amenable to leverage, resources that could be shared or shifted, and coincidental availability of appropriate funding opportunities.

Evaluating public health action

Examining progress relative to goals and targets and the monitoring of process indicators will enable you to assess the success of an action plan. Time pressures and political imperatives will make rigorous evaluation difficult[19,20] but there are many published examples for reference and guidance when developing an evaluation framework in such circumstances.[14,15]

There is also an ethical imperative to design action plans so that they can be the object of valid, unbiased evaluation. Although pragmatism may dictate the conduct of retrospective evaluations these are often limited in scope and restricted in validity. In planning evaluations it is important you allow sufficient time for changes in health outcomes to be observed, especially if interventions are very complex.[21,22]

Successful evaluation requires upfront planning and budgeting. The evaluation plan should be formulated *before* putting the interventions in place, allowing for the compilation of baseline data and detailed documentation of the implementation process. The concept of realist review[22] is especially helpful and aims to identify what works, for whom and in what circumstances, and why (on realist approaches see also 📖 Inference, causality, and interpretation).

Case study: implementing a national strategy

In the course of public affairs, health interventions are sometimes carried out as components of broader political initiatives. A recent Australian example was the Northern Territory Intervention, described in Box 4.4.2. Although unsuccessful in various ways this case offers useful learning points in relation to what can go wrong on the journey from goals, indicators, and targets to public health action.

Box 4.4.2 The Northern Territory Intervention (NTI)

Background

The indigenous people of Australia are highly disadvantaged compared with other Australians. They have poorer health outcomes, lower life expectancy, higher levels of socio-economic disadvantage, and lower school completion rates. Alcohol abuse and violence, including self-harm, are particularly common in the more isolated communities.[23,24]

A cycle of increasing Indigenous disadvantage—so called 'cumulative causation'—has occurred over many generations.[25] In response to discoveries about child abuse[26,27] the Australian Government announced a reform strategy recognizing that abuse of children in remote communities was an issue of national importance.

The resulting intervention had national and local aspects. It aimed to provide urgently needed protection for children and simultaneously announced a much wider reform agenda. The NTI was implemented via legislation that also suspended existing anti-discrimination laws and blocked the right of appeal to the social security appeals tribunal. The new legislation applied to 87 prescribed Aboriginal communities within the Northern Territories. In addition, substantial government funding was provided for health and new housing.

Specific actions implemented at a local level included alcohol restrictions, pornography bans, quarantining of welfare payments (so that they could only be spent on ways deemed socially responsible and were tied to child school attendance), compulsory child health checks (including for signs of abuse), appointment of government business managers, and support to enable community stores to deliver healthier and cheaper food.

The intervention split communities nationally and locally. There was widespread criticism of its paternalistic orientation and the overriding of individual and community preferences. Equally vocal were those who hailed the intervention as a long overdue step to protect those at greatest risk of harm. International agencies, including the United Nations Committee on the Elimination of Racial Discrimination (CERD) were highly critical.[28]

Results to date

It would be fair to say that the intervention has not resulted in a dramatic improvement in the living circumstances, health and well-being of the indigenous communities it was designed to benefit. Data on the health outcomes are patchy and difficult to interpret. Preliminary data analysis suggested income management had no beneficial effect on tobacco and cigarette sales nor on soft drink or fruit and vegetable sales—purchases have not become healthier.[29] Other data suggest health outcomes such as childhood hospitalizations and ear and eye infections may have improved.[30]

The NTI highlights some of the difficulties in implementing complex programmes with multiple interlinked goals. Problems arise with data quality, and interpretation, in particular when increased reporting might indicate increased care and awareness rather than changes in the phenomena being measured. In the NTI the programmes were implemented without time to prepare an evaluation framework or define appropriate indicators. Debate on the outcomes of the Intervention is therefore beset with intractable differences of interpretation. The NTI experience also emphasizes the risks associated with designing and implementing an intervention without appropriate and adequate local consultation and ownership.

Further resources

Commission on Macroeconomics and Health. (2001). *Macroeconomics and health: investing in health for economic development*. World Health Organization, Geneva.

Gostin LO, Powers M. (2006). What does social justice require for the public's health? Public health ethics and policy imperatives. *Health Affairs (Millwood)*, **25**, 1053–60.

Human Rights and Equal Opportunity Commission. *Close the gap: national indigenous health equality targets, outcomes from the National Indigenous Health Equality Summit*, Canberra, March 18–20, 2008.

Jenkin R. Frommer M. (2005). *A framework for developing or analyzing health policy*. University of Sydney, Sydney.

NHS Good Indicators Guide plus other resources on the UK Association of Public Health Observatories website (www.apho.org.uk).

Nutbeam D, Wise M, Bauman A, Harris E, Leeder S. (1993). *Goals and targets for Australia's health in the year 2000 and beyond*. Australian Government Publishing Service, Canberra.

References

1 Marlow P. (2005). *Literature review on the value of target setting*, HSL/2005/40 Sheffield: Human Factors Group, Health & Safety Laboratory, Sheffield.

2 United Nations (2000). *United Nations millennium declaration*. United Nations, New York.

3 Lancet/London International Development Commission (2010). The Millenium Development Goals: a cross-sectorial analysis and principles for goal setting after 2015. *Lancet* **376**, 991–1023. Available at: ℘ http://www.thelancet.com/mdgcommission.

4 Oxman A, Lavis JAF. (2007). The use of evidence in WHO recommendations. *Lancet*, **369**, 1883–9.

5 Leeder S. (2005). Setting goals for health in a time of prosperity. *Medical Journal of Australia*, **183**, 232–33.

6 Child and Youth Health Intergovernmental Partnership (2004). Healthy children—strengthening promotion and prevention Across Australia; developing a national public health action plan for children 2005–2008. National Public Health Partnership, Melbourne.

7 Council of Australian Governments. (2007). National Healthcare Agreement. Australian Government Printing: Canberra. Available at: ℘ http://www.federalfinancialrelations.gov.au/content/national_agreements/downloads/IGA_FFR_ScheduleF_National_Healthcare_Agreement.pdf (accessed 31 May 2011).

8 National Preventative Health Taskforce. (2009). *The healthiest country by 2020—national preventative health strategy—the roadmap to action*: Australian Government, Canberra.

9 Australian Institute of Health and Welfare (AIHW) (2008). A set of Performance indicators across the health and aged care system. Australian Government Printing: Canberra

10 Commonwealth Department of Health and Aged Care and Australian Institute of Health and Welfare (1999). *National health priority areas report: diabetes mellitus 1998*, AIHW cat. No PHE 10. AusInfo, Canberra

11 Hunter B. (2007). Cumulative causation and the productivity commission's framework for overcoming indigenous disadvantage. *Australian Journal of Labour Economics* **10**.

12 Hunter B. (2007). Conspicuous compassion and wicked problems. *Agenda*, **14**, 35–51.

13 National Public Health Partnership. (2000). *Deciding and specifying an intervention portfolio*. National Public Health Partnership, Melbourne.

14 Rychetnik L, Frommer M. (2002). *A schema for evaluating evidence on public health interventions, version 4*. National Public Health Partnership, Melbourne.

15 Hasson H. (2010). Systematic evaluation of implementation fidelity of complex interventions in health and social care. *Implementation Science*, **5**, 67. Available at: ℘ http://www.implementationscience.com/content/5/1/67.

16 Jorm C, Banks M, Towhill S. (2008). The dynamic of policy and practice. In: Sorenson R, Iedema R, eds, *Managing clinical processes in the health services*. Elsevier, Sydney,

17 McCaughey D, Bruning N. (2010). Rationality versus reality: the challenges of evidence-based decision making for health policy makers. *Implementation Science*, **5**, 39.

18 Jorm C, Banks M, Towhill S. The Dynamic of Policy and Practice. In: Sorenson R, Iedema R, editors. Managing Clinical Processes in the Health Services. Sydney & London: Elsevier, 2008.

19 Shepperd S, Lewin S, Straus S, et al. (2009). Can We Systematically Review Studies That Evaluate Complex Interventions? *PLoS Medicine*, **6**, e1000086.

20 Greenhalgh T, Russell J. (2005). Reframing evidence synthesis as rhetorical action in the policy making drama. *Healthcare Policy*. **11**, 31–5.

21 MacKenzie M, O'Donnell C, Halliday E, Sridharan S, Platt S. (2010). Do health improvement programmes fit with MRC guidance on evaluating complex interventions? *British Medical Journal*, **340,** c185.

22 Pawson R, Greenhalgh T, Harvey G, Walshe K. (2005). Realist review—new method of systematic review designed for complex policy interventions. *Journal of Health Services & Research Policy.* **10(Suppl. 1),** 21–34.

23 Have M. (2010). An overview of ethical frameworks in public health: can they be supportive in the evaluation of programs to prevent overweight? *BMC Public Health.* **10,** 638.

24 Hunter B. (2007). Cumulative causation and the productivity commission's framework for overcoming indigenous disadvantage. *Australian Journal of Labour Economics,* **10.**

25 Hunter B. (2007). Conspicuous compassion and wicked problems. *Agenda,* **14,** 35–51.

26 Report of the Northern Territory Board of Inquiry into the Protection of Aboriginal Children from Sexual Abuse (2007).

27 Ampe Akelyernemane Meke Mekarle (2010). *Little children are sacred.* Available at: ℘ http://www.inquirysaac.nt.gov.au/pdf/bipacsa_final_report.pdf

28 CERD (2010). *Concluding observations of the Committee on the Elimination of Racial Discrimination. Australia, 2010,* UN Doc CERD/C/AUS/CO/15-17. Available at: ℘ http://www2.ohchr.org/english/bodies/cerd/cerds77.htm.

29 Brimblecombe J, McDonnell J, Barnes A, *et al.* (2010). Impact of income management on store sales in the Northern Territory. *Medical Journal of Australia,* **192,** 549–54.

30 Department of Families, Housing, Community Services and Indigenous Affairs. (2009). *Closing the Gap in the Northern Territory, Whole of Government July-June 2009 Monitoring Report.* Australian Government, Canberra.

4.5 Media advocacy for policy influence

Simon Chapman

Objectives

Many public health interventions are controversial or potentially controversial. The way the media handle such issues can strongly influence public
and policy maker attitudes towards them and effective media advocacy
can be a powerful way of taking forward public health initiatives.

After reading this chapter you should have a better understanding of:
• how the media deal with public health issues
• how the way in which an issue is framed influences whether and how
  it leads to changes in policy
• what you can do when a public health issue is framed in an adverse or
  harmful way.

Why is this an important public health skill?

A simple yet vital lesson about influencing politicians is to understand the
centrality of news media in their lives. From the moment of waking, politicians are exposed more than most to how the news media are covering
issues relevant to their portfolio. A clock radio may wake them; a newspaper is read at the breakfast table; news is consumed on the car radio on
the way to work; on arrival, press secretaries brief them about opportunities and threats in the news media that day. Politicians also spend many
hours in hotel rooms with their main companion the television set and
they will often focus on news programmes.

Many public health advocates put great energy into trying to secure
face-to-face appointments with health ministers so they can put the case
for a particular proposal. However, if a health minister has never encountered the issue in the news previously it is likely a low priority will be
given to meeting with people representing the issue. Politicians and their
staff devote a great amount of effort to trying to get difficult issues out of
news pages and to backing high profile issues they believe will advantage
them politically.

Public health advocates' tasks are therefore bound up with both keeping
their issues in the news as unavoidable issues for politicians while doing all
that can be done to avoid framing the politicians who need to take action
as the problem. Like everyone else, politicians tend not to be attracted to

people or movements who are constantly critical of them and prefer to deal with people who can frame them in a good light. Attacking a politician who is the person who needs to take political decisions is generally a step of last resort and one that destines a proposal to be considered by a future (rather than the current) government.[1]

The importance of understanding the media

Potent public health advocates need to make the business of news-making part of their core business and, in doing so, acquire a thorough knowledge and understanding of the way news organizations operate and the nature of newsworthiness. Information about the size and demographics of the audience and readership of different media at different times of the day is basic, as is familiarity with news routines and deadlines. Advocates also need to know the predilections or interests of journalists in all news media. Some will have a particular interest in public health matters; others will be hostile toward some of its regulatory strategies and will therefore require careful attention.

Perhaps the most basic lesson I have learned in a 32-year career in public health advocacy is the importance of standing back from the 'text' of news and trying to understand the power of its subtexts. For example, a story about a research report on smoking in bars, and the concentration of particles inhaled by bar staff, is likely to be deemed newsworthy not because of the scientific particulars of the story, the journal in which it was published, or anything to do with the quality of the research. Journalists are typically not trained in science or epidemiology and do not run critical appraisal 'quality meters' over potential research stories in deciding to run them. What they do react to is the subtext of research, which in this case is bound up with the injustice of bar staff having to endure working conditions that other workers have long been protected from when smoking has been banned from other workplaces. The force and news values of the story lie in its implied injustice and the implications for those responsible.[2] The details and science of the exposure are simply the hook to the 'real' story.

The media are peerless as sites for public health debates in which large and often influential numbers of people will engage. If a public health issue is ignored by the news media, or if the media choose to frame its meaning from the perspectives of those working against the interests of public health, it is highly unlikely that political, public or funding support will follow. There are few, if any, examples of robust public health policy or well-funded programmes that have not been preceded and sustained by widespread and supportive news coverage. As a veteran reporter of 40 years' experience with the *Wall Street Journal* said: 'Well done investigative reporting produces public outrage (or policy maker outrage) that forces new regulations and laws or tougher enforcement of existing ones. Ten-thousand-watt klieg lights turned on a situation focuses the minds of policy makers very fast.'[3]

Framing

A core skill of effective public health media advocates is to appear to have an instinct for framing their concerns in ways that make their issues instantly comprehensible in terms of wider discourses that reach beyond the manifest or overt subject of their concerns. For example, while few people may comprehend the complexities of tobacco litigation rampant in the USA, people do understand from years of negative press reportage about the tobacco industry that the cases are being fought about allegations of negligence, cover-up, and deceit.[4] Such dimensions or sub-texts allow audiences who may not have detailed knowledge or awareness about the particulars of a given issue to identify that here is something similar to an issue they *do* understand. Frames and their sub-texts serve to link topics to familiar, wider socio-political discourses so that coverage of particular events are decoded by audiences as instances of more general themes or types of story.

Entman's classic description notes that framing 'select(s) some aspects of a perceived reality and make them more salient. . . in such a way as to promote a particular problem definition, causal interpretation, moral evaluation and/or treatment recommendation'.[5] Dominant framings can come to define what an issue is 'about' and conditions public perceptions of the appropriate political response to that issue. Work by cognitive psychologists such as Lakoff[6,7] has underscored the importance of understanding the value dimensions to framing and newsworthiness for those wishing to become potent advocates. Such analysis represents the policy process as a semiotic battle in which conflicting parties attempt to have their conceptions of policy problems, acceptable solutions, evaluation criteria, and legitimate policy actors dominate those of their opponents.[8,9] The policy process is portrayed as a social drama centered on conflict over the appropriate terms of the debate.[10]

Much news is not instructively seen as news but as 'olds'—essentially the retelling of age-old stories with new casts, circumstances, infectious agents, and so on. For example, the on-going news saga about doping and anabolic steroid use in sport is essentially the re-telling of the myth of Narcissus—a moral tale about the dangers of vanity, inflected to involve another widely understood sub-text: that cheats should not prosper. Effective public health advocates must learn to think about their issues in such terms, rather than assume that news media have an intrinsic interest in specific issues like cancer, infection, injury and so on.

There is no 'objective reality' that any platform of public health policy can be said to be *really* about. The often heated nature of news discourse about public health issues testifies to the essentially contested nature of advocacy. To injury prevention specialists, compulsory bicycle helmets might mean reduced brain injury and deaths; to indifferent parents their meaning might be framed more in terms of additional expense; and to fashion-conscious youth, the intrusion of a paternalistic state on their ability to dress as they please and thumb their nose at danger. Reality is always a socially constructed notion.

The emphasis or framing that is placed around particular events or issues and that seeks to define *what this issue is really about* will represent only one of many competing meanings that jostle for public dominance. While health interests may frame the meaning of a bill to introduce proof of immunization in terms of the protection of children's health, anti-immunizationists may choose to describe the bill in terms of the encroachment of the `nanny state', `compulsory medication' and other negative metaphors.[11]

Examples of the use of media advocacy

Politics, and therefore the progression of public health policy, is largely about the problem of competing interest groups seeking to advance multiple definitions of the same events. In public health, policy advocacy is ultimately the process by which advocates for different positions and values seek to define what is at issue for the public, media gatekeepers and policy makers and legislators.

For example: are compulsory fences for backyard swimming pools in Australia:[12]

- A blight on garden aesthetics and evidence of big brother, regulatory bureaucracy stepping ever closer into our personal lives?
- The use of a sledgehammer to crack a walnut (since any given pool has a very low probability of 'hosting' a drowning, should every pool owner—particularly those with no children—bear the cost of installing a fence?)

Or

- A safety net to prevent drowning, the leading cause of death in 1–5 year olds?

To take another example, are gun deaths:

- The occasional, unfortunate 'blood price' communities with liberal gun laws pay for the freedom to defend their homes from malevolent intruders?
- Perpetrated by criminals and the mentally ill who are beyond the reach of law?

Or

- Preventable carnage, capable of reduction as with any other public health problem?

When a lone gunman shot 35 people dead within a month at Port Arthur, Australia, in April 1996,[13] all political parties united in support of the Prime Minister's call for semi-automatic rifles and shotguns to be banned, for all guns to be registered, for self-defense to be explicitly excluded as a legitimate reason to own a gun, and for gun ownership to be limited to only those who satisfied a limited number of reasons to own a gun. These policies had been promoted by Australian gun control advocates for years and Port Arthur was a watershed event that overnight made gun law reform politically compelling.

Both before and after Port Arthur, the gun lobby sought to define gun control in ways that would minimize political interest in its implementation. The task for gun control advocates, of course, was to do the opposite. Over the years, we had collected many examples of their key arguments and with hindsight came to see that we had subjected these to a process of analysis amenable for use in media advocacy planning. Rather than responding off-the-cuff to gun lobby efforts to frame gun control as misguided folly, hundreds of media opportunities were disciplined by strategic attempts at framing and reframing the debate[14] to achieve particular objectives. We approached this by using a process that considered the following questions:

- What was our public health objective?
- What frame put around this objective would most neatly and clearly define what was at issue?
- What symbols, metaphors or visual images could be referenced that would trigger this frame in audiences?
- What 'sound bites' (typically, about seven seconds of speech[15] or two to three sentences in newsprint) could encapsulate the essence of the frame?

Table 4.5.1 illustrates two examples of how this process is an adaptation of an approach suggested by Charlotte Ryan[16] and subsequently applied by the Berkeley Media Studies Group to the study of the way that gun control is debated in the US press. Gun lobby 'definitions' of what was at

Table 4.5.1 Contrasting framings of gun control debates

	Gun lobby position (1) 'Why don't you ban knives, axes, and baseball bats too?'	Gun lobby position (2) 'Guns don't kill people, people kill people"
Public health objective	To comunicate that guns are especially dangerous because they are so effective at killing. They kill and injure many more than other weapons so they merit special restrictions	To refocus on the lethality of guns
Frame	Guns as ultra-lethal	• To pull guns back inside the frame defining directions for solutions. • Guns as controllable, people as less controllable
Symbol, visual image or metaphor	• When a gun is available during an argument it's like throwing petrol on a fire • Fist fight vs. gun fight • With guns, minor altercations can lead to death	A violent/disturbed/upset person with an ultra-lethal means of expressing anger
Sound bite	• Gun + criminal intent = 35 dead (Port Arthur). Gun + criminal intent equals 68 dead (Utøya). Machete + criminal intent = 7 injured (Wolverhampton) • 'Guns are a permanent solution to a temporary problem.' • 'I've never heard of a drive-by stabbing'	• People kill—guns make it possible • This is like saying 'bare wires don't kill, electricians do'. • Guns don't die—people do!

issue are shown, together with a reframing strategy encompassing the four questions listed above.

References

1 Chapman S. (2007). *Public health advocacy and tobacco control: making smoking history.* Blackwell Publishing: Oxford.

2 Champion D, Chapman S. (2005). Framing pub smoking bans: An analysis of Australian print news media coverage, March 1996- March 2003. *Journal of Epidemiology and Community Health.* **59,** 679–84.

3 Otten AL. (1992). The influence of the mass media on health policy. *Health Affairs,* **11(4),** 111–18.

4 Carter SM, Chapman S. (2003). Smoking, health and obdurate denial: the Australian tobacco industry in the 1980s. *Tobacco Control.* **12(Suppl. 3),** iii23–30.

5 Entman RM. (1993). Framing: toward clarification of a fractured paradigm. *Journal of Communication,* **43,** 51–8.

6 Lakoff G. (2004). *Don't think of an elephant. Know your values and frame the debate.* ChelseaGreen Publishing, Vermont.

7 Lakoff G. (1996). *Moral politics: what Conservatives know that Liberals don't.* University of Chicago Press, Chicago.

8 Schon DA, Rein M. (1994). *Frame reflection: toward the resolution of intractable policy controversies.* Basic Books: New York.

9 Majone G. (1989). *Evidence, argument and persuasion in the policy process.* Yale University Press, New Haven.

10 Greenhalgh T. (2006). Reframing evidence synthesis as rhetorical action in the policy making drama. *Healthcare Policy,* **1,** 34–42.

11 Leask J, Chapman S, Cooper S. (2010). 'All manner of ills': attribution of serious disease to vaccination. *Vaccine,* **28,** 3066–70.

12 Carey V, Chapman S, Gaffney D. (1994). Children's lives or garden aesthetics? A case study in public health advocacy. *Australian Journal of Public Health,* **18,** 25–32.

13 Chapman S, Alpers P, Agho K, Jones M. (2006). Australia's 1996 gun law reforms: faster falls in firearm deaths, firearm suicides, and a decade without mass shootings. *Injury Prevention,* **12,** 365–72.

14 Chapman S. (1998). *Over our dead bodies: Port Arthur and Australia's fight for gun control.* Pluto, Sydney.

15 Chapman S, Holding S, Ellerm J, et al. (2009). The content and structure of Australian TV reportage on health and medicine: a guide for health workers. *Medical Journal of Australia,* **191,** 620–24.

16 Ryan C. (1991). *Prime time activism.* South End Press, Boston.

4.6 Influencing international policy

Tim Lang and Martin Caraher

Objectives

This chapter will help you understand:
- the relationships between international policy and local policy action
- why public health practitioners should build an international dimension into their work
- how you can influence and advance public health internationally, including through local action.

Why is this an important public health issue?

Delivering public health requires an understanding of different actors, bodies, and processes, and how they interact at regional, national, and global levels; it also requires support and co-ordination between actors at each level. This co-ordination function can test your negotiation skills as tensions between local, national, regional, and global levels of health governance are exposed.

The international dimension of public health work is essential; the drivers and shapers of health may be remote both physically and in terms of the policy drivers. Even the most local actions can have international ramifications and even the best local or national interventions can be improved by outside perspectives.

Many of the policies influencing health are not directly health-related. Health-related issues such as food, transport, housing, water, energy, air, and climate may be shaped by the actions and interactions of distant companies, countries, and other institutions. For example, trade regulations may influence tobacco and food availability just as much as national policies. Because of these complexities public health needs strong advocates and cross-border organization. Public health proponents have to think and act both internationally and locally.

International causes, local effects

Even more than in the past, actions in one place can have unforeseen, and major, impacts elsewhere. For example, healthy eating campaigns in developed countries need to take into account the impact of supply chains. In Germany, advice to drink fruit juice meant an increase in long-distant fruit transport, particularly oranges from Brazil: an estimated 80% of Brazilian orange production is consumed in Europe. Annual German consumption occupied 370,000 acres of Brazilian productive land, three times the land given over to fruit production in Germany. If this level of German orange juice consumption was replicated world wide, 32 million acres would be needed just for orange production. Most of the profits went to intermediaries such as wholesailers and retailers: the incomes of orange growers in Brazil remained low and crops for local consumption were replaced by crops for export.[1] What began as a simple health education message—drink more fruit juice!—had complex and far-reaching consequences.

Infectious diseases migrate, carried by people or other vectors, without regard to national borders. There is nothing new about this: the mediaeval plagues in Europe were fearsome, one of the worst killers in the 20th century was influenza, and HIV/AIDS has caused millions of deaths. Non-communicable diseases (NCDs) cross borders in different ways and through different mechanisms, typically involving social and economic changes that have an impact on new lifestyle decisions and changes. Coronary heart disease, stroke, diabetes, and cancers have increased in incidence worldwide, often associated with changes in diet, and physical activity as populations shift towards a more 'Western' lifestyle—eating different foods, taking less exercise, spending time in front of screens and not just aspiring to, but achieving, western patterns of consumption.[2] Obesity now co-exists with malnutrition in developing countries, while in developed countries obesity rates have created a culture where historically abnormal body mass indices are accepted as normal.

Prevention strategies require the sharing and spreading of knowledge. Swinburn and Egger have argued that population weight gain is shaped by changes in the environment far beyond the immediate control of health actors.[3] WHO now also relates the increase in mental disorders to increases in poverty, urbanization, aging populations, and the pace of life, all factors shaped by international forces—economic, political, and cultural.[2]

These complexities raise questions for public health:

- Are your local and national public health systems tapped into international health organizations that monitor and share best practice on disease?
- Does your planning system include measurement of international health or social impacts?
- Have you any means for feeding data and thinking back into national and international public health systems?
- Have you created or got access to early warning systems?
- Do you have multi-disciplinary networks which give broad-based sources of information at the international level? Conversely, is your information available beyond your area to add to international intelligence?
- Do you know how your locality's profile compares not just nationally but internationally?

The scaling up of economic activity has implications for health

The acceleration of international economic activity has increased various forms of cross-border movement, all of which have health implications:

Movement of goods

The removal of barriers to trade at the 1994 General Agreement on Tariffs and Trade (GATT) talks accelerated emerging patterns of trade and a new body, the World Trade Organization (WTO), became the international secretariat to facilitate the spread of goods and services. Food came under this international economic regime for the first time; as a result, the Nutrition Transition was accelerated. For developing countries, this led to increased access to western fast food chains and soft drinks and for rich consumer societies it has meant retailers sourcing globally. This has restructured power relations between health organizations, governments, companies, and consumers (see the example above on orange juice). The effects can be debated—some see it as progress, others as subversion of national health governance.

Most immediately, these changes altered and exposed the interdependency of quality and hygiene controls. Failures in one country may have consequences far away. International frameworks become ever more important for health. As goods travel further, supply chains become longer and more complex. For public health, there must be systems of traceability and accessible paper-trails to enable audits in case of break-downs and product recalls. These extended and mass scale supply chains introduce many more points for possible contamination or error and have led to the introduction of risk assessment and management systems, such as Hazards Analysis Critical Control Point (HACCP) approaches.

Movement of ideas

Human progress has depended on the spread of ideas but the consequences of such spread can be unpredictable. Advertising, marketing, and the internet can be media by which human understanding is increased or the means by which behaviour change occurs without countervailing health infrastructure or balances in place. Multi-media sources of information give opportunities for evidence to be made more widely available but also allow urban myths and misinformation to 'go viral'.

Movement of people for leisure

In 2008 there were an estimated 922 billion tourist trips taken worldwide, up from 639 billion in 2001. Tourism generated receipts of $944 billion in 2008[4] but for international health what matters is that approximately one seventh of humanity is crossing borders annually and potentially both spreading and catching diseases. It has been estimated that tourists run a 20%–50% risk of contracting a food-borne illness.[5] Travel itself is a significant contribution to environmental damage and air transport is associated with atmospheric pollution (see 📖 Health, sustainability, and climate change).

Movement of people for economic reasons

Flows of labour across national boundaries have considerable social, cultural, and economic impact and migration is one of the key public health issues of the twenty first century. Migration of skilled labour from the global south to the global north has many implications for health care, not the least of which is the denuding of a country of its health care skills and expertise. Migration within countries from rural to urban areas also has many public health implications including the loss of land, work and income.

A seat at the table

Health considerations are often not represented at the policy table where critical decisions are taken. Public health practitioners must ensure they are able to play an active part in proceedings. We cannot assume political and institutional frameworks for addressing the 'trans-nationalization' of health patterns are adequately resourced and fit to keep abreast of economic, social, and cultural change. Public health work and institutions tend to be locally and nationally focused and based, partly due to funding and tax-collection systems, but economic and social changes are increasingly trans-national.

The long struggle to achieve some leverage over international trade in tobacco is an important case study of the value of international work (see Box 4.6.1). There is much to learn from the long, frustrating process of trying to control tobacco, from which key lessons are that a local focus is often insufficient to achieve change, that messages must be consistent, and that being well organized internationally helps the process of incremental change: a gain in one country can be replicated and exceeded elsewhere.

At the time of writing, attempts to introduce plain packaging on cigarette packets are facing legal challenges. The irony is that the challenges are economic and framed within a barrier-to-trade argument, not in relation to public health. This is similar to food and nutrition areas where companies rarely use or challenge public health initiatives in the courts, although they may well lobby about them. For example, in the late 2000s attempts to get optimum front-of-pack nutrition labeling failed in the EU

Box 4.6.1 Case study—tobacco control

Improving tobacco control has been a public health success but has required extended effort, very strong evidence, and clarity of purpose and strategy. The history of tobacco control has been slow: half a century from the first firm evidence to 'leaps' such as bans on smoking in public places and the Framework Convention on Tobacco Control (FCTC). While national campaigns restricted tobacco promotion, international funding has been used to tackle structural issues such as growing practices and health education in tobacco-producing countries, and to subsidize changes in growing practices to help farmers transition from tobacco to other cash crops. The FCTC, which came into force in 2005, was the first international treaty driven and negotiated through the WHO and is one of the most widely embraced treaties in UN history.[6] The Convention is an evidence-based treaty reaffirming the right of all people to the highest standard of health and represents a milestone for health promotion that provides new legal dimensions for international health co-operation.

following heavy and sustained lobbying by some (but not all) giant food industry interests.

Public health practitioners learned, when the GATT 1987–94 negotiations were underway, health could be seen as a 'threat' while trade is perceived as an 'opportunity'.[7] Too often, health lags behind forces driving economic restructuring.

In Europe, years of negotiation preceded the creation of the 1987 Single Market but it was not until bovine spongiform encephalopathy (BSE) 'jumped' to humans in the mid 1990s that the EU recognized and implemented stronger public health measures. A Food Safety White paper was created in 2000 and the European Food Safety Authority came into being in 2002, under Regulation EC 178/2002. A Rapid Alert System was created alongside a new Directorate-General for consumers and health (DG Sanco). In this case almost two decades passed between the facilitation of cross-border trade and the creation of public health measures and institutions to ensure health protection.

The point here is about the opportunism of public health in times of crises to lever policy change. While the BSE crisis was one of food safety and public confidence it also provided an opportunity for discussions on broader remits of food policy at all levels from the local to the global.

Alliances to help deliver change

Alliances are essential for effective championing roles in the public health. They may take different forms: within professions, between professions, in wider society, e.g. with civil society and NGOs, across government, and with pro-public health sections of commerce (see also 📖 Partnerships).

Key issues for effectively influencing international policy include:

- How to develop potential allies—who might help?
- Ongoing analysis of barriers—where might difficulties or opposition come from?
- How to combine short- and long-term perspectives.
- Building up trust relationships across borders.
- Creating trusted teams and networks.
- Accommodating diverse languages, traditions, cultures, expectations, and styles.

One way of influencing global policy involves you or your organization joining campaigning groups or non-governmental organizations and becoming part of regional and global networks. See Case Study in Box 4.6.2 on Baby Milk Action for an example of such an approach; for further examples see 📖 Activism and 📖 Media advocacy for policy influence.

Global institutions: what levers do we have?

Many institutions—governmental, non-governmental, and commercial—operate on a global level (see Table 4.6.1). You could create your own list of key bodies for your interests, and build contacts with and within them, either yourself or through a professional body.

Table 4.6.2 illustrates some conventions and international agreements supporting public health action. There are many others. Some are 'soft' commitments and not given binding power at national or legal level (e.g. Declarations). Some have been criticized as remote or undemocratic.

Box 4.6.2 Case study: international baby foods action network

The International Baby Foods Action Network (IBFAN) involves over 150 citizen groups in over 90 countries. In 1977 a boycott of Nestlé was launched in protest at the company's selling of breast milk substitutes. IBFAN came together in 1979 to promote the boycott, to monitor company infractions, to deliver policy commitments to promote breast-feeding, and to reduce ill-health and deaths from inappropriate infant feeding. It spawned moves among Health Ministries to create the International Code of Marketing of Breastmilk Substitutes (ICMBS). This was Resolution WHA34.22, adopted by the World Health Assembly in 1981 as a 'minimum requirement' to protect infant health. The WHA, WHO's democratic meeting of Member States, agreed the ICMBS should be implemented 'in its entirety'.

Since then IBFAN has become an active global network to strengthen independent, transparent, and effective controls on the marketing of baby foods. Where water is unsafe, a bottle-fed child is up to 25 times more likely to die as a result of diarrhoea than a breast-fed child and the WHO and UNICEF estimate 1.5 million infants die every year because they are not breast-fed. Companies continue to violate the provisions of the ICMBS and IBFAN's work is a reminder of the need for public health vigilance and good monitoring, as well as the value of having NGOs that can concentrate on full-time campaigning and work with professionals. IBFAN helps national campaigns by providing illustrations of best-practice, lobbies international forums, and has helped deliver resolutions at WHA every two years. It won the Right Livelihood Award (often called the alternative Nobel Prize) in 1998 for this work. (See Further resources, below, for more details.)

Table 4.6.1 Global institutions involved in health

Remit	Examples of Organizations
Public health	WHO, Food and Agriculture Organization (FAO),
Children and health	UNICEF, UNESCO
Global economic bodies with health impact	World Bank, International Monetary Fund, World Trade Organization (WTO), Organization for Economic CO-operation and Development (OECD)
Intergovernmental Agreements with a health impact	Bio-safety Convention, International Conference on Nutrition, Basel Convention on hazardous waste
Emergency aid	World Food Programme, International Committee of the Red Cross/Crescent
Environmental health	Global Panel on Climate Change, UN Conference on Environment & Development (UNCED), International Maritime Organization

(Continued)

Table 4.6.1 (Continued)

Remit	Examples of Organizations
Commercial interests	Transnational corporations, International Federation of Pharmaceutical Manufacturers Associations, World Economic Forum
Regional bodies with health role	European Union, Regional Offices of WHO and FAO
Trade Associations	International Hospitals Federation
Networks to promote public health	Healthy Cities Network [WHO], International Baby Food Action Network (IBFAN), Pesticides Action Network, Tobacco Free Initiative [WHO]
Professional associations	Health Action International, International Union of Health Education, World Public Health Association
Non-Governmental Organizations	Friends of the Earth, Oxfam, Médecins sans Frontières, World Federation of Public Health Associations.

Table 4.6.2 Examples of international commitments with public health relevance

Occasion	Date	Relevance
Universal Declaration of Human Rights	1948	Right to health
Stockholm Conference on the Human Environment	1972	Environmental protection
World Food Conference (Universal Declaration on the Eradication of Hunger and Malnutrition)	1974	Eradication of malnutrition
Ottawa Charter on Health Promotion 'Health for All'	1986	Health promotion
Convention on the Rights of Child	1989	Children
Innocenti Declaration on Breastfeeding	1990	Breastfeeding
Kyoto Protocol	1997	Climate change
Millennium Development Goals	2000	Global poverty and inequality reduction targets by 2015.

Others have been made important by being used as yardsticks for health improvement (e.g. binding agreements are ratified by national governments and turned into national laws). They can legitimate local or national actions and people working inside organizations set up to service international commitments can be useful allies.

In relation to any such agreement it is important to ask:
• How strong is it? Is it binding?
• Has your national professional body a position or statement on the issue?
• Has your government ratified it (i.e. put it into national law)?
• If not: why? What are the lessons to be learned? Was it how it was done? Who did it? Find out!

Good public health depends on practitioners and researchers finding new ways to win arguments, build evidence, and improve policy and practice. International links can help generate new methods and approaches. An example of how methods can be refined and improved is the growth of Impact Assessments, including Health Impact Assessments and Environmental Impact Assessments (HIAs/EIAs; see 📖 Assessing health impacts and 📖 Environmental health risks). If HIAs and EIAs were accompanied by Social Impact Assessments public health might have the information needed to tackle multi-level, multi-sectoral problems.

Conclusions

The international dimensions of public health will continue to be addressed by organizations such as the United Nations but there are now many international bodies competing for policy attention and influence on health. They include commerce, sectoral/special interests, professions, and civil society organizations. Sound public health practice can get lost as interests tussle so public health practitioners need to be— and to remain—well organized, informed, and funded internationally. This must not be an afterthought. It is not a luxury.

The causes of health problems are complex. Having an international perspective was always useful; today it is essential. Alliances, across sectors as well as regions, are key ingredients for success.

Influencing health at the international level means:
• combining the local, national, regional, and global
• allowing time for good advocacy and building the international case
• being well resourced and organized
• using existing international health institutions while strengthening, supporting, and sometimes cajoling them
• being prepared to enter complex terrain where there are existing powerful interest groups
• thinking and working in alliances.

Further resources

Lee K. (2003). *Globalization and health: an introduction.* Palgrave, London.

Labonte R, Laverack G. (2008). *Health promotion in action: from local to global empowerment.* Palgrave, Basingstoke.

Lang T, Barling D, Caraher M. (2009). *Food policy: integrating health, environment and society.* Oxford University Press, Oxford.

Rayner G, Lang T. (2012). *Ecological public health: re-shaping the conditions for good health*. Earthscan-Routledge, Abingdon.

UNICEF. (2005). *1990–2005 Celebrating the Innocenti Declaration on the protection, promotion and support of breastfeeding: past achievements, present challenges and the way forward for infant and young child feeding*. UNICEF, Innocenti Research Centre, Florence.

References

1   Kranendonk S, Bringezau, B. (1994). *Major material flows associated with orange juice consumption in Germany*. Wupperthal Institute, Wupperthal.

2   WHO/FAO. (2003). *Diet, nutrition and the prevention of chronic diseases*, Report of the Joint WHO/FAO expert consultation, WHO Technical Report Series, No. 916 (TRS 916). WHO/Food and Agriculture Organization, Geneva.

3   Egger G, Swinburn B. (2010). *Planet Obesity: How we're eating ourselves and the planet to death*. NSW: Allen and Unwin.]

4   Conrady R, Buck M. (2009). *Trends and Issues in Global Tourism 2010*. Springer: Berlin.

5   Käferstein FK, Motarjemi Y, Bettcher DW. (1997). *Foodborne disease control: a transnational challenge*. Emerging Infectious Diseases. **3**, 503–10.

6   WHO FCTC. (2010).*Framework Convention on Tobacco Control*. Geneva. WHO: Geneva. http://www.who.int/fctc/en/ [accessed 20 December 2010]

7   Lee K. (2003). *Globalization and Health: An Introduction*. Palgrave, London.

4.7 Public health in poorer countries

Nicholas Banatvala and Eric Heymann

More than a third of the developing world's people still live in poverty (as measured by the Multidimensional Poverty Index[1]). According to the 2010 Human Development Report around 1.75 billion people live in poverty of whom nearly 1.5 billion live on less than $1.25 a day.[2] This chapter looks at the broader determinants of health and current approaches to tackling public health in poor countries.

Objectives

Reading this chapter will help you understand:
- the major public health issues among the poor populations of the world
- the approaches used to tackle them.

Why is this an important public health issue?

Health is a long-recognized human right. Better health is associated with decreased poverty because it enables people to secure better livelihoods. This is true at both a micro (family) level (less time caring for the sick means more time to earn and learn) and at a macro level (less sickness leads to regional and national economic growth).

The World Bank's Global Burden of Diseases and Risk Factors highlights the fact that low- and middle-income countries account for a comparatively large number of premature deaths.[3] The report also notes that, worldwide, one death in every three is from communicable disease, maternal and perinatal conditions, or nutritional deficiencies. Communicable diseases remain the most important reason for the existence of the 'poor–rich' gap (world's poorest 20% to richest 20%) but nearly 80% of non-communicable deaths occur in low and middle-income countries and are the most frequent cause of death in most countries, except in Africa.[4] Even in African nations the prevalence of non-communicable diseases is rising rapidly and they are projected to exceed communicable, maternal and perinatal, and nutritional diseases as the most common causes of death by 2020.

There is huge variation in health not only between the poor and the rich globally but also within developing countries. Examples of health inequities between countries are:
- infant mortality in Iceland is 2 per 1000 live births but over 120 per 1000 live births in Mozambique

- the risk of maternal death during or shortly after pregnancy is 1 in 17,400 in Sweden but 1 in 8 in Afghanistan.

Examples of health inequities within countries include:

- Bolivia, where babies born to women with no education have infant mortality over 100 per 1000 live births while the infant mortality in babies born to mothers with at least secondary education is below 40 per 1000.
- In some countries, women in the richest 20% of the population are up to 20 times more likely to have a birth attended by a skilled health worker than poorer women.

WHO recommends using prepay mechanisms (e.g. insurance and/or taxes) to raise funds and then pooling funds to ensure equity of access and spread financial risks. There have been attempts to quantify the costs of a basic package of health care, such as that by the 2001 Commission on Macroeconomics and Health, and recent work by the WHO estimated for 2014 an annual cost of US $54 per person in 49 low-income countries.[5] Estimating these costs is very difficult and there is no universally accepted figure.

The health care budget in most developing countries is inadequate to meet health needs. There is good evidence that investing in healthcare has a positive impact on both the health and wealth of a nation, but typically 20% to 40% of health spending is wasted. Overpaying is one form of waste: for example, medicine prices can be up to 67 times the international average price.[6] In addition, in many countries resources are often inappropriately directed at expensive hospital care rather than more cost-effective primary care.

How do we define important tasks?

Targets are required to provide milestones against which progress towards the goal of eliminating poverty can be measured. A prominent set of targets is based on recent UN Conventions and Resolutions. The MDGs and their targets are described below.

Objectives for eliminating poverty

Four primary objectives can be considered when poverty elimination is the objective in poorer countries:

- promoting sustainable livelihoods through policy and action (pro-poor policies, development of efficient and well-regulated markets, access of poor people to land, resources, and markets, prevention and resolution of conflicts)
- improving access to health, education, water, and sanitation[7]
- empowering women and marginalized groups and communities
- protecting, and improving management of, the natural and physical environment (sustainable managing of physical and natural resources, using of productive capacity efficiently, protecting the global environment).

Current key areas for *health gain* include:

- infant and child mortality
- maternal mortality

- reproductive health
- HIV, TB, malaria, and other communicable diseases—including preparing for and responding to emerging diseases and pandemics
- non-communicable diseases.

HIV remains a continual threat to global development. In some areas it has overturned many decades of development investment and has affected both rich and poor countries economically, socially, politically, and culturally. More recently, poorer countries have had access to increased resources to tackle HIV and AIDS and in many countries there has been remarkable success in tackling the epidemic. There has also been progress in tackling malaria and TB. More action is required in these areas and renewed focus needed to tackle maternal and child health and start tackling non-communicable diseases.

Responding to these challenges requires the delivery of effective health care and of health systems with universal coverage. However, investment in broader areas is needed to improve health, including:

- good governance, elimination of corruption, the rule of law, and ensuring human rights are upheld
- the support of local and self-sustaining economic growth
- income and employment opportunities
- population growth
- water and food
- education
- gender inequalities
- tackling disasters and emergencies (see Chapter 3.5).

The WHO Commission for the Social Determinants of Health set out a framework for tackling the wider determinants of health.[8] The Commission was clear: it said the 'circumstances in which people grow, live, work, and age' strongly influence how people live and die.

There are four key actions that, taken together and vigorously pursued at national and international levels, would have a great impact on the health and wealth of poor populations (Table 4.7.1).

Table 4.7.1 Actions to improve the health of the poor

Priority response	Specific priorities	Examples of actions
Addressing the priority problems of the poorest billion, strengthening access to care, services, and products	Making pregnancy safer and improving reproductive and sexual services	Developing appropriate local policies and strategies, empowering communities, improving access to essential obstetric care, including abortion services, promoting availability of contraceptives, generating school-based programmes

(Continued)

Table 4.7.1 (Continued)

Priority response	Specific priorities	Examples of actions
	Controlling communicable diseases	Controlling malaria, TB, HIV/AIDS. Eradicating polio, onchocerciasis, and lymphatic filariasis. Responding to emerging infections (e.g. SARS)
	Preventing injuries and non-communicable diseases	WHO Tobacco-Free Initiative. Tackling harmful use of alcohol, unhealthy diet and physical inactivity, and mental illness[9]
Investment in strong, efficient, and effective health systems (public, private, and informal)	Supporting coherent systems rather than fracturing effort	Developing institutional and financially sustainable health systems, promoting intersectoral actions towards health improvement, utilizing public subsidies to assure equal access to health service for equal need
Creating social, political, and physical environments that empower poor people		Increasing safe shelters, road and vehicle safety. Minimizing environmental hazards, violence, pollution, and waste
A more effective global response to health and HIV/AIDS	Raising the profile	Advocacy at local national and international levels
	Enabling environment for prevention and control	Improving gender equity, programmes to reduce stigma and discrimination
	Effective health care	Improve access for poor. Improve access to medicines and technologies. Understanding social and behavioural issues such as risk behaviour
	Improving knowledge and technology	Medicines, technologies, vaccines and microbiocide development.

What is the best way of working?

No agency is able to put in place these key actions by itself. The Paris Declaration on Aid Effectiveness highlighted the importance of harmonizing and aligning aid efforts. Improving transparency in what is needed, who is willing to help, who can help, and in what way, may prevent overlap of projects and enable successful cooperation in a global effort to combat the issue at stake. Those developing strategies to implement international policy need to do four things.

Work in partnership

Partnerships between rich and poor countries can involve private and voluntary sectors, researchers, multilateral development organizations, and donors. To avoid the burden of multiple initiatives and projects, donors increasingly work with governments and other stakeholders in poor countries in a sector-wide approach so efforts are focused on agreed priorities. Public-private partnerships include the Global Fund to Fight AIDS, TB, and Malaria; the Global Alliance for Vaccines and Immunization (GAVI); and Roll-Back Malaria. There are less formal networks too, such as NCDnet. Many international NGOs have focused on generating programmes sustained by host government, private organizations, or local NGOs.

Use both multilateral and bilateral initiatives effectively

Examples of this include strengthening the technical and operational arms of UN agencies such as WHO and UNICEF and working directly on projects with governments and other partners in poor countries. The World Bank, Regional Development Banks, and the International Monetary Fund (IMF) are also key partners for development work.

Ensure local ownership of initiatives

Ensure local ownership of initiatives and local capacity development, and base activities on available evidence. The Sustainable Livelihoods approaches take a holistic view rather than just focusing on a few factors (e.g. economic issues, communicable disease, food security). The principles of sustainable livelihoods are that activities should be people-centered, responsive and participatory, multilevel, conducted in partnership, sustainable, holistic, and dynamic.[9]

Match political commitment with funding and debt relief

Maintaining funding for international development and for global health is a significant challenge. These problems become harder to promote whenever there is pressure on international financial systems, such as in times of world economic crisis. The UN MDG summits,[10] as well as the G8 and other gatherings, provide opportunities to ensure political and financial commitment is maintained. These have resulted in several initiatives, such as the International Health Partnership, that continue to work to promote public health in poorer countries. Conferences, such as the 2011 UN High Level Meeting on Non-communicable Diseases, can provide important milestones in the global effort to tackle these diseases. The ultimate aim is to turn political commitment into financing for debt relief, development, and commitment from poor countries to use aid better.

Factors essential to success

The agenda above is more likely to succeed if a number of fundamental principles are adhered to. Success is unlikely unless we can:
- address the causes rather than just the symptoms of ill-health
- remove barriers that prevent the poor accessing services
- assure public standards, accountability, and responsiveness
- strengthen state policy making, regulation, and service provision
- encourage the private sector to deliver services to poor people
- support the UN system to provide leadership for health
- fully commit to achieving the MDGs.

Nine fallacies

International public health policy is as prone to dogma as any area of domestic public health.

Fallacy 1: models focused on a single discipline are most effective in tackling public health problems in developing countries

Approaches to international health have changed over time and biomedical, economic, and institutional/governance approaches have each been promoted. The present consensus is that poverty reduction should be at the core of international development policy and addressed through a range of different disciplines.

Fallacy 2: either vertical or horizontal public health programmes are always better

Vertical programmes have been successful in areas such as immunization and useful in introducing new concepts (e.g. Directly Observed Treatment Short Course for tuberculosis (DOTS)) or the rapid roll-out of specific initiatives (e.g. insecticide-treated bed nets). In the longer term, however, sustainable services need health systems that integrate into national health systems rather than focusing on a few specific interventions and services.

Fallacy 3: the cost of action and attaining the MDGs and better health for all cannot be met

The MDG targets and wider international health commitments will not be easy to achieve—and in some areas, especially in sub-Saharan Africa, are seriously off-track—but there remains the chance of meeting them if there is effective international cooperation (the harnessing of private and public sectors and forming of global alliances including governments, NGOs, and philanthropists), maintaining (and where necessary increasing) funding for programme activity, as well as R&D, and employing principles of sustainable livelihoods.

Fallacy 4: models of health care delivery developed in Western settings can be effectively transferred to other situations

Enthusiasm for health sector reform based on management trends in Europe (decentralization, managerial autonomy, contracting, and internal market mechanisms) has been dampened by a realization that reforms must be tailored to local circumstances. Nevertheless, there are often examples where middle- and low-income countries can learn from developed countries when it comes to incentives for effective healthcare delivery and indicators that measure aspects of a successful healthcare. No single mix of policy options will work in every setting.

Fallacy 5: cost-recovery systems are an effective approach to providing long-term delivery of health services

Cost-recovery systems (self-sustaining systems financed by the local community) have fallen out of favour because of concerns about equity, with poorer patients excluded and subsidies benefiting the non-poor. In any event, revenue yields have often been minimal.

Fallacy 6: in developing countries there is no place for anything other than publically-funded and run services

The private sector should be encouraged and valued in areas of service delivery, support of health systems, research, and development, and as a policy maker and donor. In some of the most desperate countries, such as Afghanistan, private health care will form a greater component of overall health delivery than government-funded health care. The private sector cannot be ignored.

Fallacy 7: there are too many players in international health with policies muddled through the competing agendas of UN agencies, NGOs, and others

Compared with the number of agencies in developed countries, the number of agencies in development projects in resource-poor countries is often small. All the same, the number of agencies responding to global health needs has grown, leading to a co-ordination challenge, and high-profile relief events (e.g. Rwanda 1994, Kosovo 1999, South East Asia Tsunami 2004) often lead to competition between agencies for financial and media opportunities. Governments and other institutional donors have a responsibility to distribute funds to agencies with proven track records in the field of work and geographic region.

Fallacy 8: the real threat to development is globalization

Globalization is far from detrimental: there are plenty of opportunities, if harnessed appropriately, that come from a global community: economic, trade agreements, and an international response to debt relief, communication, and rapid transfer of information, maximizing flows of finance and capital, and investment, competition, and the private sector.

Fallacy 9: funding development activities is more effective than funding relief

Disaster preparedness and prevention are an essential component of development assistance. Disasters, natural and of human origin, including war, are more common in poor countries. The 'relief–development continuum' (cycles of relief and development) with agencies co-operating in different areas of expertise and 'developmental relief' (development models used in chronic relief efforts and often in complex emergencies) are both increasingly accepted approaches.

Examples of successes, failures, and lessons learnt

Readers interested in specific geographic or sector initiatives should search health databases or contact donors and implementers in these areas (see 📖 Media advocacy for policy influence). Most donors and implementing agencies produce annual reports. These often identify recent programmes—for example, annual reports produced by UN and multilateral agencies, such as WHO and the World Bank, bilateral agencies (e.g. Department for International Development (DFID) UK), and NGOs—and are widely available on the Internet.

Which criteria are most useful for measuring success?

The MDGs are a key set of measures and the focus of great attention. There are 8 MDGs and 18 targets relating to poverty, human development, environmental sustainability, and partnership (see Box 4.7.1).

Box 4.7.1 Four of the eight millennium development goals (MDGs) and associated targets

Goal 1: eradicate extreme poverty and hunger
- Between 1990 and 2015, halve the proportion of people whose income is less than $1 a day.
- Between 1990 and 2015, halve the proportion of people who suffer from hunger.

Goal 4: reduce child mortality
Between 1990 and 2015, reduce the under-five mortality rate by $2/_3$.

Goal 5: reduce maternal mortality
Between 1990 and 2015, reduce the maternal mortality rate by ¾.

Goal 6: combat HIV/AIDS, malaria and other diseases
- By 2015, halt HIV/AIDS spread and have begun to reverse it
- By 2015 halt and have begun to reverse the incidence of malaria and other major diseases.

How will we know if we have been successful?

Forty-eight indicators measure the progress of the eight MDGs. These were reviewed at the 2010 MDG Summit. Developing countries and UN agencies collect data to track their poverty reduction strategies. The development community must support improved data collection.

Improvements are being made on the health-related MDG targets in relation to child mortality, maternal mortality, access to safe drinking water, HIV infection rates, and treatment for TB.[11] Although these are promising signs, there is much more to do if we are to achieve the targets and to improve public health in poorer countries generally.

Acknowledgement

The authors alone are responsible for the views expressed in this chapter, and they do not necessarily represent the decisions, policy, or views of the World Health Organization, Global Brigades, or any other organization.

Further resources

Annual Millennium Development Goals Reports and other relevant reports, from 2005 to 2010. Available at: ℘ http://www.un.org/millenniumgoals/reports.shtml (accessed 30 May 2011).

Disease Control Priorities in Developing Countries Project. This is a collaboration of the World Bank, WHO, John E Fogarty International Center, Population Reference Bureau, US National Institutes of Health, and the Bill and Melinda Gates Foundation. There are three main publications: Disease Control Priorities in Developing Countries, Priorities in Health, and Global Burden of Disease and Risk Factors. Available at: ℘ http://www.dcp2.org/main/Home.html (accessed 31 May 2011).

MDGs. Available at: ℘ http://www.un.org/millenniumgoals/ (accessed 30 May 2011).

United Nations Development Programme. Available at: ℘ http://www.undp.org/ (accessed 30 May 2011)

UNDP. *Human Development Reports.* Available at: ℘ http://hdr.undp.org/ (accessed 30 May 2011).

World Development Reports. Available at: ℘ http://econ.worldbank.org/wdr/ (accessed 30 May 2011). Recent reports include Development and the Next Generation (2007), Making Services Work for Poor People (2004), and Investing in Health (2003).

World Health Organization. WHO, Geneva. Available at: ℘ http://www.who.int/en/.

WHO World Health Reports. WHO, Geneva. Available at: ℘ http://www.who.int/whr/en/index.html (accessed 30 June 2011). Recent reports include: Health systems financing: the path to universal coverage (2011), Primary Health Care: Now More Than Ever (2008), Working together for health (2006, focussing on the global health workforce), and Make Every Mother and Child Count (2005).

Non-governmental organizations

Centre for Global Development. Available at: ℘ http://www.cgdev.org/ (accessed 31 May 2011).

Institute of Development Studies. Available at: ℘ http://www.ids.ac.uk/ (accessed 31 May 2011).

International Health Partnership. Available at: ℘ http://www.internationalhealthpartnership.net (accessed 1st June 2011).

Médecins sans Frontières. Available at: ℘ http://www.msf.org/ (accessed 30 May 2011).

Oxfam UK. Available at: ℘ http://www.oxfam.org.uk/ (accessed 30 May 2011).

References

1 UN Development Programme. (2011). *Multidimensional Poverty Index*. Available at: ✎ http://hdr. undp.org/en/statistics/mpi/ (accessed 30 May 2011).

2 Human Development Report. (2010). *The Real Wealth of Nations: Pathways to Human Development*. Available at: ✎ http://hdr.undp.org/en/reports/global/hdr2010/ (accessed 30 May 2011).

3 Lopez AD, Maters CD, Ezzati, et al. (2006). *Global Burden of Disease and Risk factors*. The World Bank and Oxford University Press; New York. Available at: ✎ www.dcp2.org/pubs/gbd. (accessed 30 May 2011).

4 WHO. (2011). *Global Status Report on Noncommunicable Diseases 2010*. WHO, Geneva. Available at: ✎ http://www.who.int/chp/ncd_global_status_report/en/index.html (accessed 30 May 2011).

5 WHO. (2009).*Constraints to scaling up and costs*, background document for the Taskforce on Innovative International Financing for Health systems. Available at: ✎ http://www.unicef.org/health/files/MBB_Technical_Background_Global_Costing_HLTF_Final_Draft_30_July.pdf (accessed 6 June 2011).

6 WHO. (2010). *10 facts on health financing*. Available at: ✎ http://www.who.int/features/factfiles/universal_health_coverage/en/index.html (accessed 30 May 2010).

7 World Bank. (2004). *Making services work for poor people*, World Development Report, The World Bank, Washington, DC. Available at: ✎ http://www-wds.worldbank.org/external/default/main?pagePK=64193027&piPK=64187937&theSitePK=523679&menuPK=64187510&searchMenuPK=64187283&siteName=WDS&entityID=000090341_20031007150121 (accessed 31 May 2011).

8 Closing the gap in a generation (2008). *Health equity through action on the social determinants of health*. World Health Organization, Geneva. Available at: ✎ http://whqlibdoc.who.int/hq/2008/WHO_IER_CSDH_08.1_eng.pdf, (accessed 30 May 2011).

9 International Fund for Agriculture Development. (2011). *The sustainable livelihoods approach*. Available at: ✎ http://www.ifad.org/sla/index.htm (accessed 27 May 2011).

10 We can end poverty 2015. *The Millennium Development Goals*. Available at: ✎ http://www.un.org/en/mdg/summit2010/ (accessed 30 May 2011).

11 World Health Organization. (2011). *Millennium development goals: progress towards the health-related millennium development goals*. Geneva. Available at: ✎ http://www.who.int/mediacentre/factsheets/fs290/en/index.html. (accessed on 27 May 2011).

4.8 Regulation

Lawrence Gostin

Objectives

The objectives of this chapter are to help you understand:
• the impact of legislation, regulations, and litigation on the public's health
• the powers, duties, and restraints imposed by the law on public health officials
• the potential of legal change to improve the public's health, and
• the role of international law in securing public health in the face of increasing globalization.

Why is this an important public health issue?

Public health practitioners often regard law as arcane, indecipherable, and unhelpful in pursuing their objective of improving the public's health. Certainly, law can obfuscate rather than clarify, impede rather than facilitate. However, even when the law stands as an obstacle, practitioners must understand it; they may even seek to circumvent legal barriers provided it is lawful and ethical to do so. More important, the law can be empowering, providing innovative solutions to the toughest health problems. For example, most of the ten great public health achievements in the United States in the 20th century were realized, in part, through law reform or litigation:[1]
• vaccinations
• safer workplaces
• safer and healthier foods
• motor vehicle safety
• control of infectious diseases
• tobacco control
• fluoridation of drinking water.

The law—both legislation and regulation—is far more important in public health than usually acknowledged. Law creates a mission for public health authorities, assigns their functions, and specifies the manner in which they may exercise their power (see Box 4.8.1). The law is a tool to influence norms for healthy behaviour, identify and respond to health threats, and set and enforce health and safety standards. The most important social debates about public health take place in legal forums—legislatures, courts, and administrative agencies—and in the law's language of rights, duties, and justice. It is no exaggeration to say that 'the field of public health. . . could no longer exist in the manner in which we know it today except for its sound legal basis'.[2]

Box 4.8.1 Powers, duties, limitations

'Health officers must be familiar not only with the extent of their powers and duties, but also with the limitations imposed upon them by law. With such knowledge available and widely applied by health authorities, public health will not remain static, but will progress.'
Tobey (1947).[3]

Definitions

There is a subtle difference between 'public health law' and 'law and the public's health'. The former is the body of legislation that creates governmental public health agencies and enables them to carry out their activities. The latter is the wider body of law that can be used in a variety of ways to safeguard and promote the public's health.

Public health law can be defined as the legislation and administrative rules that delineate a public health agency's mission, duties, and powers to assure the conditions for people to be healthy and the limits on an agency's power to constrain the autonomy, privacy, liberty, or proprietary interests of individuals.

Law and the public's health can be defined as the legislation, regulations, and case law that can be used as a tool to safeguard and promote the public's health including altering the socio-economic, informational, natural, and built environments.

The law for public health practitioners

As a public health practitioner you should understand and obey the law. This means you must act within the scope of your legal authority, never abuse your power, treat persons with respect, and consult with community leaders. If the law is unclear, you should seek the guidance of public health lawyers. Since few lawyers have a specialized knowledge of population health, education and training programmes in public health law are needed.

Public health law: deficiencies and opportunities

Inadequacy of existing legislation

In many countries, public health legislation is so old it tells the story of health threats through time, with new layers of regulation for each page in history—from plague and smallpox to tuberculosis and polio, and now HIV/AIDS, SARS, and new forms of influenza. Legislation often pre-dates modern public health science and practice and does not conform to modern ideas relating to the mission, functions, and services of agencies. Existing laws also often pre-date advances in human rights, failing to safeguard civil liberties. These deficiencies become particularly apparent in times of crisis such as terrorism or emerging infectious diseases.

The purposes of sound public health legislation

Sound public health legislation should provide agencies with a clear and modern mission to create the conditions in which people can be healthy. The statute should enable agencies to exercise a full range of necessary functions, services, and powers. It should similarly provide funding and other structures necessary to carry out the agency's mission. At the same time, public health legislation should protect individual rights to privacy, autonomy, liberty, and non-discrimination. In particular, it should enunciate clear standards for the exercise of powers, due process, and fair treatment – see Box 4.8.2.

> ## Box 4.8.2 Model public health legislation
>
> In response to the attacks on the World Trade Center and subsequent dispersal of anthrax in the US, the Centre for Law and the Public's Health at Georgetown and Johns Hopkins Universities drafted the Model State Emergency Health Powers Act (MSEHPA). The MSEHPA was structured to reflect five basic public health functions to be facilitated by law:[4]
> * preparedness
> * surveillance
> * management of property
> * protection of persons, and
> * public information and communication.

In the US in 2003, the 'Turning Point' Public Health Statute Modernization Collaborative drafted a comprehensive public health act focusing on the organization, delivery, and funding of essential public health services, together with a full set of powers and safeguards.[5] The WHO is currently developing a model national public health law that can be used as a template by countries with different legal traditions.

Public health law: power, duty, and restraint

Public health law creates public health agencies and grants them specific powers including:
- surveillance and monitoring
- testing and screening
- vaccination and treatment
- partner notification and contact tracing
- isolation and quarantine.

The effective and careful use of these powers allows public health officials to protect and improve the public's health. The law also constrains the exercise of these powers. Public health officials should be conscious of how the exercise of these powers impacts on the enjoyment of liberties (e.g. the right to privacy and freedom of movement) and should implement appropriate limits and procedural safeguards to ensure that a proper balance between individual liberties and the public's health is reached.

Law and the public's health: regulation and litigation as a tool

If government has an obligation to promote the conditions for people to be healthy, what tools are at its disposal? There are at least seven models for legal intervention designed to prevent injury and disease, encourage healthful behaviours, and generally promote the public's health. Although legal interventions can be effective, they often raise critical social, ethical, or constitutional concerns that warrant careful consideration.

Model 1: the power to tax and spend

The power to tax and spend is ubiquitous in national constitutions, providing government with an important regulatory technique. The power to spend supports the public health infrastructure consisting of: a well-trained workforce, electronic information and communications systems, rapid disease surveillance, laboratory capacity, and response capability. The state can also set health-related conditions for the receipt of public funds. The power to tax provides inducements to engage in beneficial behaviour and disincentives to engage in risk activities. Tax relief can be offered for health-producing activities such as medical services, childcare, and charitable contributions. At the same time, tax burdens can be placed on the sale of hazardous products such as cigarettes, alcoholic beverages, and firearms.

Model 2: the power to alter the informational environment
The public is bombarded with information that influences their life choices and this undoubtedly affects health and behaviour. The government has several tools at its disposal to alter the informational environment, encouraging people to make more healthful choices about diet, exercise, cigarette smoking, and other behaviours:
- use communication campaigns as a major public health strategy (e.g. educate the public about safe driving, safe sex, physical activity, and nutritious diets)
- require businesses to label their products to include instructions for safe use, disclosure of contents or ingredients, and health warnings
- limit harmful or misleading information in private advertising (e.g. ban or regulate advertising of potentially harmful products, including cigarettes, firearms, and even high-fat or other unhealthy foods, including trans fatty acids).

Model 3: the power to alter the built environment
Public health has a long history in designing the built environment to reduce injury (e.g. workplace safety, traffic calming, and fire codes), infectious diseases (e.g. sanitation, zoning, and housing codes), and harms from the environment (e.g. lead paint and toxic emissions). As countries face an epidemiological transition from infectious to chronic diseases, environments can be designed to promote liveable cities and facilitate health-affirming behaviour by, for example:
- encouraging more active lifestyles (walking, cycling, and playing)
- improving nutrition (fruits, vegetables, and avoidance of high-fat, high-caloric foods)
- decreasing use of harmful products (cigarettes and alcoholic beverages)
- reducing violence (domestic abuse, street crime, and firearm use), and
- increasing social interactions (helping neighbours and building social capital).

Model 4: the power to alter the socio-economic environment
A strong and consistent finding of epidemiological research is that socio-economic status (SES) is correlated with morbidity, mortality, and functioning. SES is a complex phenomenon related to, amongst other things, income, education, and occupation. Some scholars have even suggested that 'justice is good for our health'.[6] By narrowing socio-economic disparities the state seeks to reduce inequities and improve the population's health.

Model 5: direct regulation of persons, professionals, and businesses
Government has the power to directly regulate individuals, professionals, and businesses:
- regulation of individual behaviour (e.g. use of seatbelts and motorcycle helmets) reduces injuries and deaths

- licences and permits enable government to monitor and control the standards and practices of professionals and institutions (e.g. doctors, hospitals, and nursing homes)
- inspection and regulation of businesses helps to assure humane conditions of work, reduction in toxic emissions, and safer consumer products.

Model 6: indirect regulation through the tort system

Attorneys general, public health authorities, and private citizens possess a powerful means of indirect regulation through the tort system. Civil litigation can redress many different kinds of public health harms:

- environmental damage (e.g. air pollution or groundwater contamination)
- exposure to toxic substances (e.g. pesticides, radiation, or chemicals)
- hazardous products (e.g. tobacco or firearms), and
- defective consumer products (e.g. children's toys, recreational equipment, or household goods).

For example, in 1998 tobacco companies negotiated a master settlement agreement with American states that required compensation in perpetuity, with payments totalling $206 billion through to the year 2025.[7]

Model 7: deregulation—law as a barrier to health

Sometimes laws are harmful to the public's health and stand as an obstacle to effective action. In such cases, the best remedy is deregulation. Consider laws that penalize exchanges or pharmacy sales of syringes and needles. Restricting access to sterile drug injection equipment can fuel the transmission of HIV infection. Similarly, the closure of bathhouses to prevent the spread of sexually transmitted infections can drive the epidemic underground, making it more difficult to reach sexually-active gay men with condoms and safe sex literature. Finally, the criminal prohibition of narcotics can often create impediments to healthcare professionals in offering pain relief to suffering patients.

Global health law: comparative and international perspectives

The use of the law to improve the public's health is also important at the international level. Health hazards—biological, chemical, and radionuclear—have profound global implications. Whether the threat's origin is natural, accidental, or intentional, the harms transcend national frontiers and warrant a transnational response. The potential scope of international public health law is vast, ranging from communicable (e.g. global surveillance and border control) and non-communicable diseases (e.g. occupational health and narcotics) and injuries to trade, environmental, and human rights concerns. This section briefly discusses three important international legal instruments.

The International Health Regulations (IHR)

The World Health Assembly adopted the revised IHR in 2005.[8] The IHR had been critiqued because of its narrow scope (applying only to cholera, plague, and yellow fever), lack of enforcement, failure to set minimum national public health capacities, and failure to provide sufficient financial and technical assistance to poor countries. The main improvements in the new IHR are:

- *Expanded jurisdiction:* covering 'all events which may constitute a public health emergency of international concern'.
- *National focal points:* for official WHO communications in each country.
- *Core capacities:* for public health preparedness in order to detect, report, and respond to public health risks.
- *Global surveillance:* by using official and unofficial sources of information and modern data systems.
- *Recommended measures:* to reduce health risks on a standing or temporary basis.

The Framework Convention on Tobacco Control (FCTC)

The WHO has turned to international law solutions in the area of chronic diseases as well as infectious diseases. Particularly remarkable is the FCTC, adopted by the World Health Assembly in 2003.[9] As of 2010, 168 states had signed the convention, 14 states had accepted it, and the FCTC had come into force. The FCTC establishes a 'framework' for ongoing diplomacy to reduce the global health threat posed by tobacco.

Human Rights Law

The effective protection of public health also rests on laws that are underpinned by, and consistent with, human rights. Human rights are legal guarantees protecting universal values of human dignity and freedom, and they define the entitlements of all human beings and the corresponding obligations of the State as the primary duty-bearer. An important human rights standard for the purposes of this handbook is the right to the enjoyment of the highest attainable standard of health, often referred to as the 'right to health'. First recognized in the WHO Constitution, it is enshrined in six core international human rights treaties, including the International Covenant on Economic, Social and Cultural Rights (ICESCR).

In order to clarify the content and meaning of the right to health, the UN Committee on Economic, Social and Cultural Rights (CESCR)'s General Comment 14 explains that the right to health is an inclusive right, extending beyond health care to the underlying determinants of health such as access to safe and potable water; adequate sanitation; adequate supply of safe food; nutrition; housing; healthy occupational and environmental conditions; access to health-related education and information, including on sexual and reproductive health; and freedom from discrimination.[10] States have an obligation to take immediate steps to progressively ensure that services, goods, and facilities are *available, accessible, acceptable,* and of *good quality.*

There is a variety of other health-related rights in international law that supports actions by government to improve the health of their populations.

These rights include the right to adequate food, clothing, and housing, and the right to 'environmental and industrial hygiene' in the ICESCR. Other rights include the right to liberty and security of the person, freedom from coerced labour, liberty of movement, and freedom from discrimination on groups including race, colour, sex, language, religion, and political opinion, as recognized in the International Covenant on Civil and Political Rights (ICCPR). Public health laws framed in ways that respect human rights are likely to be most effective in achieving the goals of disease prevention and health promotion.

Conclusion

The law is a much under-appreciated tool for health improvement. Many public health practitioners distrust the law and the law-making process; they are often not skilled in using, or reforming, the law to improve the public's health. Yet law at the national and international level can have profound effects in changing attitudes and behaviours of individuals and businesses with remarkable benefits for the health of populations.

Further resources

Books and articles

Bailey TM, Caulfield T, Ries N. (2009). *Public Health Law and Policy in Canada*. Butterworths, Markham.

Burci G, Vignes CH. (2004). *World Health Organization*. Kluwer Law International, The Hague.

Gostin LO. (2008). *Public health law: power, duty, restraint*, 2nd edn. University of California Press and Milbank Memorial Fund, Berkeley.

Gostin LO. (2010). *Public health law and ethics: a reader*, 2nd edn. University of California Press and Milbank Memorial Fund, Berkeley.

Reynolds C. (2004). *Public health law and regulation*. Federation Press, Sydney.

Websites on public health law

The O'Neill Institute for National and Global Health Law at Georgetown University. Available at: http://www.oneillinstitute.org (accessed 13 August 2010).

The Centre for Law and the Public's Health (Georgetown and Johns Hopkins universities). Available at: http://www.publichealthlaw.net/ (accessed 13 August 2010).

US Department of Health and Human Services Centers for Disease Control and Prevention. *Public health law program*. Available at: http://www2a.cdc.gov/phlp/ (accessed 13 August 2010).

World Health Organization. Available at: http://www.who.int/en/ (accessed 13 August 2010).

Commission on Social Determinants of Health (2008). *Closing the gap in a generation: health equity through action on the social determinants of health*, final report. WHO, Geneva. Available at: http://www.who.int/social_determinants/thecommission/finalreport/en/index.html (accessed 13 August 2010).

References

1 Centers for Disease Control and Prevention. (1999). Ten great public health achievements—United States, 1900–1999. *Morbity and Mortality Weekly Reports*, **48**, 241–8.

2 Grad FP. (2004). *Public health law manual*. American Public Health Association, Washington, DC.

3 Tobey JA. (1947). *Public health law*, 3rd edn. Commonwealth Fund, New York.

4 Gostin LO, Sapsin JW, Teret SP, et al. (2002). The Model State Emergency Health Powers Act: planning and response to bioterrorism and naturally occurring infectious diseases. *Journal of American Medicine Association*, **288**, 622–8.

5 Turning Point Model State Public Health Act. Available at: http://www.publichealthlaw.net/Resources/Modellaws.htm (accessed 13 August 2010).

6 Daniels N, Kennedy B, Kawachi I. (2000). Justice is good for our health. *Boston Review*, **25(1),** 6–15.

7 Gostin LO. (2007). The 'tobacco wars'—global litigation strategies. *Journal of the American Medicine Association*, **298,** 2537–2539.

8 World Health Assembly. (2005). *Revision of the International Health Regulations.* Available at: http://www.who.int/csr/ihr/en/ (accessed 23 August 2010).

9 World Health Organization. (2005). *Framework Convention on Tobacco Control*, WHO doc. A56/VR/4 (2003). Available at: ℘ http://www.who.int/tobacco/framework/WHO_FCTC_english.pdf (accessed 23 August 2010)

10 Committee on Economic, Social, and Cultural Rights. (2000). *General Comment No. 14, The right to the highest attainable standard of health*, UN Doc. E/C.12/2000/4. Available at: ℘ http://www.unhchr.ch/tbs/doc.nsf/(symbol)/E.C.12.2000.4.En (accessed 27 August 2010).

Part 5

Health care systems

5.1 Planning health services

David Lawrence

Objectives

This chapter will show you how to contribute to successful planning of health services at strategic and operational levels.

What is planning health services?

All organizations—governments, armies, for-profit corporations, not-for profit community interest companies or public service organizations—plan, whether in public service environments or market places. Health services planning is a process that converts health policy aspirations into organized practical efforts to make health services more effective and efficient. Planning aims to deliver specified health improvement objectives by examining options for change and choosing a prioritized course. Planning takes place at various levels—whole society through to local—and two overarching aspects can be categorized:

- *Technical:* effectiveness, cost effectiveness, spatial, for example, location, size of primary, secondary and tertiary care organizations, etc.
- *Organizational:* including management, financial, training and workforce.

Strategic planning is an overall approach for achieving policy objectives. It typically involves whole or large parts of health service systems and time scales of years. Operational or management planning is concerned with the specific tasks that will deliver a strategy; usually plans are shorter term and cover smaller units and individual departments of organizations.

Planning and the social/political milieu

So that your planning efforts will yield benefits, you must understand not only how a health service operates, but also its external milieu. Planning in this external milieu is usually for a whole country or state and is the subject of health policy.[1]

Planning process vary depending on a county's health care funding arrangements and the political/economic context. Funding may be from:

- taxes or subscription-based regulated social insurance, where services are usually 'clinical need'-based, free (or with a small co-payment) at the point of use
- commercial, risk-based, insurance or private fee for service, where access to services is partly or wholly on ability to pay
- a mixture of these.

Publicly-funded services often have a community needs-based planning process. Conversely, private funding systems usually have a demand-based market process.[2] In many countries there is a mixture of the two. Although these two approaches may differ fundamentally at the whole-country level, and different political values underpin them, practical planning processes at the local level often have common elements. Political context affects the way planning is carried out, but not the need for it.

Health services as systems

A health service is a system—a set of interconnected elements, where what happens in one part of the system affects the rest; they act together as a whole.[3] System approaches to planning are useful.

A health service is a complex economic input–output system. Patients with a need for care, demand (in economics usage) a service and, together with professionals and plant, are the inputs. Primary planning outputs are health outcomes—changes in patients' health status, quality of life, etc. Health services differ from most other economic systems in important ways, which will affect your ability to plan successfully:[4]

- *The usual pyramidal power hierarchy is inverted:* doctors and other frontline health care professionals are numerous, wield political and managerial power, and effectively control resource use in the system.
- Most users of health care have relatively little medical knowledge and so consumer sovereignty is limited and providers lead in making decisions.
- Health care has a special political and social position in most societies.

Conceptual frameworks for planning

One framework for health care planning is a rational system framework:[5]

- identify a future desired state
- compare it with the present state
- identify possible pathways from one to the other (options)
- implement the most cost-effective pathway.

This 'hard' system approach works best where there are well-defined, structured, and easy-to-control systems, with easily identifiable objectives, for example, in car manufacture. Health services are 'soft' systems—people-based, with complex difficult-to-define detailed objectives. Here, 'soft' systems planning is likely to be more successful.[3] This approach includes:

- intervention in an iterative cycle (with integral evaluation)
- recognizing cultural constraints
- participation in planning by most or all parties affected by the system
- approaching the problem using both systems and 'real world' (pragmatic or 'corporate') thinking.[3]

Table 5.1.1 shows various conceptual frameworks for a health care 'soft' system compared to car manufacture, a 'hard' system.

Table 5.1.1 Models and examples of input-output systems

'Input–output' model	Input	Input	Output 1	Output 2	Output 3
'Medical care' model[6]	Need	Demand	Activity	Outcome 1	Outcome 2
Donabedian model	Structure	Process	Process	Outcome 1	Outcome 2
Health services example: ophthalmology	Cataract patients, doctors, optometrists etc., manag-ers, plant	Appointments re-quested for eye examination	Cataract extractions/ lens implants performed	Change in visual functioning	Vision-related quality of life. Patient utility
Commodity production example: car manufacture	Workers, managers, materials, plant	Producers' decisions to manufacture	Cars produced	Cars sold	Cars used. User utility

What are the tasks in planning?

What planning approaches do you need?

Consider two policy making approaches: 'Rational satisficing'[7] is akin to 'hard' systems planning, whereas pragmatic, incrementalist policy making[8] is akin to 'soft' systems planning. Herbert Simon coined 'satisficing' in 1956. It combines 'satisfy' with 'suffice', and is defined as a decision-making strategy that attempts to meet criteria for adequacy, rather than to identify an optimal solution. In practice, planning is usually a mixture of 'rational' and 'pragmatic' processes. One key public health skill is to judge for any given planning situation how much the rational and pragmatic strands are going to influence the planning processes and outcomes—see Table 5.1.2.

The order of tasks in effective planning

Your first task is working well with the people responsible for managing health care so that they ask you to help achieve their policy/planning imperatives. You can do this by showing them how you, and the tools you use, will support and improve their decisions. The most difficult part of this task is to understand people's knowledge and perceptions: learning about the views that people have, is paramount.

You will need to work with:

- *Managers and clinicians in organizations:* who are involved in purchasing (or commissioning) and providing health care.
- *Service users and carers:* they will have experienced most of the good and bad aspects of services, but to be effective, patients need training in the planning role, just as professionals do. Citizens' panels can be a good way to do this,[9,10] but are time-consuming and expensive.
- There are likely to be existing planning groups—or you will need to help set them up—and to be effective you will need to work with these groups. To be really useful, these planning groups need to be part of the power structure, with authority over budgets.

The second task you will usually carry out is to develop specific options for implementing policy, including new 'models of clinical care', involving changes to inputs or processes (see Box 5.1.1, for example). Your role is to present to commissioners and providers: research evidence on the effectiveness of relevant clinical interventions; organizing clinical work; and imparting knowledge of the way health care systems work. Writing a business case often falls on public health professionals and includes considering finance, project management,[11] and organizing effective meetings.[12]

Box 5.1.1 Planning integrated care co-ordination in Brent, London[13,14]

The London Borough of Brent, together with health service organizations and local voluntary groups, successfully bid for a £1.65m Department of Health grant from April 2006 to March 2008, to set up an integrated care co-ordination service (ICCS) for vulnerable older people with multiple chronic illness. Referred patients were to be assessed holistically and their care co-ordinated by a dedicated team. The plan was to integrate organization and budgets across all major agencies, increase care co-ordinators and enhance the service by purchasing care and services and equipment to older people's homes. The plan aimed to:
- reduce hospital use and so save resources, which would be re-invested in preventive measures and home support, leading to even less hospital use
- improve patient well-being and independence
- improve outcomes for the socially excluded, older people, people from hard-to-reach groups, and black and minority ethnic communities.

Expected risks were:
- the service model would not reduce costs overall
- overall savings might be realized, but would not be cashable
- overall savings achieved would not be redistributed appropriately.

Factors that favoured successful implementation were:
- existing good co-operation between health service and social care agencies
- close involvement of voluntary organizations, including patient groups
- existing good leadership and collaboration between agencies
- effective project management and the availability of valid and reliable baseline needs, activity and finance data
- monitoring and evaluation, an integrated part of the project, provided crucial planning information

Factors that hindered implementation were:
- delay in recruiting new care co-ordinators
- fewer referrals from some family physicians (GPs) than expected
- less co-ordination activity than planned for.

What was achieved?
- an excellent evaluation showed that admissions and hospital bed-days were substantially reduced for these patients
- reduced costs to Brent Borough social services
- the Older People's Services (OPS) Unit workload was reduced and there were modest savings in OPS (lower unit costs through earlier intervention, reduced delayed transfers to residential care)
- people's quality of life was largely unchanged, but falls were reduced
- success in reaching certain ethnic minorities
- evidence that GP commissioning would benefit from the ICCS.

Table 5.1.2 'Rational satisficing' or 'incremental' planning. Which approach will work?

	Favorable to rational, evidence-based, planning	Favorable to pragmatic, incremental or 'corporate' planning
Use of technical information and quantitative modelling	Available, understood, believed, and used	Missing, not believed, and not used
Degree of concern about topic from powerful pressure groups in society	Topic not controversial, or little concern	Topic controversial, or great concern
Degree of consensus between most pluralist groups in the society	Much consensus	Little consensus
Local or central control	Local flexibility, good local control	Central, target-driven, little local control
Type of system: nature of objectives	'Hard' well-understood sys-tem with well-defined objec-tives	'Soft' system with difficult-to-define objectives

The third task is providing quantitative and qualitative information for planning.[15,16] This includes quantifying how the new arrangements will affect health service patterns of provision, activity, budgets, and outcomes. Models, especially when various scenarios are tested (sensitivity analysis) are useful for this,[17] supported by decision analysis.[18] The output from the above tasks is usually an implementation plan for a strategy or project proposal.

The fourth task is to work through the implications of the policy options produced in earlier tasks, including evaluation of actual changes, which should be an integral part of the planning process (see case study in Box 5.1.1).

The planning cycle then begins again, with monitoring and evaluation determining what effect planned changes are having on the health system.

Overcoming pitfalls in health services planning

Full implementation of planning decisions, especially strategic ones, usually takes years and often you will not have that time. However, the framework presented here can help produce the most benefit in the time you have. To save time, you may, for example, have to use estimates from others, rather than undertake your own needs survey. The aim of using information in planning is to show planners how changing resources will affect the system. It is a marginal process in the health economics sense.

It is often useful to develop simple spreadsheet models to support planning decision making. Planning rarely goes 'according to plan' as circumstances and personnel change.

The intended objectives in planning are usually only partially attained and there are often unintended consequences. Therefore, monitoring the effects of planning and making adjustment are crucial.

Fallacies about health services planning

- *Planning is rational and evidence based:* it is usually a mix of pragmatic and rational.
- *Planning is a one-off:* planning is continual and evolves.
- *Planning stifles creativity:* planning can help creativity by allowing an orderly process.
- *Planning is trying to predict the future—to give the 'right' answer:* planning is providing intelligence on what might happen in complex systems using trend models with scenario 'what ifs' so as to allow more effective decision-making.

Examples of success and failure in health services planning and lessons learnt

The planning of the specialist cleft lip and palate services for England is a good example of the reality of planning. The report[19] is essential reading for all would-be planners, showing the difficulties in implementing an evidence-based clinical care model.

One successful planning example is the case study in Box 5.1.1.

What are key determinants of success?

- As in many areas, a key skill is to know what is feasible and to work well with people
- Do the technical homework, but present information and detailed evidence in a way which politicians, managers, and clinicians will understand and find useful—be simple in a plain style and no jargon
- Find key authoritative evidence,[20] but also ask advice from experienced public health and other experts
- Be useful, for example, find information on the most pressing concerns managers and clinicians have.

How do you assess your success?

- *Monitoring and evaluation:* success is usually not absolute. Obviously there should be specific objectives and measurement of their attainment. However, success, like the planning process, is often iterative—it comes little-by-little. That implies that integral monitoring and evaluation are essential to successful planning.
- *Feedback:* discussions with colleagues and formal evaluations, including workshops, are important.

Further resources

Markwell S. *Health service development and planning*. Healthknowledge, Gerrards Cross. Available at: 🔗 http://www.healthknowledge.org.uk/public-health-textbook/organization-management/5d-theory-process-strategy-development/health-service-development-planning (accessed 30 May 2011).

Ozcan YA. (2009). *Quantitative methods in health care management*. Jossey-Bass, San Francisco.

Green A. (2007). *An introduction to health planning for developing health systems*. Oxford University Press, Oxford.

Search 'health care planning' at Department of Health, England. Available at: http://www.dh.gov.uk/Home/fs/en (accessed 30 May 2011).

Lawrence D, Mayhew L. (2011). *Health services planning teaching module*. Available at: 🔗 http://www.healthknowledge.org.uk/teaching/health-service-planning (accessed 30 May 2011).

References

1 Buse K, Mays N, Walt G. (2005). *Making health policy*. McGraw-Hill/Open University Press, Maidenhead.

2 Green A. (2007). *An introduction to health planning for developing health systems*. Oxford University Press, Oxford.

3 Van Wyk G. (2003). *A systems approach to social and organizational planning*. Trafford Publishing, Victoria, BC.

4 Lawrence D. David Lawrence offers some words of advice to Mr Brown. Available at: http://www.hsj.co.uk/david-lawrence-offers-some-words-of-advice-to-mr-brown/58956.article (accessed 30 May 2011).

5 Guy M. (2001). Diabetes: developing a local strategy. In: Pencheon D, Guest C, Melzer D, Gray JAM, eds, *Oxford handbook of public health practice*, p. 559. Oxford University Press, Oxford.

6 Logan, RFL .et al (1972) Dynamics of Medical Care Memoir14 London, LSHTM.

7 Wikipedia. Available at: 🔗 http://en.wikipedia.org/wiki/Satisficing (accessed 30 May 2011).

8 Wikipedia. Available at: 🔗 http://en.wikipedia.org/wiki/Incrementalism Accessed 30 May 2011.

9 Abelson J, Eyles J, McLeod CB, *et al.* (2003). Does deliberation make a difference? Results from a citizens panel study of health goals priority setting. *Health Policy*, **66**, 95–106.

10 Church J, Saunders D, Wanke M, *et al.* (2002). Citizen participation in health decision-making: past experience and future prospects. *Journal of Public Health Policy*, **23**, 12–32.

11 See example project management document at Wikiph.org (2010). Available at: 🔗 http://wikiph.org/index.php?title=Image:Project_management_document_2010.doc (accessed 30 May 2011).

12 See 'Meetings' section at web page. Available at: 🔗 http://wikiph.org/index.php?title=Organization_of_health_care (accessed 30 May 2011).

13 Mayhew L. (2008). On the effectiveness of care co-ordination services aimed at preventing hospital admissions and emergency attendances. Health Care Management Science. Available at: 🔗 http://www.nkm.org.uk/flyers/SpecialReports/HCMScifulltextpublished221208.pdf

14 Integrated Care Co-ordination Service (2008). The economic, health and social benefits of care co-ordination for older people. London: Cass Business School. Available at: 🔗 http://www.nkm.org.uk/flyers/SpecialReports/ICCS_Comp_doc_v1[1].pdf (accessed 30 May 2011).

15 Ozcan YA. (2009). *Quantitative methods in health care management*. Jossey-Bass, San Francisco.

16 Bullas S, Dallas A. (2002). *Information for managing health care resources*. Radcliffe Medical, Abingdon.

17 Sanderson C, Gruen R. (2006). *Analytical models for deci-sion-making*. Open University Press, Maidenhead.

18 Annalisa software. Available at: 🔗 http://annalisa.org.uk (accessed 30 May 2011).

19 Crown J. (2003). *Cleft lip and palate services*, Report from the Cleft Implementation Group and Cleft Monitoring Group. Available at: 🔗 http://wikiph.org/index.php?title=Health_care_strate-gic_management (accessed 30 May 2011).

20 Wiki Public Health Available at: 🔗 http://wikiph.org/index.php?title=Evidence_searches (accessed 30 May 2011).

5.2 Funding and delivering health care

Anna Dixon

Objectives

This chapter will help you become familiar with different models of funding and delivering health care, and give you some analytical tools to enable you to critically review health system policies in other countries and apply learning to your own context.

Different models of health care funding and delivery

From Bismarck to Beveridge and beyond?

Since the 19th century, western European welfare states have been dominated by two models of health care financing and delivery: Bismarck and Beveridge (see Table 5.2.1). Chancellor Bismarck introduced national health insurance to Germany in 1883. Aneurin Bevan, the British Minister of Health in 1948, is usually honoured as the founder of the NHS. However, it was the Beveridge Report which laid the foundations for the NHS. Subsequent reforms in most countries mean these models no longer exist in their original form.

In order to analyse modern health systems you need to understand the decisions that health policy makers have made about how to finance and deliver health care services (see Box 5.2.1). Finding out the answers to these questions will give you a good basis for understanding how the health system is structured and operates in different countries.

Collecting the money

Ultimately, all the money that is spent on health care comes from individuals and households. There are a number of different methods of raising revenues: general taxation (through direct or indirect taxes), social insurance contributions (compulsory levies on wages), private health insurance premiums, direct charges to patients, or charitable donations. As Figure 5.2.1 shows, most Organization for Economic Cooperation and Development (OECD) countries fund the majority of health care from either taxation or social health insurance contributions, with the exception of the USA, where about half of total expenditure on health is publicly funded.

Table 5.2.1 Key features of the Bismarck and Beveridge models of health care

	Bismarck	Beveridge
Entitlement based on. . .	Contribution status	Citizenship/residence
Revenues from…	Wage deductions, employees and employers pay half each	General taxation
Benefits covered are…	Defined (explicit rationing)	Comprehensive (implicit rationing)
Insurance provided by…	Occupational sickness fund man-aged by joint boards of workers' representatives (usually the trade unions) and the business representatives	State
Relationship with providers	Contracts or patient reimbursement	Integrated

Box 5.2.1 Dimensions of the funding and delivery of health services

- How much money is collected, and who decides this?
- Who collects the money, and from whom?
- Who and what is covered?
- How are resources pooled?
- How are resources allocated to purchasers?
- Is there choice between insurers/purchasers?
- From whom are services bought and how?
- At what price are services bought and how are services paid for?
- Where are the services delivered and by whom?

The different ways of generating revenues to fund health care have a number of associated pros and cons.[1] Taxes may be progressive (if the rich pay proportionately more than the poor), but direct taxes on goods and services, such as cigarettes, are often regressive (falling disproportionately on the poor). Social insurance contributions are usually ring-fenced for health care, but add to labour costs and can put a burden on employers. Private health insurance premiums are usually risk-rated—those with pre-existing conditions or at higher risk of ill health pay more or face exclusions, unless regulation requires them to be community-rated. Out of pocket payments and co-payments, where patients pay either the full cost or a proportion of the costs for the services they consume, mean that access to services is based on ability to pay and can result in people foregoing care because they cannot afford the charges.

% total expenditure on health

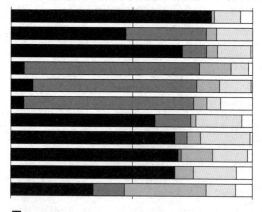

■ Taxation

Figure 5.2.1 Breakdown of expenditure on health by source of revenues, selected OECD countries and EU-15 2009 or latest available. (Source: OECD Health Data 2010.)

Deciding what services to cover

With limited public funds available, decisions have to be taken about what to spend the money on. In some countries, such as Germany and Israel, the definition of what is covered by social health insurance is explicit and set down in a defined schedule of benefits. In other systems decisions about what is covered are made locally by purchasers of health care based on the needs and priorities of the population and are not explicitly defined (see 📖 Chapter 1.5). A number of countries have established national bodies, which advise on the cost-effectiveness of new drugs and technologies. These assessments are used to make decisions nationally on whether treatments should be publicly funded (see 📖 Chapter 1.6). Where explicit decisions are taken to exclude services from public coverage, patients either have to pay out of pocket or buy supplementary insurance to cover the costs.

Allocating and pooling resources

Different organizations may be responsible for collecting the money and for purchasing services. In this case, there is a need to decide how to allocate the resources between them.

In some countries where the health system is decentralized or federalized, national revenues are allocated in the form of a block grant to the provinces, states or local governments that are responsible for health care. This central funding supplements local budgets in order to equalize access to services.

In countries with administrative devolution or local purchasers, such as the UK, resources are often allocated on the basis of a weighted capitation formula which ensures that those areas with the greatest health need receive more. In social insurance systems, resources are (re-)allocated between funds to ensure that the money they receive fairly reflects the risks of their enrollees.

To make or buy?

The third party agent, such as the state or insurance fund, responsible for providing services to patients, has several choices about how to provide health care services:

- reimburse the patient for costs incurred
- reimburse the providers for costs incurred
- contract with providers and set out agreed terms and conditions
- directly employ or own providers.

Each of these options has advantages and disadvantages, some of which are discussed elsewhere in this volume (□ Chapter 5.2).

Paying for care

How producers of services are financially rewarded has implications for efficiency (see Box 5.2.2). Financial incentives are, however, not the only factors that drive provider behaviour. Other rules and sanctions, professional ethics, and personal goals and objectives also play a role.

Box 5.2.2 Options for paying health care providers

- *Capitation:* a fixed sum per head over a defined period of time. Commonly used in primary care or integrated medical groups where doctors are responsible for a registered population.
- *Salary:* a fixed sum for working a set amount of time unrelated to activity. Used where doctors are employed by hospitals and or primary care organizations. Widely used for non-physician staff. Increasingly combined with performance-related pay.
- *Fee for service:* an amount per item of service. Used to pay hospitals and hospital doctors in some countries, more common in out-of-hospital care. Often pre-negotiated rates.
- *Budgets:* fixed sum for a fixed period unrelated to activity. Calculated on the basis of historical allocations or historical or predicted levels of activity. May be hard (any overrun or underspend is borne by the provider) or soft (an indicative budget).
- *Per diem:* a fixed amount per day. Used extensively in the past for hospital care in Europe, but incentives for excessive lengths of stay. Still used for hotel costs in some countries.
- *Per case or episode payments:* a fixed amount for each admitted patient or spell of activity. Diagnosis-related groups (DRGs) are the most commonly used. Payment associated with primary diagnosis on admission, often with case-mix adjustment for severity.

Public or private providers?

The ownership status of hospitals has become more complex with the increasing role of private finance in capital building projects, the franchising of hospital management to private companies, and the outsourcing of a number of non-clinical and clinical services. The dichotomy between public and private ownership is no longer a sufficient basis for the evaluation of hospital performance.[2] An assessment of the level of state control versus provider control over aspects of the organization, such as pay and conditions, private capital, disposal of assets, and scope of services, can give a fuller picture.

Integration

Another important dimension of health care delivery is the extent to which providers are integrated. The organizational relationships will influence the level of cooperation, coordination, and incentives. *Horizontal* integration is where groups of providers at the same level form a single organization. For example, a cooperative of general practitioners or a single company which owns a chain of acute hospitals. *Vertical integration* is where a single organization provides care at different levels. For example, a health maintenance organization, which employs family doctors, and runs its own hospitals and home-care services. Virtual integration describes providers that work together without being part of a single organization. For example, a tertiary cancer centre may be virtually integrated with oncologists and radiologists working in general hospitals and palliative care facilities as part of a cancer network.

Using this framework you will be able to understand the key dimensions of different health systems. The remainder of this chapter highlights the benefits of international exchanges and cross-national research for policy and practice.

Why learn from other countries?

Common challenges

Many of the challenges faced by health systems world-wide are the same. There are global challenges such as the HIV/AIDS pandemic, tobacco control, food security, and violence and conflict. There are also challenges common to health systems in similar political, economic, cultural, and social contexts (see Box 5.2.3). Working together to find common solutions prevents duplication of effort and increases the chances of success.

Benchmarking

By comparing health systems across a range of indicators you can highlight areas where improvements may be needed. League tables and rankings of health systems, such as that published by WHO,[3] hospitals, and individual clinical performance have been criticized.[4] Indeed, crude comparisons of inputs can be misleading. Comparing process indicators can highlight inefficiencies (see Box 5.2.4). Outcomes are the most useful, but care needs to be taken to adjust for case mix.

Box 5.2.3 Examples of common challenges to health systems

- *Political legacy:* restructuring large hospital sectors in the former Soviet Union.
- *Economic development:* allocating limited public resources to health care in low-income countries.
- *Social and cultural norms:* changing alcohol consumption patterns in Scandinavia.
- *Population profiles:* meeting the health care needs of indigenous populations in Australia and Canada.
- *Demographic trends:* funding long-term care for a rapidly ageing population in many countries.
- *Epidemiological trends:* combating childhood obesity in the USA and other industrialized countries.

Box 5.2.4 Comparing the length of stay in hospitals

A number of studies have compared the performance of the NHS in England with Kaiser Permanente (KP), a managed care organization based in California, USA. One prompted much debate about the validity of the comparison, the standardization and adjustments made to the data, and the conclusions drawn.[5] However, another study comparing hospital utilization in the over-65s by procedure has led to some interesting insights.[6] It found that the standardized length of stay for some procedures was five to six times higher in the NHS than in KP. Length of stay was consistent across age ranges in KP, whereas within the NHS length of stay increased with age. This has prompted further investigation into the use of intermediate care and intensive home care services, which enable older patients to be discharged promptly when they no longer have a need for medical care.

Avoid mistakes
Other countries have experience from which you can learn. Evaluating their policies and practices can ensure mistakes are not repeated.

Policy transfer
Looking at how another country organizes its health services may give rise to new policy ideas. Sometimes it is difficult to think creatively because of the constraints of how things have always been done.

Potential pitfalls in learning from other systems abroad

Despite the benefits of cross-national research it can easily be misused or misinterpreted.

Transferability

Even if you were to identify an apparently successful public health policy or practice in another setting, will it work in the same way? Probably not. The context in which a policy is implemented is often as critical to its success as the content of the policy. Try and be systematic about analyzing context. Table 5.2.2 sets out some of the dimensions to consider.

Table 5.2.2 Dimensions of the context of policy (based on Leichter)[7]

Dimensions of context	Definition	Examples
Situational factors	Major, but transient events	New Minister of Health appointed
Structural factors	Constant features of the political and economic system	Decentralized health care system
Cultural factors	Values and norms	Preference for professional paternalism
Environmental factors	External to the specific policy arena	Accession to the European Union

Comparability

Arguments such as 'We have too many/too few hospital beds/nurses/doctors' or 'We spend too much/too little on health compared with the rest of Europe/the world' tend to dominate policy debates. Such comparisons of crude inputs do not support informed decision-making.

International health databases, such as those produced by the OECD and the WHO, try to standardize definitions. However, national data collection procedures vary. For example, when counting beds should you include all available beds or all staffed beds or all occupied beds?

Even where a standardized measure is available what does Figure 5.2.2 tell you? If you have fewer beds than another country, is that a good or bad thing? On its own it means very little. If, for example, you were interested in efficiency then it would be important to understand how the beds are used, what the length of stay is, the re-admission rate, and the occupancy rate.

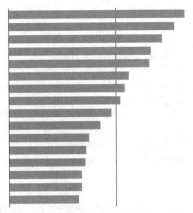

Figure 5.2.2 Number of hospital beds per 100,000 population in selected European countries 2008 or latest available. (Source: WHO Health for All database, June 2010 http://www.who.dk/hfadb (accessed 20 August 2010)).

Complexity

A danger of cross-national learning is to isolate one element of the health system without understanding the complex interactions with other parts of the system. For example, the policy to give patients the choice of going to any hospital has been credited with a reduction in surgical waiting times in Denmark. However, factors such as spare capacity in other hospitals, patients' willingness to travel, and a sufficiently generous payment transfer between county councils were also critical to its success (see Box 5.2.5; 📖 Chapter 6.9).

Box 5.2.5 Questions to ask when engaging in cross-national learning

- What is the problem I face? Which other countries are facing a similar problem?
- What solutions have other countries tried? Have they worked? Why?
- What data would help me find out? Are they available?
- Are the data comparable, up-to-date, and accurate?
- What factors contributed to the success of the policy? Are these factors present here? What adaptations or changes would be needed?
- What else was going on? How important were contextual factors?

Further resources

Useful websites

European Observatory on Health Systems and Policies. Available at: ✍ http://www.euro.who.int/observatory (accessed 13 August 2010).

European Union. Available at: ✍ http://europa.eu/ (accessed 13 August 2010).

Health Policy Monitor. Available at: ✍ http://www.healthpolicymonitor.org/ (accessed 13 August 2010).

Organization for Economic Co-operation and Development (OECD) . Available at: ✍ http://www.oecd.org (accessed 13 August 2010).

World Bank. Available at: ✍ www.worldbank.org/ (accessed 13 August 2010).

World Health Organization. Available at: ✍ www.who.int/en/ (accessed 13 August 2010).

Further reading

McKee M, Healy J, eds. (2002). *Hospitals in a changing Europe*. European Observatory on Health Care Systems, Open University Press, Buckingham.

Thomson S, Foubister T, Mossialos E. (2009). *Financing health care in the European Union: challenges and policy responses*, Observatory Study Series no 17. European Observatory on Health Care Systems, WHO, Geneva.

References

1 Mossialos E, Dixon A, Figueras J, et al. (eds) (2002). *Funding health care: options for Europe*. European Observatory on Health Care Systems, Open University Press, Buckingham.

2 Preker AS, Harding A. (2003). *Innovations in health service delivery: the corporatization of public hospitals*. World Bank, Washington DC.

3 World Health Organization (2000). *The World Health Report 2000: health systems: improving performance*. World Health Organization, Geneva.

4 Shekelle PG, Lim Y-W, Mattke S, Damberg C. (2008). *Does public release of performance results improve quality of care? A systematic review* [online] Health Foundation London. Available at: ✍ www.health.org.uk

5 Feachem RG, Sekhri NK, White KL (2002). Getting more for their dollar: a comparison of the NHS with California's Kaiser Permanente. *British Medical Journal*, **324**, 135–41.

6 Ham C, York N, Sutch S, Shaw R. (2003). Hospital bed utilization in the NHS, Kaiser Permanente, and the US Medicare programme: analysis of routine data. *British Medical Journal*, **327**, 1257.

7 Leichter HM. (1979). *A comparative approach to policy analysis: health care policy in four nations*. Cambridge University Press, Cambridge.

5.3 Commissioning health care

Richard Richards

Objectives

This chapter is concerned with the use of contracts and payments as a means of ensuring that care maximizes health at minimum cost. The chapter aims to cover the full range of health care commissioning from the simplest form, an individual patient making a private payment to an individual practitioner, through to the most complex, tax-funded, social medicine 'free at the point of delivery'.

In all health care commissioning a common set of concerns arise:
* the nature of the need, including an assessment of the (cost-) effectiveness of the relevant interventions
* examination of the services available, including inputs, quality of care, and outcomes
* the costs and efficiency of the care on offer
* the development of formal commissioning agreements.

From boom ...

The previous edition of this book was written at the height of a worldwide economic boom. In 2006 the world collectively spent $4.7 trillion ($10^{12}$) on health care, $4.1 trillion of that by the 31 OECD countries and $200 billion collectively by 3 other countries, China, India and Brazil.[1] It is very big business, consuming a huge proportion (9.8%) of world resources.

In terms of life expectancy, this expenditure seems to have little effect (Figure 5.3.1). Female life expectancy rises from about 30 to 70 years for up to $100 spent *per capita* (pc) on health care, but that spending mirrors the rise in *per capita* Gross National Income (pc GNI), resulting from the move from hunter-gatherer society to one in which the organization of society has delivered clean water, nutrition (farming), and shelter. Up to $1000 pc spend a further 10 years is added, but after that there is little or no upward trend in life expectancy amongst the countries that spend that $4.1 trillion. The USA spent $2 trillion of that world total ($7000 pc), yet has a female life expectancy less than that of Costa Rica, which spent just $400 pc. OECD data (Figure 5.3.2) paints a particularly startling situation for the USA, the highest spender, which has the 7th worst OECD life expectancy, yet those 6 worse countries also have the six lowest OECD pc health care expenditure.[2]

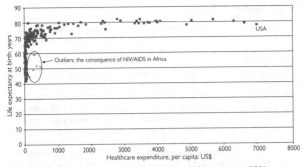

Figure 5.3.1 *Per capita* health care expenditure and life expectancy, 2006.

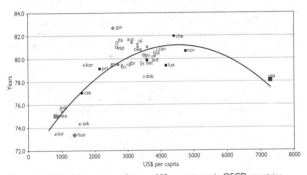

Figure 5.3.2 Health care expenditure and life expectancy in OECD countries, 2007.

.... to bust

250 years ago, Edmund Burke, politician and philosopher commented that 'Frugality is founded on the principle that all riches have limits'. With the world now in the grip of a deep economic recession, commissioning value-for-money health care that uses scarce resources wisely to maximize health and avoids diverting resources away from addressing the determinants of health is ever more important. Producing a marginal extension of life or improvement in quality of life in an OECD country, may result, through carbon emissions and global warming, significantly shortened lives in poorer countries.

Assessing need

For the individual, assessing need will usually require a diagnosis and often an assessment of the severity of the disease and associated co-morbidities. Often, there is much uncertainty about the patient's condition, introducing risk, and limiting rational behaviour in the health care 'market'.

At the population level, a variety of approaches exist to assess need (see 📖 Chapter 1.4). A centrally planned health care system requires information on the numbers of people with each type of need, to plan the extent of provision. Even entrepreneurial market systems, considered more able to change and willing to accept mistakes and failures, would first use market research to help determine the level of provision required.

Need, by definition, involves the presence of an undesirable health state plus the existence of effective interventions. In most circumstances resources are limited, so the goal is to buy the most cost-effective care to improve health.

Complex products are typically built to plans or blue prints. Health care should be no different and the equivalent is a care pathway which describes the disease progression and the interventions along that pathway: the what, when, where and by whom of health care (with whys, the evidence, by way of explanation). Ideally it should be populated with probabilities (of movement between disease states as in a Markov model), the quality of life associated with each state and costs.

Inputs

The resources needed to deliver health care are of crucial interest both to the provider and consumer/commissioner as they determine the *costs* to the former and *price* to the latter. In the situation of the private consultation, an unaffordable price represents an inaccessible treatment; in the situation of a third-party payer this situation is referred to, pejoratively, as rationing. To the consumer, be they patient or third-party payer, the input needs to be affordable and to maximize the outcomes for the available funds.

Cost containment is an inevitable goal of commissioning systems. Approaches vary from the prospective payment systems used in the US Medicare system, through removing incentives to unproductive over-activity, e.g. by placing physicians on salaries, rather than fees for service payments, and placing contracts with managed care providers. The socialized health providers in several European countries, Australia, Canada, and New Zealand operate cost containment through direct control and annual budget setting.

Inputs come in a variety of standards, quality, and availability (scarcity), which will be reflected in differences in costs and thus price. This applies to facilities, diagnostic and treatment equipment, drugs, and staff.

Quality and outcomes

The quality of health care has many dimensions, including the structures (staff, equipment, etc.), processes and outcomes. Commissioning should clearly state the quality expected in whatever dimensions seem necessary.

Whilst health technology assessments can show what treatments should be given, audit will indicate whether a unit is actually providing those treatments as intended. Often units are too small and case mixes too complex to yield definitive indications of quality of care. The lack of good information on providers' quality and outcome often means that the patient/commissioner faces significant uncertainties and cannot choose rationally between providers in the way suggested by advocates of idealized market systems.

Efficiency, the ratio of costs to outcomes, provides a measure of value for money. Commissioners seek to maximize the efficiency of services, maximizing the output for the funding they give. Providers seek to maximize funding whilst minimizing costs: where there is a relationship between quality and higher costs, this can drive down quality for the individual patient. The profit motive can further distort incentives.

Coping with risk in health care commissioning

Risks take different forms. Ask a bank manager for a loan and the manager will assess the risk compared with the likelihood of profit for the bank. From the public health perspective the 'bottom line' is not financial profit, but health gain. Each commissioning decision carries a risk that the funding will not result in health gain.

Some risk, expressed as chance or probability, is purely stochastic and can be calculated in the form of statistical significance and confidence intervals of the size of benefit described in clinical trials. However, there are more problematic determinants of risk that are systematic and difficult to quantify or even note, and many result in exaggeration of benefits and thus risk unintended inefficiencies. The most insidious of these is reflected in the term 'conflict' of interest. Such conflicts are not exclusive to research organized and funded by the pharmaceutical industry, but are seen when any interested provider of care is involved in research or the secondary analysis of research data. Public Health professionals, trained in epidemiology and thus aware of all the pitfalls of badly conducted research (clinical research being simply experimental epidemiology) are well placed to provide high quality disinterested analysis and commissioning advice that can reduce those risks.

Small organizations, be they commissioners or providers, can face significant financial risks from high-cost, low-volume interventions. These occur unpredictably in any given year. Ways for commissioners to handle that risk are based on increasing these numbers to predictable levels by:

- grouping many low-volume, high-cost interventions together in one 'basket'

- collaborating with other small organizations to increase numbers, sharing costs on a weighted capitation basis
- creating a 'higher' tier (dictated by rarity of the intervention) responsible for commissioning
- any combination of these.

Commissioners and providers can share financial risk. A provider may serve a number of small commissioners and will therefore see a larger number of the rarer interventions, which will allow risks to be shared or spread.

An agreement that includes 'floors' and 'ceilings' can also be used to share risk. A range of activity around a central estimate is commissioned and paid for: no change in funding occurs within those limits. Should activity fall below the 'floor' the provider returns funding to the commissioner and should the activity exceed the 'ceiling' the commissioner pays extra.

Agreeing costs

The amount of funding involved in commissioning a whole service depends on the concept of 'marginal' and 'step-up' cost, two sides of the same coin. Some costs to a provider are 'fixed', independent of activity levels (staff salaries, equipment, buildings, etc.). If the activity increases, these fixed costs can be spread across larger numbers of cases; the number of cases agreed determines the 'full cost' (per case) that will cover all of the fixed costs.

Once fixed costs are covered, extra activity will cost marginally less, due to the use of consumables and other non-fixed costs. Conversely, lower activity will return amounts smaller than the 'full cost'.

'Step-up' costs occur when activity exceeds the capacity of the provider, despite efficient use of facilities, requiring that extra capacity be introduced. Such capacity cannot be introduced in small amounts; it is not practicable to build a one-bedded hospital ward! It is these problems that work against change in some systems, making change very expensive for commissioners.

The chosen mechanism for sharing risk will depend on circumstances and the type of commissioning arrangement in use. There are generally four types:

- *Block:* a global sum of money in exchange for a loosely defined set of services; the provider moves money between departmental budgets; the commissioner and provider negotiate differences towards the end of the financial year.
- *Cost and volume:* specified activity levels and funding at various levels of detail (e.g. surgical, medical, etc.; by specialty; by procedure type, or groupings of procedures such as health care resource groups); monthly plans are agreed and monitored against targets.
- *Cost per case:* each episode of care is paid for; cost may vary depending on the level of activity or be fixed, independent of activity levels.
- *Fee for service:* costs for individual inputs, diagnostic, or treatment activities are separately reimbursed. This system is typically used in private insurance and parts of the US health system, and is usually

combined with a range of instruments to contain costs and limit coverage.

A cost per case system based on a set price ('tariff') for any provider can facilitate choice, and change through choice, but it can also stifle the creation of new capacity as providers have to carry the risk of additional marginal costs before activity levels use enough of the new capacity to generate the income needed. Despite a supposedly fixed cost, a commissioner may be forced to agree a higher price per case if extra capacity is needed.

In free markets for consumer products, increased sales typically result in lower costs, generating greater consumption as goods become more affordable, although the total amount of money spent in the market increases. In health care, higher volumes can also generate lower costs. However, extra consumers (patients) can only be generated by reducing treatment thresholds (to lesser severities) or treating a different condition. This will change benefit/risk and cost/effectiveness ratios, especially at the margins of this extra activity. The funding needed to cover this activity might be more effectively directed elsewhere. Commissioners need to understand the total cost and benefits, and resist simplistic claims of reduced treatment costs making a treatment more widely available.

The six basic elements of a commissioning agreement

So what would a contract or service level agreement look like? It should have at least six elements:

- *Parties to the contract:* typically one or more commissioners and a provider. A complex pathway may require several providers but this could be addressed by requiring the main provider to subcontract.
- *What treatments and services are to be provided?* Ideally, this should be described by the patient pathway and encompass 'hotel services' (nutrition, shelter, and comforts) as well as details of the diagnostic and treatment processes based on evidence of effectiveness. A good contract should be composed of many such pathways relating to the many diseases to be treated (though there are examples of providers doing a single procedure) covering both emergency care and planned care. What is excluded may also be specified.
- *Quantity of care:* the number of patients to be treated within the contract. This may be just one or in the case of block contracts undetermined except by historical patterns. Ideally each pathway should have a number established by the epidemiology of incidence/ prevalence and treatment thresholds. The provider will be expected to report activity levels regularly to the commissioner.
- *Standards to be achieved:* the quality of care must be clearly specified along with the mechanisms of monitoring. Such standards could and should include nutrition ('five portions of fresh fruit or vegetables a day', free access to fluids), the environment (clean; non-smoking; access to 'entertainments' and access for visitors, especially important in paediatrics), as well as the skills and knowledge of staff, equipment,

devices, and drugs. For some conditions or treatments an individual clinician and team may be designated (even named), e.g. for breast cancer, and minimum activity levels specified to maintain skills. Standards may be specified by reference to recognized clinical guidelines and protocols such as those produced in the UK by the National Institute for Health and Clinical Excellence (NICE) in England and Wales or the Scottish Intercollegiate Guidelines Network (SIGN). Clinical governance (including audit) will be specified as the mechanism for maintaining standards within the provider. In some reimbursement systems detailed standards are set for individual patient diagnosis and treatment planning. Often there are formal requirements on providers to seek permission from payers prior to starting specified forms of care. Permission procedures may involve the reporting of detailed clinical data to the payer to prove the presence of a health care need that is covered by the patient's insurance coverage.

- *Price:* no commissioning or purchasing agreement is complete without agreement of the price. Prices may be agreed locally or fixed by the commissioner so as to allow providers to compete on quality over and above that specified.
- *Arbitration arrangements:* things rarely go to plan, contracts are rarely exactly met as specified. Contracts should therefore specify how the parties would reach agreement should, for example, the contract not be met, demand fail to reach, or exceed, the contract, the case mix differ in terms of severities or conditions from that anticipated, new treatment become available or if events occur not covered within the contract, such as a major disaster.

Who should be involved in commissioning?

The commissioning process requires a broad range of skills and experience. Genuine team work is essential (see 📖 Chapter 4.4). Sometimes

Table 5.3.1 Skills, people, and tasks needed in commissioning health care services

	Person or discipline	Tasks
Epidemiology	Epidemiologist, public health practitioner	To use data (e.g. mortality, demographic, surveys, case registers). To analyse these data to determine the actual and potential health problems in the population
Health technology assessment	Health economist, public health practitioner	To evaluate critically the (cost)-effectiveness of health care interventions. To highlight gaps in information where further research is needed

(Continued)

Table 5.3.1 (Continued)

	Person or discipline	Tasks
Negotiation and conflict management	NHS manager, all members	To negotiate skillfully matching what the commissioner believes is required and the provider wishes to offer
Financial	Accountant, NHS manager	To handle complex finances (services are rarely costed comprehensively and in a way that readily allows comparison)
Clinical	Public health clinician, GP, specialist clinician, nurse	To understand the specialist clinical aspects of the services being offered and provided. (Beware: like any input, specialist clinical advice can be biased—more general clinical advice, for example from primary care practitioners, is often equally or more important; 'experts' are almost always enthusiasts, not disinterested observers)
Experience of the wider health system	NHS manager, public health practitioner	To appreciate how the individual services fit in with the wider health care provision of the locality or region—experience and understanding of the wider health service is essential
Information	Information special-ist, operational re-searcher, epidemiologist	To understand health information systems. (Information systems are complex and not always designed specifically to serve the commissioning process.) To understand issues such as case mix measurement, relationships between case mix, costs, and prices. To understand how the provision of health care should be matched to predictions of need
Informing and supporting patient choice	Any clinician, but also anyone appropriately trained. The patient	To provide and explain information on outcomes and quality issues to patients in a way they can understand that will permit them to make choices that are best suited to their conditions and circumstances

these can all be embodied in one person, but this is rare and usually a team-based multidisciplinary process works best.

Table 5.3.1 identifies the skills, people, and tasks needed in commissioning health care services.

The concern over variations in clinical practice (see 📖 Chapter 5.10) and its implications for quality of care, along with a desire to better involve the patient in decisions around the nature of the care they should receive, has resulted in a growing interest in shared decision making. The Harvard-based Foundation for Informed Decision Making has been leading the process of moving from analyses of clinical variation through research into decision making and onto translation of this research into independent, evidence-based decision aids for patients. Under these principles, patients will become informed commissioners of their own care.

Specialized services

There is no one agreed definition of specialized services; most of what has been described above applies to specialized services, but to reiterate some important aspects, specialized services typically involve rarer conditions, thus patient numbers are *small* and *often unpredictable*.

To ensure optimum outcomes for patients (e.g. sustained training and clinical competence for specialized staff) and optimum use of resources (e.g. to ensure cost-effectiveness of provision, making the best use of scarce resources including clinical expertise, high-technology equipment, donor organs, etc.) a *critical service mass* is required at each centre and patients from a wide area must be referred to these centres to achieve minimum activity levels. As a result, the population on behalf of which services are commissioned is much larger than that of a single commissioning organization.

Specialized services may have some characteristics different from mainstream health care, one of which is *rapidly developing high technology services*. Services can develop very quickly and often involve high technology, where research and development need to be supported and where the introduction of new technologies needs to be managed. In these situations note that the evidence for effectiveness is often emerging rather than established, making commissioning decisions on the basis of complete evidence difficult. As the new technology becomes more widely adopted, additional clinicians can be properly trained in those centres initially established.

Commissioning services with prominent ethical dimensions

Difficult ethical issues can arise, for example, around equity of access, requiring commissioners of health care to balance the high cost needs of the minority against the needs of the majority. Examples are treatment of a variety of genetically determined diseases requiring extremely expensive genetically engineered replacement therapies, and the commissioning of very expensive secure psychiatric facilities to protect society.

Nonetheless, the general 'rules' of commissioning can and should be applied to specialized services. There is a danger that issues of cost-effectiveness are set aside. Whilst larger populations mean that costs are a smaller proportion of the total budget and thus appear affordable, opportunity costs remain the same: the opportunity to treat the same number of patients is lost, irrespective of the population level at which services are commissioned.

There remains a reluctance to address explicitly the issues of distributive justice in these cases and costs are rising exponentially: lifetime costs for one individual can reach £10,000,000 yet deliver only marginal benefits. The principles of distributive justice must be addressed.

Further resources

The Foundation for Informed Medical Decision Making. What is medical shared decision making. Available at: ℒ www.informedmedicaldecisions.org (accessed 10 May 2011).

References

1 The World Bank Data Catalog. (2011). *Health, nutrition and population statistics.* Available at: http://data.worldbank.org/data-catalog/health-nutrition-and-population-statistics (accessed 30 July 2011).
2 Joumard I, André C, Nicq C. (2010). *Health care systems: efficiency and institutions*, OECD Economics Department Working Papers, No. 769. OECD Publishing, Paris.

5.4 Controlling expenditures

Thomas Rice and Iain Lang

Objectives

This chapter will help you understand:
- why controlling health care expenditures is key to achieving other public health goals
- the primary reasons for rising expenditures
- how rising expenditures have been addressed at national and sub-national levels
- ways in which controlling expenditures can fit into your professional role.

A key tool in addressing rising expenditures is an understanding of health economics and you may wish to read this chapter alongside 📖 Economic assessment.

Why addressing rising expenditures is an important public health issue

It could be argued expenditure control should not be a public policy issue. Such an argument might state that good health is among the most important aspects of well-being and people should have access to whatever they need—to all available medical products, devices, and procedures—to improve their health.

In fact, expenditure control is not only important, but likely to become more important as new technologies emerge and the costs of care increase. There are two reasons for this. One relates to the economic concept of 'opportunity costs.' An opportunity cost is essentially a tradeoff. When we spend more money on health care, it means that we have less to spend on everything else, including education, housing, and social insurance. There are many compelling ways in which public resources can be productively invested and so we ought to avoid wasting resources as much as possible – all the more so when many countries are struggling with burdensome and growing national debts (see 📖 Economic assessment).

The second reason is particular to the health care sector. There are limited resources to be devoted to health care so they need to be apportioned judiciously. If, for example, excessive amounts are spent on administration of health insurance then there will be less money available for other health-related activities. Public health initiatives are often a harder 'sell' than direct medical care procedures, especially when government budgets are stressed. Focusing on rising expenditures helps ensure we use limited health care resources efficiently and that we have more left for other public health activities.

In relation to both of these factors there are tensions: in the first case this relates to pressures to reduce spending by central and local government, and in the second case to the need for public health to try to stand up to the 'health care delivery juggernaut'.[1] In the face of these tensions it is important for public health practitioners to be aware of and engage with the need to prioritize and reduce expenditure.

The causes of rising health care expenditures

There is no agreed list of the major causes of rising health care expenditures. There are three reasons why this is the case. First, although much research has been done, there is a lot we do not know—understandable given the difficulty in conducting randomized controlled studies in health policy. Secondly, much of the analysis available is influenced by political leanings, which can lead to different interpretations of the same information. Thirdly, means of expenditure control cannot necessarily be transferred from one country to another. What works in the United Kingdom, for example, might not work in Germany (to say nothing of the United States or India) an, even if it did, institutional and political factors often make it nearly impossible to transplant an idea from one country into another.

The following equation provides a model for the causes of rising expenditures:

$$E = P \times Q$$

where E = expenditure, P = the unit price of health services, and Q = the quantity or volume of health services consumed. The equation, while simplified in that it does not distinguish between different types of services, provides a key insight: increases in either or both price and quantity will result in increased expenditure. This means there are two approaches to addressing rising expenditures: controlling quantity or volume, and controlling prices.

Quantity of services

Increases in the quantity and intensity of services are responsible for much of the increase in health care expenditures.[2] This often goes under the heading of 'high-tech' medicine, and includes new and/or improved procedures and pharmaceuticals. Advances in medical technology are desirable, but concomitant expenditure increases inevitably involve an opportunity cost: unless total budgets keep growing, increasing expenditures to cover a new technology must involve cuts to other technologies and services.

The volume of services is not the same in all parts of a country. Even after controlling for the age and health of populations there is generally a great deal of variation between different geographic regions. In the United States, for example, in 2009 *per capita* spending on Medicare (the programme for senior citizens and the disabled) varied by over 50% between states.[3] There is much debate about whether higher spending leads to better outcomes and health care processes. Although one might imagine higher spending to be associated with better outcomes, regions with higher Medicare spending also had higher mortality rates following acute myocardial infarctions, hip fractures, and colorectal cancer diagnoses.[4] Examination of such variations can be used to determine 'best practice'—within particular geographic area or within hospital systems—that can be emulated and encouraged.

High levels of expenditure can be an unintentional outcome of fee-for-service medicine, which encourages the provision of more services as well as 'unbundling'—that is, billing for each component of care provided. While alternative methods such as capitation (paying a fixed fee over a specified time period for all of the care a patient receives) and salary have their own challenges they do not provide the same incentives to over-provide.

The appropriate use of primary care systems can be effective in controlling unnecessary use of expensive specialized services. Not only are specialist physicians paid more than generalists in most countries, they tend to provide a more intensive, expensive array of services. Countries with a primary care emphasis have been shown to have lower levels of health care expenditure, in large measure because primary care can prevent or manage illnesses in a more coordinated fashion.[5]

Related to this is the importance of health behaviours on health care costs. Cigarette smoking, poor nutrition and obesity, and lack of physical activity all contribute to rising health care costs. Between 1981 and 2001, for example, the percentage of people in OECD countries who were overweight doubled from about a little over 24% to more than 50%.[6] One US study found more than 25% of the increase in *per capita* health care spending over a 14-year period ending in 2001 was due to the consequences of obesity.[7]

Finally, charging patients directly for care is a way to control the quantity of services provided. This approach, called cost sharing, is used in most countries, often for prescription drugs but increasingly for hospital and physician services. It is often effective but is problematic for two reasons. First, patients are as likely to reduce their use of effective, necessary care as they are to cut down on unnecessary services and this may lead to increased subsequent costs to deal with avoidable complications.[8] For example, charging more for prescription drugs cuts down on compliance among the chronically ill.[9] Secondly, unless designed very carefully, cost sharing is hard on people with low incomes who may have to forgo other necessities in order to afford medical care services.

Price of services

The capacity to control how much is paid to providers and for products like pharmaceuticals can have a major impact of a country's expenditure levels. As one article exploring why the USA spends so much more on health care than other countries put it: 'It's the prices, stupid'.[10]

Another thing that can raise prices is high administrative costs. Another reason the USA spends twice as much per person on health care as other countries is the high cost of administering a system based on private insurance.[11] Such costs include marketing, determining eligibility for care, paperwork required for reimbursement, and profits. Such factors should be considered as other countries increase their reliance on private insurance to cover health care costs. Further discussion of prices appears in the next section.

What can be done to control rising expenditures?

Expenditure reduction is not a goal in its own right and higher spending that brings better outcomes may be welcomed. However, over recent decades, health care has come to consume an increasing portion of most national incomes and this is the catalyst for most reforms that are being attempted. There are many approaches to controlling expenditures and their use varies across countries. Here we divide the discussion into those used on national or regional levels and those employed at local levels.

National or regional level

Most countries struggle to provide health and social services at the level expected by the population so controlling rising national health care costs is generally a high priority.

We noted earlier that there are two targets—price and quantity (or volume). Regarding price, probably the most effective method is for countries or regions to take advantage of their purchasing power in bargaining prices for services and pharmaceuticals. In some countries, such as Canada, each province acts as a single payer for services. Provinces negotiate a global budget with each hospital and negotiate fees with physician representatives. The bargaining power this brings is one of the chief reasons Canada has been able to control its expenditures better than the USA.[12]

In countries with multiple payers it is possible to control expenditures by co-ordinating payments made by insurers or sickness funds to providers.[13] Germany offers an example of a setting in which prices are set by negotiations between sickness funds and provider representatives. Other countries, like France, have stronger government involvement in such negotiations.

As noted, fee-for-service medicine is inherently inflationary and alternatives have been shown to be more effective in controlling spending. On the hospital side, for example, DRGs may be used. DRGs are payments for an entire hospital stay, fixed in advanced based on the patient's diagnosis, that incentivize hospitals to discharge patients sooner. For physicians, payment methods such as capitation (used for primary care in the UK) or salary (used by some health maintenance organizations in the USA) provide potential alternatives.

Many strategies have been adopted to control the quantity or volume of services. These include encouraging the training of primary care practitioners or regulating the number of specialists; developing 'practice guidelines' to provide physicians with up-to-date, scientifically-verified recommendations on how to treat particular maladies; and reducing duplicative services and inappropriate prescription drugs by developing electronic medical records.

Another strategy, and our focus here, is on determining the cost-effectiveness of new technologies, services and prescription drugs—and paying only for those found to be worth the investment. The best known is the UK's NICE. Another is Australia's Pharmaceutical Benefits Advisory Committee (PBAC, see 📖 Case Study 1). Even where national advisory groups such as NICE or the PBAC exist, local action may be necessary to control expenditure and public health practitioners can play a central role in this. 📖 Case Study 2 describes a local group in England that performs this function.

Case study 1: Australia's Pharmaceutical Benefit Advisory Committee[14,15]

Established in 1953 as part of the National Health Act, the Australian PBAC is an independent agency that advises the Minister of Health and Ageing on which drugs should be covered by the national health benefits system. In conjunction with its sister agency, the Pharmaceutical Benefits Pricing Authority, which negotiates the price of drugs with manufacturers, it exemplifies a structure for ensuring that only cost-effective drugs are covered and that their pricing optimizes public resources. Australia was the first country to make economic analyses a prerequisite for including drugs in its pharmaceutical benefits system.

The PBAC is composed of researchers, clinicians, pharmacologists, industry, and consumers. It assesses research on both the clinical effectiveness (based, whenever possible, on evidence from randomized clinical trials) and costs of new drugs. If it concludes a new drug is more expensive than existing therapies and does not offer significant improvements in outcomes, it will either not cover the new drug or recommend its purchase only at a price comparable with existing drugs on the market – a strategy known as 'reference pricing'.

As a result of these practices, Australia pays considerably less for prescription drugs than many countries. In 2006, prices for 30 of the most commonly prescribed drugs in Australia were about half those in the United States and two-thirds what was paid in Canada and France.[16]

Case study 2: The Peninsula Health Technology Commissioning Group

The Peninsula Health Technology Commissioning Group (PHTCG) is a joint venture of the local health care commissioning organizations in the southwest of England, which cover a combined population of around 1.7 million people, and the National Institute for Health Research Peninsula Collaboration for Leadership in Applied Health Research and Care (PenCLAHRC), based at the Peninsula College of Medicine and Dentistry. (For more on commissioning see 📖 Chapter 5.3.) The PHTCG's aim is to ensure optimal use of health care resources for local patients based on a process combining clinical and cost-effectiveness analysis to inform health care commissioning decisions and reduce local variability in access to treatment. It assesses health technologies for which there is no national guidance from NICE or for which NICE guidance is awaited.

Drugs or health technologies for assessment can be proposed by clinicians or by commissioners and proposals are prioritized by a working group that looks at overall cost, population impact, and tractability. For each topic prioritized the process includes a review of clinical effectiveness, with a focus on identifying relevant randomized controlled trials, a cost-effectiveness analysis, and input from patient organizations and local specialist clinicians. Because the topics typically involve novel or emerging health technologies, a key aim of modeling is to identify and quantify clinical and financial risks so commissioning decisions are based on the best available evidence.

Representatives of the commissioning organizations take a majority, binding vote on whether, having reviewed the evidence presented, a specific technology should be routinely commissioned. Example of technologies recently assessed by the PHTCG are bevacizumab for the treatment of neovascular (wet) age related macular degeneration and sativex for the treatment of spasticity in multiple sclerosis. A review of the first two years of PHTCG estimated implementation of its recommendations had saved the local health care economy around £1.3 million.

Controlling expenditures: implications for public health practitioners

You might have two reactions to this issue: first, that this is somebody else's problem; secondly, that there is nothing you can do about it anyway. If your reaction is the first of these then bear in mind that rising health care costs tend to occur at the downstream end of health care, but to draw yet more resources away from effective upstream interventions. If we, collectively, fail to control health care expenditure a likely consequence is a squeezing of public health budgets and a reduction in our capacity to address potential health problems, in an equitable fashion, before they arise. The more resources are drawn away from public health, the more need there will be to spend money to deal with health problems that could potentially have been avoided.

Secondly, there are a number of things you can do, depending on the role you have. If you are in a senior position and able to put in place processes to assess, and approve or reject, new expenditures then the approaches described above (and there are others) may provide you with a suitable starting point for your organization or area of responsibility.

If you are not in a position to do this then you may still be able to support the efforts of others trying to control expenditures. As a public health practitioner, your understanding of health systems and evidence will be of great value to those responsible for making decisions about commissioning and providing health services, including deciding what services are and are not needed, and identifying which do or do not represent value for money. Get involved in local decision-making forums and make sure a public health voice is contributing to the discussion. Even if there is no local group that assesses effectiveness and cost-effectiveness you can use the information produced elsewhere to inform local decisions. Just as much as more obvious issues like addressing inequity or challenging known harms to health, addressing rising health care expenditures is an area where public health activism is crucial (see 📖 Activism).

References

1 Stine NW, Chokshi DA. (2012). Opportunity in austerity — a common agenda for medicine and public health. *New England Journal of Medicine*, **366**, 395–7.
2 Smith S, Newhouse JP, Freeland MS. (2009). Income, insurance, and technology: why does health spending outpace economic growth? *Health Affairs*, **28**, 276–1284.
3 Kaiser Family Foundation. (2011). *State Health Facts*. Available at: 🔗 http://www.statehealth-facts.org/comparemaptable.jsp?ind=624&cat=6.
4 Fisher E, Goodman D, Skinner J, Bronner K. (2009). Health care spending, quality, and outcomes: more isn't always better. Dartmouth Atlas Project Topic Brief. Available at: 🔗 http://www.dartmouthatlas.org/downloads/reports/Spending_Brief_022709.pdf.
5 Schoen C, Osborn R, Huynh PT. (2004). Primary care and health system performance: adults' experiences in five countries. *Health affairs*, web exclusive, October 28, W4-497–503.
6 Loureiro ML, Nayga Jr. RM. (2005). *Obesity rates in OECD countries: an international perspective.* Available at: 🔗 http://ageconsearch.umn.edu/bitstream/24454/1/pp05lo01.pdf
7 Thorpe KE, Florence CS, Howard DH, Joski P. (2004). *The impact of obesity on rising medical spending.* Health affairs, web exclusive, October 20, W4-480–6.
8 Lohr KN, Brook RH, Kamberg CJ, et al. (1986). Effect of cost sharing on use of medically effective and less effective care. *Medical Care*, **24(Suppl. 9)**, S31–8.
9 Goldman DP, Joyce GF, Zheng Y. (2007). Prescription drug cost sharing: associations with medication and medical utilization and spending and health. *Journal of the American Medical Association*, **298**, 61–9.
10 Anderson GF, Reinhardt UE, Hussey PS, Petrosyan V. (2005). It's the prices, stupid: why the United States is so different from other countries. *Health Affairs*, **22**, 89–105.
11 Pozen A, Cutler DM. (2010). Medical spending differences in the United States and Canada: the role of prices, procedures, and administrative expenses. *Inquiry*, **47**, 124–34.
12 Evans RG. (1986). Finding the levers, finding the courage: lessons from cost containment in North America. *Journal of Health Politics, Policy and Law*, **11**, 585–615.
13 Reinhardt UE. (2011). The many different prices paid to providers and the flawed theory of cost shifting: is it time for a more rational all-payer system? *Health Affairs*, **30**, 2125–33.
14 European Observatory on Health Systems and Policies. Australia: Health System Review. (2006). Available at: 🔗 http://www.euro.who.int/__data/assets/pdf_file/0007/96433/E89731.pdf (accessed 3 September 2012).
15 Morgan SG, McMahon M, Mitton C, et al. (2006). Centralized drug review processes in Australia, Canada, New Zealand, and the United Kingdom. *Health Affairs*, **25**, 337–47.
16 Squires D. (2011). *The US Health System in perspective: a comparison of twelve industrialized nations, Commonwealth Fund, July.* Available at: 🔗 http://www.commonwealthfund.org/~/media/Files/Publications/Issue%20Brief/2011/Jul/1532_Squires_US_hlt_sys_comparison_12_nations_intl_brief_v2.pdf (accessed 3 September 2012).

5.5 Using guidance and frameworks

Rubin Minhas, Gene Feder,
and Chris Griffiths

Objectives

After reading this chapter you should be better able to:
- understand, appreciate, and identify issues where guidance and frameworks could help
- identify existing and relevant guidelines
- assess their validity
- adapt them to local circumstances
- support clinicians in their integration into practice.

Why are clinical guidelines and their integration into practice important public health activities?

Inappropriate variations in care and the delivery of suboptimal care are major public health problems across health care systems. The clinical research enterprise is increasingly prolific and there are now over 625,000 trials listed in the Cochrane controlled trials database, over 30,000 biomedical publications annually and 17,000 biomedical books published annually. The result is that, as long ago as 1992, a study estimated that a physician would have to read an estimated 11 articles a day to maintain their knowledge and the challenge now is exponentially greater. Clinicians also do not have the time to go back to primary research or even systematic reviews for the majority of practice decisions; it has been estimated that in practice if a clinician cannot find the information they need within 15 seconds they will look no further.[1] Clinicians rely on easily accessible guidance on effective clinical practice.

Unfortunately, clinicians and public health professionals are now inundated by a tide of guidance and frameworks from government, national and international health agencies, professional colleges, health care funders, and the pharmaceutical industry.

Public health professionals have an important role to play in supporting the use of guidance, both in day-to-day practice, the development of clinical policy and other related systems level approaches to improving clinical practice. In this chapter we focus on the use of clinical guidelines as an example of the application of guidance or frameworks in practice and their relationships with the broader clinical or management systems.

What are clinical guidelines?

The principles of clinical guidelines (Box 5.5.1) can also be applied to health care policy guidelines. Guidelines are complex instruments; they may promote standardization of care, but their recommendations do not always represent explicit standards for care. We do not address guidance within pay-for-performance programmes that link explicit standards of care to financial rewards (e.g. the quality and outcomes framework for UK general practice) or obligatory frameworks (e.g. managed care requirements in the USA).

> **Box 5.5.1 What are clinical guidelines?**
>
> Clinical guidelines are: 'systematically developed statements to assist practitioner and patient decisions about appropriate health care for specific clinical circumstances'.

Identifying specific skills needed to integrate guidelines into practice

To bring added value to the process of integrating guidelines there are six key competencies that you need to either have yourself (unlikely) or have in the team (more likely) (Box 5.5.2).

> **Box 5.5.2 Competencies**
>
> - Collaborating with clinicians and other stakeholders to define policy issues
> - Searching for relevant guidelines
> - Appraisal of the validity of the guidelines and their applicability to the local context
> - Adaptation of guidelines
> - Analysing and addressing obstacles to their integration
> - Assessment of the impact of the guidelines.

What are the stages in integrating guidelines into practice?

Shortell et al.[2] identified two components necessary to improve the quality of medical care: advances in evidence-based medicine (EBM), which identify the clinical practices leading to better care, i.e., 'the content of providing care', and knowledge of how to put this content into routine practice. These advances in evidence-based management 'identify the organizational strategies, structures, and change management practices that enable physicians and other health care professionals to provide evidence-based care', i.e. the context of providing care. Until both components are in place—identifying the best content (i.e. EBM) and applying it within effective organizational contexts (i.e., evidence-based management (EBMgt))—consistent, sustainable improvement in the quality of care is unlikely to occur'.[3,4]

Like any complex process involving different groups of people with different perspectives, it is important to manage the process of guideline integration carefully. There are at least eight identifiable stages in the process. It is important to appreciate the potential barriers that may occur at any of these stages.

The integration perspective

Throughout this chapter we use the term 'integration', rather than 'implementation' because it expresses more fully the complexity of incorporating guideline recommendations into clinical practice in specific health care settings.

Identifying a clinical issue

Research studies demonstrate that processes of care can be improved by integrating guidelines into local practice. The number of guidelines produced is much greater than the capacity to integrate them and so to justify devoting resources to guideline adaptation and implementation, a clinical issue must be considered a priority. Ideally, at least three criteria should be fulfilled:

- the condition or issue should have a large impact on public health or health care resources
- there should also be demonstrable and unjustified variation in its clinical management
- there should be some evidence for what constitutes good practice (Box 5.5.3).

> **Box 5.5.3 Example of a suitable issue for guideline implementation**
>
> In a local audit of survivors of a myocardial infarction it was found that although 92% were using aspirin 6 months later only 30% were using beta-blockers, with a range of 12–72% in different general practices.[5] Secondary prevention of coronary heart disease is an obvious subject for guideline implementation, with a large health impact and unjustified variation in clinical management.

Although these are necessary conditions, they are not sufficient. Discussion with clinicians is crucial; they also need to think that the issue is important and so worth their commitment to an integration project. The genuine involvement of opinion leaders (which increases the likelihood of integration) is likely to be more successful if initiated at an early stage. Potential barriers to improvement should also be considered early. If these are judged to be insurmountable, then another issue should be prioritized.

Forming a local guidelines group

Choose no more than a dozen people. This should include:

- clinicians, managers, and others who will be integrating the guidelines on the ground
- 'content' experts (people who know the subject well)
- patient representatives who should ideally have experience of the condition or be able to represent the patient perspective
- someone with the competence to identify, appraise, and summarize guidelines or systematic reviews.

The group will need to have a Chair, with all the usual management skills for guiding the process, and a timetable for meetings. Objectives must be clear and not too ambitious (see Box 5.5.4).

Identifying national or regional guidelines

National and regional guidelines are increasingly accessible via the internet and may be identified on bibliographic databases, although they are not necessarily indexed in the commonly available databases. Some of the better-developed guideline websites include full text versions or abstracts (Box 5.5.5).

Appraising the validity of guidelines

When you have identified relevant guidelines you need to appraise their validity before choosing which to adapt for your own use. Adopting recommendations from guidelines of questionable validity may harm patients or waste resources on ineffective interventions. Within the UK there are now well-established guidelines programmes (Scottish Intercollegiate Guidelines Network for Scotland and the National Institute for Health and Clinical Excellence for England and Wales) using rigorous methods and formal appraisal within the programmes. If appraised guidelines are not available, you can do your own appraisal using a validated appraisal tool (Box 5.5.6).

Box 5.5.4 Realistic and unrealistic objectives for development of local guidelines

Realistic objectives
- Develop local guidelines on use of beta-blockers after myocardial infarction
- Identify national or international guidelines on use of beta-blockers after myocardial infarction
- If none found, identify systematic reviews of use of beta-blockers after myocardial infarction
- Appraise guidelines or systematic reviews. Choose most valid one
- Adapt to local context. Circulate to target clinicians for comment
- Develop integration programme with general practitioner leaders and consultant physicians

Unrealistic objectives
- Develop local guidelines on primary and secondary prevention of cardiovascular disease
- Search for relevant randomized controlled trial evidence
- Appraise individual trials and summarize
- Formulate recommendations directly based on trial evidence.

Box 5.5.5 Identifying national or regional guidelines

Search terms for common bibliographic databases
- *Medline and Healthstar* 'guideline' (publication type) and 'consensus development conference' (publication type): Healthstar includes journals not referenced in Medline and grey literature CINAHL 'practice guidelines' (publication type). Includes full text version of some guidelines
- *EMBASE* 'practice guidelines' (subject heading): this is used for articles about guidelines and for those that contain practice guidelines; the term was introduced in 1994.

Useful websites
- *National Guideline Clearinghouse* (M http://www.guideline.gov): the largest database of full text appraised guidelines in the world, sponsored by the Agency for Health care Quality and Research. Understandable bias towards US guidance, but includes guidelines from other countries (accessed 24 May 2011).
- *National Institute for Health and Clinical Excellence* (M http://www.nice.org.uk/): growing number of full text national guidelines for England and Wales, as well as guidance on individual drugs and technologies (accessed 24 May 2011).
- *Scottish Intercollegiate Guidelines Network* (M http://www.sign.ac.uk/guidelines/index.html): full text versions of guidelines and quick reference guides (accessed 23 May 2011).

Box 5.5.6 UK guidelines appraisal tool

This is a 23-item instrument that has been validated to test the methodological quality of guidelines. It is not intended to give a 'pass/fail' assessment, but does allow a judgment of validity and comparison of different guidelines on the same clinical topic (see http://fhswedge. csu.mcmaster.ca/pebc/agreetrust/).

Adapting guidelines to fit local circumstances

This is an essential part of the process. For example, if a guideline recommends a drug not licensed in your country or an investigation that is not available, then the recommendation of the guideline must be changed. Development of a local version also allows information about local services and referral pathways. If the 'source' guideline is more than a couple of years old you should update it by identifying recent systematic reviews from bibliographic databases and sources like the Cochrane Library. Finally, there is the issue of local ownership. Involving clinicians in adapting guidelines to local circumstances increases knowledge about guidelines, but not necessarily adherence to them.

Piloting and identifying barriers to integration

Once the development group has agreed on a draft guideline it is advisable to pilot the guidelines in real-life practice settings. Recommendations may turn out to be impossible to integrate locally, no matter how much thought the guidelines group has invested in them. This also gives an opportunity to identify barriers to integration. These may relate to:
* *People*: target clinicians (skills, knowledge, attitudes, rules, or norms about roles).
* *Culture*: the organizational context (e.g. style of management and willingness to change within clinical teams).
* *Structures*: structural and resource issues can stall perfectly logical guidance for purely practical reasons (e.g. lack of resources for prescribing or extra staff).

Failure to clarify and specifically address these barriers with integration strategies will result in failure or weakened impact.[6,7]

Strategies for dissemination and integration

The previous stages will be wasted if the guidelines are not used in practice. Research on the integration of guidelines and other sources of evidence gives us a basis for designing strategy at this stage. Tailor your strategy to address the barriers identified. Passive methods of giving guidelines to clinicians (e.g. just through the post) are unlikely to be effective[5–7] unless there are other drivers for change. Multifaceted programmes, especially those that explicitly tackle obstacles to implementation, engage clinicians face to face, and built in reminders or prompts into the consultation are more likely to work.[6,7] Recent research has cast some doubt over the need for multifaceted approaches for integration of all guidance.

Information technology is increasingly used to record, guide and monitor the delivery of high quality care in primary and secondary care, but there is insufficient evidence for the added value of this technology in integrating clinical guidance.[8,9] Further evidence is required on how to effectively integrate guidance into electronic medical records is required.

Monitoring the impact of guidelines

Set up some form of routine data collection to assess whether the guidelines are used in clinical practice. Where guidelines make prescribing and referral recommendations this is relatively straightforward when data are stored electronically. In the UK the introduction of clinical governance means that acute health care trusts and primary care trusts have a statutory obligation to monitor performance through these methods. Linking performance measures with evidence-based guidelines makes them more likely to seem credible to clinicians, particularly if they have been involved in the guidelines programme.

What is actually involved in getting something done?

The importance of measurement

A potential of weakness guidelines is that they may not explicitly identify what it is that clinicians should do or are able to highlight when this has been achieved. Two key principles from the quality improvement paradigm illustrate this issue, 'measurement lays the foundations for improvement' and 'what gets measured gets done'. Without associated performance measures it is not possible to identify where and when improvement has occurred and so key recommendations within clinical guidelines should be adapted into audit criteria that can be used to help implement and monitor guidelines. Other techniques that have been shown to have some effect include the public profiling of the results of performance measures and their linking with financial incentives.[10,11] There are many elements of high quality care that are not easily quantifiable and reliance only on the information provided by limited sets of reporting data should be positively avoided as this can have significant adverse consequences.

The importance of managing the process

Integrating a guideline is like any other development work: it needs to be carefully designed and managed. Regular reviews of progress are vital, perhaps by a steering group consisting of the multidisciplinary panel that adapted the guidelines. The group needs to monitor the progress of integration (particularly when a labour-intensive approach, such as outreach visits is being used), watch for new or unforeseen barriers, and check data on expected changes in practice.

Embedding into organizational structures

Always take the opportunity to embed any process of change within a larger context. Integration may be more easily achieved by including it within local organizational structures (e.g. clinical governance in UK primary care, or an integrated care pathway in secondary care).

Potential problems

Mismatch between guidance, priorities, and available resources

The competing demands on clinicians and managers resources can limit the attention that longer term guideline integration requires. Lack of resources will hinder integration if recommendations require extensive new tasks outside clinicians' usual roles or prescription of medication where clinicians may be penalized for excessive spending. Barriers such as clinicians taking on new roles and prescribing resources should be addressed at the outset. Think carefully if resources are likely to be big problem.

Insufficient attention to integration and review

Effective integration will always demand time, enthusiasm, and resources; choosing integration methods that are likely to give the best return on available investment is vital. Even when the guidance appears to be integrated, don't assume that change will follow automatically without review of progress and, if necessary, changes in strategy.

Myths

There are many myths associated with guideline development and integration, including the four most rehearsed.

Clinicians do not use guidelines

Although clinical guidelines often get a bad press—for instance, because of suggestions that they limit clinical freedom—research shows that carefully chosen strategies do result in effective adoption of guideline recommendations both in primary and secondary care settings.

Guidelines should always be developed locally from scratch to ensure local ownership

There is commonly held view that adaptations of national guidelines don't work. The validity of nationally and internationally generated guidance needs to be appraised before being adapted, but to start from scratch with guidance at a local level is grossly inefficient. Nationally developed guidelines do have sufficient credibility, especially if they are adapted to local circumstances by respected opinion leaders.

Guideline recommendations are invariably authoritative

For many clinicians the recommendations within clinical guidelines can seem to represent scientific authority particularly if they are produced by national bodies or other high status organizations. The development of high quality systematic guidelines always requires judgments, even when there is a body of good quality evidence. In fact evidence is often absent for many decisions that need to be taken; less than half of the recommendations within clinical guidelines can be based on high quality evidence.[12] Even where strong evidence exists, developers may be able to identify one of several alternate approaches to developing strategies and recommendations as illustrated by the varying recommendations within guidelines for the same conditions produced in different countries and recommendations that take account of factors such as ethnicity. Elderly patients can be put at risk of poly-pharmacy by guidelines as they are often developed in isolation from considerations such as the medication burden resulting from recommendations of multiple guidelines.[13]

Guidelines lead to litigation

Although the legal status of guidelines varies between different countries, overall they have not been used to override expert opinion in courts of law. On the other hand, if clinicians integrate faulty guidelines it is they, rather than the authors of such guidelines, who are likely to increase their liability in negligence. The relationship between guidelines and clinician liability will vary between countries and is likely to evolve in the next few years.[14]

The increasing importance of governance means that every team, clinician, and policy maker needs to be able to justify their professional practice. An evidence base and a value base should underpin every decision and action. At an individual level there may be good reasons not to adhere to a particular recommendation in the guidance in relation to a specific patient. In this case, justification for significantly deviating from the guidance needs to be explicit, preferably in the medical record.

Pitfalls

Two randomized trials of guideline integration in general practices in east London illustrate success and failure:

- Despite using a multifaceted strategy to implement diabetes and asthma guidelines (outreach visits, consultation prompts, and audit with feedback), it was found that general practices with poor organization (e.g. no practice manager) or with internal conflict between clinicians failed to integrate guidelines. The lesson learned is that chaotic practices need organizational support before guidelines can take root.
- A trial tested the use of postal reminders concerning guidelines to patients discharged after a myocardial infarct and to their general practitioners.[5] The results indicated that some general practitioners did not see it as their responsibility to address secondary prevention in patients discharged from hospital. Furthermore, whilst practice nurses

could have played a larger part in providing secondary prevention, this part of their role was poorly encouraged. The lesson here is that the roles and responsibilities of target clinicians need to be addressed before attempting to change clinician behaviour.

Key determinants of success

Six important actions are associated with successful development and implementation of guidelines:
- setting priorities clearly
- setting clear and attainable objectives
- collaborating early with stakeholders
- identifying and targeting barriers to change
- choosing the most powerful implementation strategy that resources will allow
- ensuring a rigorous project management approach is used.

References

1 Moore A, McQuay H, Gray JAM. (1999). Bandolier 61: Evidence-based health care. *Bandolier* **6**, 1–8.

2 Shortell SM, Rundall TG, Hsu J (2007). Improving patient care by linking evidence-based medicine and evidence-based management. *Journal of the American Medical Association*, **298**, 673–6.

3 Davidoff F, Haynes B, Sackett D, Smith R. (1995). Evidence-based medicine. *British Medical Journal*, **310**, 1085–8.

4 Sackett DL, Rosenber WM, Gray JA, Haynes RB, Richardson WS. (1996). Evidence based medicine: what it is and what it isn't. *British Medical Journal*, **312**, 71–2.

5 Feder G, Griffiths C, Eldridge S, Spence ℬ (1999). Effect of postal prompts to general practitioners and patients on the quality of primary care after a coronary event (POST): randomized controlled trial. *British Medical Journal*, **318**, 1522–6.

6 Grimshaw JM, Thomas RE, MacClennan C, et al. (2004). Effectiveness and efficiency of guideline dissemination and implementation strategies. *Health Technology Assessment*, **8**, iii–iv, 1–72.

7 Grimshaw J, Eccles M, Thomas R, et al. (2006). Evidence (and its limitations) of the effectiveness of guideline dissemination and implementation strategies 1966–1998. *Journal of General Internal Medicine*, **21(Suppl. 2)**, S14–20.

8 Shojania KG, Jennings A, Mayhew A, et al. (2010). Effect of point-of-care computer reminders on physician behaviour: a systematic review. *Canadian Medical Association Journal*, **182**, E216–25.

9 Wolfstadt J, Gurwitz J, Field TS, et al. (2008). The effect of computerized order entry with decision support on the rates of adverse drug events: a systematic review. *Journal of General Internal Medicine*, **23**, 451–8.

10 Shojania KG, Grimshaw JM. (2005). Evidence-based quality improvement: the state of the science. *Health Affairs (Millwood)*, **24**, 138–50.

11 Auerbach A, Landefield S, Shojania K. (2007). Tension between needing to improve care and knowing how to do it. *New England Journal of Medicine*, **357**, 608–13.

12 McAlister F, van Diepen S, Padwal RS, Johnson JA, Majumdar SR. (2007). How evidence based are the recommendations in clinical guidelines? *PLoS Medicine*, **4**, e250.

13 Boyd CM, Darer J, Boult C, et al. (2005). Clinical practice guidelines and quality of care for older patients with multiple comorbid diseases: implications for pay for performance. *Journal of the American Medical Association*, **294**, 716–24.

14 Hurwitz B. (2004). How does evidence based guidance influence determinations of medical negligence? *British Medical Journal*, **329**, 1024–8.

5.6 Health care process and patient experience

Diana Delnoij

Objectives

This chapter will help you to analyse the health care process and, in particular, the quality of this process and its outcomes from the patient's perspective. You will read how you can measure quality from the patient's perspective, how to interpret the findings, and how to take action based on the results.

This chapter provides hands-on guidance with respect to the development and implementation of surveys measuring patient experiences. However, keep in mind that this is only a first step in the quality cycle. The results of such a survey give you a 'diagnosis' of the quality of care from the patients' perspective. It does not really tell you what you should do to improve patient experiences, however. To find effective remedies for negative experiences, often you will have to do additional research.

Definitions

Health care process

The health care process is essentially a business process. A business process is defined as a complete, dynamically co-ordinated set of activities or logically-related tasks that must be performed to deliver value to customers or to fulfill other strategic goals.[1] In health care, this process consists of all the things done for and to the patient by health care providers in the course of diagnosis and treatment, from the moment a patient enters the health care system until the moment that he or she is discharged, leaves, or dies.

Quality of care

Quality of care refers to the level of performance that characterizes the health care provided.[2]. Measures of quality of care consist of various ingredients, including, for example, measures of effectiveness[2] and patient satisfaction or patient-centeredness (the degree to which health care interventions are delivered responsive to patients' needs and preferences).

Sources of information

Health care process

The health care process can be studied from various perspectives by different disciplines using different sources of information.

Economic perspective.

From an economic perspective you may want to study the health care process, for example, because you are interested in improving the efficiency of care provision and/or in cost control. In that case, the source of information will often consist of administrative and fiscal data. You look at the costs of care in relation to volumes provided.

Health system perspective

Health systems researchers can study the health care process from policy perspective, for example, designing the optimal system by strengthening primary care, or enhancing integrated care. In this case, the factors that are studied can relate to the division of tasks between the different levels in the health care system, such as the number of referrals from primary care to hospital care, number of patients discharged from hospital to nursing homes etc.

Operations management perspective

In operations management, the health care process is usually studied with the aim to redesign and improve the logistics within a health care facility. In that case you would measure, for instance, waiting times at various stages in the process, auxiliary services used, the division of tasks between back-office and front-office etc.

Quality perspective

From a quality perspective, the health care process is seen as one of the determinants of health outcomes, together with more structural factors, such as capacity (including human resources), physical equipment and facilities. This quality perspective of looking at the health care process will be elaborated in more detail in the remainder of this chapter.

Quality of care

There are two important sources of information about quality of care:
- registration of clinical data by health care providers
- patients' reports collected through population or patient surveys.

In the scientific literature, patient reports are referred to e.g. as 'patient-reported outcome measures' (abbreviated as 'PROMs'): measures of the way patients perceive their health and the impact that treatments or adjustments to lifestyle have on their quality of life. So, PROMs include measures of patient outcomes (in terms of health or quality of life) as well as measures of patients' experiences in or their satisfaction with the process of health care delivery.

In this chapter, the focus is on the latter type of measures: patient satisfaction, or—preferably—patient experiences. In the last decennia of the 20th century, patient satisfaction had become a frequently used outcome measure in clinical trials. In addition to that, satisfaction surveys were frequently used to measure the quality of care from the patient's perspective. However, in the second half of the 1990s, it became clear that, as a tool for quality improvement, patient satisfaction surveys were not very useful. This has to do with the fact that patient satisfaction is a multidimensional concept. Patients are satisfied if their actual experiences match or exceed their *ex ante* expectations. If you find that patients are not satisfied, it is unclear what the underlying reason is: were they given substandard care, or did they have too high expectations?

As a consequence, is was argued that quality assurance it would be more useful to look at the underlying components of satisfaction, namely at patients' expectations and at specific experiences. This led to the development of a new types of patient surveys. In those surveys, the emphasis is not on an evaluation of satisfaction but on collecting detailed reports of what actually happened to patients during a hospital stay or a visit to the doctor. Examples of these patient or consumer experience surveys are the American CAHPS questionnaires (Consumer Assessment of Health care Providers and Systems), the questionnaires developed by the Picker Institute for the English NHS, or the Dutch Consumer Quality Index (CQ-index).

Why is this an important public health issue?

Patients have a specific kind of so-called experiential knowledge, that is seen as crucial for the advancement of quality care. Patients know what it is to live with a specific disease and they have a lot of experience with health care providers and treatments. Information about patients' experiences is therefore vital. Reasons for studying patient experiences can differ between health care systems. Generally, the motives vary from external accountability of health care providers to enhancing patient choice, improving the quality of care or measuring the performance of the health care system as a whole. Often, surveys of patient experiences serve multiple purposes.

Apart from that, patient experiences are an important aspect of health systems research. Since the WHO published its World Health Report 2000, the quality of care as perceived by patients has been seen as an integral part of the performance of health systems. Therefore, organizations such as the Commonwealth Fund, the Picker Institute Europe and the Organization for Economic Co-operation and Development have engaged in international comparisons of patients' experiences.

How to measure patient experiences?

Patient experiences are measured through surveys, using mail question-naires, online questionnaires, telephone surveys, and face-to-face inter-views. If you want to conduct such a survey, keep in mind the following questions:

What is the unit of analysis?

Are you interested in the performance of a health care system as a whole, or of specific regions within a system; in the performance of individual health care providers; or in the experiences of patients with a certain disease or who have had a certain treatment. It is important to clearly define your unit of analysis, because it has consequences for the definition of your study population and the sampling method that you will have to use.

How do I sample respondents to participate in the survey?

Depending on your unit of analysis, you can draw samples from the gen-eral populations or you can draw samples from the patient populations of health care providers. The latter is possible only if these health care providers have an adequate administrative system that allows for queries of patients meeting certain criteria.

What is an adequate sample size?

There is no readymade answer to this question. The necessary sample size depends on factors such as the reliability of the questionnaire, the expected response rate, and the aim of the survey. In studies comparing patient experiences across countries, the sample sizes are usually 1000–2000 citizens/patients per country. Studies comparing patient experiences between hospitals work often with sample sizes of at least 500 patients. If the aim of your study is not to compare patient experiences in different countries or different facilities, but to measure patient experiences in one facility, for example, as part of continuous quality improvement- you can generally work with smaller samples (for example, $n = 200$). If possible, try to determine your sample size using power analysis. Beware of the fact that a power analysis will give you the desired number of respondents in a survey. Your actual sample size should be bigger, because you will have to accommodate non-response.

How do I collect data?

You can use face-to-face interviews, telephone interviews, self-admin-istered mail surveys, or online surveys. Which of the methods is best depends on your study population and your financial resources. Face-to-face and telephone interviews require more human resources than mail surveys and are therefore usually more expensive. Online questionnaires are comparatively cheap, but can only be used in populations with good access to and experience with the Internet. Presently, this makes online surveys less adequate for use in an elderly population.

How do I choose a questionnaire?

In several countries, there are 'families' of standardized patient experience questionnaires that you could use if they fit the topic of your study. English language questionnaires that you may want to look at are the American CAHPS surveys (Consumer Assessment of Health care Providers and Systems) and the surveys developed by the Picker Institute Europe:

- https://www.cahps.ahrq.gov/default.asp
- http://www.pickereurope.org/patientsurveys

If you cannot find an existing questionnaire in your own language, you can either translate a questionnaire that has been developed elsewhere, or develop your own questionnaire. There are certain scientific 'rules' for translating questionnaires. You will have to have the questionnaire translated forward and backward by different translators and the translation should not be purely technical, but also include a cultural validation and adaptation to your own health care system. If you need to develop your own questionnaire, follow the steps described in the next section.

Who should be involved?

Stakeholder involvement is a prerequisite for collecting information once and for using it for multiple purposes. When using patient experience surveys, you should pay specific attention to the involvement of patients and patient organizations. It is essential that measurement and reporting of patient experiences takes place about those quality domains that matter most to patients.

Developing your own questionnaire

The development of these measurement instruments consists of the following phases:

- qualitative research
- psychometric research
- analyses of discriminative power.

Qualitative research

You measure patient experiences because you are interested in the quality of care evaluated from the patient's perspective. Therefore, your measurement instrument should contain quality items that are important to patients. We already know a lot about things that are important to patients. Coulter[3] lists the following patient priorities:

- fast access to reliable health advice
- effective treatment delivered by trusted professionals
- participation in decisions and respect for preferences
- clear, comprehensible information and support for self-care
- Attention to physical and environmental needs
- Emotional support, empathy and respect
- Involvement of, and support for, family and carers
- Continuity of care and smooth transitions.

This list covers more or less what patients expect from health care in general. However, we also know that these priorities differ between various patient groups. For that reason, the development of an instrument measuring patient experiences should preferably start with qualitative research of the preference of the specific patient group that is studied.

You can do this through a so-called focus group: a small convenience sample of people brought together to discuss a topic or issue with the aim to ascertain the range and intensity of their views.[2] A focus group discussion leads to an operationalization of quality of care from the patients' perspective and are aimed at ensuring the content validity of the questionnaires. Ideally, some 8–12 patients should participate in a focus group and you may need more than one focus group. Ask patients how they define good quality of care, and ask them about their concrete experiences with distinct aspects of health care quality.

Questionnaire construction

Focus groups can result in long lists of possible questionnaire items; mostly process aspects of health care quality such as information, communication, and interpersonal contact. In subsequent group discussions, you try to reduce this long list of items to a short list that forms the basis of your questionnaire.

There are two ways to formulate questions about patient experiences. You can ask about:

- the degree to which experiences met quality standards
- the frequency with which experiences met quality standards.

For example:

- *Degree:* in the past 12 months, did doctors listen carefully to what you had to say (response categories e.g.: yes, completely or yes, definitely; yes, to a certain extent; no)?
- *Frequency:* how often in the past 12 months did doctors listen carefully to what you had to say (response categories e.g.: never, sometimes, usually, always)?

In both types, the quality of care from the patient's perspective is usually measured on an four-point ordinal scale.

From the point of view of patients, quality of care should be improved primarily with respect to aspects that are extremely important to them, but with which they have relatively negative experiences. The importance that patients attach to the various experiences can be measured by designing an 'importance questionnaire' to go along with your patient experience questionnaire. In an 'importance questionnaire' respondents are asked to score the importance of the same set of items that are also included in the 'experience questionnaire'.

For example:

- *Experience:* how often in the past 12 months did doctors listen carefully to what you had to say (response categories e.g.: never, sometimes, usually, always)?
- *Importance:* how important is it that doctors listen carefully to what you have to say (response categories, for example, not important, important, very important, of the utmost importance)?

Psychometric research

After you have constructed a draft questionnaire on the basis of qualitative research, you want to examine this questionnaire more quantitatively through psychometric research. For this type of research you need to test your questionnaire in samples that are big enough to allow for psychometric analyses. Aim for at least $n = 600$, but preferably more.

Psychometric analyses include:

- item analyses
- inter-item analyses
- analyses of the underlying structure (factor and reliability analyses).

Item analyses

Item analyses consist of, for example, looking at the skewness of the distribution of the answers to questions about respondents' experiences and problems, and looking at the non-response to questions.

Inter-item analyses

An examination of the overlap in the pattern of answers for different items. You can do that using correlation coefficients.[2] If you find considerable overlap in the pattern of answers between two different items and if the items also deal with the same subject, this means that one of these two items could be deleted. If a correlation coefficient exceeds 0.85, there is no statistical reason to keep both items in the measurement instrument. You can delete one of the two.

Factor and reliability analyses

Factor analyses are carried out in order to estimate, describe and measure the fundamental dimensions that underlie the observed data.[2] We advise you to carry out an exploratory factor analysis using Principal Component Analysis with oblique rotation (because of the assumed interrelationships between the factors). After determination of the number of factors, you will have to examine the size of the factor loadings. The rule of thumb here is that an item's factor loading for a particular factor should be more than 0.3 if a quality aspect is to be assigned to the factor in question. If an item has factor loadings of 0.3 or more for several factors, it is assigned to the factor for which it has the highest factor loading.

Furthermore, you should examine the internal consistency reliability of a measurement instrument using Cronbach's alpha[2]. A scale is sufficiently reliable if Cronbach's alpha is greater than 0.70. Typically, the scales you will find in patient experience surveys correspond to the themes listed above under patient priorities: timely access, clear information, participative decision-making, etc.

Discriminative power

If the purpose of your survey is to *compare* the performance of health care providers with respect to patient experiences, than there is one last step that you will have to take in developing your own questionnaire. In that case, namely, you will have to assure that your questionnaire is able to detect meaningful and statistical differences between health care providers.

Multilevel analyses

An adequate way to test this is by using hierarchical analysis, also called multilevel analysis: a method that allows for integration of contextual, group, or macrolevel factors with individual-level factors.[2] This method allows you to examine the variance components through the so-called intraclass correlation.[2] If the intraclass correlation is not statistically significant, this implies there is only variance on the level of patients (in other words: health care providers do not contribute to the variance in patient experiences). In multilevel analyses you can compare the scores of health care providers on the various scales in your questionnaire through empirical-Bayes methods.[2]

Case-mix adjustment

If the purpose of your survey is to compare the performance of health care providers, you want to be sure that you are making a 'fair' comparison. In general, the elderly, people with a lower level of education and people with a worse self-reported health status report more positive experiences with health care than younger people, people with a higher level of education and people with a better self-reported health status. There are a number of other patient characteristics that may be systematically related to the responses in patient experience surveys. If those patient characteristics are beyond the control of health care providers and if the populations of the health care providers you are comparing vary on these patient characteristics, it is necessary to correct for systematic differences in response tendencies (so-called case-mix adjustment).

Analysing data and interpreting results

As mentioned earlier, the motives for measuring patient experiences vary from external accountability of health care providers to enhancing patient choice, improving the quality of care or measuring the performance of the health care system as a whole. This implies that the audience that you wish to address with your findings may vary from individual health care consumers (patients), to health insurers or other purchasers, managers and health care professionals, and policy makers. These various audiences have different information needs (see Table 5.6.1). Those differences can have consequences for your analyses and the way you present your findings.

Table 5.6.1 Information needs of different stakeholders: Who wants to know what?[4]

Who	What
Individual consumers	*Maximizers:* Who is the best provider for me (in terms of outcomes or in terms of trust)? Where can I find this provider? Do I have access (in terms of waiting times, insurance coverage etc.)?
	Satisficers: How does my usual provider perform compared to others?
Patient/ consumer organizations	Do providers meet quality standards as defined by patient/consumer organizations? Which areas of performance are lagging behind? How can we help members/patients to make an informed choice?
Health insurers	Do providers meet predefined quality standards (pay-for-performance)? Whom shall we (not) contract from the quality perspective (preferred providers)?
Health care providers	What are best practices? Which areas of our performance need improvement? What do patients and insurers expect from us?
Inspectorate for Health Care	Which providers perform below a minimum quality level (and therefore need further inspection)?
Ministry of Health	What is the overall level of quality of care in the Netherlands and how does it develop over time?

Taking action

Surveys of patient experiences often serve multiple purposes. In general, the emphasis has shifted from only using data as internal feedback for quality improvement towards also publishing this information for external accountability or to facilitate consumer choice. It is difficult to develop questionnaires that serve both internal, as well as external purposes. If you seriously strive to improve the quality of care from the patient's perspective, however, it is the only way. A review article by Fung et al.[5] suggests that individual consumers do not often use these public report cards to select better performing providers over worse performing ones, but that publicly releasing performance data stimulates quality improvement activity at the hospital level. Therefore, the instruments used for external accountability and consumer choice should also be useful for internal quality projects. This asks for stakeholder involvement in the development of questionnaires, the design of surveys, and the interpretation of survey findings. This is a complex and time-consuming process. However, the resulting standardization enables all stakeholders to move away from discussions about the validity of indicators and instruments towards discussions about the quality of care.

It is important that you realize that measuring patient experiences is only a first step in the quality cycle. It gives you a 'diagnosis' of the quality of care from the patients' perspective. But it does not really tell you what you should do to improve patient experiences.

To find effective remedies for negative experiences you will have to dig deeper, for example, by:

- going back to the targeted patient population and organize discussion groups or open interviews about the survey results, their interpretation of these results and suggestions for improvement
- identifying health care providers whose clients have very positive experiences, find out what they do differently and try to copy that in your own organization
- looking for inspiration in improvement guides that have been developed e.g. by the American Agency for Health care Quality and Research (the CAHPS Improvement Guide[6]) or the Picker Institute Europe.[7]

Potential pitfalls

Mismatch between study purpose and information products

Various audiences have different information needs and those differences have consequences for your analyses and the way you present your findings. State-of-the art analysis methods using case-mix adjusted, empirical-Bayes methods to compare the relative performance of health care providers are the best way to guarantee a fair comparison between providers. However, the statistics used in this method are relatively complicated, particularly for an audience of health care professionals. So if you use these statistics in internal feedback reports, professionals and managers may find it difficult to understand the information and recognize the 'crude' performance data that they usually work with. If this results in distrust of the information, they will not use it for quality improvement.

How to avoid bias?

High non-response is a potential source of bias in patient surveys. Therefore, you should make sure that your method of data collection is suitable for your target population:

- online surveys are less suitable for use in an elderly population. In addition, both mail
- online surveys may be inadequate tools for data collection in a population with a low level of literacy
- make sure you use easy, unambiguous language and short sentences in all cases
- resort to face-to-face or telephone interviews if you expect literacy to be a problem
- test your draft questionnaire among a few patients from your target population

- ask them to explain what they think that the questions mean and invite them to think aloud while filling out the draft questionnaire (cognitive testing)
- you can make patient surveys more inclusive by offering migrants access to questionnaires in different languages.

Ethical issues and privacy of respondents

It is not possible to measure patient experiences without the help of patients who are willing to serve as respondents in qualitative research or surveys. However, depending on the legislation in your country you may need the approval of an ethics committee before you are allowed to send out questionnaires to patients.

Apart from that, sometimes you need to draw samples from administrative data based on medical records. If necessary, seek legal counselling to make sure that you do not violate medical confidentiality or other privacy legislation.

Further resources

Dattalo P. (2007). *Determining sample size. balancing power, precision, and practicality.* Oxford University Press, Oxford.

References

1 Trkman P. (2010). The critical success factors of business process management. *International Journal of Information Management*; **30,** 125–34.
2 Porta M. (2008). *A dictionary of epidemiology.* Oxford University Press, New York.
3 Coulter A. (2007). Finding out what patients want. *ENT News*; **16,** 65–7.
4 Delnoij DMJ, Rademakers JJDJM, Groenewegen PP. (2010). The Dutch Consumer Quality Index: an example of stakeholder involvement in indicator development. *BMC Health Services Research*, **10,** 88.
5 Fung CH, Lim YW, Mattke S, Damberg C, Shekelle P. (2008). Systematic review: the evidence that publishing patient care performance data improves quality of care. *Annals of Internal Medicine*; **148,** 111–23.
6 CAHPS. (2011). Quality improvement. Available at: ℗ http://www.cahps.ahrq.gov/qiguide/default.aspx (accessed 17 May 2011).
7 Picker Institute Europe (2011). Patient reviews. Available at: ℗ http://www.pickereurope.org/usingpatientfeedback (accessed 17 May 2011).

5.7 Evaluating health care technologies

Ruairidh Milne and Andrew Stevens

Objectives

Reading this chapter will help you to:
- explain what Health Technology Assessment (HTA) is
- understand the importance of HTA to public health
- make the best use of HTA
- know the basics of how to do HTA.

What is HTA?

Health technologies

'Health technology' is the established term for any element of health care. It includes all treatments and tests used to promote health, prevent and treat disease, and improve rehabilitation and long-term care.

The purpose of labelling elements of health care (whether as 'technologies' or anything else) is to make them open to evaluation. To evaluate anything, it has to be well-defined. The elements of health care that we define as technologies are those that it is useful to evaluate. So wherever there are choices to be made in planning individual patient treatments or preventative measures (public health), in collective patient treatments (public health), or in health care infrastructure, the evaluable elements become health technologies. The following are, therefore, all health technologies:
- devices and drugs (from sticking plasters to genetically engineered anti-cancer drugs)
- diagnostic techniques (from dipsticks to PET scanners)
- surgical and other procedures (from acupuncture to transplantation or dialysis)
- programmes and settings of health care (from co-ordinated stroke care to emergency department staffing schedules).

Health technology evaluation and health technology assessment

Remember the generic definition of health care evaluation: '... the formal determination of the effectiveness, efficiency and acceptability, of a planned intervention in achieving stated objectives.'[1]

HTA is the most sophisticated manifestation of health care evaluation and it has two key characteristics:

- It aims for a formal evaluation of techniques and drugs with well-defined comparators.
- It is evaluation with an explicit purpose, that is to improve the ability of health services to meet the objectives of decision makers. These decision-makers may be patients, clinicians, managers, policy makers or the public. Their objectives commonly include efficiency, humanity, choice and equity.

Four questions and four components of HTA

HTA asks four fundamental questions (Box 5.7.1).

Box 5.7.1 the four questions of HTA

- Does the technology work?
- For whom?
- At what cost?
- How does it compare with alternatives?

The key steps of assessment are described in detail in Part 1 of the Handbook, 📖 Assessment, and outlined later in this chapter. The main components are:

- a clear description of the technology, with an analysis of its current use and the decision problem(s) facing decision-makers
- a systematic review of evidence, typically using a hierarchy of evidence (where the issue is effectiveness, this places randomized controlled trials at the top and opinion at the bottom)
- an economic assessment, typically using a decision model incorporating costs, relative effectiveness, and valuations of health states (utilities) for different treatment modes.
- together often with consideration of the organizational, social, legal and ethical implications of the technology.

Why has HTA become important?

Three main forces have driven the development of HTA over the last 25 years:

- a combination of concerns about the adoption of unproven technologies
- rising health service costs
- a steady rise in consumer expectations.[2]

At its best, HTA offers the prospect of helping health services both manage demand and budgets and also provide the best value care to the populations they serve.

Assessment and appraisal

There is an important distinction between assessment and appraisal – between the scientific process of gathering evaluation knowledge about a technology and the political process of deciding what to do about it. Technology appraisal (the political process) is, of course, based on HTA (the scientific process), but other factors come into play as well, such as local priorities, values and resources.[3]

In some countries, both steps fall under the heading of HTA; but in the English NHS the distinction is made between health technology assessment and appraisal. (At the national level in England, assessment is undertaken by research teams; appraisal is done by the NICE appraisal committee. At a local level, assessments are often undertaken by public health specialists, while appraisal is typically a function those responsible for commissioning health services.[4])

Real-life examples of health technology assessment

Table 5.7.1 illustrates the argument so far with two real-life examples from the UK: growth hormone for adults and drugs to prevent fractures in women with osteoporosis.

Health technologies and public health

HTA is not something in opposition to public health: it is a tool that allows public health practitioners to re-orientate health services to achieve greater health gain for patients.

There has been a debate over the last 40 years about the role of health care in improving public health. This was triggered by the publication in 1971 of medical demographer Thomas McKeown's book 'The Role of Medicine'.[5] Note that McKeown's thesis was about the role of medicine in the past: our concern here is to understand the likely role of health care in the present and near future. Recent estimates suggest that health care currently has had an important role in improving life expectancy and in relieving pain and suffering.

HTA therefore needs to be understood by public health professionals because:
- health care matters to the public and is a major determinant of the health of the public, both for good (for example, immunization or statins) and for ill (for example, MRSA in hospitals)
- health technologies are the building blocks of health care and matter to public health, either directly (their health benefits or harms), or indirectly (opportunity costs)
- as part of their job, they may have to contribute to the assessment and appraisal of health technologies

Table 5.7.1 Health care problems, health technology assessment and appraisal

	Growth hormone (GH) for GH-deficient adults	Drugs for the prevention of fragility fractures in post-menopausal women with osteoporosis
The health care problem	Some adults become deficient in GH, usually as a result of damage to the pituitary gland, e.g. after head injury	Osteoporosis is common for women aged over 50. It greatly increases the risk of debilitating hip and vertebral fractures.
The technologies	Synthetic GH is available. It is costly and requires daily injection	Alendronate, etidronate and risedronate; raloxifene; strontium ranelate and teriparatide all help increase bone mineral density or reduce bone loss.
		All have been shown to reduce fracture risk. But their mechanisms differ; their side-effect profiles differ. And their prices differ hugely ranging from £50 pa for generic alendronate to £3000 pa for teriparatide.
The HTA question	What is the cost-effectiveness of GH replacement in improving the quality and length of life for people with growth hormone deficiency?	What is the cost-effectiveness and incremental cost-effectiveness of these drugs for women with different risk profiles, e.g. according to T-score (a measure of bone density), prior fracture, age, co-morbidities (other illnesses) and family history?
The appraisal question	Should a particular health system pay for GH and if so, for whom?	Which, if any, of the drugs should be funded, and for which women, by a particular health care system?

Health technologies and public health

HTA is not something in opposition to public health: it is a tool that allows public health practitioners to reorientate health services to achieve greater health gain for patients.

There has been a debate over the last 40 years about the role of health care in improving public health. This was triggered by the publication in 1971 of medical demographer Thomas McKeown's book 'The Role of Medicine'[15]. Note that McKeown's thesis was about the role of medicine in the past: our concern here is to understand the likely role of health care in the present and near future. Recent estimates suggest that health care currently has had an important role in improving life expectancy and in relieving pain and suffering.

HTA therefore needs to be understood by public health professionals because:

- Health care matters to the public and is a major determinant of the health of the public, both for good (e.g. immunization or statins) and for ill (eg MRSA in hospitals)
- Health technologies are the building blocks of health care and matter to public health, either directly (their health benefits or harms), or indirectly (opportunity costs)
- As part of their job, they may have to contribute to the assessment and appraisal of health technologies

Using health technology assessments: key skills

Many HTA reports are complicated and long. They are also often place-dependent and time-limited and may not 'travel' well. So public health professionals using HTA need skills in three areas: finding the appropriate HTA; appraising what they find; and adapting it to local use.

Finding the health technology assessment

Medline is everyone's backstop, but specialist HTA resources are more specific and often more complete, for instance the Centre for Reviews and Dissemination HTA database,[6], the Cochrane library,[7] and NICE guidance.[8]

Appraising health technology assessment

Critical appraisal is dealt with in detail in 🕮 Chapter 2.7. In brief, the critical appraisal of HTA covers making sure that:

- you understand the focus of the report's question and that it's relevant to you
- the report has included the right studies
- they have been quality assured
- they are combined in sensible ways.

Adapting to local use

This stage is crucial. First, you need to be clear whether the report just deals with assessment or if it includes also some elements of appraisal. However, even assessments may 'travel' badly, as local circumstances are likely to differ from those in the HTA report that you have found. So second, you should consider whether:

- the comparator technology is the one you really use locally
- the costs are applicable to local circumstances
- the social and policy background is comparable.

The European Network for Health Technology Assessment (EUnetHTA) has put particular effort into adaptation in recent years and an 'adaptation toolkit' is available online to help with this.[9]

Doing health technology assessment: the key steps

This section outlines the key steps in doing HTA. (For more information, see part 1 of this Handbook and some of the comprehensive guides to HTA published recently: for instance, those from NICE in 2008,[10] from Australia in 2009[11] or from Europe in 2009.[12])

The key steps are to:
- *Define the question to be addressed clearly, including:*
  - the type of question (effectiveness? cost-effectiveness? cost-effectiveness and wider social, ethical and legal implications?)
  - the precise technology under evaluation
  - the comparator (pre-existing) technology
  - the disease and client group for which it is being assessed
  - the outcome measures of interest. (Normally HTA looks for patient-relevant rather than surrogate or proxy outcomes.)
- Search for background information
- *Generate a rough 'decision tree'*: this is a diagram used to portray the alternative intervention plus outcome options for the chosen population. Figure 5.7.1 illustrates a very simplified decision tree for the growth hormone example mentioned previously.

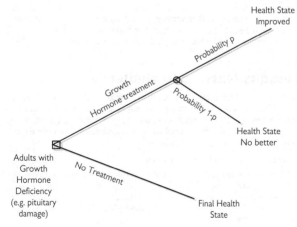

Figure 5.7.1 A simplified decision tree for the use of growth hormone.

- *Find the evidence:* being systematic is vital; being comprehensive may not be.
- *Sort and appraise the evidence:* this includes the elimination of irrelevant material, the application of study inclusion and exclusion criteria, and a full appraisal of the quality of included studies.
- *Search for cost information:* this is often difficult as it can be in the 'grey' rather than the published literature. A starting point should be any current official lists of costs. Experts can often identify useful sources.
- *Extract the data:* this includes identifying and recording key features and results of included studies. Such data needs to be summarized clearly, comparably and consistently. Statistical summary estimates can be used to synthesize data where appropriate (meta-analysis).
- *Perform an economic evaluation:* The synthesis of effectiveness information is only half of a cost-effectiveness analysis: costs also need to be factored into the equation (see 📖 Economic assessment). Cost-utility analysis is needed so that comparisons can be made across different technologies in different areas of health care. This translates effectiveness information into generic units of health value, such as the cost per QALY.
- *Consider the wider ethical, social and legal implications:* the wider effects of the introduction of some new technologies may be among their most important aspects. This is a developing area within HTA and of particular interest to public health.
- Write the report.

Undertaking an HTA requires skills in systematic review techniques, health economics, statistics and modelling, as well as clinical and public health expertise. It needs to be the work of a multidisciplinary team (see part 7, 📖 Organizations). Nobody is perfect, but a team can be!

Lessons learnt and challenges

HTA emerged first in the USA less than 30 years ago.[3] It is closely linked with evidence-based health care and health economics, the other components of the effectiveness revolution, and has great potential for improving the public health. We suggest below two lessons learnt from this experience and two challenges for the future.

Lesson 1: a colourful patchwork

HTA is never a tidy system: everywhere in the world, it is a multicoloured patchwork, with a mix of uses, funding arrangements, geographical levels and decision makers (see Table 5.7.2). However, they should all contribute to the essential goal of HTA: meeting the information needs of decision-makers in health care.

Lesson 2: the sequence of HTA

HTA is part of a sequence of research-based information collection (see Box 5.7.2). Typically, the sequence over time of HTA data gathering and synthesis looks like this:

- horizon scanning for new technologies that are likely to emerge and diffuse within a year or so

- assembly of primary randomized trial data sufficient for licensing by a manufacturer/pharmaceutical company (typically phase II and III trials)
- brief reports (such as bulletins, editorials and vignettes) on the pros and cons of the new technology
- a mainstream HTA report—typically rapid systematic review and cost-effectiveness modelling
- a longer term HTA or Cochrane systematic review (again mainstream HTA)
- pragmatic randomized controlled trials.

Table 5.7.2 The patchwork of HTA

Level	Components
Uses to which HTA may be put	<ul><li>Licensing</li><li>Coverage/funding</li><li>Clinical decision-making</li><li>Informed patient choice</li></ul>
Funding of HTA reports and systems	<ul><li>Explicitly funded or not</li><li>Privately funded or publicly</li></ul>
Geographical areas at which HTA conducted	<ul><li>Local</li><li>Regional</li><li>National</li><li>International (e.g. INAHTA)</li></ul>
The decision-makers who use HTA reports	<ul><li>Patients</li><li>Clinicians</li><li>Managers</li><li>Policy makers</li><li>Public</li></ul>

Box 5.7.2 Growth hormone for adults: the sequence of HTA in the UK

- A 'quick and clean' report was produced in 1995, prior to licensing in 1996.
- A follow-up report that took account of new evidence was published in 1997.
- Continuing concerns about the clinical role and practical role of growth hormone continued and a NICE technology appraisal was set in train.
- This resulted in a full Technology Assessment Report (published in 2002) and NICE guidance to the NHS in 2003.
- The 2003 NICE guidance was reviewed in 2006 and no decision has yet been taken to update it.
- A pragmatic RCT assessing the cost-utility of growth hormone and its impact on long-term health outcomes has yet to be undertaken.

References available from authors on request.

Challenge 1: timeliness

Decision-makers often need good, understandable information in weeks or months, rather than years. This is particularly important with expensive new pharmaceuticals. The challenge for HTA systems therefore is to temper rigour with timeliness. Don't let the best become the enemy of the good.

Challenge 2: implementation

No matter how sophisticated the HTA process it, it won't on its own be enough to manage the introduction of new technologies. We also need mechanisms for ensuring knowledge of, and adherence to its findings, given the evidence of slow uptake of research findings in clinical practice.

Conclusion

HTA is not a panacea. Generating information that is useful and relevant to health service decision-makers does not of itself ensure that that information is acted upon. However, it is a necessary first step in the development of a health service that more closely meets the objectives of those who use, fund, direct or provide that service.

References

1 Holland WW. (1983). Concepts and meaning in evaluation of health care. In: Holland WW, ed., *Evaluation of health care*. Oxford University Press, Oxford.

2 Stevens A, Milne R, Burls A. (2003). Health technology assessment: history and demand. *Journal of Public Health Medicine*, **25,** 98–101.

3 Gray JAM. (2001). *Evidence-based health care*, 2nd edn. Churchill Livingstone. Philadelphia.

4 Stevens A, Milne R. (2004). Health technology assessment in England and Wales. *International Journal of Technology Assessment in Health Care*, **20,** 11–24.

5 McKeown T. (1979). *Role of medicine*. Basil Blackwell, Oxford.

6 Centre for Reviews and Dissemination, University of York. *HTA database*. Available at: ℰ http://www.crd.york.ac.uk/crdweb/ (accessed 27 August 2010).

7 The Cochrane Library. *The Cochrane Collaboration*. John Wiley & Sons, Ltd, Chichester. Available at: ℰ http://www.thecochranelibrary.com/ (accessed 27 August 2010).

8 National Institute for Health and Clinical Excellence (2010). *NICE guidance by topic*. NICE, London. Available at: ℰ http://www.nice.org.uk/page.aspx?o=cat.diseaseareas (accessed 27 August 2010).

9 Chase D, Rosten C, Turner S, *et al*. (2009). Development of a toolkit and glossary to aid in the adaptation of health technology assessment (HTA) reports for use in different contexts. *Health Technology Assessment*, **13,** 1–142.

10 National Institute for Health and Clinical Excellence, (2010). *Guide to the methods of technology appraisal*. NICE, London. Available at: ℰ http://www.nice.org.uk/media/B52/A7/TAMethodsGuideUpdatedJune2008.pdf (accessed 3 September 2012).

11 Australian Government, Department of Health and Ageing. (2009). *Review of Health Technology Assessment in Australia*. Department of Health and Aging, Canberra. Available at: ℰ http://www.health.gov.au/internet/main/publishing.nsf/Content/hta-review-report (accessed 27 .August 2010)

12 Lampe K, Mäkelä M, Garrido MV, *et al*., for European network for Health Technology Assessment (EUnetHTA) (2009). The HTA core model: a novel method for producing and reporting health technology assessments. *International Journal of Technology Assessment in Health Care*, **25(Suppl. 2),** 9–20.

5.8 Improving equity

Sharon Friel

Objectives

After reading this chapter you will:
- be familiar with the concept and extent of health inequity in high and middle income countries
- understand how the health care system can be both a cause of health inequities and a mechanism by which to improve health equity
- recognized how to address the social determinants of health inequity
- begin to systematically apply an equity lens to your daily professional practice.

Definitions and key terms

- Health inequities are avoidable inequalities in health outcomes
- Health equity is not only about health outcomes, but also about equitable exposure to factors which affect health; and prevention of disadvantage due to ill-health
- Social determinants
- Community empowerment
- Health literacy.

Why improving equity is an important public health issue

Despite the increase in global average life expectancy of more than 20 years since 1950 and improvements in health more generally, some startling differences in health experience exists between and within countries. Improving health equity requires attention to the underlying social causes in addition to more equal access to appropriate levels of quality health care. Health inequities can be best reduced through needs-based universal primary health care and intersectoral action, action which requires leadership by public health professionals.

The extent of health inequities

The World Health Organization Commission on Social Determinants of Health (CSDH) shone a global spotlight on the marked inequities in health conditions between countries and population groups.[1] For example, premature death among adults remains a major health issue in countries rich and poor, but the rates differ enormously, for example, Australia 76 per 1000 compared with Papua New Guinea 380 per 1000.[2]

If there is no biological reason for the systematic differences in life expectancy or health conditions between different regions and countries then they are not inevitable and need not exist. These avoidable health inequities occur not just between countries, but also within countries. For example, an assessment of socio-economic inequities in mortality and prevalence of health risks among 22 countries in all parts of Europe demonstrates persistent and large inequities in health conditions within developed countries in the region. People with the lowest level of education were found to be consistently at higher risk of poor health compared to those with the highest levels of education (see Box 5.8.1).[3]

Box 5.8.1 Social inequities in health: more than one measure

Differences in health within countries are stratified along lines of ethnicity, gender, age, education, occupation, income and class. Many studies (and policy and practice) concentrate on only one of these social dimensions at a time, but it is important to recognize that real people are simultaneously positioned in terms of many social strata. For example, an 18-year-old working class urban Anglo Australian girl behaves in particular ways, is engaged in certain social relationships and attracts distinct social responses because of all those elements of who she is.

Inequities in health are not just about differences between the top and the bottom of the social ladder. There is a social gradient in health that runs from top to bottom of the socioeconomic spectrum, making health inequities a whole of population issue.

The causes of health inequities

The social determinants of health inequities

Perhaps you are a primary care physician, a tobacco cessation officer or a community health worker? When a person walks through your door, you are aware of at least two things:

- *Many factors have brought the person to this meeting:* factors positively and negatively affecting health, experienced in the immediate moment and over the course of a lifetime
- *If in a health care setting:* behind the patient are many others who do not make it to your door.

By now you should be asking what it is about society that is causing such unfair differences in health outcomes (see Box 5.8.2). For health in general, people need the basic material resources for a decent life, they need to have control over their lives, and they need voice and participation in decision-making processes. The level of material, psychosocial and political resource among different social groups is influenced by the social determinants of health and health inequities. The social determinants refer to the distribution of power, income, goods, and services, globally and nationally, and immediate circumstances of people's lives, for example, their access to health care and education, their conditions of work and leisure, their homes, communities, towns, or cities.[1]

Box 5.8.2 From social determinants to health inequities, in brief

- The global context affects how societies prosper through its impact on international relations and domestic norms and policies.
- These in turn shape the way society, at national and local levels, organizes its affairs, giving rise to forms of social position and hierarchy. Most societies are hierarchical, stratified generally along lines of ethnicity, gender, age, education, occupation, income and class. Where people are in the social hierarchy affects their health differently.
- Economic and social policies generate and distribute political power, income, goods and services. These are distributed unequally among different social groups.
- This, is turn, affects the nature of the conditions in which people grow, learn, live, work and age. This means that different social groups have different exposure to, for example, quality health care and education, conditions of work and leisure, and quality of housing and built environment.
- Together these structural factors and daily living conditions constitute the social determinants of health.
- The social determinants of health can empower or dis-empower individuals, communities and even nations through their influence on material resource, psychosocial control, behavioural options and political voice afforded to different groups along the social hierarchy.
- Inequities in each of these contribute to inequities in health risks, vulnerability to ill-health and to the consequences of ill-health.

Health care systems: a determinant of and solution to health inequities

International, national, and local health care systems are both a determinant of health inequities and a powerful mechanism to reduce inequities.[4] Given the high burden of illness particularly among the socially disadvantaged groups, it is urgent to make health care systems more responsive to population needs.

Inequities in health care are systematic differences in the use or receipt of quality primary, secondary and tertiary health care services, including hospitalizations, diagnostic tests, surgical procedures, physician visits, allied health services, medications, health promotion programmes. Gender, education, occupation, income, ethnicity, disability, and place of residence are all linked to access, experiences of and benefits from health care.

The inverse care law, initially identified by Tudor Hart, in which the poor consistently gain less from health services than the better off, is visible in every country across the globe. Out-of-pocket expenditures for health care contribute to health inequities, tending to deter poorer people from using both essential and non-essential services, leading to untreated morbidity. In OECD countries the cost of most doctor visits are subsidized and there are provisions to limit out-of-pocket costs, for a given level of need. In these countries socio-economically advantaged women are more likely to use specialist medical, allied health, alternative health and dental services than less advantaged women.[5] These inequities in access and use of a range of health care services, not just the doctor, are particularly concerning in the context of chronic disease where optimal care includes use of multidisciplinary services.

However, inequities in access and utilization of health care are not only financial—inequities play out by race, gender, age, and location. In spite of near universal coverage for antenatal visits in Pelota, Brazil, the quality of care was consistently higher among women of white skin colour and high socio-economic status women than among black and poor women.[6]

Key messages
- Health care systems are socially determined and are determinants of health and health equity
- The health care system, whether publicly or privately supported, should promote health equity and should contribute to wider efforts to reduce health inequities.

What can be done to improve equity

Primary health care systems

Appropriately configured and managed health systems provide a vehicle to improve people's lives, protect them from the vulnerability of sickness, generate a sense of life security, and build common purpose within society. Health care systems contribute most to improving health equity where the institutions and services are organized around the principle of universal coverage (extending the same scope of quality services to the whole population, according to needs, regardless of ability to pay), and where the system as a whole is organized around Primary Health Care (PHC, including both the model of locally-organized action across the social determinants of health, and the primary level of entry to care with upward referral if necessary).

Levels of care

Within each level of care, there are opportunities to improve health equity. Secondary and tertiary levels of care are concerned, mainly, with the progression from disease to death. How these types of care are set up can make an important contribution to health equity.

There are four main characteristics of primary care practice: first-contact health care, person-focused care over time, comprehensive care, and coordinated care, as well as family and community orientation. In a comparison of the supply and adequacy of primary care characteristics across 13 industrialized countries, Starfield and colleagues found that the stronger a country's primary care orientation, the lower the rates were of all-cause mortality, all-cause premature mortality, and cause-specific premature mortality from asthma and bronchitis, emphysema and pneumonia, cardiovascular disease, and heart disease.[7] In state-level analyses in the USA, there were fewer differences in self-rated health between higher and lower income-inequality areas where good primary care experiences were stronger. Evidence of success of primary level services in reducing health inequities is also available from Africa (Liberia, Niger, Zaire), Asia (China, Kerala in India, Sri Lanka) and Latin America (Brazil, Cuba).[7]

Key messages
- Strengthen geographical access to care (particularly for remote rural communities)
- Reduce/remove financial barriers (both formal and informal user fees increasing direct individual and household costs of health-seeking behaviour and treatment)
- Poorer, less educated and other categories of socially disadvantaged patients may not be aware of their rights to health care nor advocate for their own health needs as effectively as do patients with higher incomes
- Ensure health care system working models are sensitive to cultural diversity.

A focus on prevention
As a public health practitioner a large part of your professional remit is to prevent disease onset and promote wellbeing. A number of the inequities in health outcomes in middle and high income countries relate to non-communicable diseases, injuries and accidents. Much of public health's prevention focus has been on individuals and their behaviours. Eating healthy diets, being physically active, limiting alcohol consumption and not smoking are each socially graded. For example, in high and middle income countries, excess body weight tends to be more prevalent among people further down the social and economic scale. Similarly, the prevalence of tobacco use decreases with increasing socio-economic status.[8] However, even if we were able to equalize lifestyle behaviour factors, health inequities are likely to persist between socioeconomic groups.

A number of interventions at the individual and community level, such as screening, healthy eating advice, smoking cessation and statin prescribing have been shown to widen socioeconomic inequities.[9] A more upstream systems approach would involve, for example, legislating smoke-free public spaces or banning dietary transfats. Similarly, obesity prevention interventions that focus on behaviour change through personal skill development, information and social marketing campaigns may perpetuate socioeconomic inequities in obesity rates, given that the uptake of message is generally greater in higher social status groups.

Obesity prevention requires approaches that ensure an ecologically sustainable, adequate and nutritious food supply; material security; a built habitat which lends itself towards easy uptake of healthier food options and participation in both organized and unorganized physical activity, and a family, educational and work environment which positively reinforces (see Box 5.8.5) healthy living and empowers all individuals to make healthy choices.[10] Very little of this action sits within the capabilities or responsibilities of the health sector. We will return to this point later.

Box 5.8.3 Some success stories

The Brazilian population-wide Agita Sao Paulo physical activity programme successfully reduced the level of physical inactivity in the general population using a multi-strategy approach including the construction of pathways; the widening and removal of obstacles on paths; walking/running tracks with shadow and hydration points; green areas and leisure spaces in permanent maintenance; bicycle storage close to public transport stations and at entrances of schools/workplaces; private and public incentive policies for mass active transport. A whole community intervention in the town of Colac in Victoria, Australia not only reduced unhealthy weight gain in children, but also did so preferentially in those from lower socioeconomic households.

A central component of health promotion and disease prevention is community empowerment. Restricted participation results in deprivation of fundamental human capabilities, setting the context for differentials in, for example, employment, education and health care. Health equity depends vitally on the empowerment of individuals and groups to represent strongly and effectively their needs and interests. Evidence from interventions for youth empowerment, HIV/AIDS prevention and women's empowerment suggest that the most effective empowerment strategies are those that build on and reinforce authentic participation ensuring autonomy in decision-making, sense of community and local bonding, and psychological empowerment of the community members themselves.

Integrated health care

The public health practitioner is a key person within a primary health care system, playing an important role in helping to ensure fair access and use of quality health care services, from health promotion through to tertiary care. Take child, adolescent, and maternal health, for example. Lawn and colleagues demonstrated that linking communities and facilities in a continuum of care is more effective in reducing maternal and newborn deaths than is focusing on either community or facility alone.[11] In the case of child and maternal health, this lifecycle integrative approach to health requires primary- and community health care workers to engage in various levels of care including

- health promotion and community mobilization (e.g. infant and young child feeding; school health; special programme areas such as HIV)
- outpatient services (e.g. family planning; malaria prevention such as bed nets)

- case management and care (e.g. childbirth; malnutrition care and rehabilitation)
- health system tasks (e.g. essential drugs supply and logistics; data monitoring; financing such as issuing vouchers for health care).

A social determinants approach through intersectoral action

A critical starting point for health equity is within the health sector itself. However, to make a fundamental improvement in health equity requires not only technical and medical solutions, but also action in the immediate and structural conditions in which people are born, grow, live, work, and age. As a social determinants lens on health equity illuminates, good health for all is not only a matter for the health sector, but must also involve sectors such as agriculture, urban planning, employment, and education.

Effective action on health equity therefore depends vitally on cross-sectoral co-ordination. This is manifested in a dynamic inter-relation between the health system and the wider system of governance through which inequity in health outcomes are produced. Through your role as a public health practitioner you can bring together the benefits of primary health care and action in the social determinants of health. This will promote health equity through attention to the needs of socially disadvantaged groups and help provide leadership in promoting coherent policies and practices in different sectors.

Let's take mental health as an illustrative case study. Promoting equitable mental wellbeing and reducing inequities in the causes and treatment of mental illness requires an intersectoral approach as outlined in Table 5.8.1 below.[12]

Improving equity: implications for public health practitioners

There are three key areas in which public health practitioners can helpfully focus their attention in such a way that will improve health equity. What follows is not an exhaustive list, but rather an illustration of different types of action that can be taken by public health practitioners

Evidence informed practice

As a public health practitioner, using sound evidence to inform your daily practice offers the best hope of tackling health inequities. Evidence informed practice requires good data on the extent of the problem and up-to-date evidence on the causes and on what works to reduce health inequities. It also requires an understanding of the evidence such that the causes of health inequities are acted on. Routine data collection and monitoring systems that collect socially stratified health information are essential for knowing the magnitude of the problem, understanding who is most affected, and whether health equity is improving or deteriorating over time, and for assessing entry-points for intervention and evaluating the impact of practice.

Table 5.8.1 Intersectoral action in relation to equity in mental health

Determinant	Intervention
Violence/crime	Violence/crime prevention programmes
Substance abuse	Alcohol and drugs policies
Social fragmentation	Promoting programmes building family and wider social cohesion
Stigma	Mental health promotion programmes
Natural disasters	Trauma and stress support programmes
Inadequate housing	Housing improvement interventions
Work stress	Protective labour policies (e.g. restrictions on excessive shift work): workplace health promotion programmes
Unemployment	Employment programmes, skills training
Financial insecurity	Welfare policies that provide a financial safety net
Social protection	Economic policies to promote financial security, and adequate funding for a range of public sector services (education, health, housing)
Lack of available health services	Improving availability of mental health services through integration into primary health care
Unacceptable health services	e.g. ensuring that mental health staff are culturally and linguistically acceptable
Economic barriers to health care	Providing financially accessibly services
Mental health policy and legislation	Strengthening mental health policy; legislation and service infrastructure
Differential vulnerability	**Intervention**
Early developmental risks	Promote early childhood development programmes
Early developmental risks, maternal mental illness, weak mother-child bonding	Mother-infant interventions, including breastfeeding
Developmental risks for adolescence	Depression prevention programmes targeting adolescents
Development risks for older adults	Education and stress management programmes; peer support mechanisms
Inaccessibility to credit and savings facilities	Improve access to credit and savings facilities for poor

(Continued)

Table 5.8.1 (Continued)

Differential consequences	Intervention
Financial consequences of impact of depression on productivity	Support to caregivers to protect households from financial consequences of depression; rehabilitation programmes
Social consequences of depression	Anti-stigma campaigns; promotion of supportive family and social networks
Financial consequences of depression treatment	Reduce cost
Lifestyle consequences of depression	Mental health promotion, including avoidance of substance abuse

Amended WHO 2010.

Practical action
- develop a national/local health equity action plan which is fully supported by an effective health equity monitoring system
- build-up, and systematically use, an information system that collects health outcome data stratified by different social groups (including sex, income, education, occupation, age, ethnic group)
- incorporate measures on the determinants of health inequities into the health monitoring system.

Action on the determinants of health inequities requires a rich and diverse evidence base, not just a quantitative monitoring system. Collaborative knowledge production between researchers and public health professionals is needed to elucidate what works to reduce health inequities in what circumstances, and how best to implement interventions, such that they contribute to a reduction of these inequities.

Practical action
Commit appropriate amounts of public health research funding into understanding how to improve health equity through action in the social determinants and health care systems, and proactively engage with relevant researchers.

People-centred practice
All members of society, including those most disadvantaged and marginalized, are entitled to participate in the identification of priorities and targets that guide deliberations underlying public health practice. That focus is stimulated by, and feeds into, local conditions of inclusion and fair representation.

Practical action
- public health practitioners should promote the inclusion of all groups and communities in decision-making that affects health, and in subsequent programme and services delivery and evaluation

- develop a statutory local health equity action plan that is regularly monitored and reviewed, and provide statutory funding to support community engagement and participation in the processes
- ensure annual monitoring and reporting against a set of specific health equity focused outcomes.

Health literacy is a critical empowerment strategy to increase people's control over their health and their ability to seek out information. The understanding of health inequity and its causes needs to be improved as a new part of health literacy. Health literacy is not just about the individual's ability to read, understand and act on health information, but also the ability of public health professionals to communicate health related information in relevant and easy to understand ways.

Practical action
- raise awareness among the public about health inequity and its causes
- improve knowledge among socially disadvantaged groups about health and health care rights
- improve awareness and knowledge among health professionals of health equity literacy.

Prevention focused practice

Action within the health sector

If public health practitioners are to improve health equity through the health care system this means a refocusing of activities towards the removal of barriers to access and use of quality primary health care, and on the conditions in which people grow, live, work, and age.

Practical action
- Expand programmes in health promotion, disease prevention and primary health care to include a social determinant of health approach. This means prioritizing services that prevent or ameliorate the health damage caused by living and growing up in disadvantaged circumstances rather than on behaviour-change and social marketing
- Focus on developing and improving good-quality, integrated local services coproduced with the public to achieve needs driven outcomes.

Intersectoral action

Bureaucratic structures, statutory requirements, limited funding and traditional disciplinary boundaries can act to impede intersectoral action. However, it is imperative that you act as a champion and facilitator to influence other sectors to take action to reduce health inequities.

Practical action
- Make the argument for intersectoral action to reduce health inequity using regularly updated evidence and increasing the visibility of social determinants of health issues
- Map all public sector mechanisms, for example, internal and external committees, that have relevance for health equity, thereby identifying points of potential overlap and collaboration

- Sensitize colleagues in non-health sectors to the relationship between what they do and the effect on health equity, through, for example, knowledge sharing, seminars, one to one briefings
- The health equity implications of actions by other sectors need to be routinely considered. Health equity impact assessment is one tool that can be used to systematically assess the potential impact of policies, programmes, projects or proposals on health equity in a given population.

Competencies needed to achieve these tasks

A competent health workforce with the necessary specialized knowledge, skills and abilities to translate policy and current research into effective action is vital for health equity. Public health professionals need to understand how the health care sector—depending on its structure, operations, and financing—can exacerbate or ameliorate health inequities. The health care sector has an important stewardship role in intersectoral action for health equity. This requires an understanding among professionals in the health care sector of how social determinants influence health equity.

Practical action

- Commit time and financial resources to the development of relevant skills and capacity among the health workforce, and provide reward structures for intersectoral working
- Explicit integration of equity values into public health workforce competencies.

References

1 CSDH (2008). *Closing the gap in a generation: health equity through action on the social determinants of health*, final report of the Commission on Social Determinants of Health. World Health Organization, Geneva.
2 Rajaratnam J, Marcus J, Levin-Rector A, et al. (2010). Worldwide mortality in men and women aged 15–59 years from 1970 to 2010: a systematic analysis. *Lancet*, **375**, 1704–20.
3 Mackenbach JP, Stirbu I, Roskam AJR, et al. (2008). Socioeconomic inequalities in health in 22 European countries. *New England Journal of Medicine*, **358**, 2468.
4 WHO (2010). *The World Health Report 2010—Health systems financing: the path to universal coverage*. World Health Organization, Geneva.
5 Korda RJ, Banks E, Clements MS, Young AF. (2009). Is inequity undermining Australia's 'universal' health care system? Socio-economic inequalities in the use of specialist medical and non-medical ambulatory health care. *Australian and New Zealand Journal of Public Health*, **33**, 458–65.
6 Victora C, Matijasevich A, Silveira M, et al. (2010). Socio-economic and ethnic group inequities in antenatal care quality in the public and private sector in Brazil. *Health Policy Plan*, **25**, 253–61.
7 Starfield B, Shi L, Macinko J. (2005). Contribution of primary care to health systems and health. *Milbank Quarterly* 83:457-502.
8 WHO (2009). *Global health risks: mortality and burden of disease attributable to selected major risks*, World Health Organization, Geneva.
9 Capewell S, Graham H. (2010). Will cardiovascular disease prevention widen health inequalities? *PLoS Medicine*, **7**, e1000320.
10 Friel S, Chopra M, Satcher D. (2007). Unequal weight: equity oriented policy responses to the global obesity epidemic. *British Medical Journal*, **335**, 1241–3.
11 Black R, Cousens S, Johnson H, et al. (2010). Global, regional, and national causes of child mortality in 2008: a systematic analysis. *Lancet*, **375**, 1969–87.
12 WHO (2010). *Equity, social determinants and public health programmes*, World Health Organization, Geneva.

5.9 Improving quality

Nick Steel, David Melzer, and Iain Lang

Objectives

This chapter will help you understand the common approaches taken to improving quality and the competencies required of organizations, teams and individuals to improve the quality of health care delivered.

Definitions and dimensions

Quality has been defined as: 'the degree to which health services for individuals and populations increase the likelihood of desired health outcomes and are consistent with current professional knowledge'.[1]

Dimensions of quality

The dimensions of quality relate to doing the right thing to the right person in the right place at the right time in the right way at the right cost. The first stage in any attempt to measure quality is to think about what dimensions of quality should be measured, and what groups of people value those dimensions. Donabedian distinguished between measures of the 'structure, process and outcome' of health care:

- structure refers to the characteristics of such resources as hospitals, clinics, and qualified staff members
- process measures consider the care delivered
- outcome is the resulting change in health status.[2]

Table 5.9.1 gives examples of quality measures adapted from a chart book on quality in the UK NHS.[3]

Table 5.9.1 Examples of quality measures in different dimensions of quality

Measure of quality[3]	Donabedian dimension	Institute of medicine dimension
Cancer mortality rates	Outcome	Effectiveness
Appropriateness of coronary revascularization procedures	Process	Effectiveness
Practicing physicians per 1000 patients	Structure	Efficiency/capacity
Adverse events	Process/outcome	Safety
Waiting times for elective surgery	Process	Timeliness
Variation in life expectancy	Outcome	Equity
Variation in low birth weight	Outcome	Equity
Involvement in decision-making	Process	Patient-centredness

Why is improving quality important?

- Health care improves outcomes: about half of the 7½ years of the increase in life expectancy seen in the USA and UK in the second half of the twentieth century can be attributed to health care improvements[4]
- Health care is not inherently safe: up to 100,000 people die annually from medical errors in hospitals in the USA[5]
- People with common chronic illnesses receive only half of the health care they need[6]
- Health care is expensive, and spending can vary without improving quality of care. The 'Dartmouth Atlas' shows twofold Medicare spending differences per person across US regions that are not related to health differences (http://www.dartmouthatlas.org/ accessed 29 September 2010)
- Patients and members of the public want better quality[7] (see also 📖 Chapter 5.6).

Tasks for quality improvement

- Define the problem or quality gap. What is the topic and which dimension(s) of quality is affected? Information on effective care is available from, for example, the Cochrane Effective Practice and Organization of Care group (M http://onlinelibrary.wiley.com/o/cochrane/clabout/articles/EPOC/frame.html, accessed 30 September 2010)
- Specify the health outcomes that need to change and clarify who wants them to change
- Obtain the support of senior leaders and build a team. Quality improvement requires commitment from the team and the wider organization
- Decide on the approach
- Identify data to establish baseline, monitor progress, and measure outcomes over time
- Quality improvement activities have a cost and a business case should be made.

Measuring outcomes for quality improvement

The dimensions of quality mentioned above require different approaches to measurement and specific quality indicators. Quality of care can be assessed using process measures (e.g. whether treatment adheres to agreed good practice) or outcome measures (e.g. changes in health status).[2] Using process measures has the following advantages:

- there are causes of changes in health status other than health care and problems in adjusting outcomes for differences in case mix
- processes are also more sensitive measures of quality than outcomes and more clearly linked to action to improve quality.[8]

The process measures chosen should be based on evidence (where it exists) to establish a link between the health care intervention and improved health outcomes. Where robust evidence is lacking there should be a formal consensus of experts that delivering the indicated care will lead to improved health outcomes.[9]

Health systems internationally assess quality with quantitative measures of the rates of delivery of effective health care processes. Delivered health care is compared with the health care that should have been delivered, sometimes referred to as indicated care or quality standards (see Box 5.9.1, for an example). Standards can be set out in guidelines such as those published by NICE (JN www.nice.org.uk) and the Scottish Intercollegiate Guidelines Network (SIGN; JN www.sign.ac.uk) in the UK and the USA Preventive Services Task Force (USPSTF) (JN www.ahrq.gov/clinic/uspstfix.htm) in the USA.

Box 5.9.1   The RAND/UCLA appropriateness method

An example of how standards of care are developed is the RAND/UCLA (RAND Corporation/University of California Los Angeles) appropriateness method.[9] This method was developed to combine the best available research evidence with expert opinion. 'Appropriate' describes a health care intervention for which the benefits are expected to outweigh the risks. The method involves:

- Identifying clinical area(s) of care for quality assessment
- Systematic reviewing the literature on care in the relevant area(s)
- Drafting quality indicators
- Presenting draft quality indicators and their evidence base to a clinical panel of 6–15 specialists for a modified Delphi process
- The process typically involves asking panel members to anonymously rate the draft indicators for validity over at least two rounds, with or without face-to-face discussion between rounds
- Approving a final set of indicators
- The indicators can then be used to measure and improve quality.

Approaches to quality improvement

Clinical audit

Clinical audit and performance feedback have constituted the dominant approach for health professionals (see also 📖 Chapter 7.1). It has produced small to moderate effects on quality improvement,[10] although some projects have failed to complete the audit cycle by acting on the results to deliver change.

Plan-Do-Study-Act

Deming's Plan-Do-Study-Act (PDSA) cycle (Figure 5.9.1) takes audit one stage further and has been widely used in health care. The PDSA cycle has four stages: first, develop a plan and define the objective (plan). Secondly, carry out the plan and collect data (do), then analyse the data and summarize what was learned (study). Finally, plan the next cycle with necessary modifications (act). The UK NHS Institute for Innovation and Improvement recommends using PDSA with three key questions (🌐 http://www.institute.nhs.uk/quality_and_service_improvement_tools/quality_and_service_improvement_tools/plan_do_study_act.html):

- What are we trying to accomplish?
- How will we know if the change is an improvement?
- What changes can we make that will result in improvement?

In the US, PDSA has been used in 'breakthrough collaboratives', developed by the Institute for Health care Improvement (🌐 http://www.ihi.org/IHI/Programs/Collaboratives/). Collaboratives involve teams working together in a structured way for 12–18 months to improve health care in a particular area.

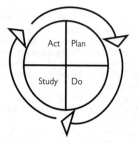

Figure 5.9.1 The Plan-Do-Study-Act cycle.

Statistical process control

Statistical process control (SPC) charts can be used to map baselines and evaluate whether projects are changing the chosen outcome measure. SPC charts add upper and lower control limits to a simple run chart to help identify unacceptable variation where there may be potential for improvement. For more information on SPC charts, including examples, see 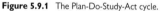 Chapter 4.3.

Six Sigma and Lean

Six sigma is a process improvement approach originally developed by Motorola and more recently used in health care. It aims to reduce variation in the customer's measure of quality using statistical techniques.[11] It has been combined with Lean, which is a set of principles developed from Toyota's approach to car manufacturing. Lean involves continuous problem solving and improvement, development of people as partners, and eliminating all forms of waste in the system.[11]

Payment for performance

Pay-for-performance programmes are increasingly common in health care, and there is limited evidence that they can improve health care.[12] Perhaps the largest quality improvement initiative anywhere is the contract entered into in April 2004 between family practitioners (GPs) and the government in the UK (Box 5.9.2).

Box 5.9.2 **Improving quality in UK general practice**

A new contract between UK general practitioners and the government came into effect on 1 April 2004. Substantial financial rewards (more than £1 billion) were linked to performance against indicators of the quality of clinical and organizational care. The aims of the contract were to reduce variations in provision of effective care and improve quality of care for ten chronic conditions.

For each condition, quality indicators described specific clinical interventions intended to improve quality of care. Financial rewards were attached to achievement of the indicators.

Example indicators for diabetes:
- % of patients for whom body mass index in the previous 15 months was recorded
- % of patients in whom the last HbA1C is <=7.4 in the last 15 months.

Who should be involved

'Desired health outcomes' is a key phrase and deliberately does not specify what outcomes are desirable, or to whom. Desired health outcomes may be different for managers (who focus on efficiency and maximizing the population health gain from a limited budget), clinicians (who focus on effectiveness and on what works for their patients), and patients (who focus on what works and how it is delivered). In addition to representatives from these three groups a quality improvement team may require input from academics or policy makers.

Competencies needed to achieve these tasks

- *Change management:* an early task in quality improvement is to show that the existing situation is a 'burning platform', and that change is essential.
- *Leadership for the project team:* supported by senior leaders in the organization.[13]
- *Networking and interpersonal skills:* to engage patients, clinicians, and managers and build a team.
- *Data skills to capture baseline data:* track progress, and communicate results to the team. SPC charts may help.
- *Systems thinking:* Berwick's law of improvement states 'every system is perfectly designed to achieve the results it achieves', shifting our understanding of performance from effort to design.[14]

Systematic performance to make action more effective

Effective care should be provided to all those who will benefit from it. Achieving this involves setting out what care will be provided to which population, providing the care, and then assessing the extent to which the care has been provided. Quality indicators (see above) are mainly used to describe effective treatment, but can also describe harmful and ineffective treatment to be prevented.

Decision aids can be used to help patients make informed choices. For many conditions, the choice between treatment options is more important than the choice between providers of the same treatment, although choice between providers receives more policy attention.

Care needs to be critically evaluated and compared with practice in other regions. This requires a local infrastructure that can support a research agenda and respond to the results. The capacity of the local health care system and follow-up rates can be compared with other regions, and with their costs if these are available. The frequency of use of services by people with chronic illness is one of the major determinants of costs in a region and more frequent care does not generally improve population health.

Ethical dilemmas

Equity is an important dimension of quality, but can suffer when new health care interventions are introduced. Disparities in access to health care are a problem in all countries and quality improvement programmes may worsen disparities unless the improvement has proportionally greater benefit for the relatively disadvantaged population. Is it acceptable to trade off a degree of equity for excellence?

Higher quality does not always mean higher cost, in fact where waste is eliminated, better care can also be cheaper. However, there will be times when higher costs need to be weighed against higher quality, and vice versa.

Potential pitfalls: analysing local variations in health care

If measurable outcomes are not chosen and monitored it will be impossible to know whether quality has improved. Good intentions and hard work are not enough; faith in an intervention needs to be backed up with data, and rigorous data collection needs to be followed up with action to improve health. Analysis of variations in health care requires a systems approach that accepts that clinicians are influenced by the capacity of the health care system, and that supported patient choice in preference-sensitive conditions can lead to better outcomes. Box 5.9.3 lists some questions to ask when you encounter activity variations.

Box 5.9.3 Questions to ask about activity variations
- Are they due to recording or classification errors?
- Do they reflect differences in need in the populations served?
- Are they due to unwarranted care, i.e. a pattern of care inconsistent with patients' preferences or unrelated to underlying illness?
- Are they due to scientific uncertainty or to medical errors and system failures?
- Are they due to differing treatment preferences? If so, does this relate to informed patient choice or physician-dominated decisions?
- Are they driven by supply of facilities? Is there an unwarranted assumption that more activity is better?

Key determinants of success
- Adequate capacity to deliver quality improvement, including organizational support, team leadership and interpersonal skills
- Collection, analysis, and dissemination of data to show effects of the quality improvement activity
- Alignment of quality improvement activities with the direction of change in the health care system
- Sustained commitment.

Quality improvement is complex, and there is no single simple solution. Most tested approaches work some of the time and none of them are guaranteed to work. Walshe and Freeman pointed out that the particular technique chosen is probably much less important than the perseverance of the people involved: 'Rather than taking up, trying, and then discarding a succession of different quality improvement techniques, organizations should probably choose one carefully and then persevere to make it work.'[15]

Key points of this chapter
- Many people experience health care that falls short of agreed quality standards
- Health care can improve population health outcomes
- The different dimensions of quality are valued differently by different people
- There are many approaches to improving quality and no one approach is always successful
- Quality improvement occurs with clear goals, sustained organizational commitment, leadership, and a team capable of delivering
- Involvement of different groups, for example patients, clinicians, and managers, is vital—user involvement is a growing force
- The risks of quality improvement should be considered. What are the opportunity costs of quality improvement? Do the benefits outweigh the costs?

References

1 Institute of Medicine Committee on Health Care in America (2001). *Crossing the quality chasm: a new health system for the 21st century.* National Academy Press, Washington DC.

2 Donabedian A (1980). *Explorations in quality assessment and monitoring. Vol 1. The definition of quality and approaches to its assessment.* Health Administration Press, Ann Arbor.

3 Leatherman S, Sutherland K. (2005). *The quest for quality in the NHS. A chartbook on quality of care in the UK.* Radcliffe, Oxford.

4 Bunker JP. (2001). The role of medical care in contributing to health improvements within societies. *International Journal of Epidemiology,* **30,** 1260–3.

5 Institute of Medicine Committee on Quality of Health Care in America (2000). *To err is human: building a safer health system.* National Academy Press, Washington DC.

6 Steel N, Bachmann M, Maisey S, et al. (2008). Self reported receipt of care consistent with 32 quality indicators: national population survey of adults aged 50 or more in England. *British Medical Journal,* **337,** a957.

7 Coulter A. (2005). What do patients and the public want from primary care? *British Medical Journal,* **331,** 1199–201.

8 Lilford RJ, Brown CA, Nicholl J. (2007). Use of process measures to monitor the quality of clinical practice. *British Medical Journal,* **335,** 648–50.

9 Shekelle P. (2004). The appropriateness method. *Medical Decision-Making;* **24,** 228–31.

10 Jamtvedt G, Young JM, Kristoffersen DT, et al. (2006). Audit and feedback: effects on professional practice and health care outcomes. *Cochrane Database of Systematic Reviews,* (2).

11 Boaden R, Harvey G, Moxham C, et al. (2008). *Quality improvement: theory and practice in health care.* NHS Institute for Innovation and Improvement, Coventry.

12 Christianson J, Leatherman S, Sutherland K. (2007). *Financial incentives, health care providers and quality improvements. A review of the evidence.* Health Foundation, London.

13 Health Foundation (2010). *Quality improvement made simple.* Health Foundation, London.

14 Berwick DM. (1996). A primer on leading the improvement of systems. *British Medical Journal,* **312,** 619–22.

15 Walshe K, Freeman T. (2002). Effectiveness of quality improvement: learning from evaluations. *Quality and Safety in Health Care,* **11,** 85–7.

5.10 Evaluating health care systems

Martin McKee, Bernadette Khoshaba, and Marina Karanikolos

Objectives

- Understand the importance of defining the boundaries of a health system in a given country
- Be able to explain the functions of a health system and how these relate to one another
- Be able to describe the goals of a health system and how to evaluate progress towards them
- Be aware of the major contemporary initiatives to assess health system performance internationally
- Recognize the limitations, including the scope for abuse, of health systems comparisons.

Defining the health system and its goals

There are two first steps in evaluating health care systems:
- define the boundaries of a system
- agree on what it is seeking to achieve.

Defining the system's boundaries is complicated by the frequent existence of multiple systems for delivering health care. Perhaps the most extreme example is the USA, where even the public sector is divided among Medicare, Medicaid, the Veterans Administration, and others. However, nearly all countries have some form of private provision alongside the statutory public system, as well as systems to care for groups such as prisoners or the armed forces. Other definitional challenges relate to:
- generation of inputs to the health system, such as research and development and training
- managing the indistinct boundary between health and social care.

Defining its goals and how to measure its performance is equally challenging. For investors on the world's stock markets, health systems provide just another investment opportunity, with performance assessed as return on capital. In contrast, campaigners for social justice may assess performance in terms of the ability to protect the poor from financial ruin in the face of illness.

Basic scientists may see performance as the ability to deliver, at least to some, advanced technology they have been working so hard to develop. Health professionals may view performance in terms of a supportive and rewarding environment for professional development. And patient groups may view performance in terms of the system's ability to respond rapidly and humanely to their physical and emotional needs.

The practical resolution of these issues emerged in the 2000 World Health Report,[1] which sought to create a means by which all of the world's health systems could be compared using common metrics. This was a major advance of anything that had been done previously and, although controversial, provided the basis for most subsequent work on health systems performance.

The report considered the 'health system', which it defined as 'all activities whose primary purpose is to promote, restore or maintain health'. This was intentionally broad and includes many activities that would commonly be seen as lying outside the health *care* system, including certain components of health promotion, although it did exclude activities, such as the promotion of female literacy, which have many other goals of which better health is only one. It also included 'selected inter-sectoral actions in which the stewards of the health system take responsibility to advocate for improvements in areas outside their direct control, such as legislation to reduce fatalities from traffic accidents.' Within the health system a number of functions were identified, each contributing to the goals of the system. The functions are:

- financing (revenue collection, fund pooling and purchasing)
- resource generation (human resources, technologies and facilities)
- delivery of personal and population-based health services
- stewardship (health policy formulation, regulation and intelligence).

The goals are:
- health improvement
- responsiveness
- fairness in financing.

The goals were operationalized to produce indicators that were then weighted and combined to create a composite measure of overall goal attainment, as well as a measure of overall performance. The latter recognized that a health system's performance would be constrained by the circumstances within which it existed and calculated a theoretical maximum value based on the country's level of economic and educational development with which it could compare its actual performance.

The remainder of this chapter looks first at the health system functions and then at the goals of the system, before concluding with examples of initiatives currently underway to measure and compare health systems performance.

Health systems functions

Financing a health system is complicated because of one key issue, the need to redistribute money. Put simply, those who have most need of health care are least able to afford it. The process of redistribution occurs both within the life course of an individual (who will typically incur most expenditure around birth and death and contribute most during working years) and among individuals (from rich to poor, well to ill and, in traditional labour markets, males to females). There are many different means of collecting money for health systems, most of which result from political decisions made many years previously. The most common sources are:

- taxation
- social insurance (where contributions are based on income)
- private insurance (where contributions are often based on risk of ill health)
- out of pocket payments.

In practice, all countries have a combination of systems so, for example, social insurance funds receive contributions from taxation for those not in employment. The second element of financing is therefore the pooling of money, prior to its redistribution and the third is the process of purchasing, whereby the funds are used to buy care for those in need.

To evaluate these elements of the financing component it is necessary to clarify their goals. This, in turn, requires clarity about the perspective being adopted as, given the scale of resources involved, decisions will have implications for the macro-economy and employment, as well as the health system and these may conflict.

From the perspective of the health system, the optimal means of collecting money will be the one that:

- is cheapest to administer
- has least scope for evasion
- and draws on the widest possible revenue base.

Often this will be taxation as it does not require a separate collection system and draws not only in income but also indirect taxes and excise revenues. The pooling element can be judged on the basis of the transfers it brings about. Out of pocket payments and some individualized approaches, such as medical savings accounts, involve few or no transfers and thus are highly regressive.

Taxation and social insurance are progressive, but to varying degrees depending on the features of the systems involved. Risk pools may be single, covering the entire population, or multiple, as is the case with competing insurance funds. In general, where it is the latter, there are systems of risk equalization. Purchasing is a recent concept that derives from the recognition that the optimal provision of care involves something more than simply reimbursing claims, regardless of the effectiveness and efficiency of the care provided. Strategic purchasing involves assessing the needs of a population and developing appropriate models of care. This can be evaluated by observing the extent to which needs are met (for example, by assessing the experience of vulnerable and marginalized groups) and by the extent to which funders encourage evidence-based models of care.

Resource generation involves the identification, creation and development of the resources required to produce health services and to build a health system. These include the workforce, health facilities, technology (including pharmaceuticals) and, increasingly, knowledge. Again, evaluation follows from the goals relating to each component.

A health system should incorporate appropriate mechanisms for training, deployment and, especially, retention of staff, with geographically equitable deployment of an optimal skill-mix. It should have mechanisms to supply modern and effective technologies, involving means of assessing their effectiveness and of ensuring their reliable distribution to where they are needed. It should have mechanisms to ensure the appropriate design, configuration, maintenance, and distribution of facilities. Finally, it should have ways of generating, synthesizing and distributing knowledge so that the care provided is based on the most relevant evidence.

Delivery of services follows on from the previous activities. Services should be provided in ways that are effective, efficient, equitable and humane. Evaluation involves a wide range of health services research methods, the choice of which will depend on the nature of the service being evaluated. It includes not only the processes by which care are delivered, but the organizational context within which it is provided.

The final component is stewardship.[2] The 2000 World Health report defined stewardship as 'the careful and responsible management of the well-being of the population'. It comprises three elements, formulating and coordinating health policy; exerting influence; and collecting and using intelligence to assure quality. Its evaluation typically involves policy research, perhaps examining the process of adopting and implementing necessary responses to a defined challenge, such as pandemic influenza or ageing populations.

Improving health

Health improvement was assessed in the 2000 World Health Report as the average level of health in a given population, measured as disability-adjusted life expectancy (DALE), and the distribution of health within the population, using data on child survival.

The measure of health adopted in the 2000 World Health Report was extremely broad. The overall DALE in a population does reflect, in part, the quality of health care delivered by the health system, but also many other factors. Thus, even in an increasingly globalized economy, dietary patterns, and consequently health, are still shaped to some extent by the predominant pattern of agriculture in a country, explaining the continuing advantage, in terms of cardiovascular mortality, experienced by the Mediterranean countries.

Exposure to vector-borne disease is also a function of climate and geography. Many diseases are the result of economic policies that impact on levels of poverty and, while the health system can pick up the pieces, the remedy lies in addressing the distribution of resources within the population. However, given the political imperative for the WHO to include all its member states in the assessment of health system performance, many of which had only rudimentary data on health outcomes (and indeed, for many countries even very limited data to calculate DALE were modelled), it was impossible to look in more detail into the specific causes of disability and premature death.

There is, however, an alternative approach. The concept of amenable mortality was proposed initially by Rutstein and colleagues in 1978.[3] It was based on the premise that deaths from certain causes should not occur in the presence of timely and effective care. Subsequent work has expanded the list of causes of death considered amenable, reflecting advances in health care and increased the upper age limit for these deaths, reflecting improvements in life expectancy.[4] The concept has also been refined to include differentiation of causes amenable to the health care system and those to public health policy, while specific causes have been partitioned into the proportion to which reductions are attributable to primary, secondary, and tertiary actions.[5]

This concept has attracted considerable attention from politicians and their advisors seeking to determine whether they are getting value from the investments they have made in healthy systems. Thus, a study showing that deaths from amenable mortality in the USA around the year 2000 had hardly changed at a time when other industrialized countries were experiencing substantial declines was cited widely in the debate on American health care reform. This methodology is now being adopted as part of the performance framework for the NHS in England, while it is also the subject of ongoing discussions within the European Union and the Organization for Economic Co-operation and Development.

It is, however, necessary to step back briefly to recall how amenable mortality was initially envisaged as being used. This was indicative of aspects of care requiring more detailed examination rather than a definitive judgement on overall performance. The latter use poses a number of problems, which illustrate more generally some of the issues that arise in assessing the performance of health systems.

The first is what is measured. Clearly, premature death is only one element of the overall burden of disease in a population. However, there are few data on disability, and even fewer that are in any way comparable, so that most published statistics are modelled from mortality data. This is of growing importance as advances in health care reduce the number of deaths amenable to health care even lower. For example, deaths from ischaemic heart disease have fallen by about half over the past three decades across Western Europe,[6] with even larger reductions in deaths arising from common surgical procedures.

Once incurable cancers, such as testicular, now have survival rates of over 90%. Thus, mortality provides an increasingly incomplete measure of overall health care performance and, specifically, misses the marked reduction in symptoms and functioning that have occurred.

A second, related problem is that of small numbers. Even apparently common conditions may cause relatively small numbers of premature deaths, making it particularly difficult to make judgements about health systems in relatively small countries.

The third is the presence of time lags. Effective treatment of, for example, an emergency such as acute appendicitis or a cardiac arrest will save a life at once. In contrast, while effective management of a chronic disorder, such as diabetes, may save a life now, in the event of, say, ketoacidosis, it may equally prevent premature death from complications many years in the future. Hence, when investigating amenable deaths, it is necessary to ascertain when any failing in the health system occurred.

The fourth is the issue of attribution. Although there are a few situations in which death can be prevented by a 'magic bullet', as occurred when penicillin was first given to patients with severe staphylococcal infections in the 1940s or when azidothymidine (AZT) was introduced to treat AIDS in the 1980s, more often health care will prevent deaths through a combination of interventions that were introduced incrementally, perhaps over decades.

It may be difficult to discern where the problem lies as there is surprisingly little evidence on the effectiveness of specific interventions in reducing death rates in the general population. First, randomized controlled trials often have limited external validity, as they often exclude both children and older people, those with co-morbidities and, in the past, women.[7] Secondly, new interventions are usually compared with best existing treatment, which is important in assessing whether the intervention should be adopted but not helpful in quantifying its effect.

Finally, it is necessary to consider the boundaries of amenable mortality. Recognizing that 'everyone must die of something', deaths designated amenable have an upper age limit. However, this is arbitrary and, although it has increased over time in keeping with lengthening life expectancy, there is a danger that the use of amenable mortality distracts attention from health care provided for older people for whom it can be extremely effective.

For all these reasons, amenable mortality can be considered as a valuable indication of how a health system is performing, provoking further investigation should it appear to be lagging compared to other countries, but it should not be seen as a definitive measure.

Responding to expectations

The 2000 World Health Report assessed responsiveness on the basis of a survey of key informants from selected countries, using a modelling approach to estimate values for the remaining ones. This was admitted to be unsatisfactory so a questionnaire-based measure was developed for use in the 2002 World Health Survey.

The WHO defined responsiveness as meeting 'the legitimate expectations of the population for their interaction with the health system'. This explicitly excludes expectations deemed to be illegitimate or unjustified, although this clearly raises questions about cultural norms. Thus, an individual in one country may expect a hospital bed to be in a single room, with access to the internet and entertainment and to a choice of high quality food while someone in another country may be grateful for a bed and clean linen. In an attempt to overcome this problem, the 2002 World Health Survey used anchoring vignettes. These are standardized descriptions of encounters that are ranked by respondents as a means of calibrating their responses. However, the multi-dimensional nature of expectations meant that this was technically insurmountable.

As noted above, responsiveness was divided into two broad categories, each with a number of dimensions. The Table 5.10.1 shows the weightings used to combine these dimensions in the 2000 report and the questions used to capture each of them in the later survey.

Table 5.10.1 Dimensions of responsiveness as defined by the World Health Organization

Category	Dimension and definition	Weighting in the 2000 WHR	Questions in the 2002 World Health Survey. How would you rate...?
Respect for persons	Dignity (respectful treatment and communication)	16.7%	... your experience of being greeted and talked to respectfully? ... the way your privacy was respected during physical examinations and treatments?
	Confidentiality (confidentiality of personal information)	16.7%	... the way the health services ensured you could talk privately to health care providers? ... the way your personal information was kept confidential?
	Autonomy (involvement in decisions)	16.7%	... your experience of being involved in making decisions about your health care or treatment? ... your experience of getting information about other types of treatments or tests?
	Communication (clarity of communication)	Not included	... the experience of how clearly health care providers explained things to you? ... your experience of getting enough time to ask questions about your health problem or treatment?

(Continued)

Table 5.10.1 (Continued)

Category	Dimension and definition	Weighting in the 2000 WHR	Questions in the 2002 World Health Survey. How would you rate...?
Client orientation	Prompt attention (convenient travel and short waiting times)	20%	... the travelling time? ... the amount of time you waited before being attended to?
	Quality of basic amenities (surroundings)	15%	... the cleanliness of the rooms inside the facility, including toilets? ... the amount of space you had?
	Access to family and community support (contact with outside world and maintenance of regular activities)	10%	... the ease of having family and friends visit you? ... your [child's] experience of staying in contact with the outside world when you [your child] were in hospital?
	Choice (choice of health care provider)	5%	How would you rate the freedom you had to choose the health care providers that attended to you?

Source: authors' compilation based on the World Health Survey instrument

Fairness of financial contribution

Fairness of financial contribution was defined in the 2000 World Health Report as the distribution of the financial burden imposed by the health system within the population. It was measured in terms of the fraction of disposable income that each household contributes to the health system (including income taxes, value-added tax, excise tax, social security contributions, private voluntary insurance, and out-of-pocket payments).

Subsequently, it has also been operationalized in terms of avoidance catastrophic payments, reflecting recognition that a well-functioning health system should prevent those falling ill from impoverishment, as exemplified by the observation that medical bills are the leading cause of bankruptcy in the USA. Both aspects are evaluated using household survey data, such as that provided by family budget surveys or the World Bank's Living Standards Measurement Studies.

Looking through the eyes of patients

The approaches described so far in this chapter involve the adoption of a macro-level perspective, looking at aggregate data on the overall system. They each provide valuable insights into the presence and, to some extent, the nature of problems but are less helpful in indicating what can be done to resolve them.

The tracer methodology offers a means to do this. It involves selecting a condition whose management requires the effective operation of multiple components of the health system and evaluating the experiences of those with that condition and their health care providers. A number of studies have used insulin dependent diabetes[8] as it has the advantage of ease of identification of those affected, as well as requiring well-functioning elements throughout the health system, including primary, secondary and tertiary care, a skilled workforce, and reliable supplies of insulin and test materials, all within a framework that is responsive to needs.

The methodology involves the use of rapid appraisal techniques, encompassing a mix of quantitative and qualitative methods, triangulating evidence from, among others, interviews with patients, providers, and policy makers, observation of facilities, assessment of supply chains, and evaluation of legislation and regulations. While its findings will be of most relevance to those suffering from the selected tracer condition, it should provide insights that are of much wider relevance. Thus, a pharmaceutical distribution system that is unable to ensure regular supplies of insulin is unlikely to be able to distribute vaccines or antibiotics.

Current developments

There are a number of important initiatives underway to take forward the methodology on health systems evaluation. The Commonwealth Fund sponsored International Working Group on Quality Indicators, which began in 1999 and that, by placing the US health system in an international context, has contributed substantially to the debate on health care reform. The European Observatory on Health Systems and Policies, at the request of the European Commission, has recently commenced a project that will complement the other programmes by looking in depth at the reasons for differences in performance. However, the most sophisticated is the OECD's Health Care Quality Indicators (HCQI) Project. It is examining the technical quality of health care, seeking to 'develop a set of indicators that reflect a robust picture of health care quality that can be reliably reported across countries using comparable data'.[9]

Indicators selected for inclusion in the HCQI project have to meet two conditions:
- they must capture an 'important performance aspect'
- they must be scientifically sound.

Importance is assessed on three dimensions:
- the measure addresses areas in which there is a clear gap between the actual and potential levels of health
- it reflects important health conditions in terms of burden of disease, cost of care or public interest
- measures can be directly affected by the health care system.

The second criterion, scientific soundness, requires indicators to be valid (i.e. the extent to which the measure accurately represents the concept/ phenomenon being evaluated) and reliable (i.e. the extent to which the measurement with a given indicator is reproducible).

The project has already identified a number of indicators that can be used to compare performance in at least some countries, but arguably its greatest achievement has been to identify and address the many problems of data comparability that exist.

Uses and abuses

The increasing interest among researchers in evaluating health systems has been accompanied by a similar increase among politicians and lobbyists. Health system evaluation is an inexact science, involving choices about the goals to be pursued, the weighting to be placed upon them, the systems to be compared, and the way to present the result.

Unfortunately, this flexibility creates scope for abuse. This may not always be apparent, as where there is selective choice of indicators, perhaps prioritizing choice over equity. Caution is always required in interpreting existing data. One of the most studied examples is cancer registration data. These have been extremely influential in a number of countries seen to achieve less than optimal results. Yet, while cancer registration covers the entire population of some countries, it is fragmentary in others.

There may also be inherent biases, as with the American SEER database, in which the poor and African-Americans are under-represented, thus tending to inflate apparent survival. It is also necessary ensure that account has been taken of methodological traps, such as lead-time bias where screening programmes result in earlier detection of cancers but confer no ultimate benefit on mortality. These issues, collectively, account in part for the often quoted cancer survival in the USA compared with Europe.[10]

References

1 World Health Organization (2000). *The World Health Report 2000. Health systems: improving performance*. World Health Organization, Geneva
2 Saltman RB, Ferroussier-Davis O. (2000). The concept of stewardship in health policy. *Bulletin of the World Health Organization*, 732–9.
3 Rutstein D, Berenberg W, Chalmers T, *et al.* (1976). Measuring the quality of medical care. *New England Journal of Medicine*, **294**, 582–8.
4 Nolte E, McKee M. (2004). *Does health care save lives? Avoidable mortality revisited*. Nuffield Trust, London.
5 Tobias M, Jackson G. (2001). Avoidable mortality in New Zealand, 1981–6.
6 Kesteloot H, Sans S, Kromhout D (2006). Dynamics of cardiovascular and all-cause mortality in Western and Eastern Europe between 1970 and 2000. *European Heart Journal*, **27**, 107–13.
7 Britton A, McKee M, Black N, *et al.* (1998). Choosing between randomised and non-randomised studies: a systematic review. *Health Technology Assessment*, **2**, 1–124.
8 Nolte E, Bain C, McKee M. (2006). Chronic diseases as tracer conditions in international benchmarking of health systems: the example of diabetes. *Diabetes Care*, **29**, 1007–11.
9 Kelley E, Hurst J. (2006). *Health care quality indicators project*, Conceptual framework paper. OECD health working papers no. 23. OECD, Paris.
10 Desai M, Rachet B, Coleman M, McKee M. (2010). Two countries divided by a common language: health systems in the UK and USA. *Journal of the Royal Society for Medicine*, **103**, 283–7.

Part 6

Personal effectiveness

6.1 Developing leadership skills

Fiona Sim

Objective

This chapter should help you to acquire the leadership competencies that are necessary to turn excellent public health technical practice into *effective* public health practice.

Definitions

Leadership
Great leaders are usually characterised as highly charismatic, high-profile individuals, e.g. Churchill or Mandela. Leaders have great power to influence, communicating a clear vision that is attractive to their followers, with the ability to deliver that vision.

Additional to this stereotype, in your workplace or community, you could probably identify someone, not necessarily charismatic, extroverted, or even very senior, who has been the architect of a substantial change and made it happen.

Public health leadership
Public health leadership is the application of leadership characteristics to the cause of improving the health of a given population or community.[1-3] Where this leadership sits organizationally is subject to political decision. For example, embedding leadership for health improvement in local government was a core proposal in English policy reform in 2010.[4]

A former Chief Medical Officer for England[5] described leadership as:
- knowing where you want to go and setting the direction of travel
- taking people with you on the journey in spite of their differences in views and methods, working background, and rates of travel
- giving sufficient time and energy to the process of changing things for the better—learning to do things in a different way.

Public health leadership should produce
- attributable improvement in the health of a population, community or service
- better collaboration at organizational and individual levels
- a higher profile for public health
- greater efficiency in health decision-making.

Is leadership different from management?

Leadership complements and differs from management in some important respects. Whilst an effective manager requires planning and problem-solving skills to produce largely predictable, desirable results, a leader will go further to *establish the vision* and take it forward, usually by motivating and developing others, to produce significant, sometimes dramatic, change. Table 6.1.1 illustrates these distinctions.

Table 6.1.1 Distinctions between managers and leaders (after Kotter[6])

Manager	Leader
Coping with complexity	Coping with change
Ensuring order and consistency	Delivering change
Planning and budgeting	Setting direction—developing a vision
Organizing and staffing to accomplish objectives	Aligning people
Problem solving	Motivating and inspiring

The relationship between management and leadership is suggested by adapting a distinction between logic and imagination made by Einstein. 'Logic (or management) will take you from A to B. Imagination (or leadership) will take you everywhere'.

Why is leadership an important public health attribute?

For a public health practitioner to be effective, technical skills, and knowledge are essential, but not sufficient. Knowing all the facts in this handbook alone will not be adequate to ensure that you are able to articulate and implement your sound professional advice, especially in the face of opposing views. It will be your leadership that prevails in ensuring your effectiveness.

In public health, as in other areas of work, it is not only those in formal leadership roles who can lead—any member of a team can adopt situational leadership if appropriate, as noted in the NHS Leadership Qualities Framework.[7]

Competencies needed by a public health leader

Virtually any piece of work in public health lends itself to scrutiny of the leadership element. For example, you are asked by the local authority to undertake a health impact assessment in relation to a proposal to set up a waste incineration facility in your locality. Review of this task, which requires you to adopt a project management role, will reveal aspects for which your leadership skills are needed:

- Clear vision as to the nature of the task and its objectives and desired outcomes
- Working across organizational boundaries to ensure engagement of all stakeholders through appropriate, effective communication
- Gaining the trust of those who may be threatened by the proposal, such as employees of existing services likely to be adversely affected by the building of the new facility
- Perseverance to complete the task despite strong opposing factions—in particular those who fear they may be disadvantaged by the HIA's conclusions
- Professional integrity—and moral courage to present your final recommendations strongly, in support of the population's health.

The evidence base for effective public health leadership is under-developed. Looking more widely, and with the exception of military leadership, most modalities of leadership have little firm evidence. Research on personality type (using Myers Briggs Personality Inventory, MBTI) shows that leaders are more likely to have certain personality characteristics than others, but there is no evidence for a causal association between personality type and leadership ability. As pointed out in relation to health services,[8] leaders are involved in enthusing, negotiating and pacifying, and must therefore have these competencies, as well as any more tangible qualifications for the job.

Box 6.1.1 shows competencies usually associated with effective public health leadership.

The leadership qualities adopted by the English NHS comprise personal, social and cognitive qualities, arranged in three clusters:

Personal qualities, setting direction, and delivering the service

These qualities may be applied in public health (Table 6.1.2) as in health care more generally.

Potential pitfalls

- Recognizing a public health challenge and producing a technically competent project plan to address it is necessary, but not sufficient.
- Neither vision nor professional expertise alone will lead to change—political skills including diplomacy, communication, and timing are just as important.
- Leadership may not always be from the front. Different styles of leadership are needed for different situations—for example, in leading

Box 6.1.1 Competencies usually associated with effective public health leadership

Knowledge
Good grasp of the core knowledge base required for public health practice

Skills
- Ability to define and articulate a clear vision
- Ability to share the vision so that others are influenced to adopt it
- Resilience and perseverance towards the vision despite difficulties
- Maintenance of professional integrity

Attitudes
- Self-esteem combined with critical self-appraisal
- A degree of humility to allow one to acknowledge that someone else is right
- An understanding and respect of others' beliefs and perceptions, which may differ from yours
- Personal values including a 'passion' for public health.

Table 6.1.2 Leadership qualities and capacities

Personal qualities	Setting direction	Delivering better population health
Self-belief	Seeing/sizing the future	Leading change through people
Self-awareness	Intellectual flexibility	Holding to account
Self-management	Broad scanning	Empowering others
Drive for improvement	Political astuteness	Effective and strategic influencing
Personal and professional integrity	Drive for results	Collaborative working

Adapted from NHS Leadership Qualities Framework, NHS Institute for Improvement & Innovation, 2006.

an outbreak control team, getting a local company to take seriously workplace health, or introducing changes to clinical practice.
- Enthusiasm may be infectious, while piety is usually not. Remember that others may not share your vision, and may need an explanation of the evidence—as distinct from the faith—on which it is based.

Dogma, myths, and fallacies about leadership

- *'Leaders are born and not made':* there is no evidence for this statement, though aptitude, intelligence, and enthusiasm are helpful attributes. An ability to learn from every situation is central for effective leadership—as President Kennedy pointed out: 'Leadership and learning are indispensable to each other'.
- *Leaders are tall or attractive or have significant physical presence:* there are plenty of high profile examples to refute this. Having said that, appearance can be important and leaders on occasion win hearts and minds by dressing respectfully for their audience.
- *Extroverts make the best leaders:* whilst there is evidence that leaders are more likely to be extrovert personalities (using MBTI), there is no evidence that other types make inferior leaders. Leaders have to deploy the most appropriate attributes at the right time.
- *'What is your leadership style?'* may be asked of applicants at interview, but the fact is that leaders have to use a range of styles to suit different situations—though most of you will have one or two preferred styles, typically on the spectrum of supportive: directive and autocratic: participative.
- *Leadership is a fancy term for management:* no, leadership and management should be considered as distinct.

Example of success and scope for improvement

National management of the 2009/10 influenza pandemic has been independently reviewed in a number of countries. A good published example comes from Canada,[5] which made particular reference to the importance of effective leadership and collaborative working across many organizations and government departments, as well as translation of the strategy to local levels for grass roots implementation.

Key determinants of success

Clarity of vision, the energy to persevere despite barriers and the humility to recognize when to adjust the vision, are all necessary. Taking people with you on the journey through implementation is essential. The successful public health leader has imagination and energy as well as professional integrity, technical knowledge and skills. And if you have passion for your subject that will be apparent in your dedication and commitment: Barack Obama was credible to many when he said 'Yes we can'.

How will you know if you have been successful?

Change in a public health context can take many years, though your vision would have been supported by a plan for implementation including measurable indicators of progress. These might comprise quantitative and qualitative measures, the latter including the extent of engagement of partner organizations, positive media coverage, or knowledge of the initiative in the local community.

However, to know if you, as a leader, have been successful, you will probably need to ask other people. You don't have to wait to do this. The concept of multi-source feedback (MSF) is now well established and the use of a validated MSF tool can provide valuable feedback about your performance. In the UK, MSF is likely to be an integral part of the evidence required for the future revalidation of public health professionals.[9]

Emerging issues

Public health increasingly requires interagency collaboration so that effective leadership across organizational boundaries is often essential (see 📖 Partnerships). So is the ability to work through others, whose job specifications—teachers, pharmacists, town planners, for example—rarely indicate public health content. To be a successful public health leader, it is worth exploring the professional practices and workplace cultures of people in quite different jobs to be able to harness their enthusiasm and energy to your common cause.

The practicalities of acquiring leadership skills

In your personal development plan, consider:

• *Taking a course in leadership development:* in England, the NHS Leadership Qualities Framework's Development Guide is accessible online.[10] In the US, the Public Health Leadership Institute has been running since 1991 and recent evaluation has demonstrated its impact.[11]

• *Ensuring you understand your own personality type and appreciate the potential impact of others:* you can study this alone,[12] although you may want to consult a personal development consultant to take this further.

• *Getting to know and learning how to work with the mass media* (see also 📖 Working with the media). The media are very effective at conveying both positive and negative health messages to the general public. Having the media, including local media, on-side for advocacy can reap rewards. Establishing a good rapport with local or national reporters can mean that next time a public health issue comes along, the story is more likely to be covered fairly and without bias. Media training is available from many sources and your organization's press office would usually be a good starting point.

• *Developing your communication skills:* different audiences will respond to different modes of communication, so it is worthwhile becoming familiar with techniques not often yet taught to professionals, such as storytelling. Humility is valuable: arrogance has no place in public health practice.

• *Knowing and respecting partners within and outside your organization:* it could be just as important to engage a key internal budget holder as forming an alliance with a Chief Executive of another body or a community leader: there is always a need for partnership working 'inside and out'.

- *Reviewing your public health competencies systematically:* for greater understanding of the local scene, not only its demography and epidemiology, but also its key players, culture, politics and priorities, of which health is, but one. All this is needed for good practice, the scope of this book.

Further resources

Adair J (1993). *Effective leadership.* Pan Books, London.

BBC World Service. *The Handy Guide to the Gurus of Management.* © BBC English/Charles Handy, Programme no.5. Available at: ℘ http://downloads.bbc.co.uk/worldservice/learningenglish/handy/bennis.pdf (accessed 22 August 2010).

Hunter D, Rayner G. (2004). Guest editorial: UKPHA and WFPHA Conference Plenary Presentations. *Public Health,* **118,** 461–87.

National Leadership Council. (2010). *NHS Leadership Qualities Framework.* Available at: ℘ http://www.nhsleadershipqualities.nhs.uk/ (accessed 20 August 2010).

National Public Health Leadership Development Network. (2005). *Public Health Leadership Competency Framework.* Available at: ℘ http://www.heartlandcenters.slu.edu/nln/about/framework.pdf (accessed 22 August 2010).

References

1 Acheson D. (1988). *Public health in England: the report of the Committee of Inquiry into the future development of the public health function,* Cm 289. HMSO, London.

2 Wanless D. (2004). *Securing good health for the whole population.* HM Treasury, London. Available at: ℘ http://www.dh.gov.uk/en/Publicationsandstatistics/Publications/PublicationsPolicyAndGuidance/DH_4074426 (accessed 21 August 2010).

3 Department of Health. (2004). *Choosing health: making healthy choices easier.* HMSO, London. Available at: ℘ http://webarchive.nationalarchives.gov.uk/+/www.dh.gov.uk/en/Publicationsandstatitics/Publications/PublicationsPolicyAndGuidance/DH_4094550 (accessed 20 August 2010).

4 Department of Health & Communities and Local Government (2010). *Liberating the NHS: local democratic legitimacy in health.* Available at: ℘ http://www.dh.gov.uk (accessed 3 October 2012).

5 Calman K. (1998). Lessons from Whitehall. *British Medical Journal,* **317,** 1718–20.

6 Kotter J. (1996). *Leading change.* Harvard Business School Press, Boston.

7 NHS Leadership Qualities Framework. (2006). *NHS Institute for Innovation & Improvement,.* Available at: ℘ http://www.nhsleadershipqualities.nhs.uk/ (accessed 20 August 2010).

8 Bohmer R. (2010). Leadership with a small 'l'. *British Medical Journal,* **340,** c483.

9 Faculty of Public Health (2010). Available at: ℘ www.fph.org.uk (accessed 19 April 2011).

10 NHS Leadership Development Framework Development Guide. (2010). Leadership development module. Available at: ℘ http://www.nhsleadershipqualities.nhs.uk/development-guide (accessed 20 August 2010).

11 Umble KE, Diehl SJ, Gunn A, Haws S. (2007). *Developing leaders, building networks: an evaluation of the National Public Health Leadership Institute—1991–2006.* North Carolina Institute for Public Health, Chapel Hill. Available at: ℘ http://www.phli.org/ (accessed 20 August 2010).

12 Myers Briggs I, Myers P. (1980). *Gifts differing, understanding personality type.* Davies-Black, Palo Alto.

6.2 Effective meetings

Edmund Jessop

Introduction

All meetings are negotiations. Whether it is a 10-minute meeting with your boss, a regular meeting with colleagues or a 20-minute presentation to a committee, you are trying to change what someone else thinks.

So there are two essentials for any meeting:
- YOU—know what you want to achieve from the meeting
- THEM—find out as much as you can about them.

Before the meeting

Think about your aims

Public health is about changing the way other people think. The best way to do that is face to face. Most people hate meetings, but part of the reason for this is that they see meetings as a chore, not an opportunity. Of course some, even many, meetings are tediously unproductive. However, for sure a meeting will waste time if you go in not knowing what *you* want out of it.

Like any negotiation, sort out in your own mind beforehand:
- What would be the best result for you (opening position)?
- What is the minimum acceptable (your fallback position)?

For example, your opening position is probably complete acceptance of your policy; but what is your fallback: partial acceptance or the decision deferred until later? What points are you willing to compromise on? How much you are prepared to change your views?

Research before the meeting

Find out as much as you can about the other people who will be there. It is especially important to find out:
- What other people believe?
- What other people want to achieve?

Of course, you need to ask these questions of yourself first.

If you are attending an unfamiliar meeting, find out about the people who will be there. Do they like the big picture or the detail? Should you be thorough or quick? Will they be impressed by government policy or dismissive of it? Sometimes quoting the opinion of a medical academy or expert society will impress, sometimes it will antagonize. Use your friends and colleagues to find out about the people who will be at your meeting.

Even if the meeting is with someone you know well, think about how are they feeling *today* about your issue.

A successful negotiation is one in which you get what you want and they get what they want—at least to some extent. Listen hard and long: find out as much as you can about what they want.

If someone is opposing you, there must be a reason. This reason is important to them. Maybe it seems trivial, irrelevant, or outrageous to you, but it impedes negotiation. So you need to find out what that reason is. Only then can you start to resolve the difference between you. Often the reason is fear—fear that something will happen if they agree with you. Unearth the fear and maybe you can remove it.

Sell the benefit not the proposal

Focus on how they will benefit, not what you want to do. And concentrate on benefits that are relevant to *them*. Of course, you can only do this if you have already found out what they want.

Remember that differences exist in the mind, not in reality

To resolve a conflict of opinion, you need to address the other person's mind, not the 'objective facts'. Scientifically trained workers find it hard to understand why people don't respond to objective data. However, if you lived next to a toxic waste dump, and your child developed leukaemia, no amount of scientific evidence on exposure, doses, and latent periods would convince you that the waste dump was safe. The same is true in any meeting, from a discussion of where to put the coffee machine to agreeing on a multimillion pound budget.

Build the relationship

Public health work takes time. The people you are meeting today will be people you have to work with again in the future:

> The relationship is more important than any one meeting.

So sometimes you need to lose gracefully and come back next time. As Dale Carnegie said 'no one ever wins an argument'. If you have an argument and 'win', the other person is left feeling bruised and battered. This is always damaging to a long-term relationship. You can't afford that kind of ill will in public health work. Your success depends on other people, so you need other people to be on your side.

Setting up your own meeting

When you set up a meeting, good administration is important. If people arrive flustered, or unprepared, or cannot attend, you will not achieve your aim.

Timing

Give people plenty of notice that you want to meet them. It is difficult to generalize, but 4 weeks' notice for a half-day meeting, and 6 weeks or more for an all-day meeting is about right for senior people. People of national importance may need 6 months' notice or more.

Be aware of committee cycles: find out regular dates, for example, budget-setting meetings. You may need to map a sequence of meetings (e.g. ethics committee before grant committee, or personnel committee before finance committee).

Venue

The venue is important, so get the best you can afford. People who are cold, sitting in uncomfortable chairs, and who have had a long, difficult journey will not be paying attention to you. Think about transport, the needs of people with disabilities, and refreshments.

Should you invite other people to your office, or go to visit them, or meet on neutral territory? For one-to-one meetings it is more polite to put yourself out by going to them; for big meetings you have to be the host. If conflict is severe, neutral territory works best.

If you are expecting conflict, avoid placing people who are likely to disagree directly opposite each other, so avoiding the feeling of 'us' against 'them'. Have everyone face a screen or board on which the problem you have in common—an outbreak, an overspend, whatever—can be described. You can do this even in one-to-one meetings: never sit across a desk from someone.

Agenda

Send out an agenda so that everyone has the chance to prepare for the meeting. Most people *will not* prepare, but if you do not send an agenda they *cannot*.

Help them to identify the important items, perhaps by indicating on the agenda how long you expect to spend on each item. It is wise to allow 10–15 minutes for people to settle in with small or routine items before tackling the major topic.

During the meeting

Meetings are the live theatre of public health: exciting, exhilarating, and unpredictable! Ok, so most meetings are pretty boring, but if you focus on what's going on, you can build up pictures of people and relationships. Remember:

Build the relationship: you'll be meeting again!

Listen: don't speak

If you are the first to speak on a topic, human nature ensures that the next two or three speakers will oppose what you have said, if only to show that they can think for themselves. So bide your time and present your ideas towards the end of discussion on an item. Sometimes this will mean not revealing your own opinion in any briefing paper you have circulated before the meeting.

Even if you've been invited specifically to give a presentation you need to listen first. So get there early to gauge the mood of the meeting, and find out who is asking what.

Words matter: use them carefully

You will not build the relationship by giving offence. If in doubt, find out beforehand from a colleague what terms are acceptable to your audience. Remember that some scientific words give offense to lay audiences—for example, 'spastic' has a clear meaning in medical meetings, but is some-times used as a term of abuse in lay language. Is it a 'case' of meningitis or a person with meningitis?

If you've achieved your objectives, stop arguing

After you've achieved your objectives, anything else you say can *only* make things worse, so shut up! Of course this means you need to be listening hard to know when you have won. However, all too often people throw away victory by continuing to argue their case and alienating people who have already been won over.

Use summary statements

With more than five people in a meeting, normal conversation is impossible and special tactics are needed. If more than eight people are present, you will not get more than one chance to speak on any topic. Often a summary statement ('sound bite')—a single phrase or sentence which puts across a message or creates an image—will be more effective than a speech in help-ing other people to change their minds or modify their views.

Read the papers before, not during, the meeting

If you are reading you are not listening. In the meeting, it is more important to concentrate hard on what is going on around you than to read some point of detail. If someone asks a detailed query the correct response is to say, 'I'll get back to you after the meeting', and carry on with more important business of listening hard to the discussion.

After the meeting

- After formal meetings, send out notes of what was decided and who agreed to take what action within 24 hours if possible. Copy this to people who did not attend.
- Even informal meetings are worth written follow-up to ensure no misunderstanding (and no reneging on agreements!) (see Box 6.2.1).

Box 6.2.1 A 'follow-up' letter

Dear Jim

This is to confirm that Fred, you, and I agreed yesterday to write a 1500-word paper together entitled 'Waiting list solutions that work' within the next 2 weeks. I will let you have the statistics by Thursday, and you will do the first draft within 5 working days. We agreed to meet next on Wednesday 30th March at 3 pm in your room.

Julie
cc. Fred

Further resources

Fisher R, Ury W, Patton B. (1999). *Getting to Yes. Negotiating agreement without giving in.* Random House, London.

McNamara C. (1999). *Basic guide to conducting effective meetings.* Available at: ⌘ http://www.mapnp.org/library/misc/mtgmgmnt.htm (accessed 06 August 2010).

6.3 Effective writing

Edmund Jessop

Introduction

The most important thing to remember when you write is that no one *has* to read what you write. Despite the importance of your writing, often people will not read it. Consider for a moment how much material you have not read in the past 2 weeks.

If what you write is difficult to read, people will simply give up. So you must do everything in your power to make reading easy for your readers. You cannot force people to read: you have to tempt them.

Objectives

This chapter will help you to make your writing more enjoyable to read. As a result, it will be more effective in initiating and sustaining appropriate change in others.

Writing has three stages: before, during, and after. The most important stage is before.

Before you write

Know who you are writing for

Are you writing for:

- Your boss?
- Co-workers?
- A committee?
- The general public?

This seems obvious, but it is the key to success. If you are going to tempt people to read, you must know who they are and what they like. Always keep the reader in mind. It is sometimes easier to think of some person you know, rather than a whole group: if writing for old people, write for your aunt. If writing a committee paper, think of one typical member of the committee and write for him or her.

Give them what they want to read—not what you want to write

Avoid the trap of thinking people *must* read what you write. Even if telling them about their own pay rise, there will always be some people who won't read your words. So give them your message in the form they want it—make it easy for them.

Most people don't want scientific methodology: so don't give it to them. If you do, they'll just give up and skip to an easier document. If *they* have stopped reading, *you* have stopped persuading.

If your readers (e.g. a grant-giving committee) have asked you to complete a form, *complete the form*. Don't leave items out. Don't add pages of extra material. If it says do it in 12-point type, don't try to cram more in by using a smaller font. Your aim is to help them to your way of thinking; and failing to heed their instructions will not achieve that aim.

Be active in finding out what your readership wants: if writing for a committee asks to see previous committee papers. Speak to the secretary of the committee.

Give it to them on time

Hit the deadline—even if it means your paper isn't perfect: as the journalists say to their editors 'You want it good or you want it Thursday?' A report or paper that arrives after the decision is made is worthless. So find out when the decision will be made. Never 'table' a paper, i.e. give the paper out for the first time at the meeting at which you want it discussed. No one can read it properly in the meeting so the only correct course of action for a chairperson if you do this is to ignore your paper completely.

Allow time for all stages of writing, review, and distribution to hit the deadline.

Remember that the formal meeting at which, say, budgets are agreed is often a formality: all details may have been sorted out long before. So you need to check if minds will be made up *before* the formal decision.

Be aware of their constraints

The usual constraints are:
- people's attitudes, prejudices, way of life
- local regulations, law, or policy
- precedent
- available funding.

Think what each may mean for your readers. You may or may not be able to alter constraints: but if not, you must at least show awareness of them.

Think before you write

If your thoughts are woolly, your writing will be woolly. Each piece of writing should have a single aim, and the whole structure of your piece should lead to this aim. Spend time thinking this out.

Write down your aim. Make it short and clear, for example
- to persuade this school to adopt a no smoking policy
- to persuade this committee to give me a research grant.

The next stage is to work out what individual messages are most likely to sell your idea. This may need further thought. For a smoking policy it could be:
1. smoking causes cancer in non-smokers or
2. smoking is a fire hazard.

Message 1 may seem more important to public health workers, but message 2 was what got the ban on smoking throughout the London underground transport system. Choose the message which will achieve your aim, not the one you most want to put.

Do all your homework before you put pen to paper (or finger to keyboard)

Typically, you need to research:
- some key statistics
- research literature
- law and government policy
- local precedents (what have they done before on this or similar issues?).

Make sure you can prove every assertion you make. You may not want to fill the text with scientific references, but truth matters: don't rely on memory! Readers increasingly want to check references online, so give an internet address (URL) when you can.

Write a framework

When you have all the facts in your head, write a framework for your piece. This needs to give:
- a major heading for each two or three pages (2000–3000 words)
- minor headings per half page (500–1000 words)
- a main point for each paragraph (100–200 words).

Start with the major headings, and then fill in the minor headings, and finally the points for each paragraph. You now have a clear line of thought for your piece, be it a one-page memo or a 10,000 word report. Without a framework, your reader will find it hard to follow your line of thought and will probably give up trying.

Make a word budget

Make a word budget for each section. For example:
- introduction, 300 words
- evidence base, 500 words
- local situation, 500 words
- recommendations, 250 words.

When you are writing

Don't write anything until you have the shape of your entire piece clear in your mind and/or sketched out on paper. Cut and paste is easy with computers, but it is lazy and destroys the clarity of thought that both you and your readers need. I find that a pencil and paper encourages structure in a way that computers often do not.

Use short words

Think what you would say in conversation: 'he had a stroke' not 'he had a cerebrovascular accident'. Sometimes the short word lacks precision—a 'heart attack' may indicate acute myocardial infarct or ventricular fibrillation; but think, does this distinction matter *to my readers*? If not choose the short word.

There is one exception to this rule: don't give offence.

Don't give offence

Words such as leper and cretin have technical meanings, but they also may give offence and should be replaced by 'person with Hansen's disease' and 'person with congenital hypothyroidism'. It may look odd, but if you give offence, people will stop reading and your writing will not achieve its aim (quite apart from common decency).

Use short sentences

Do not use a comma if a full stop and a new sentence might be better.

Avoid abbreviations

People read word groups, not individual letters or words, so in reading (unlike speaking), readers do not need abbreviations, which often make a piece difficult to read. If you must abbreviate, spell it out in full the first time, e.g. AIDS.

Use headings and subheadings

Most people don't read, they skim. So help them to skim—use headings.

If there is a house style use it. Your readers are familiar with it and anything different is a distraction. If there is no house style, keep to a standard format for the font size, underlining, etc.

Structure your piece

A good general structure for a briefing paper is as follows:
- Table of contents (if more than 10 pages long)
- Summary
- Purpose or aim
- Background
- Precedent or local/national policy
- Current issues (i.e. why now?)
- Options including implementation
- Cost
- Politics
- Recommended option and why
- Document control—authorship, reason (for info, action) sent to whom, date, version.

You should number the paragraphs in your document—this helps readers refer to particular passages in meetings or correspondence.

Use lists

Lists are easy to skim. More than three of anything demands a list. Use bullets for three or four items, but for more than that use numbers.

Use graphics

Try to put a chart, graph, or picture in to break up the text. Newspapers do it to attract readers—so should you. It is easy enough to insert graphics into text with modern software, though considerable effort may be needed to generate a good graphic.

Electronic mail

With email the message header may be the *only* thing people read, so use the header for your message not the topic. Try this sample:

- 'Read your papers before tomorrow's meeting', rather than 're: Tomorrow's meeting'.
- 'Home called: no dinner tonight', as opposed to 'Telephone message for you'.
- 'Teenage pregnancy rate lowest ever', rather than 'Latest health statistics'.

Remember that some people never read their email: if they only read hard-copy, send it.

After you write

Don't send it off

Once your paper is written, mull it over. Never send a paper out as soon as it is written: even with the most urgent deadline walk away for an hour or so. Better still; leave it overnight or over a weekend. Then come back with a fresh eye and reread your work. At this point you will always see something that could have been said better!

Get some feedback

Always ask a colleague to read your document. Make clear that you want comments on big issues not minor errors of spelling or grammar. Ask specifically for:

- material that just looks wrong (e.g. statistics for circumcisions that exceed the number of male births in your locality)
- important issues that have been missed (e.g. abortion clinics, as well as maternity units in a study of conception).

If possible, though this is often difficult, ask someone like the intended reader to review it for clarity. Don't get defensive when people point out errors and inconsistencies. Be grateful.

Consider the distribution list carefully

Send it to your intended readership, but also think 'Who else should see this?' This is particularly important for correspondence. Do a mental check of people in your own organization and in other agencies. Other organizations won't distribute it internally to everyone you think should see it, so mail them directly. In general anyone who will be affected by what you write should see it.

Offer to meet the individual or group you have sent it to

Offering your time shows your commitment to the cause, as well as giving an opportunity to lobby, and to remove any misunderstandings.

Summary

These rules may seem daunting, but as with so much in life they become easy with practice. Writing well is one of the best ways to improve your personal effectiveness.

Further resources

Easy reading

Bryson B. (1987). *Troublesome words*, 2nd edn. Penguin, Harmondsworth.

Truss L. (2003). *Eats, shoots and leaves*. Profile Press, London.

Tim Albert Training. *Effective written communications*. ℘ http://www. timalbert.co.uk/ (accessed 06 August 2010).

Reference works

Burchfield RW. (ed.). (1999). *Fowler's modern English usage*, 3rd edn. Clarendon Press, Oxford.

Economist style guide. Profile Books, London, 1999 (see ℘ http://www. economist.com/research/ StyleGuide/) (accessed 06 August 2010).

Strunk W, White EB. (1979). *The elements of style*, 3rd edn. Allyn and Bacon, Boston, MA. Full text available at ℘ http://www.bartleby.com/141/ (accessed 06 August 2010).

Writing for publication in the medical literature

Albert T. (1996). Publish and prosper. *British Medical Journal*, **313**(7070), classified supplement.

Albert T. (2000). *A–Z of medical writing*. BMJ Books, London.

Albert T. (2000). *Winning the publications game*, 2nd edn. Radcliffe Medical Press, Oxford.

How to do graphics

Tufte E. (1983). *Visual display of quantitative information*. Graphics Press, Cheshire.

6.4 Working with the media

Alan Maryon-Davis

Objectives

After reading this chapter you should be able to:
- develop a strategy for working with the media, both as an individual practitioner and as a representative of your team or organization
- review and strengthen your strategy, if you already have one in place
- undertake simple media tasks, such as writing a press release or being interviewed by a journalist, with more confidence.

This chapter addresses the basics of working with the print and broadcast media. 📖 Health communication addresses some of the newer electronic media, while more provocative engagement with the media appears in 📖 Translating goals, indicators, and targets into public health action.

Working with confidence

As health professionals we tend to be rather wary of working with the media. Like fire, publicity can be a great source of light—but can also be erratic and risky. Besides, it often takes an awful lot of matches just to get it started. Yet the media's influence and reach are invaluable to us. We need to engage large numbers of people and convey information, change attitudes, and trigger actions for health improvement. We must therefore learn how to make the most of this potential with a few basic skills and a coherent approach.

We talk of 'the media' as a single entity. In reality of course it is very plural, not only in terms of its various modalities, like print, radio, or television, but also because it comprises a diverse collection of individual journalists and programme makers, all trying to attract readers, listeners, or viewers. Fortunately for us, health issues make good copy, and media professionals need us as much as we need them. This makes our task a little easier.

Developing a media strategy

There are generic and specific elements to a media strategy.

Generic elements comprise
- *Knowing and cultivating your media*: print, broadcast, or web-based, understanding how they can help you in your work across the board, how they operate, who they reach, what their constraints and limitations are, and what risks are attached.

- *Developing media skills:* learning how to frame a story, write a press release, how to use the different media in combination (media mix), how to be interviewed, how to take part in a studio discussion, and building a team of people who can do these things with confidence.
- *Providing media back-up:* anticipating the information or materials that might be needed by your media journalists, researchers, and producers, and being prepared to provide this at short notice.

Specific elements concern the issue you are planning to promote. This involves being clear about what you're trying to achieve and asking yourself:

- What am I trying to say? (messages)
- Who am I trying to say it to? (target audience)
- How best can I get it across to them? (media mix).

To which should be added
- What support or follow-up should I provide?
- What parallel approaches should I adopt?
- How will I know if I have succeeded?

Simple clear messages, tailored to your target group, delivered through an appropriate media mix, make for success. If you can back that up with support, for example by providing a helpline or a website address, and ensure that the relevant services are primed and ready to respond to increased demand, your intervention is likely to be even more effective.

Be clear about your messages
The fewer key messages the better—a maximum of five, preferably no more than three. These should be:
- topical and newsworthy (the 'hook')
- meaningful and relevant to the target audience (the 'angle')
- informative or motivating
- in plain language and jargon-free
- accurate, valid, and backed up by reliable evidence
- agreed by your partners or managers.

Understand your target audience
Be clear who you are trying to reach and what their needs and interests are likely to be. This is crucial for framing your story and finding the right angle. If possible, meet and talk to service users themselves to gain an understanding of how they receive messages through the media—what issues they are interested in, what papers they read, radio programmes they listen to, TV programmes they watch. You need to understand how to 'grab' their interest and enthusiasm, what is the best mix of media to use, and at what level to pitch your messages.

Cultivate the media
Be familiar with their output and look for opportunities. Talk to, and if possible meet with, reporters and producers. Focus on those who usually cover health stories. Explain what you're trying to do and what you can do for them. Try to be available if they need instant public health advice or information. By and large they want to get it right.

For each issue, event, or campaign write a well-constructed press release (see 📖 Writing a press release) and follow this up with a personalized email or phone call to 'sell' your story to the appropriate editor—news editor, health editor, features editor, or programme editor. Be clear and succinct about the hook, angle, and messages. Mention any launch event or photo opportunity. Whenever possible, try to tie the story to something happening locally or nationally.

Make use of available help

Use your organization's press officer or communications manager. They can advise you on how to frame your messages and which media are best for reaching the target group. (If you don't use your organization's press officer, you may miss quality advice and your messages may be out of step with your organization's current policy.)

Always be clear, to the press and to others, on whose behalf you are speaking. Even if you claim you are speaking as an individual, it may be thought more newsworthy by journalists if they forget this. Your organization's press officer will usually have a working relationship with key journalists and producers, and perhaps a budget which can be used to set up a press conference, or pay for an 'advertorial' in the local paper. If you don't have this level of support, try to link in with a partner organization that does.

Using spokespeople and case studies

People bring news stories and features to life. The audience can identify with them and they help 'sell' your story to the editors. The spokesperson may be yourself, a colleague, or someone working for the initiative, project, or service you're promoting. You may need more than one spokesperson if there are many media slots to cover, in which case it is important to make sure they convey the same key messages. They might also benefit from the practical interview guidance below.

The case study might be a member of the general public or particular community group, or a patient, client, or other representative of the target group you are trying to reach. They, too, should be clear about the key messages and must have given their permission to be interviewed or featured.

In lining up your spokesperson or case study

- Brief them thoroughly on the purpose of the exercise
- Agree what their particular contribution should be
- Check their availability against the media slots you are trying to fill
- Give them copies of any fact-sheets, campaign, or follow-up materials
- Note their phone number in case of last-minute snags
- Do not give this to the media without permission—instead ask your spokesperson or case study either to make contact with the journalist/researcher/producer themselves or agree to be contacted by them.

Photo opportunities

Newspapers and magazines often prefer to run a 'picture-story'—a picture with a brief caption containing the essential information. This can be a good way of raising awareness of an issue, campaign, or service and can often be followed up later with more in-depth coverage. The trick is to come up with an idea that will grab the picture editor's attention—something visually interesting or amusing involving 'real' people. Using a well-known celebrity is a device that often pays off.

Staging a press event

A tried and tested approach is to set up an event such as a press briefing or campaign launch which combines a few speakers to provide different perspectives on the issue, a press pack to give the essential information (background, fact-sheet, key messages, contacts) and a photo opportunity. To carry this off successfully requires skill and experience and careful attention to organizational detail. Wherever possible, seek the assistance of any communications staff you may have access to.

Writing a press release

Unlike a paid-for advertisement or advertorial, a press release does not guarantee your story will be covered. News editors' inboxes are inundated with press releases. How can you make yours stand out?

Ten important guidelines

- Keep it short and simple—the equivalent of one side of A4 maximum.
- Devise a 'catchy' headline based on the main angle of the story.
- Use short sentences and only a few statistics.
- The introductory paragraph should summarize the whole story in a few lines—what, why, who, where, when, and how.
- The second paragraph fleshes out the detail—fuller background can be given in a 'notes for editors' section at the end.
- The third paragraph can give a direct quote from the spokesperson and a plug for any action you want taken.
- Editors are more inclined to use the story if they can lift text direct from the press release.
- Always give a contact name with daytime and evening phone numbers.
- Follow-up with a phone call offering information booklets, photographs, or photo opportunities.
- Consider putting on a formal press conference with a panel of speakers and convivial hospitality.

Responding to press enquiries

If you are rung up by a journalist

- Make a note of their name and their publication or programme
- Be open, fair, and honest. Avoid bluster or pretending to know what you do not know
- If they ask a question you are not sure about, say you will find out and call them back—and make sure you do

- Avoid saying 'no comment'. Explain why you cannot answer that particular question—perhaps because of confidentiality or because the matter is subjudice
- Avoid making 'off the record' comments—they have a habit of finding their way onto the record.

Being interviewed on radio or television

Approach each programme separately via the producer or researcher. Whether you call them or they call you, you are likely to find yourself being assessed not only on the merit of your story, but also on how well you put it across. If you seem to be saying the right things in the right way, you may be invited to take part.

Before committing yourself to being interviewed, try to find out

- What is the programme's format and style?
- What sort of audience does it have?
- How are they pitching the item?—what is the topical hook?
- In what capacity are you appearing?—personal or representative?
- Is it a one-to-one interview, or a studio discussion? If so, with whom, and what's their angle?
- Is it live or pre-recorded?
- How long will your item be? (you need to know how to pace yourself)
- What are the likely questions?
- Will it be in the studio, or will they come to you? (You may need to obtain permission for the recording to take place.)

When deciding what your messages should be

- Decide on a few key messages and get them clear in your head—you can use brief notes for radio, but not for TV. Avoid jargon.
- One or two real examples may add colour, but avoid using names unless you have been given permission to do so.
- *Quote statistics very broadly:* rather than '34.7%' say 'about a third' or 'about one in three'.
- Get your points across early—you never quite know when the item will be over.
- A light touch of humor may help, but only if appropriate. If in doubt, avoid.
- Make sure that any resource you are promoting, such as a leaflet or a service is in plentiful supply and someone is primed to provide it.

Radio interviews or phone-ins

Radio is a cosy, intimate medium so just talk naturally with the interviewer. Remember that the listeners are usually doing something else at the same time, so be upbeat, friendly, and plain speaking. If you find yourself taking part in a phone-in, here are a few more points to bear in mind:

- agree the ground you want to cover with the anchor-person so that callers are kept to the subject
- write each caller's name down and personalize your replies
- talk directly to the caller as if you were giving one-to-one advice
- avoid rambling on too long with each call, keep moving on to the next.

Television interviews

Dress simply and plainly. No glinting jewellery or jarring patterns. Avoid white, bright red, green, or blue, which can 'flare' on the screen. Go for gentle, muted colours instead.

When you are in front of the camera:

- sit up, look alert and engaging
- if your mouth is dry, have a sip from the water on the table
- maintain eye contact with the interviewer to avoid looking shifty
- don't fidget.

Measuring success

Individual feedback

At the individual level you can gauge how well you did in a radio or TV appearance by asking a few people to listen to or watch the programme and give you some honest feedback. This will be more useful if they are fairly representative of the target audience you are trying to reach. If possible, record the programme so that you can learn how to do better next time.

Media coverage

A broader assessment of the effectiveness of a press release or campaign can be obtained by auditing the coverage achieved, for example the number and reach of newspapers carrying the story or slots gained on radio and TV.

Public response

Ultimately, the key measure is the practical response achieved in terms of take-up of whatever support materials, service, or behaviour change you are trying to promote. Requests for support materials or an increase in service use are usually easy to count and can often be directly attributed to the media coverage, but behaviour change is likely to be much more difficult to assess or attribute.

Media training

As with most things, you learn best by doing. However, you can help to avoid the pitfalls by having media training. A number of educational bodies and commercial organizations offer courses to develop basic media skills. Check to see if your organization can arrange this for you and your colleagues.

Further resources

Albert T. (2000). *A–Z of medical writing*. BMJ Books, London. (A practical guide to communicating medical and health messages to various audiences in a clear and engaging way.)

Chapman S, Lupton D. (1994). *The fight for public health: principles and practice of media advocacy.* BMJ Books, London.

Easton G. (2004). Working in the media 3: Getting your message across. *BMJ Careers*, 10 April. (⅏ http://careers.bmj.com/careers/advice/view-article.html?id=116) (accessed 3 September 2010). (A basic guide writing and broadcasting for a general audience.)

Gabbay J, Porter J. (ed.). (1995). *Communication skills.* Faculty of Public Health Medicine, London.

6.5 Communicating risk

Nick Steel and Charles Guest

> Learn what people already believe, tailor the communication to this knowledge and to the decisions people face, and then subject the resulting message to careful evaluation.
>
> Morgan[1]

Objective

By reading this chapter you will be able to use an understanding of risk perception to communicate about risk more effectively.

Why is this an important public health issue?

Public health is at risk from a wide range of factors, including harmful food or medicines, poorly controlled infectious diseases, pollutants or natural environmental hazards, and poor diet. Public health practitioners are often involved in minimizing the harm from these risks, and this requires communication. There is an increasing moral and legal requirement for the public sector and private industry to inform populations about the health hazards to which they might be exposed. Risk communication is fraught with difficulty, not least because 'experts', such as policy makers, scientists, and clinicians tend to understand and perceive risks differently from the public. However, there are some predictable patterns, and an understanding of these will improve communication about risk.

Definitions

Risk

Risk is the probability that a particular adverse event occurs during a stated period of time, or results from a particular challenge.[2] It can never be reduced to zero.

Absolute risk is the probability of an event in a population, as contrasted with *relative risk*, which is the ratio of the risk of an event among the exposed to the risk among the unexposed.

Attributable risk is the rate of an event in exposed individuals that can be attributed to the exposure. Some people find the number needed to harm (NNH) more comprehensible than the attributable risk. The NNH is the number of people exposed that would result in one *additional* person being harmed over and above the background risk in the general population.

Risk assessment

Risk assessment is the qualitative and quantitative assessment of the likelihood of adverse effects that may result from exposure to specified health hazards (or from the absence of beneficial influences). It has two components, risk estimation, and risk evaluation.

Risk estimation

Relies on scientific activity and judgement. Statistics about past harmful events can be used to predict both the size and the likelihood of future harmful events, including estimates of uncertainty. It involves identifying the health problem and the hazard responsible, and quantifying exposure in a specified population.

Risk evaluation

Relies on social and political judgement. It is the process of determining the importance of the identified hazards and estimated risks from the point of view of those individuals or communities who face the risk. It includes the study of risk perception and the tradeoff between perceived risks and benefits. The term 'outrage' has been used to describe the things that the public are worried about that experts traditionally ignore.[3]

Risk communication

Risk communication is the way in which information about risk is communicated to various audiences. It is a two-way process that needs to be considered at all stages of risk management (Figure 6.5.1).

Tasks for effective risk communication

Identify and involve relevant stakeholders

The first step is to identify all those within the organization who will be involved, in order to:
- agree a line to take to avoid sending contradictory messages
- identify who will lead the communication process
- involve public affairs or a press office if available
- consider legal advice
- consider the timescale.

The next step is to involve external stakeholders early. These might be the media, professional groups, experts, special interest groups, the local community, patients, politicians, manufacturers, environmentalists, and health officials. Early involvement and acceptance as partners in risk communication will build trust and allow the exchange of information.

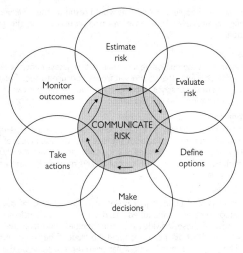

Figure 6.5.1 The risk management cycle[4].

Clarify objectives

With whom are you trying to communicate? Do you want to warn, reassure, or inform? You are unlikely to resolve all conflict over a controversial issue, but may clarify disagreements, minimize conflict, and improve decision-making. Extra care is needed when you wish to both reassure (the risk is tolerable) and at the same time to warn (but if, in the unlikely event that the situation changes, the following emergency action will be necessary), as sometimes required with infectious disease management. If behaviour change is desired, consider the wider influences on behaviour.

Anticipate potential pitfalls

Check the source of your information. Is it consistent with other knowledge? Is it peer reviewed? Expert overconfidence is a common cause of failure in risk communication. It can be countered by explicitly seeking to uncover uncertainties, and by seeking different views to expose assumptions about your scientific evidence. Listen to the language and signs of concern of all persons involved. Pilot messages before release:

> One should no more release an untested communication than an untested product.[5]

Resist the temptation to offer bland reassurance where there is real uncertainty. If the news is bad, share the burden with other stakeholders. Distinguish between scientific knowledge and value judgement, and accept that science may not change values and emotions.

Consider the target audience's risk perceptions

Analyse the different perspectives of, for example, politicians, the media, and scientists. Consider the relative importance of evidence from different domains, such as health and environment. Produce written materials and other information sources if needed.

Monitor and review each communication routinely

Keep records of decisions taken and the resulting outcomes, and identify learning points.

What are the competencies needed to achieve these tasks?

Effective risk communication requires:

- commitment to openness and acceptance of the need to share uncertainty
- familiarity with the language of risk
- understanding of risk perception
- recognition of the benefit of continual learning from experience.

Commitment to openness

Openness is a matter of principle which also produces practical benefits. Early and ongoing open and honest interaction is an essential component of effective and ethical risk communication, even though there may be strong disincentives to early openness.[6] Uncertainties should be addressed openly, if only because subsequent events may show that a risk prediction was flawed, or result in a contradictory message. People find it difficult to judge between experts when they disagree, and hard-won trust can be easily lost. Openness helps maintain trust in the source as well as the message.

The language of risk

The range of magnitudes of risk that we face is so wide that the extremes can be hard to grasp. A logarithmic scale can span this wide range and provide a basis for describing risk. Such a scale can be anchored to the size of human communities, or use the analogy of a 1 m 'risk stick' in a certain distance (Table 6.5.1). A potential problem of using risk comparisons is that people tend to over-estimate the risk of death from dramatic causes such as lightning, and under-estimate the risk from common problems such as stroke.

Risk perception

Risk perception involves people's beliefs and feelings within their social and cultural context. A particular risk or hazard means different things

Table 6.5.1 Risk scales (from Calman and Royston[7])

Risk	Risk magnitude	Unit in which one adverse event would be expected ('community risk scale')	Distance containing one 'risk stick' 1 m long ('distance analogue risk scale')	Example (based on number of deaths in Britain per year)
1 in 1	10	Person	1 m	
1 in 10	9	Family	10 m	
1 in 100	8	Street	100 m	Any cause
1 in 1000	7	Village	1 km	Any cause, age 40
1 in 10,000	6	Small town	10 km	Road accident
1 in 100,000	5	Large town	100 km	Murder
1 in 1,000,000	4	City	1000 km	Oral contraceptives
1 in 10,000,000	3	Province or country	10,000 km	Lightning
1 in 100,000,000	2	Large country	100,000 km	Measles
1 in 1,000,000,000	1	Continent	1,000,000 km	
1 in 10,000,000,000	0	World	10,000,000 km	

to different people, and different things in different contexts. An understanding of risk perception underpins all effective risk communication.

Framing

The way information about risk is presented affects the choices that will be made. For example, both patients and doctors prefer treatment with a 90% *survival* rate to treatment with a 10% *mortality* rate, although the measures are equivalent.[8]

Absolute and relative risk

It is important to distinguish between absolute and relative risk. The anxiety generated in the UK over the doubling of the relative risk of venous thrombosis with third-generation oral contraceptives compared with second-generation ones obscured the message that the absolute risk was minimal.[9] Estimated reduction in relative risk gives a more favourable impression of the benefits of medical treatment than reduction in absolute risk.

Acceptability

It cannot be assumed that a risk is acceptable just because it is smaller than another risk that people already take. The qualitative aspect is more important than the quantitative aspect in risk perception. Risks are usually considered less acceptable if they:

- are involuntary (e.g. genetically modified food or pollution) rather than voluntary (e.g. skiing or smoking)
- arise from a novel or human-made source
- cause hidden damage, perhaps through onset of illness many years after exposure
- pose a danger to small children or pregnant women
- are poorly understood by science
- damage identifiable rather than anonymous victims
- are close—concern diminishes with distance
- threaten a form of illness arousing particular dread (e.g. death from cancer rather than a sudden heart attack).[10]

Working with the media

Journalists are constrained by the nature of their work to convey complex information about health risks simply, unambiguously, and dramatically: 'terribly dangerous' is more newsworthy than 'perfectly safe'.[3] Public health practitioners cannot afford to exaggerate, and need to acknowledge the uncertainty of many health risks. 'Possibly dangerous' may be nearer the truth.

The following are indicators of potential media interest:

- questions of blame
- secrets and 'cover-ups'
- conflict (between experts or experts vs. public)
- links to sex or crime
- human interest through identifiable heroes or villains
- links with existing high-profile issues or personalities
- strong visual impact
- signal value, or suggestion that the story is a sign of further problems.[10]

Continual learning from experience

Routine and honest review of experiences and dissemination of learning points improves future risk communication.

Examples of success and failure in risk communication

Success

Singapore showed good risk communication during the outbreak of severe acute respiratory syndrome (SARS) in 2003, when the Prime Minister acknowledged that it made sense for other countries to restrict travel to Singapore until SARS was under control. In contrast, China urged people not to cancel trips to Guangdong Province, Hong Kong asserted that Hong Kong was absolutely safe and did not have an outbreak, and Toronto was slow to take action. Singapore also communicated well over the decision to close schools, which a minister explained was not on medical grounds, but because teachers and doctors reported that parents were concerned about risks to their children.[11,12]

Failure

The World Health Organization was accused of a lack of transparency in its decisions about the swine (H1N1) flu pandemic in 2009-2010, with some loss in the credibility of WHO and trust in the global public health system.[13]

Success and failure

The complex saga of bovine spongiform encephalopathy (BSE) in cattle and its possible links with a new variant of the human disease Creutzfeldt–Jakob disease (vCJD) aroused considerable public concern (Box 6.5.1).

Box 6.5.1 Communicating the BSE–CJD epidemic in the United Kingdom and Australia

United Kingdom

The Ministry of Agriculture was perceived to be secretive, and was criticized for denying the possibility of a link between BSE in cattle and vCJD in humans. The Minister for Agriculture denied risks of human infection from BSE, but later a group of 'eminent scientists' reported that they had stopped eating British beef. Articles in the press contained estimations of wildly differing numbers of people who may have contracted vCJD.

Australia

The government provided easy access to information via the media and a telephone information line to prevent the release of contradictory information and to acknowledge that there were risks involved, although small. Co-ordinated media liaison between government agencies helped to promote balanced reporting by the Australian media. It is not possible to say whether the government's media strategy would have been as effective if BSE had been discovered in Australia.

Key points

Avoid secrecy, the denial of risk, and contradictory messages. Acknowledge uncertainty promptly.

Adapted from Banwell and Guest[14]

How will you know if your communication about risk has been successful?

Success means reaching a shared understanding of risk with the relevant target audience. This can be assessed in terms of how close you have come to fully meeting your objectives about the purpose of the communication. Absence of outrage is usually the desirable outcome, and, as usual, this attracts little attention or gratitude!

Further resources

Sandman PM, Lanard J. (2010). *The 'fake pandemic' charge goes mainstream and WHO's credibility nosedives.* Available at: ℘ http://www.psandman.com/col/swinecomm.htm. (accessed 6 August 2010).

Sunstein CR. (2002). *Risk and reason: safety, law, and the environment.* Cambridge University Press, Cambridge.

Zeckhauser R, Kip Viscusi W. (2000). Risk within reason. In: Connolly T *et al.* (eds) *Judgement and decision making: an interdisciplinary reader.* Cambridge University Press, Cambridge.

References

1 Morgan MG. (1993). Risk analysis and management. *Scientific American*, July, 24–30.
2 Royal Society Study Group. (1992). *Risk: analysis, perception and management.* Royal Society, London.
3 Sandman PM. (1993). *Responding to community outrage: strategies for effective risk communication.* American Industrial Hygiene Association, Fairfax, VA.
4 The Presidential/Congressional Commission on Risk Assessment and Risk Management. (1997). *Framework for environmental health risk management*, Final report volume 1. Washington, DC. Available at: ℘ http://cfpub.epa.gov/ncea (accessed 28 August 2012).
5 Morgan MG, Fischhoff B, Bostrom A, Lave L, Atman C. (1992). Communicating risk to the public. *Environmental Science Technology*, **26**, 2048–56.
6 National Research Council. (1989). *Improving risk communication.* National Academy Press, Washington, DC. Available at: ℘ http://www.nap.edu/openbook.php?record_id=1189&page=1 (accessed 6 August 2010).
7 Calman KC, Royston GH. (1997). Risk language and dialects. *British Medical Journal*, **315**, 939–42.
8 McNeil BJ, Pauker SG, Sox HC, Tversky A. (1982). On the elicitation of preferences for alternative therapies. *North England Journal of Medicine*, **306**, 1259–62.
9 Calman KC. (1996). Cancer: science and society and the communication of risk. *British Medical Journal*, **313**, 799–802.
10 Department of Health. (1997). *Communicating about risks to public health: pointers to good practice.* Department of Health, London. Available at: ℘ http://www.dh.gov.uk/prod_consum_dh/groups/dh_digitalassets/@dh/@en/documents/digitalasset/dh_4039670.pdf (accessed 6 August 2010).
11 Sandman PM, Lanard J. (2003). Fear is spreading faster than SARS—and so it should! ℘ http://www.psandman.com/col/SARS-1.htm (accessed 6 August 2010).
12 Fung A. (2003). SARS: how Singapore out managed the others. *Asia Times*, 9 April. Available at: ℘ http://www.atimes.com/atimes/china/ED09Ad03.html (accessed 6 August 2010).
13 Cohen D, Carter P. (2010). WHO and the pandemic flu 'conspiracies'. *British Medical Journal* **340**, c2912
14 Banwell C, Guest CS. (1998). Carnivores, cannibals, consumption and unnatural boundaries: the BSE-CJD epidemic in the Australian press. In: McCalman I, Penny B, Cook M. (eds). *Mad cows and modernity: cross-disciplinary reflections on the crisis of Creutzfeldt-Jakob disease*, pp. 3–36. National Academies Forum, Canberra.

6.6 Consultancy in a national strategy

Charles Guest

Objectives

This chapter introduces the steps for developing a public health strategy. It should assist you to play a constructive role as a public health consultant (see definition below), working closely with government officials, policy advisers, and other stakeholders in the creation of a major strategy.

You will consider:

- the definition of a public health problem and the development of a strategy as a response to it
- the need to create and clarify objectives
- the need to collect and analyze relevant information
- the development of proposals and options, with appropriate balance between brevity and comprehensive detail
- the importance of a detailed study of options, which should include the case against, as well as for, the options favoured by the consultant
- consultation, one activity for improving a draft of the strategy.

Implementation and evaluation of the strategy are addressed only briefly.

Definitions

In this chapter, the word *consultant* is used in a general sense to indicate a provider of independent professional advice or services, on a contractual basis. An independent consultant working alongside government agencies will have a quite distinct role from that played by employees of those agencies (public servants). Also, distinguish the role played by medical specialists as salaried officers of a health service (e.g. consultants in public health medicine).

A public health strategy is an organized programme for public health activity at a local, regional, or national level. In this chapter 'strategy' comprises the development and documentation of a specific agenda in public health. 'Policy', a more general term, refers to a course of action, expedient or prudent, that may be 📖 less adequately documented than a specific public health strategy (see 📖 Policy arenas).

Development of a strategy should include many of the same evidence-based steps that apply to the development of guidelines. This chapter assumes some familiarity with the latter process and addresses additional steps and departures from the more circumscribed activity of developing guidelines.

Why is this an important public health activity?

Strategies represent tangible public health activities that often have large associated budgets. Most people are affected by a number of public health strategies. At some time, most practitioners will participate in the development or implementation of a public health strategy.

Methods, stages, and tasks of developing a public health strategy

Initial clarification

Whether or not to develop a major public health strategy is usually a decision taken at a high level in a government department after politicians, special interest groups, or journalists have moved an issue onto the national agenda. People in the public health field may have participated in that process, or their influence may have been slight. As the consultant, you should appreciate the circumstances that produced the requirement for a strategy, such as changes in:

- population health status
- health services
- perspectives in sectors other than health (e.g. environment or transport)
- financing
- economic and performance pressures
- alliances.

A potential for improvement in at least some of these variables may justify the development of a strategy. If you are contributing to early decisions about the possible development of a public health strategy, your advice should:

- provide structure to promote systematic thought and action about a major problem that has been poorly understood
- gather the minimum necessary information, with appropriate analysis
- indicate a range of options for public health action
- communicate results of this work to the client in a timely and understandable way.

Other stages may then follow

Defining the scope of the public health problem

A more formal definition will usually be required, in consultation with a reference group of senior officials and stakeholders, referred to in this chapter as the steering committee. A review of the relevant epidemiology and potentially effective interventions is usually required, with reference to the current position. Public opinion survey data may be available: they should be considered early in the strategy process. (Alternatively, surveys may be planned as a research activity, noted below.)

Establishing the policy framework

This includes identification of guiding principles (including, but not restricted to, 'government policy') and appropriate key partners, and then, according to the circumstances, contributing to the:

- establishment of priorities
- definition of roles and responsibilities
- planning of research and development
- scope of intervention—tools for the strategy, e.g. guidelines, standards, regulation, legislation, grants, subsidies, tax credits
- development of a work plan for some or all of these tasks (implementation)
- planning of the evaluation (measurable achievements and other outcomes).

Consultation with stakeholders

You may play a role in the conduct of consultations, of possible relevance at several phases in the development of a strategy. These may serve to obtain critical information and to foster a receptive attitude among stakeholders to the development of a strategy. Include views from a wide range of individuals and organizations by such methods as focus groups, interviews, and written submissions.

Drafting the strategy

This will then be informed by:

- views of the government (the client) and the steering committee
- results of the consultations
- review of the literature
- your own observations.

The draft strategy is then usually subject to further consultation and revision before approval at senior levels.

Managing the strategy's development

Assemble essential resources

Influence with policy makers, peers, and the public, for any activity in public health, has to be earned and cannot be granted by fiat. You will have earned at least some influence if you play a major role in the development of the strategy. If you do not also have it, ensure that your contract[1] enables you to obtain the necessary:

- legal authority
- convening power
- information
- scientific and technical expertise (e.g. for community health assessments, epidemiology, health education campaigns, or detailed policy analysis)
- advocacy, lobbying, and public relations skills.

The development of many strategies requires simultaneous attention to inputs and process.[2]

Inputs

Management

Good management is essential for the development of a strategy, including:
- competent leadership and senior management
- effective communication of objectives and priorities by the executive to all staff
- openness that seeks positive external linkages
- performance guidelines that adequately define success and failure, with due reference to integrity and ethical standards.

Staff

Appropriately qualified and motivated staff may need to be recruited and retained. Time must be allowed for this. Training may be relevant to the development of staff in major national policy activity, but you may not have time for this during the more constrained schedule for developing a new strategy.

Information technology

Is your equipment adequate? For example, do you have enough storage and processing power and software to perform tasks efficiently in the field?

Process assessment

The public health consultant needs to rapidly identify and use networks in government (within and between portfolios) and outside it. The views of those likely to be affected should be sought actively and carefully incorporated in the development of the strategy.

Detailed analysis should establish:
- the successes and failures of previous and related programmes
- possible consequences, intended and unintended, of options for the strategy
- the institution's capacity to implement the strategy, including the support at middle and lower levels necessary for the achievement of objectives.

Outputs

An immediate output of a strategy's development is represented by its publication. The published strategy may be accompanied by other background or technical reports.

The publication should specify:
- the problem to be addressed, with adequate analysis
- the scientific basis on which the strategy was developed
- who will do what, when.

Desirable features include:
- creative approaches to options and their implications
- coherence with other programmes and strategies
- practicality
- cogent advocacy of the preferred options.

A background report[3] could specify:
- how the need for the strategy was identified
- how the strategy was developed
- how strategy development has been funded, and the resources available for implementation
- who was responsible for development of the strategy
- who was consulted
- possible—as well as probable—outcomes of the strategy
- cost-effectiveness of solutions identified
- the time-frame for evaluation.

Dissemination and implementation require much greater attention than previously accorded to many major strategies. Approaches now include:
- summaries on the Internet and elsewhere
- mass media
- professional and consumer organizations
- incentives.

Engaging people in the importance of a strategy

The whole spectrum of public interests, government, and management must be engaged if a public health strategy is to achieve its goals. You should promote the development of goals that all health and other sectors can share.

As with any collaborative venture:
- seek the early involvement of partners
- identify reasons (additional to the public health concerns) for others, including representatives of industry or the private sector, to become actively involved
- expect and listen to a wide range of opinions about the development of the strategy
- obtain influential endorsements.

Potential pitfalls

Under-estimating complexity

Public health strategies may require the participation of various government departments. Identify the complexity and constraints early, to ensure that resources match the task.

Inadequate communication

For example, lack of awareness and understanding of the strategy among the target population or failure to engage all relevant professionals and sectors may lead to people ignoring or undermining the new approach.

'We have the minister's full support'

Continued support from within government should not be assumed, even if the development of a public health strategy was the minister's initiative. Choosing not to decide about possible government projects is sometimes the preferred option for politicians and their advisers. They will sometimes go to extremes to avoid association with an initiative that could fail.

The development of a strategy distorts the political process, while the real questions remain undebated

From the citizen's perspective, this may be the worst problem. Technical issues should not be allowed to obscure political questions, while the public health consultant cannot and should not assume the responsibilities of the elected representative.

The independent consultant should avoid
- arrogance
- self-censorship (tell clients what they need to know, not what you think they want to hear)
- creating problems rather than solving them
- neglect of current clients while chasing new ones.[4]

What are the key determinants of success?

- Political support
- Committed, adequate financial resources
- Collaboration across sectors
- Community participation.

How will you know when/if you have been successful?

Development of the strategy

Desirable qualities of the process and outputs of the strategy include:
- comprehensiveness
- timeliness
- responsiveness (e.g. evidence of adequate consultation with interested parties)
- clarity
- practicality
- relevance
- fairness (e.g. recommendations are balanced and equitable, as well as objective)
- cost-effectiveness (comparative costs for various solutions should be provided).

Subsequent evaluation

- Were the objectives of the strategy met?
- Did the original objectives remain in place?
- What has actually been implemented?[5]
- Has the public health problem itself changed?
- What relevance does the strategy now have?
- What were the outcomes? Were they anticipated or not?

Your role as consultant

- Was your analysis of the problem accurate?
- If the strategy was developed according to your plans, did you predict the outcome?

Also assess your efficiency, e.g. the timeliness of preparation and real costs of your input to the strategy. The measurement of effectiveness assumes a causal link between your role as a consultant and the outcome of the strategy. This will probably remain a matter only for speculation.

Conclusion

Like any project in public health, a strategy requires:
- collaboration that may be broad, while retaining sufficient focus for effectiveness
- adaptability to local and regional needs
- careful attention to the allocation and use of resources, including government and other infrastructure.

This chapter has addressed strategy as a product, while other parts of this book present strategic processes.

A parting thought

> No matter how beautiful a strategy might be, it is wise, occasionally, to see what it achieves.
>
> Attributed to Winston Churchill, 1874–1965

Further resources

Block P. (2007). *Flawless consulting: A guide to getting your expertise used.* Pfeiffer, Amsterdam.

Harvard Business School. (2004). *Harvard business essentials. Manager's toolkit.* Harvard Business School Press, Boston.

Kaplan R, Norton D. (2001). *The strategy-focused organization.* Harvard Business School Press, Boston.

Swayne LE, Ginter PM, Duncan WJ. (1996). *The physician strategist.* Irwin, Chicago.

Walt G. (1994). *Health policy.* Zed Books and Witwatersrand University Press, London.

References

1 Lasker RD, Committee on Medicine and Public Health. (1997). *Medicine and public health: the power of collaboration.* Academy of Medicine, New York.

2 Uhr J, Mackay K (ed.). (1996). *Evaluating policy advice: learning from Commonwealth experience.* Federalism Research Centre, Australian National University and Commonwealth Department of Finance, Canberra.

3 National Health and Medical Research Council (Australia). (2009). *A guide to the development, implementation and evaluation of clinical practice guidelines.* National Health and Medical Research Council (NHMRC), Canberra.

4 Nelson B, Economy P. (1997). *Consulting for dummies.* IDG Publications, Foster City.

5 Rist RC. (1994). Influencing the policy process with qualitative research. In: Denzin NK, Lincoln YS, eds, *Handbook of qualitative research*, pp. 545–57. Sage, Thousand Oaks.

6.7 Improving your professional practice

Caron Grainger

Overview

Many aspects of daily work provide opportunities for improving practice, most of which will come under the broad heading of governance, including:

- appraisal, assessment, and continuing professional development (CPD)
- audit
- complaints management and risk management.

In educational terms, learning needs would be identified by formative appraisal, but the reality is that we have to deliver against organizational objectives and the majority of our CPD will be undertaken through (and paid for by) our employing organizations. As such I focus on the process loosely termed 'performance review' (including appraisal and assessment) and CPD, enabling you to:

- understand the role of performance review in improving performance
- understand the principles of setting, and recording, a personal development plan (PDP)
- understand the principles of mentorship.

Why is this an important public health area?

Public health practitioners work in a rapidly changing environment. Practitioners must be able to constantly update skills, recognize opportunities for development in their professional portfolios, and know how to access training and development to meet these needs. Demonstration of competence and evidence of CPD are now integral to revalidation for doctors registered with the General Medical Council in the UK. This is likely to extend to specialists from other disciplines, and in many other countries, in due course.

Definitions

Performance review is a formal process, usually between employee and their line manager, of assessing performance against agreed objectives, identifying training and development needs, and setting objectives for the next work period. It encompasses elements of both:

- *Appraisal:* a non-threatening two-way dialogue exploring and agreeing objectives to be attained, or progress in attaining agreed objectives,

and the individual development needs of the appraisee, enabling them to maximize their experience.
- *Assessment:* a formal one-way process, assessing performance against pre-set competencies, standards, or objectives.

A PDP is a method of identifying gaps in professional knowledge, skills, or attributes, and planning how to address these deficits, often performed with another professional, e.g. boss, mentor, colleague. The aim should be to identify training needs for individual development and to support the individual in the role they play in meeting the organization's requirements. It may also be known as a personal learning plan.

A *learning need* is the gap between your current and your desired or optimal level of competence required to undertake a task.

Continuing professional development is learning and development which occurs after the formal completion of postgraduate training, and is defined as 'purposeful, systematic activity by individuals and their organizations to maintain and develop the knowledge, skills, and attributes which are needed for effective professional practice.' [1]

The process of performance review

Any system of performance review (Figure 6.7.1) should be focused on motivating staff through unbiased, objective feedback in *both* directions between manager and staff member. Successful performance review is a cyclical activity, which takes a joint problem-solving approach, reviewing personal, career, and organizational goals through: [2]
- assessing performance against agreed objectives and standards of competence
- a two-way appraisal reviewing and reflecting upon personal, educational, and job-related achievements, and training/development needs
- recognition of the contribution of an individual towards organizational goals, including the collaborative setting of standards for future work in the context of the local business plan.

All organizations have differing systems for performance review, often very simplistic. Work with your system, but adapt it to meet your needs. It can be particularly helpful to reflect on the following types of questions before your appraisal:
- How good a public health practitioner am I?
- How well do I perform? (How do I know this? How do I compare?)
- How up to date am I?
- How well do I work in a team?
- What resources and support do I need?
- How well am I meeting my service objectives?
- What are my development needs?

It is important to recognize that good performance review includes consideration of the wider development needs of an individual beyond the immediate job, for example developing them for a new job, or with-in their wider professional activities. Similarly, there must be recognition that

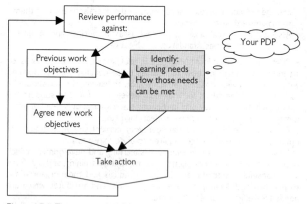

Figure 6.7.1 The process of performance review.

duties and responsibilities, and the environment in which we work, and therefore learning needs, change over time. These elements should all be considered as parts of performance review.

The process of developing PDPs

PDPs should provide the blueprint for continuing professional development. Developing a PDP requires:
- identifying learning needs—often as part of performance review
- designing learning experiences and locating resources for learning
- evaluating the outcome of learning
- recording learning objectives.

This process requires critical awareness, an appreciation of the context in which knowledge and skills will be applied, an understanding of a practitioner's personal learning style, and reflection. Many individuals find it helpful to review their learning needs, and identify means of meeting them, with another practitioner, e.g. boss or mentor, who provides an external, balanced view of both strengths and weaknesses.

Identifying learning needs

This can be carried out in three parts:
- A self-assessment of learning needs, reviewing your development needs in four main areas:
  - to fulfill the duties of your current role
  - to meet the requirements of a change in duties or role, e.g. a new job
  - general keeping up to date
  - specialist interest or personal development needs.
- Reviewing your self-identified development needs with another practitioner or mentor. The Johari window[3] (Figure 6.7.2) can help with this process, encouraging you and your mentor to look at

your skills and competencies. Through disclosure and feedback, and subsequent development, the unknown area is reduced and the arena (known to self and other) increased.
- Prioritizing learning needs, by considering:
  - corporate vs. departmental vs. personal work objectives
  - how big the learning need is
  - how urgent the need to close this gap is
  - whether resources are available
  - the commitment of the individual/department/organization to meeting the need.

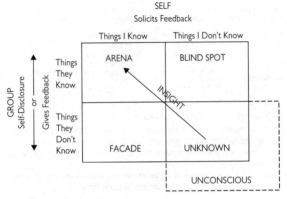

Figure 6.7.2 The Johari window.

Designing learning experiences and locating resources for learning

To identify the most appropriate learning experience, consider your learning style (see list below) and the settings in which learning can take place. Honey and Mumford's[4] learning cycle comprising 'Having an experience', 'Reviewing the experience', 'Concluding from the experience' and 'Planning the next steps' identifies 4 learning styles:
- *Activists (do):* learns best from 'having a go', often in adverse or pressured situations.
- *Reflectors (review):* learns best from assimilating information prior to action, and having the opportunity to review what they observe without the pressure to perform.
- *Theorists (conclude):* needs to understand the theoretical framework before participating in complex situations. Requires structured situations, logical frameworks, and clear purpose.
- *Pragmatists (plan):* learns best from practical/real life situations, often following a role model. Takes a 'common sense' approach.

Matching the learning setting to the learning preference of an individual will enable them to process new information as quickly as possible. There are four main settings for learning (Table 6.7.1), planned and unplanned, on the job (internal CPD) and off the job (external CPD). Within these four main categories are a variety of learning opportunities, e.g. didactic lectures, learning sets, one-to-one training, self-directed learning, distance learning, etc.

Table 6.7.1 Learning settings

Planned	
External	Internal
For example, attend a 1-day course on improving chair-manship skills	For example, observe chair-manship skills in others
For example, have someone assess your chairmanship skills at the beginning and end of a learning process	For example, noting styles of chairmanship on a TV documentary
Unplanned	

Evaluating the outcome of learning

As part of setting learning objectives, it is important to recognize how you will evaluate the impact of your learning. Evaluation criteria can be either:
• qualitative, e.g. your perception of change, your insight as a result of learning
• quantitative, e.g. the use of an objective assessment tool, such as an examination, or external assessment of performance.

It is worth noting the difference between output, i.e. the knowledge or skill that has been acquired, and outcome, or how you are applying this knowledge and skill to greater effect. A simple way of assessing outcome is to ask whether what you have learned has resulted in change in practice.

Recording learning objectives

Having identified learning needs and potential outcome indicators, it is possible to set a learning objective according to SMART criteria:
• specific
• measurable
• achievable
• realistic/relevant
• timed.

A template for recording your PDP is given in Table 6.7.2.

Table 6.7.2 A template for a PDP

What development needs do I have?	Expected outcome	How will I address them?	Timescale completed?
Explain the need	How will your practice change as a result of the development activity?	Explain how you will take action, and what resources you will need	
To improve chairmanship skills (specific)	All meetings have a clearly defined agenda, adequate time for discussion involving all parties, and clearly agreed decisions/ actions which are appropriately recorded (achievable, measurable)	Observe chairmanship skills in three others. Read a book on chairing meetings. Attend a 1-day course on improving chairmanship skills. Have someone assess my chairmanship skills at the beginning and end of the 6 months' learning	6 months period (timed, realistic)

Reflective practice

Donald Schön[5] in 1983 suggested that the capacity to reflect on action in order to continuously learn was one of the defining characteristics of professional practice. However, Schön noted a particularly critical point—that learning should not only be about doing something the right way (single loop learning), but also about doing the right thing (double loop learning). There are many models of reflective practice, but I find it easiest to use Honey and Mumford's[4] learning cycle:

- having an experience
- reviewing the experience
- concluding from the experience (which I modify to take account of double loop learning and ask both 'Did I do this the right way?' and 'Did I do the right thing?')
- planning the next steps.

The process of keeping reflective notes both to support CPD and prove engagement in CPD is now well established in medical practice, with many of the Royal Colleges making use of such schemes, by providing standard templates for reflection. These templates attempt to take you through Kolb's learning cycle in its entirety. Table 6.7.3 shows how reflective notes relate to Kolb's learning cycle, and the sorts of prompts that are helpful to maximize benefit from reflection.

Remember that it is worth recording your new knowledge too in a reflective note, so that it is easily retrievable. You may also find that you have a new learning need identified too, which can be added to your PDP. The Faculty of Public Health website includes an electronic diary for recording your CPD, constructed around reflective notes (http://www.fph.org.uk/).

Table 6.7.3 Reflective notes

Honey and Mumford's learning stage	Prompts for reflective notes
Having an experience	Why was I there? What prompted your involvement? What was your role in the situation? What were you trying to achieve? How did others respond? What were the consequences? Did something make you reflect on your practice? What piece of feedback prompted reflection and why?
Reviewing the experience	What were the most important things I learnt? What was useful for me? What was good/bad about the experience? What does this tell me? About me? About my attitudes? About my relationships? What knowledge/skills did you acquire? How does this relate to other knowledge? Are there patterns to your behaviour? Have you made a judgment about practice (good or bad)? Is there evidence of learning how cause and effect are interrelated? Has a theoretical construct been provided which explains your experience?
Concluding from the experience	How will my learning influence/change practice? What is my new understanding of the situation? Did I do this the right way? Did I do the right thing? What should I do differently to improve/resolve the situation/feel better? Or would I do the same again? Can I generalize from a single experience? Are there any broader issues I need to take account of? Can I apply this learning in a different setting or to a different problem?
Planning the next steps	What is the most important thing for me to do as a result of this activity? Have I discovered something I need to find out more about? Will you try something different? What, when, and how? What might the consequences of this be? Has a new way of working been tried? Any impact?

Mentors[6]

A mentor (literally 'wise one') can be a useful source of support in identifying and planning personal development. A good mentor will help you consider your roles and responsibilities 'in the round', i.e. the balance of work and home, development needed in the current job and for future jobs, and will play a variety of roles (see Box 6.7.1). Key issues for managing a mentoring relationship include:

- Agree a mentoring contract, i.e. how long the relationship will last for, how often the meetings will be held, confidentiality, and boundaries
- Give thought to who you approach as a mentor. Whilst they are not necessarily friends, they must be a trusted and respected individual you can relate to easily
- Look for someone who can translate his or her personal experience into generic 'how tos'
- Learning needs will vary over time. One individual may not be able to provide all the help you need, but should be able to direct you to others as appropriate. Similarly, consider whether one individual should be used on an ongoing basis, or should be picked for particular skills to help resolve a short-term training need, or a mixture of the two
- Mentors are usually senior to you and usually work in a different organization. Mentors may come from the same organization, although this can be sensitive, particularly if they are your boss's boss and you are seen to be going above your boss's head!

Box 6.7.1 Roles in mentoring

- Sounding board
- Joint problem solver
- Ratifier
- Mirror
- Coach
- Repository
- Flaw finder
- Connector and networker
- Empathizer
- Guide
- Referee

Further resources

The Faculty of Public Health website. Available at: Ꭻ http://www.fph.org.uk/ (accessed 19 April 2011). Includes information about professional standards, appraisal for medical consultants, and information for CPD, including an electronic register for recording your learning.

Some excellent online learning resources are available at: Ꭻ http://group.bmj.com/products/learning (some are charged for non-members) and Ꭻ www.doctors.net.uk/ (only for doctors). Both of these sites tend to be focused around clinical topics. More specialized resources for both practitioners and specialists are available at Ꭻ www.healthknowledge.org.uk/e-learning, and are free. There are many resources for broader professional and personal development on the web. Search and you will find! Try Ꭻ www.google.com

References

1 Mackie A. (2008). *Continuing Professional Development (CPD)*. Faculty of Public Health, London
2 Standing Committee on Postgraduate Medical Education (SCOPME). (1999). *Doctors and dentists. The need for a process of review*, a working paper. SCOPME, London.
3 Luft J, Ingham H. (1955). *The Johari-window: a graphic model for interpersonal relations*. University of California, Western Training Laboratory, Los Angeles.
4 Honey P, Mumford A. (1982). *The manual of learning styles.*. Peter Honey Publications, Maidenhead.
5 Schon D. (1983). *The reflective practitioner: how professionals think in action*. Temple Smith, London.
6 Grainger C. (2002). Mentoring—supporting doctors at work and play. *BMJ Career Focus*, **324**, S203.

6.8 Activism

J. A. Muir Gray

One person is a crank, two people are a pressure group, three people are public opinion

Objectives

After reading this chapter, you may better appreciate how lobbying and direct action can raise the profile of a public health issue.

Case study

The first report of The Royal Commission on Environmental Pollution was published in the UK in 1971. It had highlighted the problems of the illicit dumping of toxic waste—known as 'fly tipping'—at sites, such as waste ground, not registered to receive it. Although the problem had first been identified in 1963, the government had not acted. Through 1971, the Royal Commission lobbied the government to act on this matter, because of the potential danger to water supplies and the risk to public health, but to no avail. One day, however, a Midlands lorry driver called Lonnie Downes took the matter into his own hands. He had discovered that fellow drivers were being given a bonus of £20 a week to dump toxic waste (which was described as 'suds oil'). After complaining to the management, he was threatened with dismissal. Several weeks later, he was offered a promotion: Lonnie declined. Lastly, he was offered £300 to leave the firm; again Lonnie declined. Instead, he went to the local branch of the Conservation Society, which then sent a detailed report to the Secretary of State for the Environment. Despite this, the government still decided not to act.

The Conservation Society then sent its findings to the press. The story was published in the Birmingham *Sunday Mercury* on 10 January 1972. On 24 February that same year, 36 drums of sodium cyanide were found on a derelict piece of ground near Nuneaton where children were known to play. The government finally acted. A Bill was drafted and passed into law by 30 March 1972.

On this occasion, the evidence alone, even that from a scientifically respectable government report, was not enough to determine policy. Decisions taken by policy makers and managers can be made either in response to public pressure or from an ideological position in which the scientific evidence may play only a negligible part.

Making and amending laws

The process by which law is made or amended is sometimes weird and wonderful, but you can make an impact by doing one or more of the following:

- raising the public awareness of an issue
- lobbying politicians personally
- lobbying politicians through pressure groups
- becoming a politician
- breaking the law.

Political action can be very exciting and seductive, so it is wise to pause and reflect (see Box 6.8.1) before suddenly embarking on the campaign.

> **Box 6.8.1 Five points to ponder before getting politically active**
>
> - Could present legislation be enforced more effectively?
> - What do the public think about this problem and the proposed legislation?
> - What is the current best evidence about the need for, and benefits of, legislative change?
> - What else should I stop doing to create time for political action?
> - What will my boss and my employer think about my getting involved?

Raising the issue with the public

This is the first step. The fact that some change is required, and the reason for that change, needs to be raised within the consciousness of the electorate, either as a new idea or as an issue that is more important than they previously considered. It may be sufficient to say something must be done, but it is more effective to describe what should be done.

Issues can be raised by press releases and other means of getting coverage in the media (see 📖 Media advocacy for policy influence 📖 Working with the media). However, as in so many aspects of life, it is insufficient by itself and other steps must be taken to change the law.

Lobbying politicians personally

A lobby is an open space in a house of legislature, open in architecture and open in style, for politicians and the public to meet. Lobbying is the process of influencing the members of a legislature and it is the right of every citizen to influence their representative. Lobbying is an art, not a science, and there is no evidence on which to base guidelines other than experience, but it is possible to identify ways of lobbying that appear to be more effective (see Box 6.8.2).

It is essential to lobby the representative of the population concerned even though they appear to be powerless or even though they are known to be opposed to the desired course of action. Even if lobbying does not change the politician's mind it has an impact on the vehemence of their feelings and this may be very important.

Box 6.8.2 Guidelines for effecting lobbying

- *Focus:* don't lobby politicians on everything, but let them know you are willing to give information on any public health issue
- *Aim at the right level:* start locally and work up
- *Don't rely on letters alone:* make an appointment for an interview
- In an interview, listen, and leave a note of your main points
- *Don't embarrass your employer:* keep people informed about your political activities.

Lobbying politicians through pressure groups

In the United States the word 'lobby' has come to mean the pressure group itself. For example, the gun lobby works with highly paid consultants running sophisticated campaigns to influence politicians by a wide variety of methods, usually stopping just short of corruption by money. Corruption is 'the perversion of integrity by money or favours'; in many countries favours are used by those promoting goods or services hostile to public health.

There have been pressure groups for health for many years, but it was in the 1960s that consumer pressure groups blossomed, as attitudes changed and leaders emerged. Ralph Nader, who took on the American car industry on the issue of safety, became an icon of this activity. There are now hosts of health pressure groups. Public health professionals who wish to influence policy should ask the questions presented in Figure 6.8.1.

ASH (Action on Smoking and Health), Greenpeace and Amnesty International are all examples of pressure groups who are powerful forces for health improvement. They usually have highly skilled and committed staff who may have some reservations concerning the public health professional who wants to get involved. Pressure group workers are usually on low pay and shorter contracts, so it is wise to approach with humility and an eagerness to learn from very effective operators.

Becoming a politician

If many of the causes of ill-health can be tackled effectively by political action, it could be argued that every public health professional should become a politician; if some do, then why not all?

There is no formal study of this, but consider these issues:

- a politician has to sign up to a broad range of party policies, some of which require the individual to compromise
- policies are often based on ideology not evidence, because politics is based on values: the person who likes evidence-based decision–making may find this unsatisfactory
- politicians in power have power; those who are not may have less power than the public health professional managing a budget
- the politician has to cover many issues other than those which directly affect health; the public health professional can focus on health issues.

Is there an effective pressure group?

No | Yes

- What would be the risks, costs and benefits of starting one?

- Who could help?

- What should be its constitution? Informal or formal, charity or company?

- Could any resources from my organization be used or should it be entirely within my free time and resources?

- Would the pressure group put me in conflict with my employer?

- What would be the risks, costs and benefits or getting involved?

- Should I get close or use it as an external agency for change?

- If I get close, should I join or have observer status?

- Would it be better to put my energies into a national or local pressure group?

- What would my employer think?

Figure 6.8.1 Pressure groups.

Even the public health professionals who become successful politicians may find that they are steered away from health jobs for fear they will fail to do what politicians are there to do: bring values to decision making and challenge the professionals. The politician's role has been most eloquently described by Enoch Powell in his book *A new look at medicine and politics*[1] in which he argued not only that doctors were not necessarily better Ministers of Health than others (and could be less effective), but also that any politician in a post for more than 2 years started using the jargon of their officials and had lost the edge they contributed to a department before they became institutionalized.

Breaking the law

Most public health professionals break the law frequently, but usually in a way that endangers the public health rather than protecting it. Speeding is one of the most common offences and has a significant effect on mortality. However, the type of law-breaking that might protect the public health—an environmental protest that triggers police action, for example—is less commonly committed by public health professionals, particularly if they are employed, directly or indirectly, by a government. Law-breaking may be necessary to improve the public health, but law-making and enforcement has had an even greater impact and the skills of the public health professional are best used in this activity.

Personal survival amongst organizational change

Structural change in government and health-care organizations is frequent. In times of structural change in an organization, the job of the orthopaedic surgeon is relatively secure. The public health practitioner, however, is more exposed, often because of our inability to describe what we do quickly and clearly and concisely.

The following experience-based survival tips I pass on, gleaned from those people who have survived a series of organizational changes.

● *Never try to guess the future:* always do the job you are currently paid to do to the best of your ability.
● *Never put your faith in institutions:* only in individuals.
● *Make sure you can describe public health* and your own contribution to the service in one minute if someone asks you to do so.
● *Keep fit:* constantly attend training courses, and keep a good record of the training and the professional development that you have done, and plan to do.
● *Watch your back:* only the paranoid survive. Be careful how you use your official position and email. To be secure use your personal email and set up your own web site. It is a bold employer who tries to discipline what someone does in their own time.

Finally, know what would be a resignation issue for you. In a democracy values trump evidence and a politician has the right to make a decision that goes against an officer's advice. When this happens the good professional either accepts it, or resigns, both with a good grace.

Further resource

Machiavelli N. (1998) *The Prince*. Penguin, Harmondsworth.

Reference

1 Powell JE. (1976). *Medicine and politics: 1975 and after*. Pitman Medical, London. (How to work with full-time politicians and senior civil servants.)

6.9 Innovation

J.A. Muir Gray

More of the same is not always the answer. More data, more staff, more analyses, more reports—these activities will not necessarily solve the problems faced by the public health professional. Different approaches to problem solving have been developed in other disciplines and can be used by public health professionals.

Resolving disputes using linguistic techniques

The public health professional is often entangled in endless debate where different individuals and organizations are arguing about what should be done about a particular problem such as health inequalities. Each party has their own argument, which they pursue with commitment and precision, but make little progress. In this situation the public health professional can unlock problems and make progress by ensuring agreement on the terms being used and the propositions for change being put forward.

Agreeing to the meaning of terms

Much of the effort involved in solving problems, and sometimes all of the reasons for failing to do so, are due to the failure to define the terms being used. Words such as 'plan', 'strategy', 'consulting', 'engaging', 'inequality' or 'inequity', can be a source of confusion, impair problem solving, and may become a problem in their own right unless steps are taken to reach a common understanding of the way in which the term will be used in this particular public health context. This is best done not by consulting the *Shorter Oxford English Dictionary*, although this, and Porta's *Dictionary of Epidemiology*,[1] may help, but by asking all the key stakeholders to work together to develop the meaning that will be used, for example by:

- Assembling key stakeholders
- Asking them to work in pairs for 3 minutes to agree the words that they associate with the term being discussed; the term 'quality', for example, could elicit the words 'standards', 'goodness', 'efficiency' and 'safety'
- Writing these on a board or flip chart
- Asking the stakeholders to group the words into sets. (For example, 'standards' and 'goodness' emerge as being central to the meaning of quality; at this stage a definition such as that developed by Avedis Donabedian—'the quality of a service is the degree to which it conforms to preset standards of goodness'[2]—can be introduced. 'Efficiency' and 'safety' can then be pointed out as being aspects of a service, each of which have its quality appraised.)
- Writing down the meaning developed and agreed by the group.

Sometimes it is necessary to take steps to discontinue the use of a term which is consistently and frequently the cause of confusion and as such prevents understanding and progress. This is less frequently necessary in management than in clinical practice because management decision making involves many terms, which are created and enter widespread use until they themselves become displaced by later fashions. 'Benchmarking' and 'modernizing' are examples of such terms, and the same fate may, heaven forefend, befall 'evidence-based decision-making', but if it does cause more confusion than clarity then it should be dropped from decision-making discourse. Even in clinical practice, however, terms can cause confusion and may need to be deleted from debate.

In his highly praised biography, Ray Monk[3] describes how Ludwig Wittgenstein, when a technician in a research laboratory in Guy's Hospital in 1941, joined a Medical Research Council team whose leader had observed that 'there is in practice a wide variation in the application of the diagnosis of 'shock' without an agreed meaning of the term' which was harmful to patients and 'renders it impossible to assess the efficacy of the various methods of treatment adopted.' He argued that there is good ground, therefore, for the view that it is better to avoid the diagnosis of 'shock' and to replace it by an accurate and complete record of a patient's state and progress, together with the treatment given.

Clarifying the meaning of propositions

It is not only single terms that cause confusion; sometimes the problem is created by failure to agree the meaning of propositions, for example, 'community engagement will increase the sense of empowerment of those whose health is worst.' Resolution of this type of problem is best done not by analysis of the individual words, but by using the techniques developed by the logical positivists and most clearly articulated by A.J. Ayer.[4]

We use the criterion of verifiability to test the genuineness of apparent statements of fact. We say that a sentence is factually significant to any given person, if, and only if, he knows how to verify the propositions which it purports to express; that is, if he knows what observations would lead him, under certain conditions, to accept the proposition as being true, or reject it as being false.

With regard to a question the procedure is the same. We enquire in every case what observations would lead us to answer the question, one way or the other; and, if none can be discovered, we must conclude that the sentence under consideration does not, as far as we are concerned, express a genuine question, however strongly its grammatical appearance may suggest that it does.

The logical positivists believe that no term should be examined in isolation—a study of the term 'efficiency' would be pointless—but investigated in the context of propositions, such as 'this hospital is more efficient than that hospital'. To define the meaning of this proposition a logical positivist would not have recourse to a dictionary, but instead seek to agree on the data that would need to be collected to confirm or refute it. Thurs, for this particular proposition, the debate immediately becomes: 'How would you measure efficiency?'

The meaning of propositions can be elucidated by:
- asking stakeholders to work in pairs for 3 minutes
- recording the criteria suggested on a flip chart or board
- asking the group to assess the validity and feasibility of each criterion to agree how the impact, if any, of the proposed change could be measured.

This approach can irritate those whose basic training is in the social sciences because they may see this as a positivist, reductionist, or medical approach. It is therefore sensible and correct, to adopt this approach not only for vaguer statements, but also for propositions that appear to be self-evident, such as 'our objective is to reduce the prevalence of smoking'.

Resolving linguistic differences can solve many public health problems, but significant obstacles can remain because the different disciplines that have to combine to solve a public health problem can have different views of reality.

Resolving multiple realities

Reality is a social construct.[5] What a person takes as reality is constructed by their upbringing and their professional training and created by the language they used. The view of reality held by the professionals and the public involved in tackling the problem is determined by their world view: to the anthropologist the problem is one of cultures and beliefs; to the sociologist the problem is one of social class or gender, to the politician the problem is one of values and beliefs; and to the community worker the problem is one of empowerment and disadvantage.

The public health professional needs to reconcile these views, and one method is to use the metaphor of the lens. Each professional can be asked to describe how the problem looks through their lens. This model, for example, 'the public health model', implies that the reality must fit the model; the lens implies that there is a focus on part of a whole, just as the lens in an optician's spectacle frame may be placed in front of other lenses, each focusing on a part of the whole.

A second technique is to use John Rawl's 'veil of ignorance,'[6] that is, to ask each professional to look through the veil of ignorance to imagine they do not know who they will be in the next life, imagining if possible that they are powerless and poor, rather than seeing the problem through their confident view of reality. For this approach to be successful requires each professional to accept not only that they have a biased view of a problem, but also that the reality of the problem they see is itself constructed by their concepts and described by their esoteric language.

Narrative-based public health

A story can help an individual or group leave a fixed position.

Age brings some consolation for the public health professional because the number of personal stories of successes (and, even more useful, failures) accumulates. If there is not an apposite personal story then the stories of others can be used, and two excellent sources are the collections of anthropological essays on public health failures: *Health, Culture and Community* by Benjamin Paul[7] and *Anthropology in Public Health* by Robert A. Hahn.[8]

The content of the story is important, but so too is the manner of its telling. One objective can be to induce a state of trance in the audience. Trance induction can be brought about by the tone of voice and by the choice of words, and should start with the opening sentence. In a shared state, individual professionals can safely leave their bunkers and mingle in a common understanding of a problem and are more likely to find the means of mitigation, if not solving it. The use of theatre could also be useful and might play a part in helping a whole community come to terms with a problem and its solution, but such an approach requires a major commitment of resources. Mild trance induction, on the other hand, is relatively easy to achieve with practice, although you will need sufficient insight to be able to distinguish between trance and sleep induction!

References

1 Porta M. (2008). *A dictionary of epidemiology*. 5th edn. Oxford University Press, Oxford.
2 Donabedian A. (1980). The definition of quality: a conceptual exploration. In: *Explorations in quality assessment and monitoring. Volume 1: The definition of quality and approaches to its assessment*. Health Administration Press, Ann Arbor.
3 Monk R. (1991). *Ludwig Wittgenstein: the duty of genius*. Vintage, London.
4 Ayer AJ. (1936). *Language, truth and logic*. Penguin, London.
5 Berger PL, Luckman T. (1967). *The social construction of reality*. Anchor Books, New York.
6 Rawls J. (1971). *A theory of justice*. Harvard University Press, Boston.
7 Paul B. (1955). *Health, culture and community*. Sage Foundation, New York.
8 Hahn RA (1999). *Anthropology in public health*. Oxford University Press, Oxford.

Part 7

Organizations

7.1 Governance and accountability

Virginia Pearson

Objectives

Reading this chapter will:
- improve your understanding of the principles of governance and accountability
- help you recognize potential shortcomings in systems that may result in risk to individuals
- improve your knowledge of how to reduce risk through creating assurance that those systems are working effectively.

Definitions

Governance is the process by which an organization safeguards the interests of its stakeholders and delivers its objectives through a monitored framework of rules and procedures (from the Greek *kubernao*, to steer).

Governance may be sub-divided into different types, all commonly found within both public and private sector organizations, including:
- corporate governance
- clinical governance
- research governance
- information governance.

These different types may be combined and described as 'integrated governance'. Each type of governance forms a building block of integrated governance and assures an organization that its interests in each of these areas are being safeguarded through the use of tools including risk assessment and an assurance framework.

Why is this an important public health issue?

You will be undertaking needs assessments and reviewing determinants of health and provision of services to determine how to improve health and wellbeing and the quality of care. To assess how well an organization is meeting its objectives you will need to understand how those objectives are defined and how the organization assures itself that they are being met.

To do this and to be able to make change and deliver improvements you will need to know how, and how well, that organization is governed and made accountable. If you are using your public health skills to assess quality of care, knowledge of the organizational approach to governance in clinical systems is essential.

As an employee of an organization you should be aware of how your organization governs itself, how your personal work objectives contribute to the organization's, and what policies and procedures you must follow as part of your contract of employment.

Integrated governance

Integrated governance is a term often used to describe the interlinking elements of good governance. This ensures, irrespective of the type of governance, the underlying principle is co-ordination. One definition of integrated governance is:

> Systems, processes and behaviours by which [organizations] lead, direct and control their functions in order to achieve organizational objectives, safety and quality of service and in which they relate to patients and carers, the wider community and partner organizations.[1]

The governance function of a board relies on it defining, within the organization's overall goals, its own purpose and strategic direction, with clarity of purpose, objective setting and planning of the annual business cycle. Successful integrated governance includes risk assessment and assurance arrangements, the use of 'intelligent' information, and committee structures and supporting arrangements that has clear terms of reference and clarity about expected actions and behaviours.[1] Behaviours are important because the culture of the board drives that of the organization: a board-level commitment to openness, transparency, honesty and accountability will help embed those values in the organization.

How do I assess organizational governance arrangements?

To assess how well an organization is assuring itself it is delivering its objectives, you should look to see whether these core components of governance are in place:

- a defined group of people, or person, responsible for the delivery of the organizational objectives (such as a board of directors, a chief executive officer, or an 'accountable officer')
- a written contract or similar document between the organization and its stakeholders or (for the public sector) the relevant government department (for example a Department of Health)
- rules or procedures by which the organization operates
- systems for collecting, monitoring and acting on information about the delivery of the organization's objectives.

It should be possible for any individual working within an organization to track his or her responsibilities through the management structure directly to the accountable officer—this is the line of accountability. When the line of accountability is unclear an organization cannot be confident that failures in the system can be escalated to a higher managerial level, and ultimately to the Board, for resolution. The process by which the Board assures itself that its objectives are being delivered will rely on these lines of accountability and escalation arrangements working properly.

Corporate governance

Corporate governance is the mechanism by which an organization can demonstrate it has systems in place to manage its corporate functions, such as its financial and business processes, and its assurance systems. One example of recommended best practice in corporate governance is contained in the seven principles of public life documented in the Nolan Report in the UK:[2]

- *Selflessness:* holders of public office should act solely in the public interest. They should not act in order to gain financial or other benefits for themselves, their family, or their friends
- *Integrity:* holders of public office should not place themselves under any financial or other obligation to outside individuals or organizations that might seek to influence them in the performance of their official duties
- *Objectivity:* in carrying out public business, including making public appointments, awarding contracts, or recommending individuals for rewards and benefits, holders of public office should make choices on merit
- *Accountability:* holders of public office are accountable to the public for their decisions and actions and must submit themselves to whatever scrutiny is appropriate to their office
- *Openness:* holders of public office should be as open as possible about the decisions and actions they take. They should give reasons for their

decisions and restrict information only when the wider public interest clearly demands
- *Honesty:* holders of public office have a duty to declare any private interests relating to their public duties and to take steps to resolve any conflicts arising in a way that protects the public interest
- *Leadership:* holders of public office should promote and support these principles by leadership and example.

Putting good corporate governance in place

If you are undertaking work for an organization, for example a health needs assessment, service review, or research, you should be able to define the *line of accountability* for the work through to the top of the organization.

You may need to put these structures in place to ensure adequate ownership and accountability. You will need to understand whether you or your group have *delegated authority* to make decisions. Your group could be a working or steering group that reports to a formal subcommittee of the organization's board of directors or management board. You should write *terms of reference*, which include the following:
- name of group or committee
- purpose of group (including any delegated powers or executive function) and whether it has a defined lifespan
- membership (including who will chair the meeting)
- accountability and reporting arrangements (if the structures are complicated a diagram may be appended to the terms of reference showing the links through to the board of directors)
- frequency of meetings
- how many members and of what type will be required for a decision, for example, 'three out of five members of the group, of whom one must be clinical'
- administrative arrangements (for example, who will take the minutes; how far in advance of meetings papers will be sent out; when draft minutes will be made available after the meeting)
- when the terms of reference will be reviewed (for example 'annually from the date of adoption').

You should ensure you have sufficient information to assess the issue and make sensible recommendations. You must also ensure there is sufficient challenge in the process so you do not produce work that may be unduly criticized.

Understanding the timescale is important as your own work plan may need to be constructed backwards from a particular date, for example when the board receives your work. You should be clear what action you expect of them. Will they be approving it? Does it have financial or wider service implications that need to be considered?

Good quality minutes with clear action points will help in providing an audit trail for actions and ensuring that all tasks are completed by the deadlines set. Action points should define:

- the action to be undertaken
- who will be responsible for completing the action
- the date by which the action needs to be completed.

(See also 📖 Developing leadership skills, 📖 Effective meetings.)

Clinical governance

Clinical governance provides 'a framework through which [health care] organizations are accountable for continually improving the quality of their services and safeguarding high standards of care by creating an environment in which excellence in clinical care will flourish'.[3] Lack of effective clinical governance can have dire consequences (see Box 7.1.1).

Box 7.1.1 Case Study: Independent Inquiry into care provided by Mid Staffordshire NHS Foundation Trust, England, January 2005 – March 2009, chaired by Robert Francis QC[4]

Robert Francis QC was asked by the UK Secretary of State for Health to chair an inquiry into the poor standard of hospital care at Mid Staffordshire NHS Foundation Trust during the period 2005–2009. He noted the appalling experiences of patients were the result of problems that had existed in the Trust for a long time and were known about by those in charge. A constant theme at the Trust was the perception it had lacked effective clinical governance. One comment from a witness (page 244 of the report) indicates the lack of proper governance in place in the Trust:

... there was no effective governance. There was a very poor flow of information. It was very poor information anyway, there was muddled data collection, there were very complicated incomprehensible structures of committees and it was very unclear which committee reported to which or what the functions were. There were few terms of reference. I mean I could go on.

Good clinical governance relies on clarity of strategic direction, clinical and managerial leadership, and reliable systems in just the same way as corporate systems. Clinical governance has a number of components:

- clinical effectiveness
- clinical audit
- risk management (including learning from incident reports and complaints)
- continuing personal development
- user/patient experience
- value for money
- research and development.

Quality can drive change and clinical governance sits at the heart of the integrated governance agenda.[5] Some components of good clinical governance involve monitoring or supervision to ensure the quality of services is measured including assessing the nature of the interventions, the performance of the staff carrying out those interventions, and the environment in which interventions are delivered. It should be possible to detect both good and poor performance through data monitoring. Structure, process and outcome measures may all be useful but you should remember that some of the most significant failures in clinical governance occur when insufficient emphasis is placed on outcome monitoring.

In addition to regular monitoring there is a developmental aspect to clinical governance that applies the principles of continuous quality improvement to the system. The cycle of improvement occurs when repeated learning is applied to the system, and this includes staff members demonstrating improvements in their own practice.

Clinical effectiveness

Clinical effectiveness is the application of evidence-based practice and relies on an understanding by the practitioner of the quality of evidence for a particular intervention or technology and its generalisability on the basis of the reasearch to that particular setting. The quality standards may take the form of guidelines but still form the basis of expected good practice by a particular professional.

Clinical audit

Clinical audit is the process of measuring clinical practice against a given set of standards for clinical care. The audit cycle is the mechanism by which adjustments are made to achieve these standards and re-measurement can occur to demonstrate the improvement in care. A link can be made with health equity audits, which measure, on a regular basis, the closure of the gap in unmet need to achieve equity in health status as defined by a health needs assessment (see 📖 Improving equity and 📖 Assessing health needs).

Continuing personal development

Linked to clinical audit, continuing personal development (CPD) is the process by which professionals or practitioners are able to apply their learning to ensure safe practice and drive improvements in quality. CPD incorporates incorporating training, education and learning from incidents or complaints

User/patient experience

No assessment of quality of service provision is possible without an understanding of the perception of the customer (see also ▣ Health care process and patient experience). Dimensions that should be assessed include being treated with respect, being given sufficient information about the service, and meeting expectations in relation to the intervention and to any personal care received. There are standard tools available for the measurement of patient experience, such as those produced by the Picker Institute (⅍ www.pickerinstitute.org), whose principles for patient-centred care are:

• respect for patients' values, preferences and expressed needs
• co-ordination and integration of care
• information, education and communication
• physical comfort
• emotional support and alleviation of fear and anxiety
• involvement of family and friends
• continuity and transition
• access to care.

Value for money

Any judgement about the quality of a service must take into account value for money. An integrated governance approach links this directly to financial objectives.

Research and development

As part of a quality improvement process, research and development adds to the knowledge base and influences future practice, improving the quality of care. It is subject to its own governance arrangements, as there is an ethical dimension to research which requires additional safeguards (see the ▣ Research governance).

Research governance

Research governance involves a series of principles, requirements and standards for research, and how those standards will be monitored and assessed. The intention of research governance is to safeguard the public and researchers by enhancing ethical standards for research, reducing adverse incidents and generating learning opportunities, promoting good practice, and forestall any problems which might arise through poor performance or misconduct.[5]

Information governance

Information governance provides safeguards and systems for personal and patient information and has four main components:

• information governance management
• confidentiality and data protection assurance
• information security assurance
• information quality assurance.

Information governance will incorporate legal frameworks for the use of information and be defined in codes of practice that govern how those data are managed and accessed. It will include the storage and handling of personal and patient information, on paper or electronically, including the transfer of information by email.

Confidentiality is a cornerstone of health records management. Personal and private information should only be shared on a 'need to know' basis – see Box 7.1.2 for an example of how this has been handled within a health system.

Box 7.1.2 Ensuring confidentiality in the English NHS: Caldicott Guardians

In 1997 Dame Fiona Caldicott chaired a committee that made recommendations for regulating the use and transfer of person identifiable information between NHS organizations in England and to non-NHS bodies.[6] Health organizations must have a board member (known as a Caldicott Guardian) who has a specific responsibility for ensuring that patient confidentiality is safeguarded. The Caldicott Guardian works strategically to support the sharing of information where it is legally and professionally appropriate to do so and the functions of the role are set out in the Caldicott Guardian Manual.[7]

The *Caldicott principles* are:

- justify the purposes(s) of using confidential information
- only use it when absolutely necessary
- use the minimum required
- access should be on a strict need-to-know basis
- everyone must understand his or her responsibilities
- understand and comply with the law.

Risk and assurance

When setting organizational objectives the responsible body—for example, the board of directors—should regularly review the risks to achieving those objectives. To do this a process of risk assessment is used in which a judgement is made about the level of risk. This level of risk is assigned a numerical value which is the product of the product of the probability and the impact of the event. For example, being hit by a car when crossing a road as a pedestrian has a low probability but if it were to happen the impact would be high: it could result in death or serious injury. On a scale of 1–5 (where 5 represents the greater probability or impact), a probability of 1 and an impact of 5 would give us an overall risk score of 5.

Risk register

A risk register contains all the risks identified in relation to a project or an organization's functions. It can be ranked according to the product of the probability and the impact. The higher the risk score the more important it is to put in place measures to manage that risk. Not all risks on the risk register need to be reviewed by the highest level in the organization—it is common for a board of directors to only review risks that fall into a category of high or very high risk, relying on managers within the organization to review risks on a regular basis and to increase the risk score if necessary. This then escalates the risk to the appropriate level within the organization for review and, if necessary, management action. Effective systems of incident reporting and monitoring are also an important component of risk assurance.

Assurance framework

An assurance framework contains information about controls and mitigating factors that reduce either the likelihood or impact of the risk. An organizational control describes the part of the governance framework in place to help manage the risk, such as, a monthly report to the board of directors. A mitigating factor will be something that diminishes the risk (for example, plans to install a pedestrian crossing). A further assessment of risk can then be made according to the revised assessment of the controls and mitigating factors on the original risk. This is defined as the residual risk, and it is the residual risk that indicates the significance of the risk to the organization. The risk threshold is the level at which risks are escalated and each organization can define its own threshold depending on how risk averse it is.

Audit committee

Audit committees are a cornerstone of good governance. They are the place where the assurance framework is reviewed, including both the risks to the organizational objectives and the management action in place to control and to mitigate the risks. Internal and external auditors scrutinize aspects of the organization's functioning and produce independent assessment of compliance with any legal or organizational duties and of standards of conduct.

What questions should I ask about governance?

You can assess governance arrangements by asking questions about the organization, service (or function), for example:

- What organizational objectives relate to the service?
- Where does responsibility lie and what are the lines of accountability through to the highest level in the organization?
- How does the board assure itself that it knows what the service is doing and how well it is doing it?
- How is the service managed?
- What types of data are being reviewed?
- How reliable are these data and what do they really tell us about the service?
- Do they focus sufficiently on outcomes?
- How regularly does the board see this information?

- Are additional data available but not routinely reviewed (such as comparative data from elsewhere—'benchmarking'—or any trend analyses)?
- Have there been internal or external audits of the service or peer reviews that add to the knowledge we have?
- How is user or customer feedback about the service obtained and how is this taken account of in the board's assessment of the service?
- Does the organization regularly review the risks in this area? How does it do this?
- What evidence is there of action taken by the organization to control or mitigate (that is, reduce) risks? Are they effective?

References

1 Department of Health (2006). *Integrated governance handbook: a guide for executives and non executives in health care organizations*, Gateway reference 5947. Department of Health, London.
2 Lord Nolan (Chair) (1995). *First Report of the Committee on Standards in Public Life*. Public Appointments Commission, London.
3 Scally G, Donaldson LJ. (1998). Clinical governance is here to stay. *British Medical Journal*, **317**, 61–5.
4 Francis R (Chair) (2001). *Independent Inquiry into care provided by Mid Staffordshire NHS Foundation Trust January 2005 – March 2009*. Department of Health, London.
5 Department of Health (2005). *Research governance framework for health and social care*. Department of Health, London.
6 Caldicott F. (1997). *Report of the review of patient-identifiable information*. Department of Health, London.
7 Department of Health. (2010).*The Caldicott Guardian Manual 2010*. Department of Health, London.

7.2 Programme planning and project management

John Fien

Objectives

Programme management, through the coordinated development, implementation, and evaluation of a series of related sub-programmes or projects, is central to the efficient delivery of all public health services. This chapter draws from the project management and programme/project evaluation fields to provide a practitioner's guide to programme planning and project management. You may find it useful to read this chapter alongside 📖 Business planning.

This chapter covers:
- the relationship between programmes and projects
- the components of effective programme and project planning
- how to develop a programme theory and logic model for a project, and how to implement it
- ways of developing an evaluation strategy
- managing projects as part of a programme
- the attributes of an effective programme planner and project manager.

Definitions

You may hear any undertaking that requires people to organize effectively to a plan and achieve specific objectives loosely defined as a project and the terms 'project' and 'programme' are often used interchangeably. Here, we distinguish between them and refer to a project as a smaller and more discrete activity than a programme, which is a set of activities or projects, usually with multiple levels and work across two or more organizations. In other words, in a public health context:-
- a *project* has objectives for a particular group of people in a particular place in relation to a particular health target, often using a specific strategy
- a *programme* comprises an integrated suite of related projects for a wider group of people and often across a wider region, over a longer period of time, and involving multiple strategies and projects.

A programme may have a series of projects within it, and each project may need to have its own set of objectives and activities to ensure it is planned well and implemented effectively. Table 7.2.1 compares programme and project management.

Table 7.2.1 A comparison of programme and project management

Program Management	Project Management
Whole-of-organization focus	Section or department focus
Aligned to strategic vision and goals of the organization	Aligned to the strategy and objectives of the programme
Focuses on the interdependencies between projects and the complementarity and scheduling of deliverables across projects	Focuses on the deliverables, milestones and activities of a single project
Ensures consistent use of common processes across projects	Focus on application of programme processes within a single project
Risk spread across projects	Risks contained within a single project
Broad range of management, leadership and project management skills needed	In-depth project management skills required

Programme planning

Programme planning is key to successful public health campaigns. It involves identifying the most critical needs of stakeholders and partners and determining priority responses to them and may be based on the outcome of a health needs assessment (see 📖 Assessing health needs). When involved in such priority setting you will need to decide:
- what are most important activities to undertake
- how to complete these activities, and the steps involved
- how much time to spend on them
- what staff, financial and other resources will be allocated to them.

After priority setting

Following needs assessment and priority setting, the basic steps in programme planning include:
- Preparing a rationale or business case for the programme
- Developing a goal statement or aim for the programme
- Determining objectives by analysing the goal statement and breaking it down into workable 'chunks' around which projects and activities can be organized. Objectives describe the intended results for the targeted need and, as far as possible, should be measurable
- Designing projects by developing and resourcing specific methods and activities for projects that will lead to the desired results
- *Project scheduling*: this is normally the responsibility of individual project managers but programme managers are responsible for coordinating the development of project implementation plans to complement each other—the outputs and outcomes of one project can be the inputs to a related or subsequent project.

- *Programme evaluation:* making plans for monitoring and evaluating the programme on four levels (and sometimes more): as an on-going process within each project; as a summative or concluding assessment of each project; as an assessment of whether the overall outcomes and impacts of the projects have achieved the programme goal; and as a synthesis of the appropriateness of all projects and activities in the programme.

Managing a programme

Effective programme management structures and processes enable programme directors to support successful project managers.[1] Programme planning is the first step in programme management. Other aspects of programme management include:

- *Governance:* defining roles and responsibilities; ensuring an appropriate culture across the programme team; and co-ordinating oversight and feedback (see 📖 Governance and accountability).
- *Administration:* ensuring appropriate and rigorous processes for documenting all programme and project activities.
- Financial management and accountability.
- Personnel management and programme team culture (see 📖 Workforce)
- *Infrastructure:* ensuring appropriate workspaces, technology and related facilities to support the programme effort.

You will find these fundamentals of programme management discussed in more detail in programme management textbooks and other resources (see 📖 Further Resources, this chapter). You may find the *Gateway Review* materials produced by the UK Office of Government Commerce particularly useful.[2]

Project management

The logic of a project

Project management begins with the development of a logic model—or theory—of what will make the project work. Figure 7.2.1 shows the logical links between the original problem, our inputs, and the outputs, outcomes and impacts you seek.

You need to think about evaluation at the same time you plan a project because this helps clarify:

- *Inputs:* the resources of time (labour), funds and other resources you have to invest in a project
- *Outputs:* the activities you plan and implement to achieve your results and the participation level that is needed
- *Outcomes:* the short- and medium-term results you seek. *Short*-term outcomes are usually expressed in terms of what people will learn from their participation in activities; *medium*-term outcomes are usually expressed in terms of changes in what participants will be able to do following their learning.

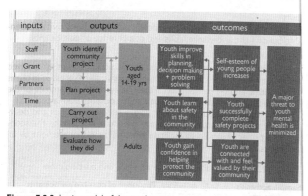

Figure 7.2.3 Logic model of the youth community engagement and emergency management project.

Project evaluation

Many people think project evaluation occurs when a project has been completed. This can be the case but to improve project and programme quality evaluation should occur throughout the project and provide information about progress. Projects are not linear and you need to monitor whether the logical causal links between inputs, outputs (activities and participation levels) and outcomes and impacts are performing as anticipated.

Logic models are helpful here as they can help you to:
- match evaluation to the planned results of the project
- understand what and when to measure. For example, are you primarily interested in process, outcomes, or both?
- focus on obtaining important information by prioritizing where you spend your limited evaluation resources.

The purpose of evaluation is related to its focus and timing. A number of related processes can be considered part of this, including needs assessment, system evaluation, and impact assessment (see 📖 Assessing health needs, 📖 Assessing health impacts, and 📖 Evaluating health care systems).

Potential pitfalls

Several conceptual and practical issues make programme and project management more complex than you might anticipate. First, the vernacular use of the terms 'programme' and 'project' often results in confusion when discussing specific professional activities – even books dedicated to these topics often use the terms interchangeably.

Second, a belief you should challenge is that programme planning and project management are common tasks that everyone can do. This is true in that we do use these skills every day but we are not all equally capable

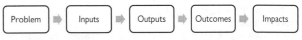

Figure 7.2.1 Steps in the logic of a project.

- *Impacts:* the long-term goals you seek to attain through the project. These are usually achieved at the programme level, rather than the individual project level because impacts take longer to achieve (and may not be realized during the lifespan of a project) and require the combined outputs and actions from several related projects (i.e. a programme).

Paying attention to these distinctions will help you ensure the causal relationships between outputs, outcomes and impacts are carefully thought through as a *hierarchy of objectives* that clarifies exactly what the project will need to achieve and in what sequence. These relationships are usually represented in a logic model, which is a visual or diagrammatic way of explaining why and how you believe a project will work as you plan, implement and evaluate it. Figure 7.2.2 illustrates the 'logic' of a youth leadership project through a series of 'if-then' relationships.

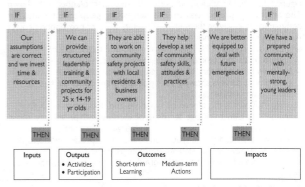

Figure 7.2.2 The 'if-then' relationships in a logic model of a youth leadership project in the area of emergency management.[3]

Constructing a logic model

Problem analysis

The key skill in problem analysis is distinguishing between the causes and symptoms of a perceived problem. Many projects fail because they focus on symptoms rather than causes. For example, one symptom of youth disengagement in a community—a growing concern in youth mental health—might be increased levels of anti-social behaviour (such as vandalism and petty crime). If a community perceives this as a problem and initiates a campaign to prevent anti-social behaviour it risks failing to recognize root causes and may increase youth disengagement and anti-social behaviour.

Research involving social mapping, surveys and focus groups as well as regular and honest community engagement is an important tool for identifying root causes and planning activities to address them rather than put Band-Aids on the symptoms (see 📖 Engaging communities in participatory research and action).[4,5]

Assumptions

These logical relationships depend upon the *assumptions* you make about the resources available, the commitment brought by organizations and clients to a project, and your reasons for believing the planned activities will work in a particular community. For example, the logic model in Figure 7.2.2 is for an adolescent mental health project planned in MyTown. The aim of the project was to integrate young people better into the community by engaging them in a community disaster prevention project. Assumptions involved include:

- many adolescents in MyTown feel isolated due to the lack of opportunities for community engagement and service
- MyTown lacks a history of organized youth volunteering despite local government surveys showing young people want opportunities to show community leadership
- while MyTown is threatened by typhoons and flooding every wet season, and climate change seems to be increasing their severity, most households and small businesses lack emergency evacuation plans
- easily accessible, donated space can be found for project workshops and emergency services staff are available as trainers
- young people have time to be involved during long summer holidays.

External influences

As well as being aware of our own assumptions about a project you need to take stock of the social, economic and political factors in the community that can act as positive and negative external influences. This is the context of the project, and involves seeking answers to questions such as: What are the potential barriers and/or supports that might impact the change you hope for? What skills and assets in the community can be drawn on? Are there policies or other factors that could affect the programme?

Inputs

Project inputs include everything you need to invest in the activities tial to building the knowledge, skills and competence of participants.

Outputs

Project outputs are the staged activities for particular groups of invo people that you plan and implement. Outputs are usually expressed in ter of (i) activities, and (ii) participation. Table 7.2.2 provides examples of t wide range of activities that could be part of the outputs from a project.

You can express outputs as a work plan, a set of milestones and deliv erables, or a Gantt Chart. Such tools are important not just for the scop ing of the project but also to facilitate effective time-management by all participants.

Table 7.2.2 Project outputs: sample activities and participation

Sample activities	The range of possible participants
Survey community attitudes	Clients
Conduct a workshop	Business associations
Make a website	Service clubs
Network with others	Neighbourhood groups
Build coalitions	Government agencies
Meet with politicians	Decision makers
Train staff and volunteers	Policy makers

Outcomes and impacts

As explained above, the logic of a project requires a connection between short-, medium- and long-term results (see Table 7.2.3). A sample logic model of the youth project described above is shown in Figure 7.2.3.

Table 7.2.3 The logical connections between short-, medium-, and long-term results of the youth engagement project

Short-term outcomes	Medium-term outcomes	Long-term impacts
Young people improve skills in planning, decision-making and problem-solving	Young people demonstrate leadership skills	We have a prepared community with mentally strong, young leaders
Young people learn about community emergency management	Young people successfully complete safety projects	We are better equipped to deal with emergencies
Young people gain confidence in helping protect the community	Young people are connected with and feel valued by their community	Community cohesion and neighbourhood social capital are built

at planning and logistics. When you have had the benefit of working with a professional project manager a few times you may wish you could have one as a life-coach! Developing a programme theory and a logic model based upon a hierarchy of objectives for a project, all held together by a strategy for evaluation, involves specialized rather than intuitive skills.

Finally, the best advice on programme planning and project management comes out of the evaluation literature. This means the most effective programme and project planning often begins with thinking first about evaluation. This is because thinking about the results you want is the only real way of planning a strategy for achieving them. As the famous baseball catcher and coach Yogi Berra once said, 'If you don't know where you're going, how are you gonna know when you get there?'

Conclusion

Getting programme planning and project management right is central to effective public health practice. Ensuring a sound and feasible hierarchy of objectives and a logic model that relates needs assessment to inputs, activity, and participation outputs can help ensure the desired outcomes and impacts are achieved and are logical consequences of all you do.

The 📖 Further Resources section, below, deals with ways of using the logic model approach to project management as well as issues of project initiation and scheduling, building staff capacity for effective implementation, financial controls, process and output monitoring, and project closure.

Further resources

Centers for Disease Control and Prevention (multiple dates) *Manuals/assistance with specific evaluation steps – logic models.* Available at: ℘ http://www.cdc.gov/eval/resources/index. htm#logicmodels (accessed 18 November 2011).

Centre for Health Services and Policy Research (2004) *A results-based logic model for primary health care.* University of British Colombia, Vancouver, Available at: ℘ http://www.ncbi.nlm.nih.gov/ pmc/articles/PMC2906214/pdf/policy-05-033.pdf (accessed 12 November 2011).

University of Wisconsin (2010) *Enhancing program performance with logic models.* A free introductory e-course (and downloadable PDF version also). Available at: ℘ http://www.uwex.edu/ ces/lmcourse/#

WK Kellogg Foundation (2004). *Evaluation handbook.* Available at: ℘ http://www.wkkf.org/knowledge-center/resources/2010/W-K-Kellogg-Foundation-Evaluation-Handbook.aspx   (accessed 18 November 2011).

References

1 For more on programme planning and management, especially in public health organizations: McNamara C. (2003). *Field guide to non-profit design, marketing and evaluation.* Authenticity Consulting, Minneapolis.

2 Office of Government Commerce (OGC). (2010). *UK successful delivery toolkit; and OGC gateway review pack.* Available at: ℘ http://webarchive.nationalarchives.gov.uk/20100503135839/ http://www.ogc.gov.uk/programmes_and_projects.asp (accessed 18 November 2011).

3 WK Kellogg Foundation (2004) Using logic models to bring together planning, evaluation, and action—logic model development guide, p. 3. Available at: ℘ http://www.wkkf.org/knowledge-center/resources/2006/02/WK-Kellogg-Foundation-Logic-Model-Development-Guide.aspx (accessed 18 November 2011).

4 Wadsworth Y. (2011). *Do it yourself social research*, 3rd edn. Allen & Unwin, Sydney/Left Coast Press, San Francisco.

5 Wadsworth Y. (2010). *Building in research and evaluation: human enquiry for living systems.* Allen & Unwin, Sydney/Left Coast Press, San Francisco.

7.3 Business planning

Mike Gogarty

Objectives

This chapter will help you:
- understand the fundamentals of business planning
- develop an effective business case.

Why is this an important public health issue?

To be an effective public health practitioner you need to be able to secure funding for initiatives and interventions as well to influence and support proposed developments likely to impact on the wider determinants of health. This includes understanding and fully participating in cross-agency corporate thinking; if public health is not central to this it is unlikely it will be effective.

Definitions

Business planning or operational planning is the way an organization agrees how it will use the limited resources entrusted to it. The resulting plan usually covers a single financial year. New investment in the plan is often the sum of business cases that determine how and why developments should be resourced.

What informs the content of the business plan?

An organization should have a very clear strategy of which staff are aware and that has a few clear high-level goals defining the organization's direction of travel. Public health practitioners need to be aware of the strategy and work to secure its goals.

Departments of public health may be part of organizations that commission health services, provide health services, or have some other function. Whatever the case, business planning is crucial to determining how public health objectives are to be delivered within available resources.

The business plan defines how resources will be used over the next year to deliver services, health gains, and outcomes, and is informed by:
- the strategic goals of the organization
- national targets, plans and objectives the organization must deliver
- formally agreed prioritization that will be more or less robust
- political considerations
- pressures and demands arising from changing political and health needs and emerging technologies
- the level of resources available.

Developing a business plan

Identify 'must do's'
The things an organization 'must do' may arise from national political imperatives, unavoidable service pressures, and changes essential to accommodate shifting demand for services. Financial commitments made in previous years are usually considered in this growth but resource-constrained organizations need to identify non-essential areas where disinvestment may free up resources to be used elsewhere.

Consider the opportunity to deliver the organizational strategy
Delivering organizational strategy is of key importance but you will often find deliberate progress tempered by the need to achieve a plethora of 'must do's' within very limited resources. Often there are few resources left to progress schemes in this area, although every effort should be made to deliver strategy and align resources with this.

Work with providers/budget holders
You should share, as early as possible, information about how much money is available, what the likely cost pressures are within the system, and what developments you wish to see. A clear understanding of the organization's strategy, priorities, and financial pressure will help you develop a realistic plan.

Decide the priority of discretionary developments
The organization should have a robust, widely shared and widely owned prioritization process that has been developed with local stakeholders. Public health is well placed to lead on this work. This prioritization process should be applied to any proposals for development that may be funded in addition to the 'must do's'. These could be prioritized before you know what resources are available but often need to be revisited to 'reality check' in the light of available funds.

Be clear about the realities of investment and disinvestment

Your business plan must be financially robust. You may encounter pressure, particularly when resources become tight, to move investment from current 'tried and trusted' (but potentially inefficient) services into more innovative cost-effective models of care. This is appropriate but you need to be clear about what resources will actually be released and how they will be used. There is a potential danger that savings will be over-estimated and not realized from the service where disinvestment occurs and that the assumptions around the promise of the new service may be optimistic.

Consult

Consulting with those likely to be involved with implementing a service change, or affected by it, is good practice. Failure to consult with the right groups or individuals may lead to barriers to or delays in the implementation and uptake of service change (see also 📖 Partnerships). In addition, consulting with stakeholders on changes in services is often required by local or national policy.

Developing a business case

Unless ideas and thoughts can be turned into health gains for the population you serve, public health will be ineffective. Skills in writing and presenting a business case are crucial to securing resources to deliver changes (see also 📖 Effective writing).

Your business case explains what you propose and why it should be funded. You will need to set out clearly how your proposal will deliver health improvement, release resources, and/or improve the quality of services. You will need to make the best case you can to secure limited resources in competition with other business cases. Your case is most likely to be successful if the following issues are addressed.

Relevance to organization

Your business case should:
- fit with the organization's strategy—and this link should be made explicit
- complement the evolving business plan in terms of delivering a national 'must do' or addressing an identified recognized gap in service or poor quality service
- recognize the broader financial climate:
  - when resources are plentiful services can be more focused on optimal target achievement and health improvement
  - when resources are tight a focus on ideas that produce a return on investment by releasing resources elsewhere will be required.

Robustness of the case

Effective public health business cases should:

- Be supported by evidence of effectiveness or a consideration of generalizability. This is certainly not always the case within organizations and public health practitioners have a role in challenging colleagues around these issues to ensure best use of limited resources
- Define the problem to be addressed. Public health practitioners are well placed to define and quantify population health needs using available data
- Be affordable and represent value for money. This may be defined in terms of cost of adverse health events prevented or release of resources elsewhere in the system such as hypertension management in older people to prevent cost of stroke admissions.

Ownership

It is important you have support for your case from key decision makers and opinion formers, including clinicians and politicians:

- Clinical support is always helpful in developing a business case; depending on the subject of your business case, it may be crucial to developing the case and securing its success. Support may come from clinicians in primary or secondary care. You may find it helpful to identify clinical champions and ensure they are engaged and informing the proposals
- Engaging with politicians will play a greater or lesser role in the preparation of your business case depending on the context in which you are working. In some public health organizations key decisions on policy, strategy, and direction are developed and agreed by elected politicians; if this is the case where you are then engaging them appropriately is likely to be important to the success of your business case.

Flexibility

To be successful flexibility is helpful—it may be that certain points of your case require reworking, or less funding may be available than you require. Sometimes there are ways to work around such difficulties: for example, if funding is inadequate a simple solution would be to try and negotiate a later start in the year for the full scheme with the understanding that all costs are available the following financial year. You may have to consider whether reducing the size of your scheme may be possible while still realizing many of the benefits.

Content

The business case should include:

- strategic context
- health needs

- evidence base
- objectives and benefits
- costs, capital and revenue
- workforce implications
- timetable—what will be achieved by when
- wider impact and implementation
- evaluation and outcomes
- possible sources of funding, e.g. national bid, local funding, grants
- risk assessment, e.g. funding, recruitment
- procurement process.

Appraisal of other options will be required if major investment is undertaken.

How will you know if you have been successful?

In the short-term it will be clear if you have been successful: you will have secured funding for public health work or been able to influence other proposed developments in a way likely to have a positive impact on the broader determinants of health. In the medium- or longer-term the initiative or intervention should be evaluated in order to inform and improve future business plans.

Further resources

Bryson JM. (2011). *Strategic planning for public and nonprofit organizations: a guide to strengthening and sustaining organizational achievement*, 4th edn. Jossey-Bass, London.

De Geus A. (1997). *The Living Company*. Nicholas Brearley Publishing, London.

UK Local Government Improvement and Development Agency. (2011). *Developing a Business Case for Health*. Available at: ✏ http://www.idea.gov.uk/idk/core/page.do?pageId=14121508 (accessed 12 October 2011).

Flanagan N, Finger J. (2003). Planning. In: *The management bible*. Plum Press, Toowong, Queensland.

Gericke C, Kurowski C, Ranson MK, Mills A. (2005). Intervention complexity—a conceptual framework to inform priority setting in health. *Bulletin of the World Health Organization*, **83,** 4.

Handy C. (1993). *Understanding organizations*, 4th edn. Penguin, London.

7.4 Partnerships

Julian Elston

Objectives

This chapter should help you understand:
- what is meant by partnership
- how national and local contexts influence partnership
- what processes and interactions are key to partnership success
- how to develop partnership and achieve collaboration
- key elements of success and the signs of a faltering partnership.

Why this is an important public health issue?

Partnership working has become a way of life in public health in recent years. It seems there is no escape from the many policy documents, directives and dictates encouraging, if not mandating, health organizations, local government, and the voluntary sector to work together to improve population health, reduce health inequalities, and enhance the quality of health and social care services.

Working in partnership is seen as an alternative to bureaucratic or market modes of delivering services, improving the co-ordination, effectiveness and efficiency of services whilst increasing their responsiveness to users' needs. Working in partnerships also has the potential to generate novel approaches to public health problems. Their participative approach to decision-making enhances legitimacy of solutions and provides greater local accountability.[1]

Many organizations and agencies have an important role to play in improving population health but may not recognize their role or see it as within their remit. Services provided by government-funded agencies are often designed around the needs of agencies rather than users or populations with the result that services are fragmented and unresponsive. Partnership working recognizes solutions to health problems are complex and cannot be solved by any single organization. It provides a means of joining up perspectives and resources from the outset in a co-ordinated and collective effort to improve outcomes.

Definitions

Partnership
- Is a mutually beneficial process by which stakeholders or organizations work together towards a common goal
- Involves the joint development of structures in which decisions are made, resources shared, and mutual authority and accountability exercised.

Partnerships differ with respect to the number and type of partners involved, the centrality of common goals to member organizations, the formality of structures and governing rules, the scope and quantity of resources mobilized, the degree of information sharing and reframing of the problem under scrutiny, the type of decision-making, and the extent of each partner's influence over decisions and the types of outcome attained. Table 7.4.1 sets out key criteria by which to distinguish different forms of partnership.

The objectives of partnership can be considered in terms of outcome and process objectives and it is important objectives are clear from the outset so appropriate structures and processes are developed to support them. Failure to do so may create unrealistic expectations, lead to dysfunctional relationships, weaken commitment and undermine performance. Table 7.4.2 compares the suitability of the different forms of partnership with achieving different types of outcome and process objectives.

Types of partnership

Partnerships may involve individuals, teams, professional groups, health and social care providers, and health and well-being organizations. They may:
- develop a project to tackle a specific health concern
- formulate a joint local health and well-being policy or strategy
- improve the co-ordination of information and human resources between providers
- improve the supply of goods and materials to support services
- improve service quality and responsiveness to user needs
- co-ordinate and govern a number of smaller partnerships.

Motivation for partnership working

Individuals, agencies or organizations need to recognize two key factors before engaging in partnership:
- their interdependence in tackling a health problem
- the potential mutual benefit arising from working together .

Without these, commitment to working in partnership will be weak, as partners cannot see the relevance to their work, only the immediate costs associated with participating. Partnerships mandated by government, in particular, face this difficulty, although this may be mitigated by the provision of incentives such as funding or greater freedoms and flexibilities to act, or sanctions for non-compliance such as reduced financial autonomy.

Influence of national context on partnership

The context of the partnerships in which you work is important. Health service and local government departments, for example, are subject to external influences at a national level with the potential to affect not only the structure and functioning of partnership but also its outputs and outcomes. Partners need to be aware of the impact of four influences: policy, resource flows, incentives and sanctions, and performance management.[2]

Policy

National policy is often incoherent, multi-themed and fluid, and thus can be detrimental to working in partnership. It is not unusual for government departments to work in 'silos' (rather than in partnership) and develop conflicting policy goals or multiple policy priorities. The focus of policy may shift as politicians respond to emerging social issues, leaving partners struggling to join up policy imperatives and targets or to decide which policies should take priority and which are no longer relevant.

Resource flows

The conditionality of resources, particularly (additional) funding, may influence the focus and outcomes of partnership. Ring-fenced funding may protect resources from being redirected but restrict the funding of innovative initiatives outside the usual remit of what would be considered 'health'. Pressure to spend funds within a financial year may lead to hasty decision-making while short-term funding may result in difficulties in recruiting and retaining suitable staff. Funding is rarely available to support partnership itself.

Incentives and sanctions

Incentives and sanction can enhance or undermine motivation to work in partnership and distract from shared aims. Relaxing organizational statutes or providing additional resources may entice more agencies into partnership but this risks attracting partners whose only interest is getting a piece of the funding pie, may require lengthy negotiations between multiple competing interests, and can lead to tokenistic involvement.

Table 7.4.1 Types of partnership working by key dimensions.

Type of partnership	Organizational vision	Goals congruity	Structural linkages	Rules and formality	Information/knowledge sharing	Resource sharing	Threat to autonomy	Decision-making	Mutual activity
Co-existence / competition	Individual perceptions	Own goals	None or market price signals	Own rules	Independent use	None	No threat	Independent	Non-mutual activity
Networking	Some shared perceptions	Own goals although some crossover	Transient, as required	Informal; based on cultural norms	Some knowledge sharing	Limited – on individual basis	Little threat	Consultative	Some mutual activity
Co-operation	Some shared perceptions	Own goals although some crossover	Few linkages in areas	No formal rules	Some knowledge sharing	Relatively few – requires lower grade officers	Little threat	Consultative	Some mutual activity
Co-ordination	Shared perceptions	Overlapping goals and aligned activities	Some vertical or horizontal linkages	Some formalization of rules	Sharing and joint interpretation	More resources involved – requires higher grade officers	More threatening	Joint (possibly unequal)	More mutual activity
Collaboration	Joint perception	Joint goals and supporting activities	Stronger vertical or horizontal linkages	Formal rules agreed	Sharing and reframing of problem	Resources pooled – requires senior officers	Significant loss	Participative (equal)	Novel, mutual activity

Table 7.4.2 Comparison of the suitability of different partnership forms to achieving different partnership objectives

Purpose	Partnership form			
	Networks	Co-operation	Co-ordination	Collaboration
Outcome objectives				
Information exchange or joint agreements	✓	✓✓	✓✓	✓✓✓
Developing a shared task or vision			✓✓	✓✓✓
Advancing a novel solution			✓	✓✓✓
Process objectives				
Empowerment and participation		✓	✓	✓✓✓
Power relationships		✓	✓	✓✓✓
Addressing conflict			✓	✓✓✓

Key: ✓ – well suited; ✓✓ – moderately suited; ✓– less well suited; blank – not well suited.

Performance management

Following the decentralization and privatization of many state services, many governments have turned to performance management as a means to influence the implementation of their policies by local agencies (see 📖 Translating evidence to policy on indicators and targets). In the context of partnership working, the scope, degree, and alignment of performance monitoring by different organizations may detract resources (time, effort, and energy) away from partnership, often at the expense of relationship building, problem-solving and decision-making. The pressure to report performance at set times can come at the expense of developing creative solutions.

Influence of local context on partnership

At a local level you will find partnerships are subject to five contextual influences that affect their development and functioning, and potentially their outputs and outcomes.[2]

Professional

Partnership working often involves multiple professional groups. Each will have its own perspective on health that shapes how its members think about an issue and propose solutions. The opinions of some professional groups may carry greater weight than others in discussions due to their higher status. Initial educational work with partners may be required to ensure partners understand why they have been invited, what they can contribute, and how they stand to benefit.

Cultural

Public, private, and voluntary sector organizations often have different cultures of management, decision-making, and public involvement. Health services typically have top-down, managerial, or professional decision-making structure. Local government organizations are influenced by local politicians in relation to deciding priorities and allocation of resources. Officers involved in partnership, although more used to democratic decision-making processes, may have limited capacity to act without consultation. Political elections can also result in a change in political leadership and policies, which may or may not favour partnership or its aims. Voluntary sector organizations, on the other hand, tend to have flat decision-making structures that facilitate consultation with their memberships. Partners need to understand decision-making may be slow, referential and protracted, otherwise expectations will be unrealistic and frustrations will arise.

Financial

Partners often have different financial arrangements and planning cycles. This can be challenging when determining budgets (which may be subject to different financial pressures and change) and planning actions. Larger, statutory organizations are more likely to absorb the human and financial costs of working in partnership whilst smaller, voluntary sector organizations may struggle, limiting their capacity to participate fully.

Relational

Besides working in partnership to tackle public health issues local organizations may have other relationships that make them dependent on each other for resources (i.e. goods and services). The symmetry of resource dependencies can influence how partners interact. The relative size of the resource exchange to the organization and the presence of alternatives may weaken a partner's influence and lead them to avoid conflict for fear of jeopardizing future access to resources. Voluntary sector organizations may be particularly vulnerable to this influence.

Structural

Organizations have different boundaries, procedures and financial arrangements. In some locations these are coterminous; in others, typically rural areas, they do not coincide. This may result in many more organizations having to be involved in the partnership, each with their own priorities and timelines. This can hinder consensual decision-making, particularly the development of a shared vision and joint actions.

Process in partnership

You will find partners are constrained by their own organizational contexts and have their own priorities and interests. Understanding the outcomes of partnerships means understanding three key elements relating to process in partnership:

- *Cognitive:* developing a joint appreciation of the problem (possibly involving reframing perspectives and understanding) and developing appropriate solutions.
- *Social:* understanding the social order of the group, i.e. the perspectives and interests of each partner (individually, organizationally and professionally) and the resources they bring
- *Managerial:* directing interaction in a systematic and purposeful way to achieve the aims of the partnership. This will involve jointly agreeing ground rules and governance mechanisms, as well as employing problem-solving techniques (such as brainstorming or more sophisticated techniques from operational research and systems science).

The nature of interaction

To work effectively in partnership you need to be able to influence others in relation to what should be done, who is going to resource, and how. Understanding how partners interact and how relationships develop is key to progress. In particular, you need to understand the nature and influence of power and trust in partnership and their influence on decision-making.

Power

There are three dimensions of power, each of which can be active in partnership.[3] The *first dimension* of power is influencing others to do what you want them to do, without coercion. The *second dimension* is limiting membership and/or what is discussed in partnership. The *third dimension* relates to wider social and economic forces that condition thinking about what could and should be done. Box 7.4.1 illustrates how and when power can manifest itself in partnership.

Box 7.4.1 Examples of power in partnership

- Who is invited or excluded from the partnership
- Who sets the agenda
- Which issues are 'kept off' the agenda
- How issues are conceptualized or framed
- Who decides how resources are allocated and who does not
- How decisions are made
- What type of solutions are developed and whose interests are served (individual, professional, organizational).

There are three key elements to the first dimension of power which need to be understood:[4]

- *Formal authority:* a partner's legitimate right to convene a partnership and influence decisions crucial to partnership, without directing others. This is particularly evident in partnerships mandated by government
- *Control over critical resources:* partners that provide critical resources can exert control over their use. These organizations can often dictate terms, the nature of interaction, and the type of partnership developed
- *Discourse legitimacy:* partners that speak on behalf of others (e.g. users' organizations or community groups) often have discourse legitimacy; that is, their influence comes from being seen as a legitimate voice of marginalized stakeholders or of a specialist body of knowledge.

How partners use these elements determines the structure and process of partnership and the nature of interaction. In partnerships with diffuse resources or symmetrical resource dependencies, decision-making is more likely to be marked by negotiation, compromise and resource pooling. If critical resources rest solely with one partner or dependencies are unbalanced, debate may be biased and decision-making imposed. This may lead to strife, disillusionment and withdrawal from the partnership (particularly if dependencies are imbalanced or weak).

Trust

Trust is the degree of assuredness that partners will do what they say they are going to do, and do it well. You must nurture trust for a partnership to perform.[5] Without trust, partners may fear others will exploit them opportunistically, leading to defensive behaviour. Lack of certainty or ignorance about how others will behave may lead to partners taking fewer risks and can impact on the development of innovation.

There is rarely a complete absence of trust between partners but levels may be low when a partnership is formed, particularly if partners have had a poor experience of working together previously. However, some partners may bring *goodwill trust*—an open commitment to keep to promises—or *competence trust,* a willingness to accept others will not only complete their actions but do so to a required standard. Organizational reputation is important for both but this initial baseline of trust can be diminished by poor performance, perceived lack of commitment, or inappropriate use of power.

The building and maintenance of trust is an on-going endeavour whereby small, successful outcomes reinforce trust, which in turn encourages partners to take greater risks. To achieve this you will need not only resources, but active management of:

- *Purpose of partnership:* clarity of aims, objectives, and partners' roles
- *Power imbalances:* sometimes not easy to recognize
- *Leadership:* without one party trying to taking over
- *Time:* for relationships and understanding to develop between partners
- *Workload:* it is shared evenly, i.e. partners do not feel exploited
- *Commitment:* differences in levels are resolved
- *Credit sharing for achievements:* important issue in the public sector.

Acceptance that working in partnerships takes some time before it starts performing – typically two to three years.

Pathway to developing partnership

There are four distinct steps to developing partnerships (see Box 7.4.2), during which each different process element will come to the fore and need to be managed. In reality, you may find individual steps need to be revisited at different stages of the journey.

Active participation by partners in debating the problem from a variety of perspectives is key. Conflicting views can lead to a reframing of perspectives and the development of a joint appreciation of the problem—a key process in the development of novel solutions. Ensuring conflict plays a positive role in partnership requires the process of interaction to be non-judgmental so views can be expressed openly and critiqued constructively without ridicule or personal comments, and all members must have an equal opportunity to contribute.[6] Having a trained, impartial facilitator can aid this process; conversely, abuse of power by individual partner can undermine it.

Achieving collaboration

This is the most difficult type of partnership to achieve, although potentially the most rewarding, as it can lead to synergy and innovation.

Box 7.4.2 Pathway to successful partnership

- Assessing the need for partnership:
  - Identifying stakeholders
  - Recognizing common interests and developing shared goals
- Building the partnership: clarifying roles and constructing relationships (trust, commitment, empowerment)
- Managing negotiations and social relations: agreement, implementation, and delivery
- Evaluating the partnership (processes and impact):
  - Feeding back and learning from the experience
  - Termination if successful.

Role of leadership

Effective leadership is essential to partnership working, helping to forge the vision, letting people know why they are there, and ensuring the process of partnership is managed effectively. Unlike organizations where leaders can use formal authority to get things done, leadership in partnership relies heavily on persuasion, charisma, temperament, and interpersonal skills. Networking abilities are important. Because of the potential for disruptive personality clashes to emerge, good facilitation and agreement on ground rules are important (see also 📖 Developing leadership skills).

Voluntary sector participation in partnership

Voluntary sector organizations are often key stakeholders and can provide insights into the nature of health problems. Most voluntary sector organizations operate on tight budgets with few resources so power to influence decision-making often resides in their discourse legitimacy. Voluntary sector involvement in partnerships can be undermined by:
• lack of resources and organizational capacity to engage
• partners not responding to their input—perceived lack of action can lead to disillusionment and disengagement ('consultation fatigue')
• lack of partnership/networking skills of non-experts/lay participants
• lack of skills of other partners to recognize these limitations
• lack of a long-term, public-sector strategy to develop the voluntary sector and support its involvement in partnership.

How will you know if you have been successful?

Look for the following:
• recognition of interdependence
• recognition of a stake in the outcome (mutual interest)
• development of and belief in shared vision and goals
• sense of commitment to the group and its objectives
• full participation and decision-making by consensus
• open expression of feelings and disagreements
• free flow of information and avoidance of jargon
• feeling of mutual trust/dependency
• resolution of conflict by members themselves
• mutual support and problem-solving
• 'enabling' and 'can do' approach
• implementation and delivery of actions to achieve outcomes
• critical and constructive self-evaluation.

What goes wrong with partnership working?

You may find working in partnership is ineffective or unproductive if:

- the wrong people attend i.e. people who cannot influence resource use in their organization or do not have a stake in the outcome
- too many people attend, making it difficult to manage a large number of conflicting views positively
- key partners lack partnership skills—problem-solving, negotiation, and management skills
- partners adopt defensive behaviour resulting in 'turf wars' over professional roles and boundaries
- discussions focus on resources, not outcomes
- performance is not periodically evaluated and deficits are not recognized or addressed.

📖 Case study: strategic health partnerships describes a case in which an attempt at partnership working was unsuccessful.

Case study: strategic health partnerships

Metrocity (anonymized location) is an urban area in England with a deprived and multi-ethnic population. In the decade following a change in government in 1997, national policy was to encourage local health partnerships to improve joint working across health and social wellbeing organizations and to provide 'joined-up' services. Areas with poor health were encouraged to bid for Health Action Zone (HAZ) status, which brought additional funding and greater legislative and administrative flexibility. Partnership was accompanied by a strong government emphasis on performance and delivery.

Metrocity, which had a history of joint working, secured this additional funding but development of the HAZ stagnated when senior managers turned their attention instead to addressing other demands stemming from national policies. Appointing a HAZ Director and secretariat re-energized the initiative and led to the development of structures, governance mechanisms, and some clarity of purpose. The Director provided leadership and the secretariat helped co-ordinate and administer the partnership. A review of progress identified a need to engage 'absent' stakeholders (voluntary sector, community organizations, and local hospitals) and this was achieved through workshops that improved understanding about partners' pressures, priorities, and ways of working.

A number of overlapping problems arose. Discussions about tackling local health issues were thwarted by government pressure to spend funds quickly. More time was spent fulfilling reporting requirements to secure continued funding than developing innovative initiatives. Some partners lost interest and became disengaged when their project ideas were not funded. Work to develop a local vision that incorporated the multiple and sometimes incoherent strands of national policy, partnership initiatives, and health targets proved complicated and challenging.

Efforts were also hindered by poor communication and a lack of clarity about decision-making and governance, a consequence of the large umbrella-style partnership structure designed to accommodate the broad agenda. Voluntary sector engagement was limited by a lack of resources (staff and time), despite their keenness to shape local services. A pre-election commitment by the majority local political party to reduce voluntary sector funding limited wider involvement and raised suspicion about partners' real commitment to listening to alternative viewpoints and developing innovative solutions. Partnership performance was also challenged as pressure to align spending towards national priority areas created disillusionment and a questioning

The Director responded by, first, developing a communication strategy intended to convey purpose and transparency to the governance structures and, second, organising further relationship-building events to bolster trust and commitment and to ensure all key stakeholders were still engaged. Despite these efforts, two years after formation the partnership was still struggling to identify and implement innovative initiatives, let alone deliver outcomes.

Misconceptions about partnership working

- Partnership is best for everything
- Partnerships are substantively different to other organizational forms
- Partnerships mean lots of multi-agency projects
- Partnership can be successful without specific resourcing.

Conclusion

You will find working in partnership to be a challenging, long-term enterprise but it has the potential to provide innovative approaches to public health problems. Partnerships work when partners commit time and resources, are open and transparent in their relationships, and seek to resolve conflict constructively.

Further resources

Guides

Wilson A, Charlton K. (1997). *Making partnerships work. A practical guide for the public, private, voluntary and community sectors.* York Publishing Services, The Joseph Rowntree Foundation, York.

Evaluation frameworks

Funnell R, Oldfield K, Speller V. (1995). *Towards Healthier Alliances. A tool towards planning, evaluating and developing healthier alliances*: Health Education Authority and Wessex Institute of Public Health Medicine ℛ Available online at: http://www.nice.org.uk/niceMedia/documents/towardshealthall.pdf (accessed 4th September 2012)

McCabe ALV, Skelcher, C. (1997). *Partnerships and networks. An evaluation and development manual*. Joseph Rowntree Foundation, York.

References

1 Glasby J, Dickinson H. (2008). *Partnership working in health and social care*, Better Partnership Working. Policy Press, Bristol.

2 Bridgen P. (2003). Joint planning across health/social services. *Local Government Studies*, **29**, 17–31.

3 Lukes S. (1974). *Power: a radical view*. MacMillan, London.

4 Hardy C, Phillips N. (1998). Strategies of engagement: lessons from the critical examination of collaboration and conflict in an inter-organizational domain. *Organization Science*, **9**, 217–30.

5 Vangen S, Huxham C. (2003). Nurturing collaborative relations. building trust in interorganizational collaboration. *Journal of Applied Behavioral Science*, **39**, 5–31.

6 Eden C, Ackerman F. (2001). Group decision and negotiation in strategy making. *Group Decision and Negotiation*, **10**, 119–40.

7.5 **Knowledge transfer**

Jeanette Ward, Jeremy Grimshaw, and
Martin Eccles

Objectives

Effective research transfer will ensure patients and populations benefit
from evidence-based best practice. While there is an increasing rigor
with which to approach research transfer in health care settings, greater
demand among those responsible for research transfer for a more scientifically sound knowledge base will accelerate development of the discipline.
There is greater recognition that research transfer requires sophisticated,
theoretically informed and phased designs.[1] Practitioners who seek to
transfer evidence into practice must work with these epistemological deficits as best they can.

Reading this chapter will help you to:
- identify and respond to situations that require research transfer
- apply a systematic approach to research transfer, learning from the
  work of others and planning locally in context
- contribute to a growing body of evidence about research transfer
  itself.

You may find it useful to read this chapter alongside 📖 Translating evidence to policy, which is focused more on the producers of research and
offers a complementary perspective.

Why is research transfer an important public health responsibility?

There is an increasing evidence base to inform and define 'best practice'
in public health. Unless health care professionals and public health practitioners know and apply evidence relevant to their work consistently, the
promise of health and medical research will not deliver better population
health. Information overload, pressures of work, contradictory policies and
other factors can result in troubling lag times between definitive research
findings and their consistent delivery in practice (Box 7.5.1). The population health gain inherent in more effective and efficient research transfer
affords public health a unique leadership role in getting research into practice wherever aspects of the health system are under-performing.

Box 7.5.1 Examples of failure in research transfer

Clinical[2,3]

Studies in different countries have compared current practice with best evidence. Treatments shown to improve survival are not always received by patients and there is persistent evidence that 20–30% of patients may receive unnecessary interventions or care that might be potentially harmful with no promise of benefit. Sub-groups of patients may miss out systematically on best-practice treatments such as women presenting with chest pain (gender bias in care) or ethnic minority patients diagnosed with cancer (see also 📖 Improving quality).

Public health[2]

Even in high-income countries, rates of participation in cervical screening can be as low as 55% in certain population groups. Studies of the frequency and quality of smoking cessation advice given by primary care providers to smokers repeatedly show poor preventive practice.

A systematic approach to research transfer

You should endeavor to take a systematic approach to reducing the gap between 'best practice' based on evidence and the care actually delivered. There are three interrelated stages to such an approach:

- *identifying* the magnitude and importance of this gap and prioritizing research transfer within your organization
- *developing* an implementation plan for research transfer with particular reference to 'research about research transfer' relevant to your circumstances
- *evaluating* the impact of research transfer and publishing your results to help others.

Identifying and prioritizing gaps between evidence-based 'best practice' and current practice

Situations where deliberate research transfer is needed include:

- suboptimal or inequitable population health outcomes shown by surveillance, performance or health equity audits, or needs analyses to reflect inadequate uptake of evidence
- critical event analysis suggesting specific problems in health care delivery
- stakeholder or professional opinion perceives discrepancies or gaps between evidence and current practice that can be confirmed
- publication of definitive new evidence, systematic reviews, or evidence-based guidelines that invite improvement on documented current performance.

To prioritize your efforts to get research into practice consider these questions:

- What is the magnitude and distribution of suboptimal population outcomes? Does this arise from available knowledge not implemented in practice or other decisions in policy or resource allocation?
- Could research transfer achieve better population outcomes?
- Where is health gain most likely if research transfer is effective?
- What are the local, regional, and national health priorities?
- Is there sufficient momentum for local initiatives to enhance research transfer?

Answering these questions will help you to prioritize manageable topics for local research transfer. Once prioritized, a systematic approach to implementation can proceed.

Developing an implementation plan for research transfer

Creating local coalitions for action

From the outset, research transfer requires collaborative leadership, a mandate for change and coordinated action by a range of local organizations and health care professionals at relevant levels.[4,5] If you can create a local multidisciplinary coalition of stakeholders and engage them actively in planning you will improve the chances of achieving successful research transfer. Such coalitions may not already exist – and may require significant commitment to engender (see 📖 Partnerships). Creative thinking with due attention paid to local politics, power-bases, and steady champions for 'best practice' is critical.

Developing local evidence messages

Clearly answer the question 'What is the evidence that should be transferred?' Doing this will force you to articulate the evidence-based best practice that you seek to promote in a clear, compelling message. Be ready to be challenged about the level of evidence and interrogated about why this research needs to be applied in practice. Be clear about benefits for patients and communities, sharing how you envisage successful research transfer in terms of behaviour and outcomes.[5]

Systematic reviews summarize entire bodies of evidence relevant to a clinical condition or public health challenge. As research evidence synthesized in a systematic review is usually not presented in a format easily accessible to professionals, consider derivative formats such as guidelines, decision aids, or actionable messages for local consumption that remain 'true' to the evidence collected and synthesized in the systematic review. Local adaptation of a systematic review can be undertaken by an engaged multidisciplinary group with adequate technical and administrative support and this is the kind of group your local coalition might aim to mobilize (for an example, see Box 7.5.2).

Box 7.5.2 Example of a local multidisciplinary coalition to implement guidelines about referral of patients with microscopic haematuria

- General practitioners
- Urologist
- Nephrologist
- Anaesthetist
- Theatre nurse
- Specialist nurse
- Public health specialist
- Manager
- Patient (consumer) representative(s).

Identifying barriers, readiness for change, and previous approaches to research transfer relevant to your context

Thorough analysis of local barriers and facilitators alongside an enumeration and description of target audiences will be needed to inform your implementation plan. By establishing the primary target audience you will have identified the relevant professional groups whether clinicians, public health practitioners, or senior health bureaucrats. Bear in mind there are likely to be different barriers and facilitators operating at distinct levels (Box 7.5.3). Individual professionals in any target group may vary in their preparedness for change and face different barriers and facilitators. Furthermore, different 'segments' of the target audience may be identified and need different implementation approaches.

A variety of methods can be used to elicit information about barriers to evidence-based practice, such as informal discussions with key professionals, purposeful qualitative research (focus groups), and representative surveys.[3,6] Accurate assessment of barriers to evidence-based best practice is crucial.[6]

Box 7.5.3 Barriers to evidence-based practice

Determine barriers by considering five organizational levels:
- *Within the health care system:* for example, methods of reimbursement may inadvertently present perverse incentives to professionals counter to evidence-based best practice.
- *Within the health care organization:* for example, inappropriate skill mix in the hospital or an organizational culture that does not embrace purposeful change.
- *Within local professional peer groups:* for example, desired behaviour change counter to prevailing norms and attitudes.
- *Within individual professionals:* for example, individuals are not up-to-date, lack skills to perform a procedure, or have little awareness of better referral pathways and others' skill sets.
- *Within professional–patient consultations:* for example, within busy consultations professionals may overlook important items of care.

Choosing strategies

An evidence base has emerged over the last several decades that, while less complete than we might wish for, is an essential first reference point from which strategies can be identified and selected for research transfer. Continual updates of evidence to inform how best to transfer research in different contexts are produced globally through the Cochrane Effective Practice and Organization of Care Group[7] (Box 7.5.4).

Box 7.5.4 Cochrane Effective Practice and Organization of Care (EPOC) Group[7]

This international group undertakes systematic reviews of the effects of:

- professional interventions (e.g. continuing professional development, quality assurance strategies, audit, and feedback)
- organizational interventions (e.g. multidisciplinary teams, practice systems)
- financial interventions (e.g. reimbursement mechanisms)
- regulatory interventions (e.g. statutory requirements).

Reviews and the specialized register are published in the Cochrane Library. Abstracts are open access.

There are no 'magic bullets' in research transfer: interventions might be effective in some circumstances and none are effective under all circumstances.[8] Thoroughly research your strategies, interrogating the existing evidence for their effectiveness in a manner akin to that of a clinician interrogating the evidence base for a new drug or treatment before offering it to a patient. The risk of harm is considerable.[2] Other useful sources of strategies include the Canadian Health Services Research Foundation and the Institute of Knowledge Transfer (UK). Read relevant journals, such as *Implementation Science*.

Myths, fashions, and fads plague research transfer. For these reasons, efforts are underway to provide taxonomies, descriptors and standardized terms for strategies that might be used in research transfer (see ⅋ www.interventiondesign.co.uk). Be explicit in your implementation plan about your theoretical approach, your assumptions about the professional mind-set and your choices (are they theoretically driven, pragmatically determined, or simply selected according to what is affordable at the time?). In general, your choice of strategy should reflect your analysis of barriers (see Box 7.5.4), the available evidence about the effectiveness of strategies if tested in circumstances comparable to your own, resources available to you, and other practical considerations.

Consider:

- Political and macro-policy interventions for reform may be necessary if the barriers relate to the overarching health care system
- Specific organizational interventions may be necessary if the barriers relate to the local health care organization
- Approaches involving social influence (local consensus processes, educational outreach, opinion leaders, marketing, etc.) may be useful when barriers relate to local professional peer groups

- Audit and feedback may be useful when health care professionals are unaware of suboptimal practice and to reinforce change
- Traditional educational approaches may be useful where barriers relate to health care professionals' knowledge, skills, and attitudes; in general, interactive educational activities are more likely to lead to research transfer
- IT solutions such as electronically generated reminders as tested in highly computerized academic health science centres show promise in chronic disease management
- Patient-mediated interventions when barriers relate to information processing within consultations, especially tools for sharing evidence such as patient decision aids
- 'Push' strategies deliver to practitioners whereas 'pull' strategies are those whereby practitioners themselves seek out research. Long-term partnerships between practitioners and researchers have also been recommended as a platform for research transfer[9]
- Strategies used to transfer research to public health practitioners and policy makers include evidence portals and 'knowledge brokers' but should be adopted with caution.[10]

Research transfer requires adequate resources for the development of local evidence messages and implementation activities so you will benefit from seeking out others who share your goals. For example, quality improvement units or departments within hospitals may include individuals with appropriate technical skills to support development and implementation of local guidelines. Performance management in large organizations can reinforce fundamental principles such as evidence-based practice. Document your choices, your reasons and your trade-offs. Your implementation plan should be a succinct, engaging document from which roles and responsibilities can be tasked.

Evaluating impact and contributing to a better understanding of research transfer

Metrics by which to evaluate research transfer ought to encompass both process and outcome indicators. You might evaluate participation and activities, or intermediate outcomes such as practitioner knowledge or changes in clinical behavior such as treatments, prescribing, or counseling practices in recognition of the longer-term, downstream population outcome. Resources and access to large population datasets might permit measures of 'downstream' population outcomes. This is especially useful if measures are unobtrusive and routinely collected.

Adopt a constructive, collaborative approach when developing the evaluation section of your implementation plan, explaining why you have selected specific outcomes for tracking and evaluation. Invest time to find or create sound instruments for evaluation; explore academic interest in your work; include quantitative and qualitative methods. Wherever possible, consider sophisticated evaluation designs as you will likely find others who share the continuing frustrations of the limited evidence currently available to inform research transfer. Implementation research is the scientific study of methods and strategies to promote the uptake of research findings.[6] This body of scholarship must grow if population health is to improve and, as part of this, evaluation design should aim to produce results that will be locally or generally applicable.

Key points

- Public health practitioners are well placed to facilitate implementation of research findings.
- Systematic reviews which convey the totality of evidence are better foundations for 'best practice' than enthusiasm for individual studies.
- Implementation strategies used in research transfer should align, with insights garnered from previous implementation research, local contingencies, and available resources.
- Reference to 'implementation research' is crucial and implementation of evidence, for public health as in all sectors, should itself be evidence-based.
- Greater reference to theory and a systematic, disciplined approach will deliver better research transfer by building its own evidence base.

References

1 Michie S, Fixsen D, Grimshaw J, Eccles M. (2009). Specifying and reporting complex behavior change interventions: the need for a scientific method. *Implementation Science*, **4**, 40.

2 Muir Gray J. (2009). *Evidence-based healthcare and public health: how to make decisions about health services and public health*, 3rd edn. Elsevier, London.

3 Grol R, Wensing M, Eccles M (eds) (2005). *Improving patient care. The implementation of change in clinical practice*. Elsevier, London.

4 Grol R, Baker R, Moss F (eds) (2004). *Quality improvement research: understanding the science of change in health care*. BMJ Publishing, London.

5 Nutley SM, Walter I, Davies HTO. (2007). *Using evidence: how research can inform public services*. Policy Press, Bristol.

6 Straus S, Tetroe J, Graham I. (2009). *Knowledge translation in health care: moving from evidence to practice*. Wiley-Blackwell, Oxford.

7 Cochrane Effective Clinical Practice and Organization of Care Group. (2010). Available at: ℘ http://epoc.cochrane.org/epoc-reviews (accessed October 2010).

8 Grimshaw JG, Thomas RE, MacLennan G, *et al.* (2004). Effectiveness and efficiency of guideline dissemination and implementation strategies. *Health Technology Assessment*, **8**, 1–72.

9 Lavis JN. (2006). Research, public policymaking, and knowledge-translation processes: Canadian efforts to build bridges. *Journal of Continuing Education in the Health Profession* **26,** 37–45

10 Mitton C, Adair C, McKenzie E, Patten SB, Perry BW. (2007). Knowledge transfer and exchange: review and synthesis of the literature. *Milbank Quarterly*, **85,** 729–68.

7.6 Health, sustainability, and climate change

David Pencheon, Sonia Roschnik, and
Paul Cosford

If not us, who? If not now, when?

(Attr. various)

Objectives

This chapter will help you understand the relationships between health, health care, sustainability, climate change, and carbon reduction, locally and globally.

The specific objectives of the chapter are to help you:

• *Make the case for action* by showing how health, health care, sustainable development, and climate change are linked positively such that what is good for mitigating climate change is also good for health and health care today

• *Translate science into policy and practice* and help move research and action about climate science into policy and practice

• *Engage a wide range of stakeholders* and appreciate that, as in much public health practice, appropriate action comes from involving a diverse group of people through genuine engagement.

Our generation has a duty of care to people in our own communities and elsewhere in space and time and this involves addressing identifiable needs and promoting social justice. This chapter aims to help you fulfill that duty at a personal, organizational and professional level.

Definition of key terms

Sustainable development

This is 'development that meets the needs of the present without compromising the ability of future generations to meet their own needs.'[1] This definition should be extended to refer not just to time (the future), but also to place (people elsewhere in the world now).

Climate change, carbon reduction, and *sustainability* are not synonymous. Climate change is happening as a result of the use of natural resources with too little attention paid to the consequences, especially in terms of the greenhouse gases (predominantly carbon dioxide) emitted as a result.

We live in an increasingly resource-constrained world in an unsustainable way and the additional threat of irreversible and chaotic climate change only adds to urgency around this matter. Because this can add to the sense of hopelessness, denial and inaction, it is important to be positive about the future and ensure serious and coordinated action is taken *now*.

Why is this an important public health issue?

Like many threats to public health, climate change and lack of sustainability have the greatest adverse health impact on the most vulnerable communities.[2] Such communities often lack resilience and people there are particularly susceptible to disease and premature mortality. In a world where there are differences in life expectancy between countries such as Japan and Chad of 35 years[3,4] we should not tolerate health threats that increase this inequity. Older people are often the most vulnerable to sudden climate related events in countries where physical frailty is combined with poor care systems;[5,6] in poorer countries, children are particularly at risk.[7]

Sustainability is now framed as one of the pillars of health (care) quality, alongside and related to other dimensions such as safety.[8] The public health opportunity involves quantifying the benefits of taking action on health, security and prosperity in order to make the broad case for taking action, aligning environmental sustainability with financial and social sustainability: the 'triple bottom line'.[9]

Sustainable development is as much a way of thinking and behaving as it is a discrete set of interventions. To make it part of your public health practice means integrating it into health protection, health improvement and service delivery. How (rather than why) you can do this is contested and we need to ensure the uncertainties and research issues are acknowledged and addressed openly, honestly, and systematically (e.g. by continuing to develop and deliver an explicit research agenda).

Box 7.6.1 summarizes the key issues you should understand in relation to health, sustainability, and climate change.

Public health competencies needed

There are two important public health skills you will need to make the case for rapid and meaningful progress towards a sustainable world:
• generating, analysing, and presenting data and research
• engaging people in addressing the consequences and opportunities.

In practice this means being able to frame and reframe the challenges, the opportunities and uncertainties, and the definitions of success.

> **Box 7.6.1 Key issues for public health practitioners to understand:**
>
> - Mechanisms of anthropogenic climate change:
>   - energy from fossil fuel or renewables
>   - the role of food and water
> - Health effects of climate change on human health:
>   - direct local effects (heat wave, drought, flood)
>   - global effects (migration, biodiversity)
> - Relationship between adaptation and mitigation
> - Practical steps that can be taken at an:
>   - individual level
>   - organizational level
>   - national/international level
> - What health professionals[10,11] and health services[12–14] can do.

Measuring progress consistently and repeatedly is a crucial part of the process. We tend to value what we can measure rather than measure what we value, and we need to measure at regular intervals to assess the rate of progress. We often use metrics such as life expectancy, QALYs, and DALYs (see 📖 Economic assessment), but sometimes we need to use other equally (and often more) meaningful indicators of progress. Success criteria may include dignity, community engagement, participation, and empowerment (see also 📖 Assessing health impacts). Some measures exist (such as the Happy Planet Index, which 'reveals the ecological efficiency with which human well-being is delivered'[15]) and are being seriously considered by world leaders.[16]

To be successful in all of this you will need to use techniques to frame the issues in ways that make sense to a broad range of people (on framing see also 📖 Media advocacy for policy influence). This requires you to understand issues of concern to stakeholders and that there are many perspectives from which issues can be seen, including:

- individual, community, business, government
- funder, regulator, commissioner, provider
- organizational, professional, patient, public.

You also need to understand issues of change management in relation to behavioural change or cultural change; top-down, bottom-up and from middle management; incentivization; and emotional reactions to evidence and need for change.

You will find it easier to help people and organizations change if you can present them with a compelling vision of how much better things can be. This emphasizes the importance of a vision of what this better future can look like and narratives of how we can get there. Such scenarios are not predictions but descriptions of trends that help people ask good questions, address the most important uncertainties (e.g. via research), and frame realistic plans.[17]

People do not take the threat of climate change and the opportunities of sustainable development seriously if respected people like health professionals do not do so visibly themselves. Health professionals need to show they consider this to be one of the if not the pre-eminent health risks of the twenty first century in visible ways.[11,18] Health care may be getting less carbon intensive but there is much more health care happening so the absolute impact is greater. Moreover, many of the gains (e.g. via combined heat and power plants in large hospitals) are hidden from view. Just as in the changing role of tobacco in the more industrialized world, health professionals can make a significant contribution through research,[19] direct, peaceful action, and through example.

From our experience of engaging health care organizations in England we have found the priorities that appeal to leaders in large health care organizations, and which a sustainable approach can help deliver, are:

- saving resources (human capital and money[20])
- improved governance (complying with regulation and legislation)
  (see 📖 Governance and accountability)
- protecting and enhancing reputation
- delivering resilient services (the capacity of a system to absorb sudden and unpredicted disturbance and still function)
- protecting and improving health (especially exploiting the opportunities of health co-benefits).

Three key areas on which to focus in sustainable approaches to public health

Focus on promoting early action by multiple groups

Sustainable development is related to other major public health issues such as inequalities and social justice. The issue of sustainability and health resembles emergent public health challenges of the past in that:

- it is relatively new
- it is rapidly developing and has a contested evidence base
- it involves closely interrelated technical, policy, and behavioural issues
- action is needed before the whole picture is clear
- there is no obvious end point of success.
- there is no magic bullet and it is not a single issue.

There are multiple opportunities to be exploited and risks to be avoided through early action by professionals, by governments, by individuals, and by health services.[21] In addressing these you should remember two important principles:

- Do not focus all your effort in one area (e.g. policy or practice or research). Those embarking on programmes of large scale change must recognize that large organizations, such as those in the health sector, are complex adaptive systems that behave in unpredictable ways.[22]
- Do not focus on efficiency gains alone. There is a limit to what you will be able to achieve in this way. Improving efficiency is necessary but insufficient. It is important to have a broad approach to both efficiency (doing the same things with fewer resources) and transformational

change (revisiting the objectives of the organization and meeting them in radically different ways).[23]

Focus on co-benefits and common interests

Public health action is rarely successful if its practitioners are seen to be pointing fingers and instilling guilt. Fortunately, in the area of health and sustainability there are multiple co-benefits for health. You should address these as a priority instead of focusing entirely on trade-offs and compromises. Co-benefits for health from work on sustainability and climate change exist at three levels: individual health, health care organizations, and global health (see Box 7.6.2).

> ### Box 7.6.2 Three levels of health co-benefits from addressing sustainability and climate change
>
> - *For populations:* more physical activity, better diet, improved mental health, less road trauma, less air pollution, less obesity/heart disease/ cancer, greater social inclusion.
> - *For patients and the health care system:* more prevention, care closer to home, more empowered / self care, better use of drugs, better use of information and IT, better skill mix, better models of care.
> - *For people in poorer and less resilient societies:* the adoption of economic systems such as Contraction and Convergence that distribute resources (such as carbon credits) equitably amongst the world's populations.

At each level there are both short- and long-term benefits. The most obvious examples are in the ways we eat (a low-carbon diet, low in intensively raised animal products, and high in fruit and vegetables is good for human and environmental health, now and in the future) and the way we move (a more active lifestyle improves physical and mental health now, reduces air pollution and transport trauma, improves social cohesion, and reduces reliance on high carbon transport systems) (see also 📖 Influencing international policy).

Focus on adapting, mitigating and developing resilience

If you want to play a part in preparing your health system for future opportunities and challenges (especially those relating to sustainability and climate change), it is important that you understand the role of adaptation and mitigation, the relationship between them, and the need to address both of these intimately inter-related approaches. If adaptation is managing the unavoidable then mitigation is avoiding the unmanageable.

Mitigation involves acting to reduce our contribution to the causes of climate change. Adaptation (*preparing* for the impact of climate change) is equally important and not just complementary but integral. It is dangerous to view the approaches as separate: they are both important parts of the same strategy. While individual disasters or incidents can never be specifically attributed to climate change there is good evidence climate change leads to increases in incidents of flooding, heatwaves, and changes in patterns of infection.

Flooding incidents create significant harm economically, physically, and especially psychologically to those affected. Heat waves, such as the one in central Europe in 2003 in which 30,000 excess deaths occurred,[5] have a particular impact on the elderly and most vulnerable who are least able to adapt physiologically, rely on robust social networks, or access equipment that will help them to cope with such stresses. Similarly, the potential for increases in infectious diseases (especially vector-borne diseases) such as malaria and dengue fever all require a public health response that predicts the likely impact, future pattern of diseases, and those most likely to be affected. Emergency preparedness must include sound planning to mitigate the impact of severe weather events, flooding, and heatwaves and their consequences (see 📖 Managing disasters and other public health crises).

Health systems and health professionals should be clear about their responsibility to maintain population size within the limits the available resources can support. Average family size should mean the total population does not exceed available resources, now and in the future. Although health professionals and systems should not prescribe family size they should make clear, through their policies and actions, that population size is a crucial determinant of our ability to maintain health for all, now and in the future.[24]

Sustainability and quality

Rather than seeing sustainability as an issue to be balanced and traded off against other issues such as money, safety and convenience, you should appreciate that it is the one dimension of quality that competes least with, and reinforces most of, the other dimensions (see 📖 Improving quality).[25] 'Any quality aims that cannot be maintained with the resources available to us are set up to fail. It is important to realize that working to improve sustainability will seldom be in conflict with the other dimensions of quality; in particular, low carbon health care is likely to improve cost efficiency and patient empowerment.'[26]

Quality (and change to achieve it) does not necessarily cost more. The initial investment may involve shifting cultures more than shifting budgets. Although there are inevitable transition costs these can often be absorbed by making savings elsewhere, for example from energy-saving or service re-design programmes.

Summary

As a public health practitioner you are well placed to bring about change by engaging stakeholders positively in a system-wide journey that exploits the robust evidence on the health co-benefits of making sustainable development a crucial principle of public health research and action in the 21st century.

Further resources

Charlesworth A, Gray A, Pencheon N, Stern N. (2011). Assessing the health benefits of tackling climate change. *British Medical Journal*, **343**, d6520.

Faculty of Public Health (2009). *Sustaining a healthy future: its time to take action on climate change.* Available at: ℜ http://www.fph.org.uk/sustaining_a_healthy future (accessed 30 October 2010).

Griffiths J, Rao M. (2009). Public health benefits of strategies to reduce greenhouse gas emissions. *British Medical Journal* **339**, b4952.

Hanlon P, Carlisle S, Hannah M, Lyon A, Reilly D. (2011). Learning our way into the future public health: a proposition. *Journal of Public Health (Oxford)*, **33**, 335–42.

Haines A, Wilkinson P, Tonne C, Roberts I. (2009). Aligning climate change and public health policies. *Lancet* **374**, 2035–8.

IPCC (Intergovernmental Panel on Climate Change) (2007). *Assessment Report 4 (AR4)*. Available at: ℜ http://www.ipcc.ch/ipccreports/ar4-wg1.htm (accessed 30 October 2010).

Pencheon D. (2009). Health services and climate change: what can be done? *Journal of Health Service Research and Policy*, **14**, 2–4.

Roberts I, Edwards P. (2010). *The energy glut: the politics of fatness in an overheating world*, Zen Books, London.

Stott R. (2006). Healthy response to climate change. *British Medical Journal*, **332**, 1385–7.

UCL Health Commission/The Lancet (2009). *Managing the health effects of climate change*, 15 May 2009. Available at: ℜ http://www.thelancet.com/climate-change (accessed 30 October 2010).

References

1 Brundtland GH. (1987). *Our Common Future*, The Brundtland Report: World Commission on Environment and Development.

2 Costello A, Abbas M, Allen A, *et al.* (2009). Managing the health effects of climate change. *Lancet* **373**, 1693–733.

3 World Health Organization. (2011). *World Health Statistics Report, 2011*. WHO, Geneva.

4 World Health Organization (2009). *World Health Statistics Report 2009*. WHO, Geneva.

5 Dhainaut J, Claessens Y, Ginsburg C, Riou B. (2004). Unprecedented heat-related deaths during the 2003 heat wave in Paris: consequences on emergency departments. *Critical Care* **8**, 1–2.

6 Semenza JC, Rubin CH, Falter KH, *et al.* (1996). Heat-related deaths during the July 1995 heat wave in Chicago. *New England Journal of Medicine*, **335**, 84–90.

7 UNICEF. (2011). *The $100 billion question: how do we secure a climate resilient future for the world's children?* UNICEF.

8 Wilkinson P. (2008). Climate change & health: the case for sustainable development. *Medical Conflict Survival*, **24(Suppl. 1)**, S26–35.

9 Elkington J. (1997). *Cannibals with forks: the triple bottom line of 21st century business*. Capstone, Oxford.

10 Gill M, Stott R. (2009). Health professionals must act to tackle climate change. *Lancet*, **374**, 1953–5.

11 Coote A. (2008). How should health professionals take action against climate change? *British Medical Journal*, **336**, 733–4.

12 Coote A. (2006). What health services could do about climate change. *British Medical Journal*, **332**, 1343–4.

13 NHS Sustainable Development Unit. (2008). *Carbon Reduction Strategy for NHS England*. NHS Sustainable Development Unit, Cambridge.

14 NHS Sustainable Development Unit. (2010). *Saving carbon, improving health; UPDATE NHS Carbon Reduction Strategy*. NHS Sustainable Development Unit, Cambridge.

15 nef (2009). *The Happy Planet Index*. Available at: ℜ http://www.happyplanetindex.org/ (accessed: 1 August 2011).

16 Cameron D. (2007). In praise of general well-being. In: Simms A, Smith J, eds, *Do good lives have to cost the Earth?* Constable, London.

17 NHS Sustainable Development Unit (2009). *Forum for the future. fit for the future. Scenarios for low-carbon healthcare 2030*. NHS Sustainable Development Unit, Cambridge.

18 Stott R, Godlee F. (2006). What should we do about climate change? Health professionals need to act now, collectively and individually. *British Medical Journal*, **333**, 983–4.

19 Doll R, Hill AB. (2004). The mortality of doctors in relation to their smoking habits: a preliminary report. 1954. *British Medical Journal*, **328**, 1529–33.

20 Coote A. (2002). *Claiming the health dividend, unlocking the benefits of NHS spending*. King's Fund, London.

21 Griffiths J, Rao M, Adshead F, Thorpe A. (2009). *The health practitioner's guide to climate change*. Earthscan, London.

22 Plsek PE, Greenhalgh T. (2001). The challenge of complexity in health care. *British Medical Journal*, **323,** 625–8.

23 NHS Sustainable Development Unit. (2011). *Route Map for Sustainable Health*. NHS Sustainable Development Unit, Cambridge.

24 Guillebaud J, Hayes P. (2008). Population growth and climate change. *British Medical Journal*, **337,** 247–8.

25 Haines A, Smith KR, Anderson D, *et al*. (2007). Policies for accelerating access to clean energy, improving health, advancing development, and mitigating climate change. *Lancet*, **370**, 1264–81.

26 O'Donoghue D. (2010). *Sustainability, the seventh dimension of quality*. Available at: ℘ http://renaltsar.blogspot.com/2010/05/sustainability-seventh-dimension-of.html (accessed 27 May 2010).

7.7 Workforce

Felix Greaves and Charles Guest

Objectives

Reading this chapter will help you:
- understand the internal and external influences on the public health workforce
- identify practical steps you can take to improve the public health workforce in your area.

Why is this an important public health issue?

Effective public health practice depends on the workforce. An adequate supply of well prepared public health professionals is essential for an effective public health system. That workforce needs education, training, development and motivation, and must be of a sufficient size and skill-mix. Maintaining and improving the workforce is an important role for public health practitioners and you should not assume this is a job for others (see also 📖 Improving your professional practice).

Definitions

- *Public health workforce* is the body of people working intentionally to improve the population's health. The workforce required to deliver public health is complicated and involves a diverse group with skills in health promotion, health protection, health systems, information management, and many other disciplines. It requires people who can work with communities at the frontline as well as those with the skills to influence decision makers in boardrooms and similar settings.
- *Public health specialists* have been through a specific training programme or accreditation process to ensure they have the relevant knowledge and skills and are regulated. There is normally a formal public health body at a national level that sets standards for membership, often through a defined training curriculum and examinations (see Box 7.7.1 for an example of a public health training system.)
- *Public health practitioner* is a more inclusive term (see glossary) that includes a wider range of workers. These workers may not be regulated or may have their regulation linked to their primary profession (such as nurse, doctor or dietician). They are essential to the running of public health systems.

- *Professionalism* is claimed by an increasing number of public health practitioners. Professional status includes responsibility for maintaining competence or skill based on scientific knowledge. Claims of professionalism also bring expectations of honesty, confidentiality, the avoidance of conflicts of interest, commitment to improving practice, and the exercise of accountability.[1]
- *Credentialling* of public health practitioners is considered differently around the world. The general aim is to increase focus on competencies that can measure work performance and educational achievement in content areas identified as central to public health practice.[2]
- *The human resources function* is the part of an organization responsible for managing the workforce. Its role is vital and wide-ranging yet it is often neglected. The human resources department is usually involved in:
  - selection and recruitment
  - training
  - monitoring staff performance
  - organizational design, including change management
  - employee relations
  - succession planning and leadership development
  - workforce analysis and planning
  - developing policies on pay and other issues.

Effective public health practice requires optimizing our partnership with and input into the human resources function.

Box 7.7.1 How does public health training in the UK work?

Public Health Specialists are recruited into a training programme from both medical and non-medical backgrounds. Trainees follow a defined curriculum and must demonstrate competence in a number of stated technical disciplines, as well as in particular knowledge and skills.

Training usually takes four to five years and may include an MPH degree. Progression is by yearly assessment of competences against this framework, and by passing examinations set by the Faculty of Public Health. Training takes place in a range of institutions, including local health care organizations, in health protection, in national organizations and in academia.

A national body, the Faculty of Public Health, sets out the competency-based curriculum. Qualified specialists engage in continuing professional development after their initial training.

Professional standards are maintained by registration with the General Medical Council for medical graduates and UK Public Health Register for individuals from other backgrounds.

What influences the workforce in your organization?

- *Politics:* national and regional governments play a role in determining the size of budgets, the degree of autonomy, and organizational structures in the public sector. Public health involves making controversial decisions about scarce resources and this attracts the attention of politicians. Although politicians often claim to support public health, the slow return on investment makes it vulnerable to cost cutting.
- *The changing demography of the workforce:* over time, the make-up and expectations of workforces change in response to broad cultural forces. Family and school experiences shape what we anticipate in our careers and how we expect to work. In many high-income countries Baby Boomers (born between 1945 and 1960) have a different perspective to Generation Y (born between 1980s and the early 1990s). The needs of the workforce will shift in keeping with these demands.
- *The changing demography of the population:* the nature of the local population affects the work of the public health workforce. Populations are changing and will continue to do so. In some countries, there are changes in the urban-rural distribution and ageing is a major cross-national challenge for the twenty-first century. With these changes come differences in disease distribution, such as increasing chronic disease prevalence. The local workforce must adapt to meet these needs.
- *Changes in the expectations of the population:* the health care sector is seeing an increase in consumer behaviours, rising expectations of customer service, and a reduction in respect for traditional professions. There is also a trend towards increased transparency of information, including availability of knowledge around performance of health systems and decision-making processes.
- *Reorganizations:* public health workforces and institutions are prone to frequent reorganizations and restructurings. The workforce may develop 'change fatigue' because of constant changes and this can lead to a loss of motivation and innovation.
- *Internationalization:* there is a tension between human rights and national and international interests for the public health workforce. In poor countries, valuable trained staff are often tempted abroad by the offer of salaries and better opportunities. Wealthy countries, aware they do not have to pay the cost of training these individuals, may actively recruit and welcome staff from abroad (see Box 7.7.2 and 📖 Chapter 4.7).
- *The public-private sector divide:* the limited public health workforce faces competing demands from the public and private sectors, and increasingly from NGOs. There are different levels of resources between sectors and thus different working conditions. This may lead to a drain of valuable human resources from one sector to another, with the public sector most at risk.
- *Regulation:* there is a move towards stronger regulatory structures in health care in many countries. These may affect public health workers, often in the form of increased workforce assessment (e.g. revalidation) and requirements for continuing professional development.

- *Internal culture:* the internal culture of an organization, including the values, beliefs, norms and customs contributing to its unique character, has a profound effect on the workforce. Some of this culture may be clear, such as expectations in a mission statement, but unwritten organizational rules, language and activities may be more important.
- *Workforce in related sectors:* the health care workforce in other sectors has seen changes in working practice, with working time regulation reducing working hours in many countries and a trend towards multi-disciplinary working. Traditional roles are changing across the sector with, for example, specialist nurses taking on increasing levels of responsibility.
- *Models of care:* the way health care services are delivered is changing. Increasing chronic disease prevalence and health care costs are leading to new models of care provision, including providing more treatment in the community. Technology offers opportunities for long-distance monitoring and improved communication. In many areas, there are changes in health insurance coverage and use, and other funding models for care are emerging. The public health workforce needs to respond to these changes and to build structures and skills that allow us to work across organizations and disciplines.

Box 7.7.2 The World Health Organization Workforce Practice Code

There is considerable variation in the supply of trained health care personnel in different countries. There is one doctor per 50,000 people in Malawi and one for every 405 people in Australia.[3]

In May 2010, WHO and its member states formally adopted a code on the international recruitment of health staff[4] that states:

Member States should strive, to the extent possible, to create a sustainable health workforce and work towards establishing effective health workforce planning, education and training, and retention strategies that will reduce their need to recruit migrant health personnel.

WHO Global Code of Practice on the International Recruitment of Health Personnel, May 2010

The adoption of this code, with its collection of procedural and institutional mechanisms for monitoring workforces, has been described by Taylor and colleagues[5] as a significant step towards improving international cooperation and maintaining the capacity of health systems worldwide. The practical effects of the code remain to be seen.

How can you improve the workforce in your organization?

Plan your workforce and think about succession

- *Think ahead:* study the workforce age profile and anticipate future shortages. Co-ordinate your training programmes to fill these gaps.
- *Plan succession:* continuity is important because it allows knowledge to be built up about an organization and how it works. Large corporations go out of their way to organize a planned transfer of power when people leave important positions. This should happen at every level of the organization. If you know people are planning to leave, create a plan to ensure handover of knowledge and skills.

Ensure opportunities for training and development

- *People value training and development opportunities:* training and development opportunities mean people are more likely to stay and help them do their jobs better. Training budgets are often limited and vulnerable to cuts. Use these budgets, protect them, and make sure time is available for training.
- *Consider developing a mentoring scheme for your staff:* this involves matching a less experienced member of the team with a more experienced mentor. The development of a long-term, two-way relationship is an excellent opportunity to provide transfer of skills and knowledge, and can be useful for both parties (see 📖 Improving your professional practice).
- *Coaching* for team members can provide guidance around skills and ways of working.
- *Think about alternative pathways to educational opportunities* such as short courses, continuing education programmes, and distance learning.
- *Ensure training is relevant:* some professional training is narrowly conceived and out-dated, and does not prepare those being trained to work in an increasingly multi-disciplinary and independent world.

Allow new ways of working

- *Think about how you can allow people to work flexibly:* allow your team the freedom to manage their own time as long as they deliver what is expected of them.
- *New technology provides opportunities to make health workers more efficient:* consider holding meetings by teleconference or allowing people to work from home.

Create an attractive organizational climate

- *People want to work somewhere pleasant:* Do junior team members feel able to speak up at meetings? What are the unwritten rules about how people behave? Identify the positive attributes of your organizational culture and enhance them. Identify the negative aspects and consider why they developed and how they can be removed (see also 📖 Developing leadership skills).
- *Work on your induction programme:* induction presents an opportunity to promote the positive aspects of your organizational culture.

Think more widely about the pool of available people

- *You may need to look outside the usual places to find the people you need:* there may be a 'hidden' workforce you might otherwise miss.
- *Try actively recruiting more mature candidates or those returning to the workforce after a career break:* bring in people from other sectors with relevant experience. If people have portfolio careers make the most of their range of experience. Wherever you find people, make sure you support them in their transitions to new roles.
- *Engage mature staff in dialogue* about how best to use their skills and knowledge and support them to plan their career path and retirement.
- *Think about adapting or offering different roles to more mature staff:* roles may need review and redesign to suit older people, which could include reduced hours, with more emphasis on training other staff.
- *Volunteers* present a potentially useful resource but must be carefully managed and resourced. They need administrative support, funds for continuing education, access to information, regular communication, and formal recognition programmes.[6]

Inclusive management

- *Ensure management involvement and support:* co-ordinating support from senior management through to middle and line managers across an organization allows access, opportunity and support to all workers, regardless of position or job type.
- *Communicate the aims and purpose of the organization consistently and effectively:* keep staff updated about changes or developments.
- *Make sure your team is involved in the planning process:* a participatory approach to project planning and implementation helps to create employer and worker ownership and longer-term success.

Promote staff health and wellbeing

- *Think about workplace health promotion programmes:* can you change the workplace to encourage the ideas we promote to the population? Could you introduce, for example, a cycle-to-work scheme or a healthy eating campaign in your workplace cafeteria?
- *Multi-component programmes* covering a variety of health-related issues ensures many behavioural risk factors are addressed and engages a greater number of workers with different preferences and health needs
- *Work with occupational health and safety initiatives* within your organization.

Rowe and Kidd[7] set out useful ideas for resilience that would promote health and wellbeing for us all. For example, we should:

- make home a sanctuary
- value strong relationships
- have an annual preventive health assessment
- control stress, not people
- recognize conflict as an opportunity
- manage bullying and violence assertively.

Motivation

Different people are motivated by different things. Theoretical models may be useful in thinking about what you can do to encourage your staff and keep them motivated – it's not just pay (although that is important). Use these theories to consider what aspects of working life could become sources of enthusiasm for your team (see also 📖 Developing leadership skills).

Maslow's hierarchy of needs[9]

This theory suggests there is a hierarchy of needs we seek to fulfill. These can be seen as a pyramid with the most basic needs at the bottom and social and intellectual needs closer to the top. Once one set of needs is fulfilled, according to the theory, people seek to fulfill the set above (Table 7.7.1).

Table 7.7.1 Maslow's Hierarchy of needs

Level of need	Example	What it might mean at work
Self-actualization	Self-realization, personal growth	Being innovative and creative
Esteem	Social recognition, self-esteem and accomplishment	Receiving that cherished promotion
Social	Being part of a group, friendship and intimacy	Having a group of friends to talk to every day in the office
Security	Protection, security, law	Having a contract and getting paid regularly
Physiological	Food and shelter	Having an office that is warm and dry

Herzberg's Motivation Hygiene hypothesis[10]

Herzberg distinguished between positive factors that motivate people and hygiene factors that need to be present or people will be dissatisfied. This theory is also called the 'two-factor model' of motivation.

The *positive factors*, or motivators, include responsibility, recognition, and challenge. These may make people actively enjoy their role.

Hygiene factors do not necessarily create satisfaction but their absence will lead to dissatisfaction. Examples include wages and job security.

In practice, employers need to think about getting both factors right. You need to provide the basics—job security, a decent workplace, and payment—but you also need to challenge your staff, make sure they feel respected, and validate their work in some way.

Team working

Public health practitioners rarely work in isolation and need to be able to work effectively in teams. These may be formal teams working within or between organizations or informal groups of people coming together to think about a problem.

Developing teams

Belbin[11] described a series of different team roles characterized by clusters of behaviour people adopt while working in groups. Each of these roles has its own strengths and weaknesses and to be successful Belbin suggested teams need the correct balance of these skills.

The team roles are:
- *Completer finisher:* makes sure things are polished and completed to a sufficient standard. A details person.
- *Coordinator:* focuses on objectives, delegates work, and achieves group consensus, often with a chairing role.
- *Implementer:* creates practical, workable plans and gets things done.
- *Monitor evaluator:* watches the process from an impartial perspective and makes rational decisions on objective data.
- *Plant:* comes up with bright ideas and creative thought.
- *Resource investigator:* networks and engages with individuals outside the team to get what is needed.
- *Shaper:* provides drive and challenge to make sure goals are achieved.
- *Specialist:* has specialist knowledge related to the subject area.
- *Team worker:* uses interpersonal skills to help the team work together as an effective unit.

To build an effective team, make sure you fill all these roles. Try to make sure there are no gaps, bearing in mind individuals can take on more than one role.

Team development

Truckmann[12] described a set of stages groups go through as they develop. You may find it useful to consider these as you work with people in a group:

- *Forming:* when a group first comes together aims are established and background information is shared.
- *Storming:* different ideas and solutions to the task are put forward and discussed.
- *Norming:* the team settles on an agreed goal and plan.
- *Performing:* the team works together to achieve the stated aim.

Future challenges

The actions of individual public health practitioners, choosing how we work and whom we recruit, will remain critical in defining our workforce. There will be significant future challenges, particularly in adapting the workforce to suit emerging models of health care. These will come from changes in demography, expectations, and technology.

It is important we continue to demonstrate the value of the public health workforce so we can ensure a constant supply of people for the many and varied roles required.

The ongoing problem of global health workforce stability poses a challenge of sustainability. An increased awareness of the issues, and acceptance of the ethical and logistic complexity involved, has led to significant steps forward from global institutions. The workforce presents a relatively neglected area in public health practice but is now subject to greater attention. (See Box 7.7.3 for an example of some of the challenges that arise when the workforce needs of a health care system are inadequately addressed.)

Box 7.7.3 A work force conundrum: NHS Commissioning in England

A substantial challenge in England for the public health workforce has been to commission local services for the NHS. Local commissioners have been responsible for spending more than £80 billion a year and the public health community is supposed to play a vital role in this process.

Many criticisms have been made about the underperformance of the system, including a lack of technical ability, silo working, and unnecessary duplication. A report by the Health Select Committee[8] in parliament found:

> Weaknesses are due in large part to PCTs' [Primary Care Trusts] lack of skills, notably poor analysis of data, lack of clinical knowledge and the poor quality of much PCT management. The situation has been made worse by the constant re-organizations and high turn-over of staff.

Paying insufficient attention to workforce planning, organizational design and staff training has, presumably, been part of the problem.

Summary

The existence of an effective public health workforce is vital to ensuring good public health. To create the public health workforce of the future you must understand and work with your colleagues in human resources. Public health practitioners will need the skills of leaders, managers, planners and team members to play a full part in delivering this workforce.

Further resources

Beaglehole R, Dal Poz MR. (2003). Public health workforce: challenges and policy issues. *Human Resources in Health*, **1**, 4.

Crisp N, Gawanas B, Sharp I. Task Force for Scaling Up Education and Training for Health Workers (2008). Training the health workforce: scaling up, saving lives. *Lancet* **371**, 689–91.

Website of the Global Health Workforce Alliance. Available at: ℗ http://www.who.int/workforcealliance/en/ (accessed 8 April 2011).

World Health Organization (2006). *The World Health Report 2006—working together for health*. WHO, Geneva.

References

1 Thistlethwaite JE, Spencer J (2008). *Professionalism in medicine*. Radcliffe, Oxford.

 2 Goldstein BD. (2008). Credentialing in public health: the time has come. *Journal of Public Health Management Practice*. **14**, 1–2.

 3 Mills EJ, Schabas WA, Volmink J, *et al.* (2008). Should active recruitment of health workers from sub-Saharan Africa be viewed as a crime? *Lancet*, **371**, 685–88.

 4 World Health Organization (2010). *Global Code of Practice on the International Recruitment of Health Personnel*. WHO, Geneva.

 5 Taylor A, Gostin L. (2010). International recruitment of health personnel. *Lancet*, **375(9727)**, 1673–5.

 6 Prabhu VR, Hanley A, Kearney S. (2008). Evaluation of a hospital volunteer programme in rural Australia. *Australian Health Review*. **32**, 265–70.

 7 Rowe L, Kidd M. (2010). *First do no harm: being a resilient doctor in the 21st century*. McGraw-Hill, London.

 8 House of Commons Health Select Committee (2010). *Commissioning*. Stationery Office, London.

 9 Maslow AH. (1943). A Theory of Human Motivation. *Psychological Review*, **50**, 370–96.

10 Herzberg F, Mausner B, Snyderman BB. (1959). *The motivation to work*, 2nd edn. John Wiley & Sons, New York.

11 Belbin J. (1981). *Management teams*. Heinemann, London.

12 Truckmann BC. (1965). Development sequence in small groups. *Psychology Bulletin*, **63**, 384–99.

7.8 Effective public health action

Chris Spencer Jones

Objective

This aim of this chapter it to help you to measure your progress towards creative and sustainable public health practice. It is intended to address the absence of criteria and standards against which to audit much of the wide spectrum of public health work and to help you improve your delivery of public health when faced with this absence.[1]

Definition

Effective public health action is the work you do to achieve desired public health outcomes. These outcomes must include some measurable improvement in health or a clear indication of likely possible benefit in terms of process. This handbook contains many useful and well-described tips on effective practice but competent work that does not lead to health improvement or improved health protection may not add value.

Many of us are measured already: academics in terms of publications, civil servants in terms of policy development, and practitioners in local settings through changes in routine population measures.

The tools offered to help us to be effective in achieving health improvement are generic. Though often well conceived they may lack an evidence base to justify them and public health practitioners need to be able to access and use a range of valid outcome measures, making use of peer review and external assessment. For commissioners of public health, effective public health needs to have an impact on a perceived problem.

Understanding success criteria in public health will help you not just evaluate what you do but also help you shift your efforts to where they are most beneficial. A useful question to ask ourselves and each other, when setting our agenda, is: 'If this endeavour were to be successful, how would we know?'

Deconstruct to reconstruct

Right task, right person, right time

You are responsible for ensuring the work you do will improve health. Your relationship with the objectives of the organization is two-way. You need to *shape* the objectives in the longer term as well as *meeting* them in the shorter term (see also 📖 Business planning). It is not unusual to be asked to take on ill-defined tasks that present a problem to somebody in a powerful position.

You need to ensure the right task is being performed (in the right way) by the right person at the right time. Use the check lists from Tables 7.8.1, 7.8.2, and 7.8.3.

The politics of effecting change is not something to be avoided in public health. Part of the work of public health practitioners is to change people's understanding, attitudes, opinions, and actions in a way that improves health.

Wherever you are working, as a capable practitioner you will need to be able to work effectively in a wide diversity of environments, with a wide variety of people and organizations, and with public health objectives kept in mind and prioritized over other objectives. This requires turning problems into tasks that are possible and that will create outcomes that are beneficial and definable (see Table 7.8.4).

Table 7.8.1 Right task?

Consider	Essential	Desirable
Opportunity cost	The work is likely to bring health benefits	There are health benefits available that can and will be measured
Management support	The work is supported explicitly by the public health department you are associated with	The organization you work for requests a plan, agrees on the plan, and supervises the plan
Work programme	The task fits into a portfolio of work that offers job satisfaction	At completion you will meet both personal and organizational objectives
Allies (see 📖 Chapter 7.4)	The people affected by the work expressed willingness to support the work	The people affected by the work are part of the commissioning process
Whether it can be done	There is an end-point that can be identified	The task is to change something specific—not the world!

Table 7.8.2 Right person?

Consider	Essential	Desirable
Your engagement	You were asked to become involved because you have competencies essential to progress the issue	You were consulted about the nature of the work from an early stage and are able to comment upon your contribution
Skill-mix (see 📖 Work-force)	The work can only be done if you possess or can access the required skills or can develop them effectively on the job	The task requires public health skills in proportion to the time you are requested to invest
Politics	Your involvement in this work strengthens your links with the people who make decisions affecting health	Your contribution is likely to be appreciated

Table 7.8.3 Right time?

Consider	Essential	Desirable
Timing	Your involvement is welcomed by key individuals	You do not have to push the door hard—somebody is holding it open for you
Timetable	Something is going to happen within an explicit timescale and this piece of work will influence events	A timetable is agreed at the start—that takes account of relevant external constraints
Timing of engagement	There is time to consider the value of your contribution	You can weigh up the benefits of involvement in the context of your own and your department's overall work programme
Product	The outcome of the work is anticipated by an audience	The product is of wide interest and perhaps publishable

Table 7.8.4 Criteria for excellent execution

Steps	Essential	Desirable
Problem into tasks	Definable blocks of achievable work	Every person relevant identified
Project planning (see 📖 Business planning)	A structured project plan endorsed by your department	Project plan endorsed by your organization
Engagement	Identify people who share common objectives	Share project planning with possible partners in action
Consultation	Project plan shared with key players following approval	Project plan agreed with key players in advance
Communication	Ensure everybody in your organization who acts in the same field is aware of develop-ments	Define a network of key players and interested parties and keep them informed
Project monitoring	Regular reports on progress to your department	Supervision by trusted colleague or mentor
Time keeping	Complexity of task matches timetable	Other relevant timetables identified
Record keeping	Details of all work undertaken kept separately	Annual report on activity of individuals

Organization for excellent execution

Achieving positive change requires careful forethought and preparation. Whenever a piece of work seems set to last more than a few weeks or take more than a few hours it is useful to define the work in terms of a project. When we are 'consulted' a less formal approach will suffice. A project should have a project plan, and be managed accordingly (see 📖 Programme planning and project management).[2]

Effective public health action is creative and proactive. Many of us work in a reactive environment with pressures that push us towards consultancy and away from defined projects. Whatever the circumstances you have to make the best of them, carrying a positive message and remaining focused on our objectives.

Even with careful commissioning, precise and careful planning, and deployment of adequate personal skills a piece of work may be unsuccessful. The major pitfalls and ways of reducing the risk of encountering them are shown in Table 7.8.5.

Table 7.8.5 Preventive action against pitfalls

Pitfall	Prevention
Under-estimation of complexity	Achieving change is complex. Detail the stages required to make change happen and the complexity soon emerges
Taking on too much oneself	Remember: in public health the highest standard is to involve others fully, not to do well only what you can do. We will have optimal impact when we work to gain the understanding and commitment of others
Expectations too high	A clear project plan with agreed aims, objectives, and methods overcomes this if circulated to all key people. It will tell them something useful is going to happen—even if it will not do all they seek
Lack of focus	Talk over what you are trying to achieve with somebody else. If it is still unclear then start from scratch. If it is somebody else's project then go back to them for clarity. If it still isn't clear then downgrade this work quietly, quickly
Undermining	Let facts, reason, and logic solve this one. Remain resolute!
Impossible	Look through the files and find out how many people have been involved in the recent past. If more than two other people have had a go already then assume you will do no better. Fresh soil is generally more fertile, though it may look harder to dig over!
Hurry and fudge	Difficult tasks can be done quickly, but complex tasks cannot. Differentiate and spell out complexity through a project plan. It is worth spending a couple of days to prevent taking on a complex task with inadequate time or resources
The boss mucks it up	It is his or her prerogative. Take it well and find a way of entering the event into the vocabulary of the department. It helps if you understand your boss. Do you always get it right? Humour sometimes helps!

What went wrong?

All these pitfalls cause us strain and stress. They are all common and you need to have the humility to take responsibility for our contribution. When you feel stress you need to identify the source and address it. In particular, when you are away from our known competencies it is best to consider yourself more as a trainee than as a practitioner, taking cautious steps under supervision.

If things are not working well you need help:
- Tell somebody it's not working—but not just anybody. Tell somebody who is in a position to help.
- Start asking people about their success stories. Ask them for tips.

- Identify on which criteria you are failing and on which competencies you are light.
- Consider whether you would benefit from supervision (or different supervision!).
- Is it you? If you think everybody around you is OK then it probably is not but if everybody else looks bad: what about you? Consider finding a mentor or paying a professional listener to listen to your story (see also 📖 Improving your professional practice).

Formal public health audit, with other members of your department or within a looser affiliation, is helpful. Together with self-reflective learning it is the best way to increase your effectiveness.[3]

Competencies

To fulfill the criteria for successful public health action you need all the public health competencies. In particular you need to be able to:
- deconstruct and reconstruct an issue
- plan in detail
- work with others—and make them work with your agenda
- win over other people
- reflect on your own work with honesty.

Key determinants of success

What really matters is that you make yourself useful or, ideally, indispensable. You have to contribute to agendas shaped by, and which matter to, the communities you serve. You must have a sense of responsibility for the work that you do; a sense not only that it matters but also a certainty it will achieve health benefits.
    Key determinants are:
- the right task at the right time
- planning and execution of plans avoiding pitfalls
- patience
- prioritization
- partnership working
- participation in the execution of one's own plans
- explicit goals
- reflection incorporated in action.

Personal effectiveness is very important, particularly leadership skills and complementary management abilities (see 📖 Developing leadership skills, plus 📖 Further Resources below).

How will you know when you have succeeded?

Public health outcomes are diverse. They can be 'hard', such as community action to address deprivation. They can be 'soft', such as clarifying what may need to be done to make specific improvements. They may be highly organized, such as instigation of a preventive programme. They may be *ad hoc*, such as clarifying evidence on effectiveness. They may be concerned with the wider public health agenda, such as advocacy on behalf of excluded communities. They may be concerned with the biomedical model, such as health service reviews. Table 7.8.6 summarizes the criteria of success.

Table 7.8.6 Criteria of success

People indicators	Activity indicators
Commissioners increasingly ask for work that seeks to achieve public health goals	Information and ideas developed by you and your colleagues are adopted by other people or agencies
Partners from other agencies build public health into their work programmes	Measurable health gains are linked to your initiatives
Our colleagues and seniors feedback, through a formal process of review, that we are working well	Acceptance by peer-reviewed journals of outputs from your work. Positive coverage in the media and successful input to radio or television

It is helpful to hold regular reviews, discussing issues using an agreed, structured approach. The preparation and implementation of an annual public health report provides a good opportunity to reflect on successes and failures.

Further resources

Landrum L, Baker S (2004). Managing complex systems: performance management in public health. *Journal of Public Health Management Practice*, **10**, 13–18.

Riley WJ, Parsons HM, Duffy GL, *et al.* (2010). Realizing transformational change through quality improvement in public health. *Journal of Public Health Management Practice*, **16**, 72–8.

Umble KE, Baker EL, Diehl SJ, et al. (2011). An evaluation of the National Public Health Leadership Institute—1991–2006: Part II. Strengthening public health leadership networks, systems, and infrastructure. *Journal of Public Health Management Practice*, **17**, 214–24.

Umble KE, Baker EL, Woltring C. (2011). An evaluation of the national public health leadership institute—1991–2006: part I. Developing individual leaders. *Journal of Public Health Management Practice*, **17**, 2–13.

Wright K, Rowitz L, Merkle A, *et al.* (2000). Competency development in public health leadership. *American Journal of Public Health*, **90**, 1202–7.

References

1 Richardson A, Jackson C, Sykes W. (1992). *Audit guidelines in public health medicine: an introduction.* Nuffield Institute for Health Services Studies, University of Leeds, Leeds.

2 Kerzner H (2009). *Project management: a systems approach to planning, scheduling, and controlling,* 10th edn. John Wiley & Sons, Hoboken.

3 Jacobs R, Gabbay J. (1994). *An action research report on audit in public health departments.* Faculty of Public Health Medicine of the Royal College of Physicians of the United Kingdom, London.

A chronology of public health practice

Charles Guest, Katherine Mackay, and
Felix Greaves

This book has sought to identify effective methods for modern public
health practice, building not only on past success, but also learning from
failure. Some past highlights are gathered here. Any historical summary has
an unavoidable arbitrariness: selection criteria for the following list cannot
be precise. The items included are, or were, clearly significant for practice, rather than the possibly simpler documentation of scientific advance.
Some dates are approximate: we have tried to avoid spurious precision.

- c. 2600 BC: evidence of covered drains in the cities of Mohenjo-Daro
  and Harappa in the Indus Valley
- c. 1500 BC: Old Testament (Leviticus): religious practices of the
  Hebrews, including cleanliness, disinfection, food and water protection,
  hygiene of maternity
- c. 700 BC: Assyrians build a 50-km aqueduct to provide water to the
  city of Nineveh
- c. 460–375 BC: Hippocrates, Greek physician (descendant of a
  hereditary guild of magicians), insisted on scientific methods, including
  clinical observation; prolific author whose Aphorisms and Airs, Waters
  and Places recognize the importance of climate, environment, and diet.
  The Hippocratic Oath still provides a widely observed ethical code
- c. 430 BC: first European account of a widely fatal epidemic (in Athens).
  Resignation and stoicism was the contemporary response, although the
  role of contagion was recognized
- AD c. 60: Pliny the Elder proposes, in his Natural History, the use
  of respirators to avoid dust inhalation (a hazard as ancient as the
  manufacture of stone tools)
- Medieval: lepers (probably including many without true leprosy)
  isolated from the general population, with uncertain public health
  effect
- 900s: hospitals established in the East
- c. 1000: early recorded systematic use of variolation (the induction of
  mild smallpox to reduce mortality) in China
- 1215: Magna Carta provides the foundations of human rights
- 1347–51: the Black Death spreads across Europe, with high mortality
  and social disruption
- 1377: initiated by Ragusa, Italian city-states are the first to develop
  practical methods to reduce contagion, including quarantine, isolation
  of the sick, and waste disposal
- 1500s: syphilis spreads rapidly through Europe. Sexual nature of
  transmission recognized; control measures include the examination of

prostitutes and social exclusion of sufferers. Rubbish collectors employed to clear away rubbish on the streets in a number of municipal authorities, a strategy that spreads across Europe by 1700

- *1546:* Fracastoro publishes his treatise *On Contagion*, clearly presenting the notion of infection as caused by minute infective agents
- *1556:* Georg Agricola publishes a treatise on mining, describing occupational diseases and possible prevention strategies
- *1600s:* filtration of water in France in households and the army. Variolation spreads to Africa, Europe, the Ottoman Empire, and the Americas
- *1662:* John Graunt analyses population data, publishing *Natural and Political Observations . . . on the Bills of Mortality*
- *1691:* William Petty publishes *Political Arithmetic*, including calculations of regional needs for hospitals and physicians
- *1700:* Ramazzini publishes the first comprehensive treatise on the health of workers
- *1717:* Giovanni Maria Lancisi links malaria with exposure to swamps, and particularly to mosquitoes
- *1742:* John Pringle claimed that disease was caused by the chemical emanations from decaying human wastes (miasma) and advocated the 'Sanitary Idea'
- *1753:* naval surgeon James Lind publishes *Treatise on Scurvy*, describing citrus fruit as effective prevention, based on empirical work
- *1765:* Manchester forbade the practice of drowning cats and dogs and washing dirty linen in its Shute Hill water reservoir
- *1775:* Percival Pott describes scrotal cancer in chimney sweeps, probably the first cancer associated specifically with an occupational exposure
- *1787:* Association for the Abolition of the Slave Trade formed
- *1796:* Jenner immunizes James Phipps with cowpox virus, demonstrating protection against smallpox, thus initiating vaccination
- *1830s:* cholera arrives in Europe
- *1839–42:* first Opium War in China, ending with the treaty of Nanjing. Western domination of China's treaty ports begins
- *1844:* Royal Commission on Health in Towns
- *1847:* Semmelweiss shows that child-birth fever is preventable by medical attendants washing their hands with chloride of lime, confirming the observations of Oliver Wendell Holmes and others
- *1847:* Edwin Chadwick's sanitary campaign results in the English Public Health Act
- *1851:* First International Sanitary Conference, Paris. European countries attempt consensus on international quarantine regulations
- *1854:* John Snow shows that cholera spreads through contaminated drinking water, developing theories from Thomas Shapter and others
- *1854:* Florence Nightingale and Mary Seacole's reform of nursing practice during the Crimean War reduces the death rates of wounded soldiers
- *1864:* Henri Dunant founds the Red Cross; first Geneva Convention
- *1870:* Pasteur devises the process for killing bacteria in milk
- *1882:* Koch discovers the bacillus causing tuberculosis. Subsequently, Koch, Pasteur, and others identify bacterial causes of many diseases, including cholera, diphtheria, and pneumonia

- *1899:* London School of Tropical Medicine founded, later expanded to include 'Hygiene' in all climates. Many schools of public health established during the twentieth century
- *1914:* Goldberger begins studies of pellagra in Alabama, eventually showing the disease is caused by nutritional deficiency
- *1914:* Ernest Codman evaluates the outcomes of surgical care in his hospital. He is later ostracized by the medical community in Boston
- *1918–19:* Spanish influenza pandemic
- *1921:* Marie Stopes establishes a birth control clinic
- *1925:* Ronald Fisher introduces the concept of significance testing in statistics
- *1928:* Fleming discovered the antibacterial effect of penicillin
- *1930s:* Eugenic extremism of the Nazi party in Germany
- *1939:* publication of the first major medical paper proposing a link between cigarette smoking and lung cancer in Germany by Dr F. H. Muller
- *1940:* Florey, Chain, and Heatley purify penicillin and demonstrate its clinical effect
- *1940s:* USA and Britain fortify foods such as margarine and flour with various vitamins and minerals, including vitamins A and D, calcium, thiamine, iron, riboflavin, and niacin
- *1945:* intervention trial, fluoridation of water to reduce dental caries
- *1946:* 61 countries approve the constitution of the World Health Organization, becoming a branch of the United Nations in 1948
- *1946:* United States Public Health Service establishes the Communicable Disease Centre, later the Centres for Disease Control and Prevention
- *1948:* National Health Service begins in Britain. Later many other European and Commonwealth countries institute state-provided assistance for medical care. Universal Declaration of Human Rights
- *1949:* Framingham Study—probably the best known cohort study of heart disease—begins, focusing attention on risk factors and prevention of chronic disease
- *1950s:* mass spraying of DDT in many countries initially proves a dramatic success in reducing malaria rates
- *1953:* Watson and Crick discover the structure of DNA
- *1954:* polio vaccine introduced
- *1958:* WHO launches the Eradication of Smallpox Program
- *Mid-20th century:* spread of hepatitis associated with the reuse of syringes
- *1960s:* developments in injury control, including seatbelts for motor vehicle occupants
- *1961:* cholera strain *eltor* appeared in Indonesia, eventually leading to crises in Asia, Africa, and the Americas
- *1962:* *Silent Spring* by Rachel Carson, an early influence on public understanding of environmental degradation
- *1964:* US Surgeon General's report *Smoking and Health*
- *1965:* Bradford Hill publishes criteria for epidemiological assessment of the causes of disease, developing postulates from David Hume, John Stuart Mill, Robert Koch, and others
- *1966:* Donabedian introduces the concepts of structure, process and outcome in healthcare evaluation

- *1970s:* Yaws (*Framboesia tropicana*) largely eliminated by massive treatment programmes with penicillin
- *1971:* Julian Tudor Hart describes the inverse care law in which need and supply of healthcare are inappropriately matched
- *1972:* Cochrane's *Effectiveness and Efficiency: Random Reflections on Health Services* argues for more use of evidence in clinical practice and initiates the modern approach to evidence based medicine
- *1974:* Lalonde Report, *A New Perspective on the Health of Canadians*, launches a worldwide effort for health promotion
- *1974:* WHO launches the Expanded Program of Immunization to protect all children of the world from six diseases
- *1976:* swine flu outbreak (with only one confirmed death) in the United States of America. President Ford launches a national immunization campaign, which allegedly had adverse effects on many recipients
- *1977:* WHO declares the worldwide eradication of smallpox—last indigenous case in Somalia. WHO resolution 'Health For all by the Year 2000'
- *1978:* Alma Ata declaration for health-care workers, governments, and the world community to protect and promote the health of all the people of the world through primary health care
- *1981:* Rose describes the prevention paradox, in which the majority of cases of a disease may come from a population at lower rather than higher risk (see Glossary), altering approaches to preventive health programmes
- *1983:* isolation then culture of the human immunodeficiency virus
- *1986:* The Ottawa Charter for Health Promotion
- *1988:* Californian voters pass Proposition 99 (Tobacco Tax and Health Promotion Act 1988), for a comprehensive tobacco control program. By 2004 this is credited with reducing California's smoking rates to among the lowest in the United States at 15.4% (from 22.8% in 1988)
- *1990s:* decline in sudden infant death syndrome, following educational campaigns about unsafe sleeping position
- *1991:* public disclosure of mortality rates associated with individual cardiac surgeons in New York State, promoting transparency of health service outcome. Dahlgren and Whitehead publish their 'rainbow' model of the determinants of health, describing successive layers of determinants of health radiating out from the individual
- *1992:* HIV epidemic in China caused by unsafe needle practices while taking blood donations
- *1993:* foundation of the Centre Francois Xavier Bagnoud, Harvard School of Public Health, an academic centre to focus exclusively on health and human rights
- *1993:* program of Universal Salt Iodization established. Cochrane Collaboration established to undertake systematic reviews of all aspects of health care
- *1998:* following the Jakarta Declaration, reaffirming principles and practice of health promotion, the World Health Assembly passes its first resolution on health promotion, with strategies to: build healthy public policy, create supportive environments, strengthen community action, develop personal skills, and reorientate health services

- *1999:* WHO launches global tobacco-free initiative
- *2000:* United Nations Millennium Goals, for improvements in health, education, environmental sustainability, and reduced poverty
- *2001:* Human Genome Project completed. Anthrax apparently deliberately spread through US mail system, following the attacks on the World Trade Centre, New York City, provoking global concerns about bioterrorism not seen since the Cold War
- *2003:* severe acute respiratory syndrome (SARS)
- *2005:* WHO Commission on Social Determinants of Health established to help countries address the social factors leading to ill health and inequities
- *2008:* World Health Assembly passes resolution on climate change and health, reflecting broader concerns by public health community
- *2009:* wild polio virus identified in 21 different countries, despite efforts to eradicate the disease over last 50 years. H1N1 influenza pandemic causes global concern, but has lower mortality than expected
- *2010:* millennium development goals await achievement.

Further resources

Cochrane AL (1971). *Effectiveness and Efficiency: Random Reflections of Health Services,* 2nd edn. Nuffield Provincial Hospitals Trust, London.

Detels R, McEwen J, Beaglehole R, Tanaka H. (eds) (2004). *Oxford Textbook of Public Health,* 4th edn. Oxford University Press, New York.

Gray S, Pilkington P, Pencheon D, Jewell, T. (2006). Public health in the UK: success or failure? *Journal of the Royal Society for Medicine,* **99**, 107–11.

Lewis MJ, Macpherson KL. (2008). *Public health in Asia and the Pacific: historical and comparative perspectives.* Routledge, New York.

Porter R. (1997). *The greatest benefit to mankind. A medical history of humanity from antiquity to the present.* HarperCollins Publishers, London.

Rosen G. (1993). *A history of public health.* Johns Hopkins University Press, New York.

Rose G. (1981). Strategy of prevention: lessons from cardiovascular disease. British Medical Journal, **282**, 1847–51.

Stoto M. (2002). The precautionary principle and emerging biological risks: lessons from swine flu and HIV in blood products. *Public Health Reports,* **117**, 546–52.

The United Nations (2000). *UN millennium development goals.* Available at: ℘ http://www.un.org/millenniumgoals/ (accessed 10 October 2010).

The US National Library of Medicine (2002). Smallpox, the great and terrible scourge. Available at: ℘ http://www.nlm.nih.gov/exhibition/smallpox/sp_variolation.html (accessed 10 October 2010).

Public health organizations, websites, and other resources

These lists are highly selective, and, due to the volatile nature of the Internet and public health reorganizations, susceptible to change.

National public health associations

National bodies that represent the views of public health professionals in countries. Examples include:
- American Public Health Association. Available at: ℘ www.apha.org
- Australasian Faculty of Public Health Medicine. Available at: ℘ www.racp.edu.au/page/racp-faculties/australasian-faculty-of-public-health-medicine
- Canadian Public Health Association. Available at: ℘ www.cpha.ca
- Indian Public Health Association. Available at: ℘ www.iphaonline.org
- Japan Public Health Association (English version). Available at: ℘ http://www.jpha.or.jp/jpha/english/
- Public Health Association of South Africa. Available at: ℘ http://www.phasa.org.za/
- United Kingdom Faculty of Public Health. Available at: ℘ www.fph.org.uk.

National government organizations

Organizations that perform public health functions on behalf of national governments:
- The Centers for Disease Control and Prevention (CDC) is the main federal agency responsible for health protection and promotion in USA. Available at: ℘ www.cdc.gov
- The Chinese Centre for Disease Control (China CDC) is the country's leading public health agency . Available at: ℘ http://www.chinacdc.cn/
- The Centre for Health Protection of the Hong Kong special administrative region is under the Department of Health of Hong Kong. Available at: ℘ http://www.chp.gov.hk/en/index/7.html
- The Health Protection Agency (HPA) is a semi-independent body that is responsible for health protection in England. Available at: ℘ www.hpa.org.uk
- The Oswaldo Cruz Foundation (Fiocruz) promotes health and social development through scientific and technological knowledge in Brazil. Available at: ℘ http://www.fiocruz.br/cgi/cgilua.exe/sys/start.htm?User ActiveTemplate=template%5Fingles&sid=185 (English version)

- The National Institute for Communicable Disease. The South African agency for control of infectious disease. Available at: ℘ www.nicd.ac.za
- The Robert Koch Institut (RKI) is Germany's central federal authority for disease control and prevention. Available at: ℘ http://www.rki. de/cln_151/nn_216264/EN/Home/homepage__node.html?__nnn=true (English version)
- The Public Health Agency of Canada .The government agency in Canada responsible for public health. Available at: ℘ www.phac-aspc. gc.ca
- The Swedish National Institute of Public Health (SNIPH) is a state agency under the Ministry of Health and Social Affairs. Available at: ℘ http://www.fhi.se/en/ (English version).

International organizations

- The European Centre for Disease Prevention and Control (ECDC) is an EU agency for infectious disease control. Available at: ℘ www. ecdc.europa.eu
- International Association of National Public Health Institutions. A collection of the various national public health institutions. Available at: ℘ www.ianphi.org
- International Federation of the Red Cross and Red Crescent. One of the oldest and largest health-related NGOs. Available at: ℘ www.ifrc. org
- UNICEF, the United Nations Children's Fund, which is active in paediatric public health. Available at: ℘ www.unicef.org
- World Health Organization. A specialized agency of the United Nations that acts as a coordinating authority on international public health. Available at: ℘ www.who.int

International data sources

- WHOSIS Statistical Information System. A database containing health statistics for the 193 WHO Member States. Available at: ℘ www.who. int/whosis/en/
- European Health For All Database. WHO database containing more detailed health information for Member States of the WHO European region. Available at: ℘ www.euro.who.int/en/what-we-do/data-and-evidence/databases/european-health-for-all-database-hfa-db2
- Cancermondial. Links to several databases containing information on the epidemiology of cancer worldwide. Managed by the International Association on Research on Cancer, Lyon, France. Available at: ℘ www-dep.iarc.fr
- OECD Health Data. Comparative data health system performance from the respected international economic organization that aims to stimulate economic progress and world trade. Available at: ℘ www.oecd.org/statistics

National data sources

UK

- Hospital Episode Statistics. Data on all hospital admissions in England. Available at: ℘ http://www.hesonline.nhs.uk/
- NHS Information Centre. The central repository for health data in England, including comparative NHS organizational performance data (NHS comparators), pay for performance data (Quality and outcomes framework), screening and workforce data. Available at: ℘ www.ic.nhs.uk/
- Office for National Statistics. The national statistical agency for the UK, including data on populations and societal trends. Available at: ℘ www.statistics.gov.uk/hub/index.html

USA

- CDC Data and Statistics. The CDC's collection of health data, including information on infectious and chronic diseases. Available at: ℘ www.cdc.gov/DataStatistics/
- Partners in information access for the public health workforce. A collaboration of US government agencies, public health organizations and health sciences libraries, including a section on public health data available across different agencies. Available at: ℘ www.phpartners. org/health_stats.html

Clinical effectiveness

- The Agency for Healthcare Research and Quality (AHRQ) is the lead US agency charged with improving the quality, safety of health care. Available at: ℘ www.ahrq.gov
- The Cochrane Library. A database of systematic reviews of clinical effectiveness. Available at: ℘ www.thecochranelibrary.com
- National Guideline Clearinghouse. The AHRQ's public resource for evidence-based clinical practice guidelines. Available at: ℘ www.guideline.gov
- The National Institute for Health and Clinical Excellence (NICE) is the English organization responsible for national guidance on effective health care, including clinical guidelines and cost effectiveness analysis. Available at: ℘ www.nice.org.uk
- New Zealand Guidelines Group. A national organization producing evidence based healthcare guidance. Available at: ℘ www.nzgg.org.nz
- NHS Evidence. The NHS's attempt to bring together health evidence in one portal. Available at: ℘ www.evidence.nhs.uk

Careers

- What is Public Health? A US website with information on public health careers in the US system. Available at: ℘ www.whatispublichealth.org
- Public Health Careers. The UK Faculties of Public Health's career advice section. Available at: ℘ www.fph.org.uk/public_health_careers
- Public healthy. A resource describing the training programme in the UK, put together by a young public health doctor, and containing links to many useful UK data sources. Available at: ℘ www.publichealthy.com

Field epidemiology training programmes

- The European Programme for Intervention Epidemiology Training (EPIET) provides training and practical experience in intervention epidemiology at the national centres for surveillance and control of communicable diseases in the EU. The programme is aimed at EU medical practitioners, nurses, microbiologists, and other health professionals in a two year programme. Available at: ℘ ecdc.europa.eu/en/epiet/Pages/HomeEpiet.aspx
- The Epidemic Intelligence Service (EIS) is a 2-year post-graduate training programme of service and on-the-job learning for health professionals interested in the practice of applied epidemiology, based at CDC in the US. EIS officers conduct epidemiologic investigations, research, and public health surveillance both nationally and internationally. Available at: ℘ www.cdc.gov/eis/index.html

Other perspectives

Blogs

- Blogs provide useful commentary and analysis. In the US, there are many blogs on public health and health policy, a useful cross section can be found at *Health Wonk Review*. Available at: ℘ www.healthwonkreview.com
- The UK has a smaller specialist health blogging community. A good start is *Health Policy Insight*, including regular commentary from senior figures in the UK health system. Available at: ℘ www.healthpolicyinsight.com
- Effect measure. A respected US based blog on epidemiology, and more broad-based public health discussion. Available at: ℘ www.scienceblogs.com/effectmeasure
- Badscience. The popular UK based blog that highlights examples of bad science, media misinterpretation of science and conflicts of interest in the scientific literature. Available at: ℘ www.badscience.net
- Asia Healthcare Blog. China and Southeast Asia healthcare and related challenges. Available at: ℘ http://www.asiahealthcareblog.com/
- Health Blog. The *Wall Street Journal* on health and business of health. Available at: ℘ http://blogs.wsj.com/health/

Abbreviations and glossary

This list aims to standardize some of the more frequently used terms in this book. The glossary is restricted to words or phrases with a technical meaning in the broad field of public health practice. Selected resources follow the list below, including a recommended general dictionary, a guide to usage, and, of primary importance, the *Dictionary of Epidemiology*. Many terms below are defined at greater length in the latter. While we have intended to provide a sufficient list here, the annotation '(see Porta)' indicates either that we have closely followed the *Dictionary of Epidemiology* or that it contains a more elaborate description that may be particularly helpful. Last's *Dictionary of Public Health* is also invaluable.

AAP: American Academy of Pediatrics
AF: attributable fraction
AFp: attributable fraction for the population
AHRQ: Agency for Healthcare Research and Quality (see ℘ http://www.ahrq.gov/ accessed 20 October 2010)
AIDS: acquired immune deficiency syndrome
ASH: Action on Smoking and Health
AURN: Air Quality Monitoring Network
AZT: azidothymidine
BMI: body mass index
BSE: bovine spongiform encephalopathy
CAPHS: Consumer Assessment of Health Care Providers and Systems
CAQDAS: computer-aided qualitative data analysis software
Care Quality Commission (UK): A UK body that assures, monitors and helps improve the quality of healthcare. Available at: ℘ http://www.cqc.org.uk (accessed 20 October 2010)
Case mix: an index of the type of illnesses managed in a health-care facility
CBO: community-based organization
CBPR: community-based participatory research
CDSR: Cochrane Database of Systematic Reviews, part of the Cochrane Library coordinated by the International Cochrane Collaboration. Available at: ℘ http://www.thecochranelibrary.com (accessed 20 October 2010)
CEPH: Council on Education of Public Health
CERD: Committee on the Elimination of Racial Discrimination
CESCR: Committee on Economic, Social and Cultural Rights
CI: confidence interval
Clinical governance: a framework for continuous quality improvement
Clinical indicators: measurements of aspects of clinical care related to quality
CME: continuing medical education

Cochrane Collaboration: the international organization that prepares and disseminates systematic reviews of the effects of health-care interventions. Available at: ℜ http://www.cochrane.org/ (accessed 20 October 2010)

Co-morbidity: the simultaneous presence of two or more health disorders

Cost–benefit analysis: an analysis in which the economic and social costs of medical care and the benefits of reduced loss of net earnings due to preventing premature death or disability are considered (see Porta)

CPA: Chinese Progressive Association

CPD: Continuing professional development

CQ-index: consumer quality index

CSDH: Commission on Social Determinants of Health

CVD: cardiovascular disease

DALE: disability-adjusted life expectancy

DALY: see disability-adjusted life year

DBCP: dibromochloropropane

DCIS: ductal carcinoma *in situ*

DFID: Department for International Development

DFLE: disability-free life expectancy

Diagnosis-related group (DRG): Classification of hospital patients according to diagnosis and intensity of care required, used by insurance companies to set reimbursement scales (see Porta)

Disability: temporary or long-term reduction of a person's capacity to function (see Porta)

Disability-adjusted life year: Measure adopted by the World Bank to estimate the burden of disease by combining premature mortality and disability (see Porta)

Dose: the stated quantity of a substance to which an organism is exposed

DOTS: directly observed treatment short course for tuberculosis

DRG: see diagnosis-related group

EBM: evidence-based medicine

EBMgt: evidence-based management

EC: European Commission

ECDC: European Centre for Disease Prevention and Control

EIA: Environmental impact assessment

EMBASE: An European electronic database of health-related scientific references. This database has a significant overlap with Medline, but has a more European and pharmacological emphasis

EPHIA: European Policy Health Impact Assessment

EQUATOR: Enhancing the Quality and Transparency of Health Research

EU: European Union

Evaluation: a process that attempts to determine as systematically and objectively as possible the relevance, effectiveness, and impact of activities in the light of their objectives (see Porta)

Evidence-based health care/medicine/public health: systematic use of evidence derived from published research and other sources for management and practice

Exposure: a measure of the actual contact with an agent (usually chemical, physical, or biological)

Expressed needs: needs expressed by action, e.g. visiting a doctor

FAO: Food and Agriculture Organization (of the United Nations). Available at: ℘ http://www.fao.org/ (accessed 20 October 2010)

FCTC: Framework Convention on Tobacco Control

Felt needs: what people consider and/or say they need when asked

Focus group: small, convenient sample of people brought together to discuss a topic or issue with the aim of ascertaining the range and intensity of their views, rather than arriving at a consensus (see Porta)

GATT: General Agreement on Tariffs and Trade

GIS: Geographical Information Systems

Goal: a general statement of direction and intent (usually measurable)

GP: general practitioner (family doctor)

GRADE: Grading of Recommendations Assessment, Development and Evaluation

HACCP: Hazards Analysis Critical Control Point

HALE: health active life expectancy

Handicap: reduction in a person's capacity to fulfill a social role as a consequence of an impairment or disability, or other circumstances (see Porta)

HAZ: health action zone

Hazard: the intrinsic capacity of an agent, a condition, or a situation to produce an adverse health or environmental effect

HCQI: health care quality indicators

Health: the extent to which an individual or a group is able to realize aspirations and satisfy needs, and to change or cope with the environment. Health is a resource for everyday life, not the objective of living; it is a positive concept, emphasizing social and personal resources as well as physical capabilities. Your health is related to how much you feel your potential, to be a meaningful part of the society in which you find yourself, is adequately realized (see Porta)

Healthcare resource groups: classification of patients according to severity and intensity of care required, used by insurance carriers (or equivalent) to compare resource use throughout a health system

Health impact assessment: An assessment process to look at the impact on health of government policies or other actions, completed or projected (see ▢ Assessing health impacts)

Health outcome: health status, sometimes related to the effects of health care or other interventions

HeaLYs: healthy life years. A composite indicator that incorporates morbidity and mortality into a single number (see Porta)

HES: hospital episode statistics

HIA: see health impact assessment

HIS: Health Information System

HIV: human immunodeficiency virus

HLE: healthy life expectancy

HNA: health needs assessment

HTA: Health technology assessment

IARC: International Agency for Research on Cancer

IBFAN: International Baby Foods Action Network

ICMBS: International Code of Marketing of Breastmilk Substitutes

ICC: inherited cardiovascular condition

ICCPR: International Covenant on Civil and Political Rights

ICCS: integrated care co-ordination service

ICD-10: International Classification of Disease, edition 10

ICD-9 (CM): International Classification of Disease, edition 9 (clinical modification)

ICOH: International Commission on Occupational Health

ICESCR: International Covenant on Economic, Social and Cultural Rights

IHR: International Health Regulations

IIA: integrated impact assessment

Impairment: a physical or mental defect at the level of a body system or organ. Contrast with Disability and Handicap (see Porta)

Indicator: a summary measure that describes the condition or performance of a system.

IOM: Institute of Medicine

IRA: initial rapid assessment

JSNA: joint strategic needs assessment

KP: Kaiser Permanente

LIHEAP: Low Income Home Energy Assistance Program

MBTI: Myers Briggs Personality Inventory

MCADD: medium chain acylCoA dehydrogenase deficiency

MDG: Millennium Development Goal

MDR-TB: multidrug-resistant resistant tuberculosis

MeSH: medical subject heading

MPH: Master of Public Health

Medline: an electronic database that provides citations, sometimes including abstracts, from the biomedical literature (beginning 1966)

MOU: memoranda of understanding

MSF: multi-source feedback

National Institute for Health and Clinical Excellence (NICE): NICE is the UK independent organization responsible for providing national guidance on the promotion of good health and the prevention and treatment of ill-health. Available at: ℘ http://www.nice.org.uk/ (accessed 20 October 2010)

National service framework (UK): national service frameworks set national standards and define service models for a specific service or care group, put in place programmes to support implementation, and establish performance measures against which progress within an agreed timescale will be measured

NCD: Non-communicable disease

NCI: National Cancer Institute

NGO: Non-governmental organization

NHS: National Health Service (UK)

NICE: see National Institute for Health and Clinical Excellence

NIGB: National Information Governance Board

NNH: number needed to harm

NNT: numbers needed to treat

Normative needs: needs as defined by a health professional

NPV: negative predictive value

NSW: New South Wales

NTI: Northern Territories Intervention

O/E: observed/expected

OECD: Organization for Economic Cooperation and Development

OPS: Older People's Services

OR: Odds Ratio

PA: physical activity

PAHA: Pan-American Health Organization

PBAC: Pharmaceutical Benefits Advisory Committee

pcGNI: *per capita* Gross National Income

PCT: Primary Care Trust

PDSA: Plan-Do-Study-Act

PHC: primary health care

PHCTT: Peninsula Health Technology Commissioning Group

PICO: Population or participant, Intervention or indicator, Comparator or control, Outcome

PKU: phenylketonuria

PDP: Personal development plan

PPV: positive predictive value

PROM: patient-reported outcome measures

Prevention paradox: a measure whose effect is considerable at a population level, but minimal at an individual level (see Porta)

PSA: prostate-specific antigen

PT: person time

Public health: the science and art of preventing disease, prolonging life, and promoting health through the organized efforts and informed choices of society, organizations, public and private, communities and individuals. Public health practice is the emphasis in this book, while public health may also be considered as a discipline or a social institution

Public health practitioner: In this book, includes anyone working in the broad field of public health, neither defined by formal qualifications nor restricted to a professional group.

PubMed: a service of the National Library of Medicine, provides access to over 20 million citations from Medline and additional life science journals. PubMed includes links to many sites providing full text articles and other related resources. Available at: http://www.ncbi.nlm.nih.gov/PubMed/ (accessed 20 October 2010)

PVC: polyvinyl chloride

QALY: quality-adjusted life year

QDA: qualitative data analysis

RCT: randomized controlled trial

RD: Risk Difference,

Risk: the probability that a particular adverse event occurs during a stated period of time, or results from a particular challenge. It can never be reduced to zero

RR: relative risk

SARS: severe acute respiratory syndrome

Screening: the systematic application of a test or inquiry to identify individuals at sufficient risk of a specific disorder to benefit from further investigation or direct preventive action among persons who have not sought medical attention on account of symptoms of that disorder

SIGN: Scottish Intercollegiate Guidelines Network

SIR: standardized incidence ratio

SMR: standardized mortality ratio

SPC: statistical process control

Stakeholders: persons or organizations with an interest that may affect the outcome of an activity. Responses to stakeholders may include collaboration, involvement, monitoring, or defense

Surveillance: the ongoing, systematic collection, collation, and analysis of data and the prompt dissemination of the resulting information to those who need to know so that an action can result

SWOT: (analysis of) strengths, weaknesses, opportunities, and threats

Target: a specific destination or change, intended within a given time period

ToR: terms of reference

UNCED: UN Conference on Environment & Development

UNESCO: United Nations Economic, Social and Cultural Organization

UNICEF: United Nations Children's Fund

URL: Uniform resource locator (technical name for a Web address)

USPSTF: USA Preventive Services Task Force

vCJD: new variant Creutzfeldt–Jakob disease

WHO: World Health Organization

WTO: World Trade Organization

YLL: years of life lost.

Further resources

Burchfield RW (ed.) (2004). *Fowler's modern English usage*, 3rd edn. Oxford University Press, Oxford.

Last JM (ed.) (2007). *A dictionary of public health*. Oxford University Press, Oxford.

Porta M (ed.) (2008). *A dictionary of epidemiology*, 5th edn. Oxford University Press, Oxford.

Oxford University Press (1998). *New Oxford Dictionary of English*. OUP, Oxford.

Bibliography

Abdel Aziz MI, Radford J, McCabe J. (2000). *Health impact assessment, Finningley Airport.* Doncaster Health Authority. Available at: ℘ http://www.doncasterhealth.co.uk/documents/finningley/finningley_report.html (accessed 26 August 2010).

Abelson J, Eyles J, McLeod CB, *et al.* (2003). Does deliberation make a difference? Results from a citizens panel study of health goals priority setting. *Health Policy*, **66**, 95–106.

Abrahams D. (2002). *Foresight Vehicle Initiative Comprehensive Health Impact Assessment. Executive summary.* IMPACT—International Health Impact Assessment Consortium, University of Liverpool, Liverpool. Available at: ℘ http://www.liv.ac.uk/ihia/IMPACT%20Reports/FVI_Comprehensive_-_Summary.pdf (accessed 26 August 2010).

Abrahams D, den Broeder L, Doyle C, *et al.* (2004). *EPHIA—European policy health impact assessment: a guide.* IMPACT, University of Liverpool, Liverpool. Available at: ℘ http://www.liv.ac.uk/ihia/IMPACT%20Reports/EPHIA_A_Guide.pdf (accessed 26 August 2010).

Acheson D. (1988). *Public health in England: the report of the Committee of Inquiry into the future development of the public health function*, Cm 289. HMSO, London.

Agency for Toxic Substances and Disease Registry. (2010). National Toxic substances Incidents Program (NTSIP). Document on Internet. |℘ http://www.atsdr.cdc.gov/ntsip/index.html (accessed 17th August 2010).

Agency for Toxic Substances and Disease Registry. A primer on health risk communication principles and practices. Document on Internet. ℘ http://www.atsdr.cdc.gov/HEC/primer.html (accessed 17th August 2010).

Alexander FE, Boyle P. (1996). *Methods for investigating localized clustering of disease*, IARC Scientific Publication No. 135. International Agency for Research on Cancer, Lyon.

Alexander FE, Cuzick J. (1996). Methods for the assessment of disease clusters. In: Eliott P, Cuzick J, English D, Stern R, eds, *Geographical and environmental epidemiology methods for small-area studies*, pp. 238–50. Oxford University Press, Oxford.

Ampe Akelyernemane Meke Mekarle (2010). Little children are sacred. Available at: ℘ http://www.inquirysaac.nt.gov.au/pdf/bipacsa_final_report.pdf

Anderson CA, Bushman BJ. (2001). Effects of violent video games on aggressive behavior, aggressive cognition, aggressive affect, physiological arousal, and pro-social behavior. A metanalytic review of the scientific literature. *Psychological Science*, **12**, 353–83.

Anderson GF, Reinhardt UE, Hussey PS, Petrosyan V. (2005). It's the prices, stupid: why the United States is so different from other countries. *Health Affairs*, **22(3)**, 89–105.

Anderson LM, Brownson RC, Fullilove MT, *et al.* (2005). Evidence-based public health policy and practice: promises and limits. *American Journal of Preventive Medicine*, **28(Suppl. 5)**, 226–30.

Annalisa software. Available at: ℘ http://annalisa.org.uk (accessed 30 May 2011).

Anscombe FJ. (1973). Graphs in statistical analysis. *American Statistician*, **27**, 17–21.

Ashenden R, Silagy C, Weller D. (1997). A systematic review of the effectiveness of promoting lifestyle change in general practice. *Family Practice*, **14**, 160–75.

Association of Public Health Observatories. (2007). *The HIA Gateway.* Available at: ℘ http://www.apho.org.uk/default.aspx?QN=P_HIA (accessed 26 August 2010).

Atwood K, Colditz GA, Kawachi I. (1997). From public health science to preventive policy. Placing science in its social and political contexts. *American Journal of Public Health*. **87**, 1603–6.

Auerbach A, Landefeld S, Shojania K. (2007). Tension between needing to improve care and knowing how to do it. *New England Journal of Medicine*, **357**, 608–13.

Auger N, Zang G, Daniel M. (2009). Community-level income inequality and mortality in Québec, Canada. *Public Health*, **123**, 438–43.

Australian Government. (2004). *Environmental health risk assessment—guidelines for assessing human health risk from environmental hazards.* Available at: ℘ http://www.health.gov.au/internet/publications/publishing.nsf/Content/CA25774C001857CACA2571E0000C8CF1/$File/EHRA%202004.pdf (accessed May 31, 2012)

Australian Government NHMRC/NRMMC (2004). *Australian drinking water guidelines.* http://www.nhmrc.gov.au/publications/synopses/eh19syn.htm (accessed 3 August 2010).

Australian Government, Department of Health and Ageing. (2009). *Review of Health Technology Assessment in Australia.* Department of Health and Aging, Canberra. Available at: ℘ http://www.health.gov.au/internet/main/publishing.nsf/Content/hta-review-report (accessed 27 .August 2010)

Australian Institute of Health and Welfare (AIHW) (2008). A set of Performance indicators across the health and aged care system. Australian Government Printing: Canberra

Ayer AJ. (1936). *Language, truth and logic.* Penguin, London.

Bammer G. (1997). The ACT heroin trial: intellectual, practical and political challenges. The 1996 Leonard Ball Oration. *Drug & Alcohol* Review, **16**, 287–96.

Banwell C, Guest CS. (1998). Carnivores, cannibals, consumption and unnatural boundaries: the BSE-CJD epidemic in the Australian press. In: McCalman I, Penny B, Cook M. (eds). *Mad cows and modernity: cross-disciplinary reflections on the crisis of Creutzfeldt-Jakob disease*, pp. 3–36. National Academies Forum, Canberra.

Barnes R (2004). HIA and urban regeneration: the Ferrier Estate, England. In: Kemm J, Parry J, Palmer S, eds, *Health impact assessment. Concepts, theory, techniques and applications*, pp. 299–307. Oxford University Press, Oxford.

Barratt A, Trevena L, Davey HM, McCaffery K. (2004). Use of decision aids to support informed choices about screening. *British Medical Journal*, **329**, 507–10.

Bates DW, Gawande AA. (2003). Improving safety with information technology. *New England Journal of Medicine*, **348**, 25–34.

Battersby J, Flowers J, Harvey I. (2004). An alternative approach to quantifying and addressing inequity in healthcare provision: access to surgery for lung cancer in the east of England. *Journal of Epidemiology and Community Health*, **58**, 623–5.

Beaglehole R, Bonita R. (1997). *Public health at the crossroads.* Cambridge University Press, Cambridge.

Beauchamp T, Childress J. (1994). *Principles of biomedical ethics*, 4th edn. Oxford University Press, Oxford.

Belbin M. (1981). *Management teams.* Heinemann, London.

Berger PL, Luckman T. (1967). *The social construction of reality.* Anchor Books, New York.

Berkman LF, Kawachi I. (2000). A historical framework for social epidemiology. In: Berkman LF, Kawachi I, eds, *Social epidemiology*, pp. 3–12. Oxford University Press, New York.

Berner ES, Detmer DE, Simborg D. (2005). Will the wave finally break? A brief view of the adoption of electronic medical records in the united states. *Journal of the American Medical Informatics Association*, **12**, 3–7.

Bertazzi PA, Consonni D, Bachetti S, *et al.* (2001). health effects of dioxin exposure: a 20-year mortality study. *American Journal of Epidemiology*, **153**, 1031–44.

Berwick DM. (1996). A primer on leading the improvement of systems. *British Medical Journal*, **312**, 619–22.

Bhopal RJ. (1995). Public health medicine and primary health care: convergent, divergent or parallel paths? *Journal of Epidemiology and Community Health*, **49**, 113–16.

Biggs SD. (1989). *Resource-poor farmer participation in research: a synthesis of experiences from nine national agricultural research systems.* The Hague, Netherlands.

Bilheimer LT. (2010). Evaluating metrics to improve population health. *Preventing Chronic Disease*, **7**, A69. Available at: ℘ http://www.ncbi.nlm.nih.gov/pubmed/20550827

Birley MH. (1995). *The health impact assessment of development projects.* HMSO, London.

Black AD, Car J, Pagliari C, *et al.* (2011). The impact of eHealth on the quality and safety of health care: a systematic overview. *PLoS Medicine*, **8**, e1000387. doi:10.1371/journal.pmed.1000387.

Black C. (2008). *Working for a healthier tomorrow.* TSO, London.

Black N. (2001). Evidence based policy: proceed with care. *British Medical Journal*, **323**, 275–9.

Black N, Barker M, Payne M. (2004). Cross sectional survey of multi-centre clinical database in the United Kingdom. *British Medical Journal*, **328**, 1478–81.

Black RE, Cousens S, Johnson HL, *et al.* (2010). Global, regional, and national causes of child mortality in 2008: a systematic analysis. *Lancet*, **375**, 1967–87.

Blue Ridge Academic Health Group. Advancing Value in Health Care (2008). *The Emerging Transformational Role of Informatics*, Report. Blue Ridge Academic Health Group, Atlanta.

Boaden R, Harvey G, Moxham C, *et al.* (2008). *Quality improvement: theory and practice in health care.* NHS Institute for Innovation and Improvement, Coventry.

Bohmer R. (2010). Leadership with a small 'l'. *British Medical Journal*, **340**, c483.

Bolsin S, Colson M. (2000). The use of the Cusum technique in the assessment of trainee competence in new procedures. *International Journal of Quality Health Care*, **12**, 433–8.

Bowling A (1997). *Measuring health: a review of quality of life measurement scales*, 2nd edn. Open University Press, Buckingham.

Boyd CM, Darer J, Boult C, *et al.* (2005). Clinical practice guidelines and quality of care for older patients with multiple comorbid diseases: implications for pay for performance. *Journal of the American Medical Association*, **294**, 716–24.

Bridgen P. (2003). Joint planning across health/social services. *Local Government Studies*, **29(3)**, 17–31.

Brimblecombe J, McDonnell J, Barnes A, et al. (2010). Impact of income management on store sales in the Northern Territory. Medical Journal of Australia, 192(10), 549–54.

Britton A, McKee M, Black N, *et al.* (1998). Choosing between randomised and non-randomised studies: a systematic review. *Health Technology Assessment*, **2**, 1–124.

Brotherton P, Withers M. (2010). *Health needs assessment in an English prison*. Case study prepared for OUP.

Brownson RC, Chriqui JF, Stamatakis KA. (2009). Understanding evidence-based public health policy. *American Journal of Public Health*, **99**, 1576–83.

Brownson RC, Fielding JE, Maylahn CM. (2009). Evidence-based public health: a fundamental concept for public health practice. *Annual Review of Public Health*, **30**, 175–201.

Brownson RC, Gurney JG, Land GH. (1999). Evidence-based decision making in public health. *Journal of Public Health Management and Practice*, **5**, 86–97.

Brownson RC, Royer C, Ewing R, McBride TD. (2006). Researchers and policymakers: travelers in parallel universes. *American Journal of Preventive Medicine*, **30**, 164–72.

Brundtland GH. (1987). *Our Common Future*, The Brundtland Report: World Commission on Environment and Development.

Buchanan DR, Miller FG, Wallerstein N. (2007). Ethical issues in community-based participatory research: balancing rigorous research with community participation in community intervention studies. *Progress in Community Health Partnerships*, **1**,153–60.

Bullas S, Dallas A. (2002). *Information for managing health care resources*. Radcliffe Medical, Abingdon.

Bunker JP. (2001). The role of medical care in contributing to health improvements within societies. *International Journal of Epidemiology*, **30**, 1260–3.

Burke W, Zimmern R. (2004). Ensuring the appropriate use of genetic tests. *National Review of Genetics*, **5**, 955–9.

Burkle FM Jr. (2010). Future humanitarian crises: challenges to practice, policy, and public health. *Prehospital and Disaster Medicine*, **25**, 194–9.

Burton H, Alberg C, Stewart A. (2010). Mainstreaming genetics: a comparative review of clinical services for inherited cardiovascular conditions in the UK. *Public Health Genomics*, **13**, 235–45.

Buse K, Mays N, Walt G. (2005). *Making health policy*. McGraw-Hill/Open University Press, Maidenhead.

CAHPS. (2011). Quality improvement. Available at: ℬ http://www.cahps.ahrq.gov/qiguide/default.aspx (accessed 17 May 2011).

Caldicott F. (1997). *Report of the review of patient-identifiable information*. Department of Health, London.

Calhoun JG, Ramiah K, Weist EM, Shortell SM. (2008). Development of a core competency model for the master of public health degree. *American Journal of Public Health*, **98**, 1598–607.

Calman K. (1998). Lessons from Whitehall. *British Medical Journal*, **317**, 1718–20.

Calman KC. (1996). Cancer: science and society and the communication of risk. *British Medical Journal*, **313**, 799–802.

Calman KC, Royston GH. (1997). Risk language and dialects. *British Medical Journal*, **315**, 939–42.

Cameron D. (2007). In praise of general well-being. In: Simms A, Smith J, eds, *Do good lives have to cost the Earth?* Constable, London.

Campbell R, Starkey F, Holliday J, et al.(2008). An informal school-based peer-led intervention for smoking prevention in adolescence (ASSIST); a cluster randomized trial. *Lancet*, **371**, 1595–602.

Carey V, Chapman S, Gaffney D. (1994). Children's lives or garden aesthetics? A case study in public health advocacy. *Australian Journal of Public Health*, **18**, 25–32.

Cargo M, Mercer SL. (2008). The value and challenges of participatory research: strengthening its practice. *Annual Review of Public Health*, **29**.

Carter SM, Chapman S. (2003). Smoking, health and obdurate denial: the Australian tobacco industry in the 1980s. *Tobacco Control*. **12(Suppl 3)**, iii23–30.

Catelan D, Biggeri A. (2008). A statistical approach to rank multiple priorities in environmental epidemiology: an example from high-risk areas in Sardinia, Italy. *Geospatial Health*. **3**, 81–9.

Centers for Disease Control. (1990). Guidelines for investigating clusters of health events. *Morbidity and Mortality Weekly Report*. **39**(RR-11): 1–23.

Centers for Disease Control and Prevention. (1999). Ten great public health achievements—United States, 1900–1999. *Morbity and Mortality Weekly Reports*, **48**, 241–8.

Centers for Disease Control and Prevention (2001). Updated guidelines for evaluating public health surveillance systems: recommendations from the guidelines working group. *Morbidity and Mortality Weekly Report*, **50(RR-13)**, 1–35. Available at: ⌚ http://www.cdc.gov/mmwr/preview/mmwrhtml/rr5013a1.htm (accessed 21 June 2010).

Centers for Disease Control and Prevention. (2004). Framework for evaluating public health surveillance systems for early detection of outbreaks; recommendations from the CDC Working Group. *Morbidity and Mortality Weekly Report*, **53(RR-5)**, 1–13. Available at: ⌚ http://www.cdc.gov/mmwr/preview/mmwrhtml/rr5305a1.htm (accessed 21 June 2010).

Centre for Reviews and Dissemination, University of York. *HTA database*. Available at: ⌚ http://www.crd.york.ac.uk/crdweb/ (accessed 27 August 2010).

Centres for Medicare & Medicaid Services. *Cost reports*. Available at: ⌚ http://www.cms.hhs.gov/CostReports/ (accessed 21 January 2006).

CERD (2010). Concluding observations of the Committee on the Elimination of Racial Discrimination. Australia, 2010, UN Doc CERD/C/AUS/CO/15-17. Available at: ⌚ http://www2.ohchr.org/english/bodies/cerd/cerds77.htm.

Champion D, Chapman S. (2005). Framing pub smoking bans: An analysis of Australian print news media coverage, March 1996- March 2003. *Journal of Epidemiology and Community Health*. **59**, 679–84.

Chan EY, Griffiths S. (2009). Comparison of health needs of older people between affected rural and urban areas after the 2005 Kashmir, Pakistan earthquake. *Prehospital. & Disaster.Medicine*, **24(5)**, 365–71.

Chapman S. (2007). *Public health advocacy and tobacco control: making smoking history*. Blackwell Publishing: Oxford.

Chase D, Rosten C, Turner S, *et al*. (2009). Development of a toolkit and glossary to aid in the adaptation of health technology assessment (HTA) reports for use in different contexts. *Health Technology Assessment*, **13**, 1–142.

Chaudhry BD, Wang JD, Wu SD. (2006). Systematic review: impact of health information technology on quality, efficiency, and costs of medical care. *Annals of Internal Medicine*, **144**, 742–52.

Child and Youth Health Intergovernmental Partnership (2004). Healthy children—strengthening promotion and prevention Across Australia; developing a national public health action plan for children 2005–2008. National Public Health Partnership, Melbourne.

Child Health Impact Working Group. (2007). *Unhealthy consequences: energy costs and child health impact assessment of energy costs and the low income home energy assistance program*. CHIWG, Boston.

Christianson J, Leatherman S, Sutherland K. (2007). *Financial incentives, health care providers and quality improvements. A review of the evidence*. Health Foundation, London.

Church J, Saunders D, Wanke M, *et al*. (2002). Citizen participation in health decision-making: past experience and future prospects. *Journal of Public Health Policy*, **23**, 12–32.

Closing the gap in a generation (2008). *Health equity through action on the social determinants of health*. World Health Organization, Geneva. Available at: ⌚ http://whqlibdoc.who.int/hq/2008/WHO_IER_CSDH_08.1_eng.pdf, (accessed 30 May 2011).

Cochrane Effective Clinical Practice and Organization of Care Group. (2010). Available at: ⌚ http://epoc.cochrane.org/epoc-reviews (accessed October 2010).

Cochrane Library summaries. Available at: ⌚ http://summaries.cochrane.org/ (accessed 24 May 2012).

Cohen D, Carter P. (2010). WHO and the pandemic flu 'conspiracies'. *British Medical Journal* **340**, c2912

Coker R, Thomas M, Lock K, Martin R. (2007). Detention and the threat of tuberculosis. Evidence, Ethics and Law. *Journal of Law and Medical Ethics*, **35**, 609–15.

Cole BL, Fielding JE. (2007). Health impact assessment: a tool to help policy makers understand health beyond health care. *Annual Review of Public Health*, **28**, 393–412.

Collins J, Koplan JP. (2009). Health impact assessment: a step toward health in all policies. *Journal of the American Medical Association*, **302**, 315–17.

Commission on Social Determinants of Health. (2008). *Closing the gap in a generation: health equity through action on the social determinants of health*. WHO, Geneva.

Committee on Economic, Social, and Cultural Rights. (2000). *General Comment No. 14, The right to the highest attainable standard of health*, UN Doc. E/C.12/2000/4. Available at: ⌚ http://www.unhchr.ch/tbs/doc.nsf/(symbol)/E.C.12.2000.4.En (accessed 27 August 2010).

Committee for the Study of the Future of Public Health (1988). *The future of public health*. National Academy Press, Washington DC.

Commonwealth Department of Health and Aged Care and Australian Institute of Health and Welfare (1999). National health priority areas report: diabetes mellitus 1998, AIHW cat. No PHE 10. AusInfo, Canberra

Conrady R, Buck M. (2009). *Trends and Issues in Global Tourism 2010*. Springer: Berlin.

Cook AJ, Gold DR, Li Y. (2007). Spatial cluster detection for censored outcome data. *Biometrics*. **63**, 540–9.

Cook AJ, Gold DR, Li Y. (2009). Spatial cluster detection for repeatedly measured outcomes while accounting for residential history. *Biometrical Journal*. **51**, 801–18.

Coote, A. (2002). *Claiming the health dividend, unlocking the benefits of NHS spending*. King's Fund, London.

Coote A. (2006). What health services could do about climate change. *British Medical Journal*, **332**, 1343–4.

Coote A. (2008). How should health professionals take action against climate change? *British Medical Journal*, **336**, 733–4.

Costello A, Abbas M, Allen A, et al. (2009). Managing the health effects of climate change: Lancet and University College London Institute for Global Health Commission. *Lancet*, **373**, 1693–733.

Costello A, Osrin D, Manandhar D. (2004). Reducing maternal and neonatal mortality in the poorest communities. British Medical Journal, **329**, 1166–8.

Coulter A. (2005). What do patients and the public want from primary care? *British Medical Journal*, **331**, 1199–201.

Coulter A. (2007). Finding out what patients want. *ENT News*; **16**, 65–7.

Coulter A, Ellins J. (2007). Effectiveness of strategies for informing, educating, and involving patients. *British Medical Journal*, **335**, 24–7.

Council of Australian Governments. (2007). National Healthcare Agreement. Australian Government Printing: Canberra. Available at: ℘ http://www.federalfinancialrelations.gov.au/content/national_agreements/downloads/IGA_FFR_ScheduleF_National_Healthcare_Agreement.pdf (accessed 31 May 2011).

Council on Education for Public Health. (2011). *Accreditation Criteria: Schools of Public Health*. CEPH, Washington, DC.

Crown J. (2003). *Cleft lip and palate services*, Report from the Cleft Implementation Group and Cleft Monitoring Group. Available at: ℘ http://wikiph.org/index.php?title=Health_care_strategic_management (accessed 30 May 2011).

CSDH (2008). *Closing the gap in a generation: health equity through action on the social determinants of health*, Final Report of the Commission on Social Determinants of Health. WHO, Geneva.

Daniels N, Kennedy B, Kawachi I. (2000). Justice is good for our health. *Boston Review*, **25**, 6–15.

Davidoff F, Haynes B, Sackett D, Smith R. (1995). Evidence-based medicine. *British Medical Journal*, **310**, 1085–8.

De Vito C, Nobile CG, Furnari G, et al. (2009). Physicians' knowledge, attitudes and professional use of RCTs and meta-analyses: a cross-sectional survey. *European Journal of Public Health*, **19**, 297–302.

Delnoij DMJ, Rademakers JJDJM, Groenewegen PP. (2010). The Dutch Consumer Quality Index: an example of stakeholder involvement in indicator development. *BMC Health Services Research*, **10**, 88.

Department of Families, Housing, Community Services and Indigenous Affairs. (2009). Closing the Gap in the Northern Territory, Whole of Government July-June 2009 Monitoring Report. Australian Government, Canberra.

Department of Health. (1997). *Communicating about risks to public health: pointers to good practice*. Department of Health, London. Available at: ℘ http://www.dh.gov.uk/prod_consum_dh/groups/dh_digitalassets/@dh/@en/documents/digitalasset/dh_4039670.pdf (accessed 6 August 2010).

Department of Health (2000). *The NHS plan: a plan for investment, a plan for reform*. HMSO, London.

Department of Health. (2000). *Good practice guidelines for investigating the health impact of local industrial emissions*. Department of Health, London.

Department of Health. (2004). *Choosing health: making healthy choices easier*. HMSO, London. Available at: ℘ http://webarchive.nationalarchives.gov.uk/+/www.dh.gov.uk/en/Publicationsandstatitics/Publications/PublicationsPolicyAndGuidance/DH_4094550 (accessed 20 August 2010).

Department of Health (2005). *Research governance framework for health and social care*. Department of Health, London.

Department of Health (2006). *Integrated governance handbook: a guide for executives and non executives in health care organizations*, Gateway reference 5947. Department of Health, London.

Department of Health (2010). *Equity and excellence: liberating the NHS*. HMSO, London.

Department of Health. (2010).*The Caldicott Guardian Manual 2010*. Department of Health, London.

Department of Health. Reference costs. Available at: http://www.dh.gov.uk/PolicyAndGuidance/OrganizationPolicy/FinanceAndPlanning/NHSReferenceCosts/ (accessed 21 January 2006).

Department of Health & Communities and Local Government (2010). *Liberating the NHS: local democratic legitimacy in health*. Available at: http://www.dh.gov.uk/dr_consum_dh/groups/dh_digitalassets/@dh/@en/documents/digitalasset/dh_117721.pdf (accessed 22 August 2010).

Department of Health. Health Survey for England. Available at: http://www.dh.gov.uk/PublicationsAndStatistics/PublishedSurvey/HealthSurveyForEngland/fs/en (accessed 20 March 2005).

Desai M, Rachet B, Coleman M, McKee M. (2010). Two countries divided by a common language: health systems in the UK and USA. *Journal of the Royal Society for Medicine*, **103**, 283–7.

Detels R, McEwen J, Beaglehole R, Tanaka H. (eds) (2002). *Oxford textbook of public health*. Oxford University Press, New York.

Detmer DE. (2003). Building the National Health Information Infrastructure for Personal Health, Health Care Services, Public Health, and Research. *BMC Medical Informatics and Decision-Making*, **3**, 1–40.

Detmer DE, Bloomrosen M, Raymond B, Tang P.(2008). Integrated personal health records: Transformative tools for consumer-centric care. *BMC Medical Informatics and Decision-Making*, **8**, 45–72.

Dhainaut J, Claessens Y, Ginsburg C, Riou B. (2004). Unprecedented heat-related deaths during the 2003 heat wave in Paris: consequences for emergency departments. *Critical Care* **8**, 1–2.

Dhara VR, Dhara R. (2002). The Union Carbide disaster in Bhopal: a review of health effects. *Archives of Environmental Health*, **57**, 391–404.

DiSario JA, Foutch PG, Mai HD, *et al.* (1991). Prevalence and malignant potential of colorectal polyps in asymptomatic, average-risk men. *American Journal of Gastroenterology*, **86**, 941–5. http://www.framinghamheartstudy.org/risk/coronary.html (accessed 26 March 2011).

Doll R, Hill AB. (2004). The mortality of doctors in relation to their smoking habits: a preliminary report. 1954. *British Medical Journal*, **328**, 1529–33.

Donabedian A (1980). *Explorations in quality assessment and monitoring. Vol 1. The definition of quality and approaches to its assessment*. Health Administration Press, Ann Arbor.

Donabedian A. (1980). The definition of quality: a conceptual exploration. In: *Explorations in quality assessment and monitoring. Volume 1: The definition of quality and approaches to its assessment*. Health Administration Press, Ann Arbor.

Donabedian A. (2003). *An introduction to quality assurance in health care*. Oxford University Press, Oxford.

Donal O'Donoghue (2010). Sustainability, the seventh dimension of quality. Available at: http://renaltsar.blogspot.com/2010/05/sustainability-seventh-dimension-of.html (accessed 27 May 2010).

Donaldson C, Mooney G. (1991). Needs assessment, priority setting, and contracts for healthcare: an economic view. *British Medical Journal*, 303, 1529–30.

Dorfman L, Wallack L, Woodruff K. (2005). More than a message: framing public health advocacy to change corporate practices. *Health Education & Behavior*, **32**, 320–36;

Dowie R. (1983). *General practitioners and consultants: a study of outpatient referrals*. King Edward's Hospital Fund for London, London.

Drummond MF, O'Brien BJ, Stoddard GL, Torrance GW. (1997). *Methods for the economic evaluation of health care programmes*, 2nd edn. Oxford University Press, Oxford.

Eden C, Ackerman F. (2001). Group decision and negotiation in strategy making. *Group Decision and Negotiation*, **10**, 119–40.

Egger G, Swinburn B. (2010). *Planet Obesity: How we're eating ourselves and the planet to death*. NSW: Allen and Unwin.]

Elkington J. (1997). *Cannibals with forks: the triple bottom line of 21st century business*. Capstone, Oxford.

Elliott P, Wartenberg D. (2004). Spatial epidemiology: Current approaches and future challenges. *Environmental Health Perspectives*, **112**, 998–1006.

Elliott P, Wakefield JC, Best NG, Briggs BJ. (2000). *Spatial epidemiology—methods and applications*. Oxford University Press, Oxford.

Emory University (2008). Available at: ℘ http://whsc.emory.edu/blueridge/reports.cfm#report_12 (accessed 13 April 2011).

Enthoven A. (1999). *Rock Carling Fellowship 1999. In pursuit of an improving National Health Service.* Nuffield Trust, London.

Entman RM. (1993). Framing: toward clarification of a fractured paradigm. *Journal of Communication*, **43**, 51–8.

Equator Principles (2006). *The Equator Principles.* Available at: ℘ http://www.equator-principles. com (accessed 26 August 2010).

European Observatory on Health Systems and Policies. Australia: Health System Review. (2006). Available at: ℘ http://www.commonwealthfund.org/~/media/Files/Publications/Issue%20 Brief/2011/Jul/1532_Squires_US_hlt_sys_comparison_12_nations_intl_brief_v2.pdf.

Evans RG. (1986). Finding the levers, finding the courage: lessons from cost containment in North America. *Journal of Health Politics, Policy and Law*, **11**, 585–615.

Faculty of Occupational Medicine (2006). *Guidance on ethics for occupational physicians.* Faculty of Occupational Medicine, Royal College of Physicians, London.

Faculty of Occupational Medicine, Ireland (2007). *Guidance on ethical practice for occupational physicians.* Faculty of Occupational Medicine, Dublin.

Faculty of Public Health (2010). Available at: ℘ www.fph.org.uk (accessed 19 April 2011).

Feachem RG, Sekhri NK, White KL (2002). Getting more for their dollar: a comparison of the NHS with California's Kaiser Permanente. *British Medical Journal*, **324**, 135–41.

Feder G, Griffiths C, Eldridge S, Spence ℘ (1999). Effect of postal prompts to general practitioners and patients on the quality of primary care after a coronary event (POST): randomized controlled trial. *British Medical Journal*, **318**, 1522–6.

Finnegan JR, Viswanath K. (2008). Communication theory and health behavior change: the media studies framework. In: Glanz K, Rimer B, Viswanath K, eds, *Health behavior and health education: theory, research, and practice*, 4th edn, pp. 363-87. Jossey-Bass, San Francisco.

Fisher E, Goodman D, Skinner J, Bronner K. (2009). Health care spending, quality, and outcomes: more isn't always better. Dartmouth Atlas Project Topic Brief. Available at: ℘ http://www. dartmouthatlas.org/downloads/reports/Spending_Brief_022709.pdf.

Fitzpatrick M. (2001). *The tyranny of health—doctors and the regulation of lifestyle.* Routledge, London.

Fletcher SW. (1997). Whither scientific deliberation in health policy recommendation? Alice in the Wonderland of breast-cancer screening. *New England Journal of Medicine*, **336**, 1180–3.

Flicker S, Travers R, Guta A, McDonald S, Meagher A. (2007). Ethical dilemmas in community-based participatory research: recommendations for institutional review boards. *Journal of Urban Health*, **84**, 478–93.

Flowers J. (2007). *Technical Briefing 2: Statistical process control methods in public health intelligence.* APHO, York. Available at: http://www.apho.org.uk/resource/item.aspx?RID=39445

Fox S, Jones S. (2009). *The social life of health information* [Report on the Internet]. Pew Research Center's Internet & American Life Project, Washington DC. Available at: ℘ http://www.pewinternet.org/Reports/2009/8-The-Social-Life-of-Health-Information.aspx

Francis R (Chair) (2001). *Independent Inquiry into care provided by Mid Staffordshire NHS Foundation Trust January 2005 – March 2009.* Department of Health, London.

Frankel S, Davey Smith G, Donovan J, Neal D. (2003). Screening for prostate cancer. *Lancet* **361**, 1122–8.

Frankel S, Eachus J, Pearson N, et al. (1999). Population requirement for primary hip-replacement surgery: a cross-sectional study. *Lancet*, **353**(9161), 1304–9.

Friedman DJ, Parrish RG. 2nd (2010). The population health record: concepts, definition, design, and implementation. *Journal of the American Medical Informatics Association*, **17**, 359–66.

Fung A. (2003). SARS: how Singapore out managed the others. *Asia Times*, 9 April. Available at: ℘ http://www.atimes.com/atimes/china/ED09Ad03.html (accessed 6 August 2010).

Fung CH, Lim YW, Mattke S, Damberg C, Shekelle P. (2008). Systematic review: the evidence that publishing patient care performance data improves quality of care. *Annals of Internal Medicine*; **148**, 111–23.

Gebbie K, Rosenstock L, Hernandez LM (eds) (2003). *Who will keep the public healthy? Educating public health professionals for the 21st century.* National Academies Press, Washington DC.

Gerbner G, Gross L, Morgan M, Signorielli N, Shanahan J. (2002). Growing up with television: Cultivation process (pp. 43-67). In: Bryant J, Zillmann D, eds, *Media effects: advances in theory and research.* Lawrence Erlbaum, Mahwah.

Gill M,.Stott R. (2009). Health professionals must act to tackle climate change. *Lancet*, **374**, 1953–5.

Gillam S. (2004). What can we learn about quality of care from US health maintenance organisations? *Quality in Primary Care* **12**, 3–4.

Gillam S. (2008). Is the declaration of Alma Ata still relevant to primary health care? *British Medical Journal*, **336**, 536–8.

Gillam S, Barna S. (2011). Sustainable general practice: another challenge for trainers. Primary Care Education, **22**, 7–10.

Gillam S, Meads G. (2001). *Modernisation and the future of general practice*. King's Fund, London.

Gillam S, Siriwardena N, eds (2010). *The Quality and Outcomes Framework: transforming general practice*. Radcliffe, Oxford.

Glasby J. (ed.) (2011). *Evidence, policy and practice: critical perspectives in health and social care*. Policy Press, Bristol.

Glasby J, Dickinson H. (2008). *Partnership working in health and social care*, Better Partnership Working. Policy Press, Bristol.

Goffman E. (1961). *Asylums: essays on the social situation of mental patients and other inmates*. Doubleday/Anchor, New York.

Goldman DP, Joyce GF, Zheng Y. (2007). Prescription drug cost sharing: associations with medication and medical utilization and spending and health. *Journal of the American Medical Association*, **298**, 61–9.

Goldstein BD (2008). Credentialing in public health: the time has come. *Journal of Public Health Management Practice*, **14**, 1–2.

Gostin LO. (2007). The 'tobacco wars'—global litigation strategies. *Journal of the American Medicine Association*, **298**, 2537–2539.

Gostin LO, Sapsin JW, Teret SP, *et al*. (2002). The Model State Emergency Health Powers Act: planning and response to bioterrorism and naturally occurring infectious diseases. *Journal of American Medicine Association*, **288**, 622–8.

Grad FP. (2004). *Public health law manual*. American Public Health Association, Washington, DC.

Graham H. (1993). *When life's a drag: women, smoking and disadvantage*. HMSO, London.

Graham, H (1994). Surviving by smoking. In: Wilkinson S, Kitzinger C (eds) *Women and Health: Feminist Perspectives*. Taylor and Francis, London.

Graham H. (2010). Where is the future in public health? *Milbank Quarterly*, **88**, 149–68.

Grainger C. (2002). Mentoring—supporting doctors at work and play. *BMJ Career Focus*, **324**, S203.

Gray JAM. (2001). *Evidence-based health care*, 2nd edn. Churchill Livingstone. Philadelphia.

Green A. (2007). *An introduction to health planning for developing health systems*. Oxford University Press, Oxford.

Green MC. (2006). Narratives and cancer communication. *Journal of Communication*, **56(s1)**, S163–83.

Greenhalgh T. (2006). Reframing evidence synthesis as rhetorical action in the policy making drama. *Healthcare Policy*, **1**, 34–42.

Greenhalgh T, Russell J. (2005). Reframing evidence synthesis as rhetorical action in the policy making drama. Healthcare Policy. 11(1), 31–5.

Greenhalgh T, Russell J. (2010). Why do evaluations of eHealth programs fail? An alternative set of guiding principles. *PLoS Medicine*, **7**, e1000360.

Griffiths J, Rao M, Adshead F, Thorpe A. (2009). *The health practitioner's guide to climate change*. Earthscan, London.

Griffiths S, Jewell T, Hope T. (2006). Setting priorities in health care. In: Pencheon D, Guest C, Melzer D, Muir Gray JA, eds, *Oxford handbook of public health practice*, 2nd edn, pp. 404–10. Oxford University Press, Oxford.

Grimshaw J, Eccles M, Thomas R, *et al*. (2006). Evidence (and its limitations) of the effectiveness of guideline dissemination and implementation strategies 1966–1998. *Journal of General Internal Medicine*, **21(Suppl. 2)**, S14–20.

Grimshaw JG, Thomas RE, MacLennan G, *et al*. (2004). Effectiveness and efficiency of guideline dissemination and implementation strategies. *Health Technology Assessment*, **8**, 1–72.

Grimshaw JM, Thomas RE, MacClennan C, *et al*. (2004). Effectiveness and efficiency of guideline dissemination and implementation strategies. *Health Technology Assessment*, **8**, iii–iv, 1–72.

Grol R, Baker R, Moss F (eds) (2004). *Quality improvement research: understanding the science of change in health care*. BMJ Publishing, London.

Grol R, Wensing M, Eccles ℗ (eds) (2005). *Improving patient care. The implementation of change in clinical practice*. Elsevier, London.

Guillebaud J, Hayes P. (2008). Population growth and climate change. *British Medical Journal*, **337**, 247–8.

Guy M. (2001). Diabetes: developing a local strategy. In: Pencheon D, Guest C, Melzer D, Gray JAM, eds, *Oxford handbook of public health practice*, p. 559. Oxford University Press, Oxford.

Haddow J, Palomaki G. (2004). ACCE: a model process for evaluating data on emerging genetic tests. In: Khoury M, Little J, Burke W, eds, *Human genome epidemiology*, pp. 217–33. Oxford University Press, Oxford.

Haegebaert S, Duche L, Desenclos JC. (2003). The use of the case-crossover design in a continuous common source food-borne outbreak. *Epidemiol Infect*, **131**: 809–13.

Hahn RA (1999). *Anthropology in public health*. Oxford University Press, Oxford.

Haines A, Smith KR, Anderson D, et al. (2007). Policies for accelerating access to clean energy, improving health, advancing development, and mitigating climate change. *Lancet*, **370**, 1264–81.

Hall BL. (1992). From margins to center: The development and purpose of participatory action research. *American Sociologist*, **23**: 15–28.

Ham C, York N, Sutch S, Shaw R. (2003). Hospital bed utilization in the NHS, Kaiser Permanente, and the US Medicare programme: analysis of routine data. *British Medical Journal*, **327**, 1257.

Hansen J, de Klerk NH, Eccles JL, et al. (1993). Malignant mesothelioma after environmental exposure to blue asbestos. *International Journal of Cancer*, **54**, 578–81.

Hardy C, Phillips N. (1998). Strategies of engagement: lessons from the critical examination of collaboration and conflict in an inter-organizational domain. *Organization Science*, **9**, 217–30.

Hardy LL, Okely AD, Dobbins TA, Booth ML.. (2008). Physical activity among adolescents in New South Wales (Australia): 1997–2004. *Journal of Science and Medicine and Science in Sports and Exercise*,. **40**, 835–41.

Harrington JM, Stein GF, Rivera RO, de Morales AV. (1978). Occupational hazards of formulating oral contraceptives—a survey of plant employees. *Archives of Environmental Health*, **33**, 12–15.

Harris P, Harris-Roxas B, Harris E, Kemp L. (2007). *Health impact assessment: a practical guide*. Centre for Health Equity Training, Research and Evaluation (CHETRE), University of New South Wales, Sydney.

Hasson H. (2010). Systematic evaluation of implementation fidelity of complex interventions in health and social care. Implementation Science, 5, 67. Available at: ℘ http://www.implementationscience.com/content/5/1/67.

Hatsukami D, Slade J, Benowitz N, et al. (2002). Reducing tobacco harm: Research challenges and issues. *Nicotine & Tobacco Research*, **4**, 89–101.

Have M. (2010). An overview of ethical frameworks in public health: can they be supportive in the evaluation of programs to prevent overweight? BMC Public Health. 10, 638.

Head BW. (2008). Three lenses of evidence-based policy. *Australian Journal of Public Administration*. **67**, 1–11.

Health Development Agency. (2005). *Understanding the barriers to completing health equity audit in PCTs*. NHS, London. Available at: ℘ http://www.nice.org.uk/nicemedia/documents/understanding_barriers.pdf

Health Foundation (2010). *Quality improvement made simple*. Health Foundation, London.

Health Policy. (1995). Special issue devoted to programme budgeting and marginal analysis. **33**.

Health Protection Agency. (2005). Chemical Incidents in England and Wales. HPA, Chilton.

Healthy Cities Belfast. Available at: ℘ http://www.belfasthealthycities.com/ (cited 1 August 2010).

Heart Foundation. (2010). Healthy by Design: a guide to planning and designing environments for active living in Tasmania. Available at: ℘ http://www.heartfoundation.org.au/Professional_Information/Lifestyle_risk/Physical_Activity/Active_by_Design/Pages/default.aspx (cited 3 August 2010).

Heath I. (1995). *The mystery of general practice*. Nuffield Provincial Hospitals Trust, London.

Herzberg F, Mausner B, Snyderman BB. (1959). *The motivation to work*, 2nd edn. John Wiley & Sons, New York.

Hill AB. (1965). The environment and disease: association or causation? *Proceedings of the Royal Society of Medicine.*, **58**, 295–300 .

Hills M. (1996). Some comments on methods for investigating disease risk around a point source. In: Eliott P, Cuzick J, English D, Stern R, eds, *Geographical and environmental epidemiology methods for small-area studies*, pp. 231–7. Oxford University Press, Oxford.

Holland WW. (1983). Concepts and meaning in evaluation of health care. In: Holland WW, ed., *Evaluation of health care*. Oxford University Press, Oxford.

Honey P, Mumford A. (1982). *The manual of learning styles.*. Peter Honey Publications, Maidenhead.

Hornik RC. (2002). Public health communication: making sense of contradictory evidence. In: Hornik RC, ed., *Public health communication: evidence for behavior change*, pp. 1–19. Lawrence Erlbaum, New York.

House of Commons Health Select Committee (2010). *Commissioning*. Stationery Office, London.

Huang YL, Batterman S. (2000). Residence location as a measure of environmental exposure: a review of air pollution epidemiology studies. *Journal of Exposure and Analytic Environmental Epidemiology*, **10**, 66–85.

Hulscher MEJL, Wensing M, van der Weijden T, Grol R. (2001). *Interventions to implement prevention in primary care*, Cochrane Review. *The Cochrane Library*, **Issue 1**, Update Software, Oxford.

Human Development Report. (2010). *The Real Wealth of Nations: Pathways to Human Development*. Available at: ℘ http://hdr.undp.org/en/reports/global/hdr2010/ (accessed 30 May 2011).

Hunter B. (2007). Conspicuous compassion and wicked problems. *Agenda*, **14**, 35–51.

Hunter B. (2007). Cumulative causation and the productivity commission's framework for overcoming indigenous disadvantage. *Australian Journal of Labour Economics*, **10**.

Hurwitz B. (2004). How does evidence based guidance influence determinations of medical negligence? *British Medical Journal*, **329**, 1024–8.

Institute of Medicine. (2001). *Crossing the quality chasm: a new health system for the 21st century*. National Academy Press, Washington, DC.

Institute of Medicine. (2006). *Food marketing to children and youth: threat or opportunity?* Institute of Medicine, Washington, DC.

Institute of Medicine Committee on Health Care in America (2001). *Crossing the quality chasm: a new health system for the 21st century*. National Academy Press, Washington DC.

Institute of Medicine Committee on Quality of Health Care in America (2000). *To err is human: building a safer health system*. National Academy Press, Washington DC.

Integrated Care Co-ordination Service (2008). The economic, health and social benefits of care co-ordination for older people. London: Cass Business School. Available at: ℘ http://www.nkm.org.uk/flyers/SpecialReports/ICCS_Comp_doc_v1[1].pdf (accessed 30 May 2011).

International Fund for Agriculture Development. (2011). *The sustainable livelihoods approach*. Available at: ℘ http://www.ifad.org/sla/index.htm (accessed 27 May 2011).

International Telecommunication Union (2010). *World Telecommunication/ICT Indicators Database* [Report on the Internet]. Available at: ℘ http://www.itu.int/ITU-D/ict/statistics/ (accessed 24 November, 2010).

Israel BA, Eng E, Schulz AJ, Parker EA (eds) (2005). *Methods in community-based participatory research for health*. Jossey-Bass, San Francisco.

Israel BA, Lantz PM, McGranaghan RJ, et al. (2005). Detroit Community-Academic Urban Research Center: in-depth semistructured interview protocol for board evaluation, 1996–2002. In: Israel BA, Eng E, Schulz AJ, Parker EA (eds) *Methods in community-based participatory research for health*, pp. 425–9. Jossey-Bass, San Francisco.

Israel BA, Schulz AJ, Parker EA, Becker AB. (1998). Review of community-based research: assessing partnership approaches to improve public health. *Annual Review of Public Health*, **19**, 173–202.

Jackson R, Ameratunga S, Broad J, et al. (2006). The GATE frame: critical appraisal with pictures. *Evidence Based Medicine*, **11**, 35–8.

Jacobs R, Gabbay J. (1994). *An action research report on audit in public health departments*. Faculty of Public Health Medicine of the Royal College of Physicians of the United Kingdom, London.

Jacobson B (2002). Delaying tactics. *Health Service Journal*, **112**, 22.

Jadad AR, Moore R, Carroll D, et al. (1996). Assessing the quality of reports of randomized clinical trials: Is blinding necessary? *Controlled Clinical Trials*, **17**, 1–12.

Jain A, Ogden J. (1999). General practitioners' experiences of patients' complaints: qualitative study. *British Medical Journal*, **318**, 1596–9.

James L, Matthews I, Nix B. (2004). Spatial contouring of risk: a tool for environmental epidemiology. *Epidemiology*. **15**, 287–92.

Jamtvedt G, Young JM, Kristoffersen DT, et al. (2006). Audit and feedback: effects on professional practice and health care outcomes. *Cochrane Database of Systematic Reviews*, (2).

Janssens AC, van Duijn C. (2009). Genome-based prediction of common diseases: methodological considerations for future research. *Genome Medicine*, **18**, 20.

Jones EF, Forrest JD. (1992). Underreporting of abortion in surveys of U.S. women: 1976 to 1988. *Demography*, **29**, 113–26.

Jones M. (2000). Walk-In primary care centres: lessons from Canada. *British Medical Journal*, **321**, 928–31.

Jordan J, Dowswell T, Harrison S, Lilford R, Mort ℘ (1998). Whose priorities? Listening to users and the public. *British Medical Journal*, **316**, 1668–70.

Jorm C, Banks M, Twohill S. (2008). The dynamic of policy and practice. In: Sorenson R, Iedema R, eds, *Managing clinical processes in the health services*. Elsevier, Sydney,

Joumard I, André C, Nicq C. (2010). *Health care systems: efficiency and institutions*, OECD Economics Department Working Papers, No. 769. OECD Publishing, Paris.

Jüni P, Altman DG, Egger M. (2001). Systematic reviews in health care: assessing the quality of controlled clinical trials. *British Medical Journal*. **323**, 42–6.

Käferstein FK, Motarjemi Y, Bettcher DW. (1997). *Foodborne disease control: a transnational challenge*. Emerging Infectious Diseases. **3**, 503–10.

Kaiser Family Foundation. (2011). *State Health Facts*. Available at: ℅ http://www.statehealthfacts.org/comparemaptable.jsp?ind=624&cat=6.

Kelley E, Hurst J. (2006). *Health care quality indicators project*, Conceptual framework paper. OECD health working papers no. 23. OECD, Paris.

Kerzner H (2009). *Project management: a systems approach to planning, scheduling, and controlling*, 10th edn. John Wiley & Sons, Hoboken.

Kesteloot H, Sans S, Kromhout D (2006). Dynamics of cardiovascular and all-cause mortality in Western and Eastern Europe between 1970 and 2000. *European Heart Journal*, **27**, 107–13.

Khan A, Walley J, Newell J, Imdad N. (2000). Tuberculosis in Pakistan: social-cultural constraints and opportunities in treatment. *Social Science and Medicine*, **50**, 247–54.

Khoury MJ, McCabe LL, McCabe ERB. (2004) Population screening in the age of genomic medicine. *New England Journal of Medicine*, **348**, 50–8.

Kibble A, Harrison R. (2005). Point sources of air pollution. *Occupational Medicine*, **55**, 425–31.

Kindshauer MK (ed.) (2003). *Communicable diseases 2002—global defense against the infectious disease threat*, WHO/CDS/2003.15. World Health Organization, Geneva. Available at: M http://www.who.int/infectious-disease-news/cds2002/intro.pdf (accessed 31 August 2010).

Kingsley BS, Schmeichel KL, Rubin CH. (2007). An update on cancer cluster activities at the Centers for Disease Control and Prevention. *Environmental Health Perspectives*, **115**, 165–71.

Kinmonth A-L, Marteau T. (2002). Screening for cardiovascular risk: public health imperative or matter for individual informed choice? *British Medical Journal*, **325**, 78–80.

Kirkwood BR. (2003). *Measures of mortality and morbidity. Essentials of medical statistics*, 2nd edn. Blackwell Scientific Publications, Oxford.

Kivipelto M, Rovio S, Ngandu T, *et al.* (2008). Apolipoprotein E ε 4 magnifies lifestyle risks for dementia: a population-based study. *Journal of Cellular and Molecular Medicine*. **12**, 2762–71.

Kotter J. (1996). *Leading change*. Harvard Business School Press, Boston.

Kranendonk S, Bringezau, B. (1994). *Major material flows associated with orange juice consumption in Germany*. Wupperthal Institute, Wupperthal.

Krieger N, Northridge M, Gruskin S, *et al.* (2003). Assessing health impact assessment: multidisciplinary and international perspectives. *Journal of Epidemiology and Community Health*, **57**, 659–62.

Kyffin RGE, Goldacre MJ, Gill M. (2004). Mortality rates and self reported health: database analysis by English local authority area. *British Medical Journal*, **329**, 887–8.

La Torre G, De Vito E, Langiano E, *et al.* (2003). Epidemiology of hepatitis C virus antibodies in blood donors from the province of Latina, Italy. *European Journal of Epidemiology*, **18**, 691–4.

Lakoff G. (1996). *Moral politics: what Conservatives know that Liberals don't*. University of Chicago Press, Chicago.

Lakoff G. (2004). *Don't think of an elephant. Know your values and frame the debate*. ChelseaGreen Publishing, Vermont.

Lampe K, Mäkelä M, Garrido MV, *et al.*, for European network for Health Technology Assessment (EUnetHTA) (2009). The HTA core model: a novel method for producing and reporting health technology assessments. *International Journal of Technology Assessment in Health Care*, **25(Suppl. 2),** 9–20.

Lancet/London International Development Commission (2010). The Millenium Development Goals: a cross-sectorial analysis and principles for goal setting after 2015. Lancet 376, 991–1023. Available at: ℅ http://www.thelancet.com/mdgcommission.

Lang IA, Galloway TS, Scarlett A, *et al.* (2008). Association of urinary bisphenol A concentration with medical disorders and laboratory abnormalities in adults. *Journal of the American Medical Association*, B **11**, 1303–10.

Lang IA, Guralnik J, Wallace RB, Melzer D. (2007) What level of alcohol consumption is hazardous for older people? Functioning and mortality in U.S. and English national cohorts. *Journal of the American Geriatrics Society*, **55**, 49–57.

Lang IA, Llewellyn DJ, Hubbard RE, Langa KM, Melzer D. (2011). Income and the midlife peak in common mental disorder prevalence. *Psychological Medicine*, **41**, 1365–72.

Lasker RD, Committee on Medicine and Public Health. (1997). *Medicine and public health: the power of collaboration*. Academy of Medicine, New York.

Lavis JN. (2006). Research, public policymaking, and knowledge-translation processes: Canadian efforts to build bridges. *Journal of Continuing Education in the Health Profession* **26**, 37–45

Lawrence D. David Lawrence offers some words of advice to Mr Brown. Available at: ✍ http://www.hsj.co.uk/david-lawrence-offers-some-words-of-advice-to-mr-brown/58956.article (accessed 30 May 2011).

Leask J, Chapman S, Cooper S. (2010). 'All manner of ills': attribution of serious disease to vaccination. *Vaccine*, **28**, 3066–70.

Leatherman S, Sutherland K. (2005). *The quest for quality in the NHS. A chartbook on quality of care in the UK.* Radcliffe, Oxford.

Lee K. (2003). *Globalization and Health: An Introduction.* Palgrave: London.

Leeder S. (2005). Setting goals for health in a time of prosperity. Medical Journal of Australia, 183(5), 232–33.

Leichter HM. (1979). *A comparative approach to policy analysis: health care policy in four nations.* Cambridge University Press, Cambridge.

Leukaemia Research Fund. (1997). *Handbook and guide to the investigation of clusters of disease.* Leukaemia Research Fund Centre for Clinical Epidemiology, University of Leeds, Leeds.

Levy PS, Lemeshow S. (2008). *Sampling of populations: methods and applications,* Wiley Series in Survey Methodology, 4th edn. Wiley, Hoboken.

Lilford RJ, Brown CA, Nicholl J. (2007). Use of process measures to monitor the quality of clinical practice. *British Medical Journal*, **335**, 648–50.

Lohr KN, Brook RH, Kamberg CJ, *et al.* (1986). Effect of cost sharing on use of medically effective and less effective care. *Medical Care*, **24(Suppl. 9)**, S31–8.

London Health Observatory. (2011). *Basket of Indicators.* Available at: ✍ http://www.lho.org.uk/LHO_Topics/national_lead_areas/Basket_of_indicators/BasketOfIndicators.aspx

Lopez AD, Maters CD, Ezzati, et al. (2006). *Global Burden of Disease and Risk factors.* The World Bank and Oxford University Press; New York. Available at: ✍ www.dcp2.org/pubs/gbd. (accessed 30 May 2011).

Lord Nolan (Chair) (1995). *First Report of the Committee on Standards in Public Life.* Public Appointments Commission, London.

Lorenzi NM, Kouroubali A, Detmer DE, Bloomrosen M. (2009). How to successfully select and implement electronic health records (EHR) in small ambulatory practice settings. *BMC Medical Informatics and Decision-Making*, **23**, 9–15.

Loureiro ML, Nayga Jr. RM. (2005). *Obesity rates in OECD countries: an international perspective.* Available at: ✍ http://ageconsearch.umn.edu/bitstream/24454/1/pp05lo01.pdf

Luft J, Ingham H. (1955). *The Johari-window: a graphic model for interpersonal relations.* University of California, Western Training Laboratory, Los Angeles.

Lukes S. (1974). *Power: a radical view.* MacMillan, London.

Mackenbach J, Stronks K. (2002). A strategy for tackling health inequalities in the Netherlands; *British Medical Journal*, **325**, 1029–32.

MacKenzie M, O'Donnell C, Halliday E, Sridharan S, Platt S. (2010). Do health improvement programmes fit with MRC guidance on evaluating complex interventions? British Medical Journal, 340, c185.

Mackie A. (2008). *Continuing Professional Development (CPD).* Faculty of Public Health, London

Mahoney M, Simpson S, Harris E, Aldrich R, Stewart Williams J. (2004). *Equity focused health impact assessment framework.* Australasian Collaboration for Health Equity Impact Assessment, Newcastle. Available at: ✍ http://www.hiaconnect.edu.au/files/EFHIA_Framework.pdf (accessed 26 August 2010).

Majone G. (1989). *Evidence, argument and persuasion in the policy process.* Yale University Press, New Haven.

Makk L, Delmore F, Creech Jr JL, *et al.* (2006). Clinical and morphologic features of hepatic angiosarcoma in vinyl chloride workers. *Cancer*, **37**, 148–63.

Mallinson S, Popay J, Kowarzik U. (2006). Developing the public workforce: a 'communities of practice' perspective. *Policy and Politics*, **34**, 265–85.

Marlow P. (2005). Literature review on the value of target setting, HSL/2005/40 Sheffield: Human Factors Group, Health & Safety Laboratory, Sheffield.

Marmot M. (2011). Fair Society, Healthy Lives—the Marmot Review. Available at: ✍ www.ucl.ac.uk/marmotreview

Marshall EC, Spiegelhalter DJ. (1998). Reliability of league tables of in vitro fertilization clinics: retrospective analysis of live birth rates. *British Medical Journal*, **316**, 1701–5.

Martens PJ, Roos NP. (2005). When health services researchers and policy makers interact: tales from the tectonic plates. *Healthcare Policy*, **1**, 72–84.

Maslow AH. (1943). A Theory of Human Motivation. *Psychological Review*, **50**, 370–96.

Mayhew L. (2008). On the effectiveness of care co-ordination services aimed at preventing hospital admissions and emergency attendances. Health Care Management Science. Available at: M http://www.nkm.org.uk/flyers/SpecialReports/HCMScifulltextpublished221208.pdf

McAlister F, van Diepen S, Padwal RS, Johnson JA, Majumdar SR. (2007). How evidence based are the recommendations in clinical guidelines? PLoS Medicine, **4**, e250.

McCarthy N, Giesecke J. (1999). Case-case comparisons to study causation of common infectious diseases. Int J Epidemiol, **28**: 764–8.

McCaughey D, Bruning N. (2010). Rationality versus reality: the challenges of evidence-based decision making for health policy makers. Implementation Science, 5, 39.

McDonald D, Bammer G, Deane P. (2009). Research integration using dialogue methods. Australian National University E Press, Canberra. Available at: ℘ http://epress.anu.edu.au/dialogue_methods_citation.html.

McGuire A, Henderson J, Mooney G. (1988). The economics of health care: an introductory text. Routledge, London.

McKeown T. (1979). Role of medicine. Basil Blackwell, Oxford.

McNally RJ, Alexander FE, Vincent TJ, Murphy MF. (2009). Spatial clustering of childhood cancer in Great Britain during the period 1969–1993.International Journal of Cancer, **124**, 932–6.

McNamara C. (2003). Field guide to non-profit design, marketing and evaluation. Authenticity Consulting, Minneapolis.

McNeil BJ, Pauker SG, Sox HC, Tversky A. (1982). On the elicitation of preferences for alternative therapies. North England Journal of Medicine, **306**, 1259–62.

Mercer SL, Green LW, Cargo M, et al. (2008). Reliability-tested guidelines for assessing participatory research projects. In: Minkler M, Wallerstein N, (eds) Community-based participatory research for health: from process and outcomes, 2nd edn. Jossey-Bass, San Francisco.

Mezei G, Kheifets L. (2006). Selection bias and its implications for case-control studies: a case study of magnetic field exposure and childhood leukaemia. International Journal of Epidemiology, **35**,397–406.

Michie S, Fixsen D, Grimshaw J, Eccles M. (2009). Specifying and reporting complex behavior change interventions: the need for a scientific method. Implementation Science, **4**, 40.

Midgley M. (2001). Science and Poetry. Routledge, London.

Miilunpalo S, Vuori I, Oja P, Pasanen M, Urponen H. (1997). Self-rated health status as a health measure: the predictive value of self-reported health status on the use of physician services and on mortality in the working-age population. Journal of Clinical Epidemiology, **50**, 517–28. Available at: ℘ http://www.ncbi.nlm.nih.gov/entrez/query.fcgi?cmd=Retrieve&db=PubMed&dopt=Citation&list_uids=9180644

Miké V. (2003). Evidence and the future of medicine. Evaluation and the Health Professions, **26**, 127.

Milio N. (1987). Making healthy public policy: developing the science by learning the art. Health Promotion International, **2**, 263–74.

Mill J. (1969). Utilitarianism. In: Collected Works of John Stuart Mill, Vol 10. University of Toronto Press, Toronto.

Mill JS (1869/2002) On Liberty. Dover Publications, Mineola.

Mills EJ, Schabas WA, Volmink J, et al. (2008). Should active recruitment of health workers from sub-Saharan Africa be viewed as a crime? Lancet, **371**, 685–88.

Milton, J. (1999). When I consider how my light is spent. In: Ricks, C , ed.,, Oxford Book of English Verse, p. 168. Oxford University Press, Oxford.

Mindell J. (2003). A glossary for health impact assessment Journal of Epidemiology Community Health, **57(5)**, 647–51. Available at: ℘ http://jech.bmj.com/cgi/doi/10.1136/jech.57.9.647

Mindell JS, Boltong A, Forde I. (2008). A review of health impact assessment frameworks. Public Health. **122**, 1177–87.

Minkler M, Lee PT, Tom A, et al. (2010). Using community-based participatory research to design and initiate a study on immigrant worker health and safety in San Francisco's Chinatown restaurants. American Journal of Industrial Medicine, **53**, 361–71.

Minkler M, Wallerstein N. (2008). Introduction to CBPR: New issues and emphases. In: Minkler M, Wallerstein N (eds) Community-based participatory research for health, pp. 5–24. Jossey-Bass, San Francisco..

Mitton C, Adair C, McKenzie E, Patten SB, Perry BW. (2007). Knowledge transfer and exchange: review and synthesis of the literature. Milbank Quarterly, **85**, 729–68.

Mohammed MA. (2004). Using statistical process control to improve the quality of health care. Quality Safe Health Care, **13**, 243–5.

Mohammed MA, Cheng KK, Rouse A, Marshall T. (2001). Use of Shewhart's technique. Lancet., **358**, 512.

Monk R. (1991). *Ludwig Wittgenstein: the duty of genius.* Vintage, London.

Mooney G, Gerard K, Donaldson C, Farrar S. (1992). *Priority setting in purchasing: some practical guidelines,* Research Paper 6. National Association of Health Authorities and Trusts (NAHAT), Birmingham.

Moore A, McQuay H, Gray JAM. (1999). Bandolier 61: Evidence-based health care. *Bandolier* **6,** 1–8.

Moore G. (2000). *Managing to do better. General practice for the twenty-first century.* Office of Health Economics, London.

Morgan MG. (1993). Risk analysis and management. *Scientific American,* July, 24–30.

Morgan MG, Fischhoff B, Bostrom A, Lave L, Atman C. (1992). Communicating risk to the public. *Environmental Science Technology,* **26,** 2048–56.

Morgan SG, McMahon M, Mitton C, *et al.* (2006). Centralized drug review processes in Australia, Canada, New Zealand, and the United Kingdom. *Health Affairs,* **25,** 337–47.

Moss SM. (1991). Case-control studies of screening. *International Journal of Epidemiology* **20,** 1–6.

Mossialos E, Dixon A, Figueras J, *et al.* (eds) (2002). *Funding health care: options for Europe.* European Observatory on Health Care Systems, Open University Press, Buckingham.

Muir Gray JA. (1999). Post-modern medicine. *Lancet,* **354,** 1550–2.

Muir Gray J. (2009). *Evidence-based healthcare and public health: how to make decisions about health services and public health,* 3rd edn. Elsevier, London.

Mukoma W, Flisher AJ. (2004). Evaluations of health promoting schools: a review of nine studies. *Health Promotion International,* **19,** 357–68.

Mullan F, Epstein L. (2002). Community-oriented primary care: new relevance in a changing world. *American Journal of Public Health,* **92,** 1748–55.

Myers Briggs I, Myers P. (1980). *Gifts differing, understanding personality type.* Davies-Black, Palo Alto.

Nass SJ, Levit LA, Gostin LO. (2009). *Beyond the HIPAA privacy rule: enhancing privacy, improving health through research.* National Academy Press, Washington, DC.

National Cancer Institute. (2008). *The role of the media in promoting and reducing tobacco use,* Tobacco Monograph Series 19. Department of Health and Human Services, National Cancer Institute, Washington DC.

National Centre for Health Statistics, US statistics. Available at: ⅆ http://www.cdc.gov/nchs/ (accessed 21 March 2005).

National Centre for Health Statistics. National Health Interview Survey (NHIS). Available at: ⅆ www.cdc.gov/nchs/nhis.htm (accessed 20 March 2005).

National Health and Medical Research Council (Australia). (2009). *A guide to the development, implementation and evaluation of clinical practice guidelines.* National Health and Medical Research Council (NHMRC), Canberra.

National Institute for Health and Clinical Excellence (2010). *NICE guidance by topic.* NICE, London. Available at: ⅆ http://www.nice.org.uk/page.aspx?o=cat.diseaseareas (accessed 27 August 2010).

National Institute for Health and Clinical Excellence, (2010). *Guide to the methods of technology appraisal.* NICE, London. Available at: ⅆ http://www.nice.org.uk/aboutnice/howwework/devnicetech/technologyappraisalprocessguides/guidetothemethodsoftechnologyappraisal.jsp (accessed 1 September 2010).

National Institute for Health and Clinical Excellence (2012). *How we work.* NICE, London. Available at: ⅆ www.nice.org.uk/aboutnice/howwework/how_we_work.jsp

National Institute of Health and Clinical Effectiveness. Available at: ⅆ http://www.nice.org.uk (accessed 14 January 2006).

National Preventative Health Taskforce. (2009). The healthiest country by 2020—national preventative health strategy—the roadmap to action: Australian Government, Canberra.

National Public Health Partnership. (2000). Deciding and specifying an intervention portfolio. National Public Health Partnership, Melbourne.

National Research Council. (1989). *Improving risk communication.* National Academy Press, Washington, DC. Available at: ⅆ http://www.nap.edu/openbook.php?record_id=1189&page=1 (accessed 6 August 2010).

National Statistics, Official UK statistics. Available at: http://www.statistics.gov.uk (accessed 20 March 2005).

National Telecommunication and Information Administration, United States Department of Commerce (2010). *Exploring the digital nation: home broadband Internet adoption in the United States.* [Report on the Internet]. Available at: ⅆ http://www.esa.doc.gov/DN/nef (2009). *The Happy Planet Index.* Available at: ⅆ http://www.happyplanetindex.org/ (accessed: 1 August 2011).

Nelson B, Economy P. (1997). *Consulting for dummies*. IDG Publications, Foster City.

Neutra R, Swan S, Mack T. (1992). Clusters galore: insights about environmental clusters from probability theory. *Science and Total Environment*, **127**, 187–200.

Newton J, Garner S. (2002). *Disease registers in England. Report for the Department of Health policy research programme*. Available at: ℘ www.erpho.org.uk/viewResource.aspx?id=12531 (accessed 21 January 2006).

NHS Centre for Reviews and Dissemination. Evidence from systematic reviews of the research relevant to implementing the 'wider public health' agenda. York: University of York, NHS Centre for Reviews and Dissemination, 2000.

NHS Confederation. (2005). Alternative providers of medical services—a contracting guide for primary care trusts. NHS Confederation, London.

NHS Diabetic Eye Screening Programme. National screening programme for sight-threatening retinopathy website. Available at: ℘ www.nscretinopathy.org.uk (accessed (30 November 2004).

NHS Leadership Development Framework Development Guide. (2010). Leadership development module. Available at: ℘ http://www.nhsleadershipqualities.nhs.uk/development-guide (accessed 20 August 2010).

NHS Leadership Qualities Framework. (2006). *NHS Institute for Innovation & Improvement,*. Available at: ℘ http://www.nhsleadershipqualities.nhs.uk/ (accessed 20 August 2010).

NHS Management Executive. (1993). *Health Service Guidelines HSG(93)38: arrangements to deal with health aspects of chemical contamination incidents*. Department of Health, Health Aspects of the Environment and Food Division, London:

NHS Management Executive. (1993). *Health Service Guidelines HSG(93)56: Public health responsibilities of the NHS and the roles of others*. Department of Health, Health Aspects of the Environment and Food Division, London.

NHS Sustainable Development Unit. (2008). *Carbon Reduction Strategy for NHS England*. NHS Sustainable Development Unit, Cambridge.

NHS Sustainable Development Unit (2009). *Forum for the future. fit for the future. Scenarios for low-carbon healthcare 2030*. NHS Sustainable Development Unit, Cambridge.

NHS Sustainable Development Unit. (2010). *Saving carbon, improving health; UPDATE NHS Carbon Reduction Strategy*. NHS Sustainable Development Unit, Cambridge.

NHS Sustainable Development Unit. (2011). *Route Map for Sustainable Health*. NHS Sustainable Development Unit, Cambridge.

Noji E (ed.) (1997). *The public health consequences of disasters*. Oxford University Press, New York.

Nolte E, Bain C, McKee M. (2006). Chronic diseases as tracer conditions in international benchmarking of health systems: the example of diabetes. *Diabetes Care*, **29**, 1007–11.

Nolte E, McKee M. (2004). *Does health care save lives? Avoidable mortality revisited*. Nuffield Trust, London.

Noseworthy JH, Ebers GC, Vandervoort MK, I (1994). The impact of blinding on the results of a randomized, placebo-controlled multiple sclerosis clinical trial. *Neurology*, **44**, 16–20.

Noyes J, Popay J. (2007). Directly observed therapy and tuberculosis: how can a systematic review of qualitative research contribute to improving services? A qualitative meta-synthesis, *Journal of Advanced Nursing*, **57(3)**, 227–43.

Nutbeam D, Boxhall AM. (2008). What influences the transfer of research into health policy? Observations from England and Australia. *Public Health*. **122**, 747–53.

Nutley SM, Walter I, Davies HTO. (2007). *Using evidence: how research can inform public services*. Policy Press, Bristol.

O'Carroll PW, Yasnoff WA, Ward ME, Ripp LH, Martin EL. (eds) (2003). *Public health informatics and information systems*. Springer-Verlag, New York.

O'Fallon LR, Dearry A. (1992). Community-based participatory research as a tool to advance environmental health sciences. *Environmental Health Perspectives*, **110(Suppl. 2)**, 155–9.

O'Keefe E, Scott-Samuel A. (2010). Health impact assessment as an accountability mechanism for the International Monetary Fund: the case of Sub-Saharan Africa. *International Journal of the Health Service*, **40**, 339–45.

Office of Government Commerce (OGC). (2010). *UK successful delivery toolkitTM; and OGC gatewayTM review pack*. Available at: ℘ http://webarchive.nationalarchives.gov.uk/20100503135839/ http://www.ogc.gov.uk/programmes_and_projects.asp (accessed 18 November 2011).

Otten AL. (1992). The influence of the mass media on health policy. *Health Affairs*, **11**, 111–18.

Oxman A, Lavis JAF. (2007). The use of evidence in WHO recommendations. *Lancet*, 369, 1883–9.

Ozcan YA. (2009). *Quantitative methods in health care management*. Jossey-Bass, San Francisco.

Paquet C, Coulombier D, Kaiser R, Ciotti M. (2006). Epidemic Intelligence: A new framework for strengthening disease surveillance in Europe. *European Surveillance*, **11**, pii–665. Available at: ✇ http://www.eurosurveillance.org/ViewArticle.aspx?ArticleId=665 (accessed 21 June 2010).

Parkin DM, Whelan SL, Ferlay J, Teppo L, Thomas DB. (2003). *Cancer incidence in five continents*, Vol. VIII. IARC, Lyon.

Parry JM, Kemm J. (2005). Criteria for use in the evaluation of health impact assessments: recommendations from an European workshop. *Public Health*, **119**, 1122–9.

Pasetto R, Comba P, Marconi A (2005). Mesothelioma associated with environmental exposures. *La Medicina del Lavora*, **96**, 330–7.

Paul B. (1955). *Health, culture and community*. Sage Foundation, New York.

Pawson R, Greenhalgh T, Harvey G, Walshe K. (2005). Realist review—new method of systematic review designed for complex policy interventions. Journal of Health Services & Research Policy. 10(Suppl 1), 21–34.

Pawson R, Tilley N. (1997). *Realistic evaluation*. Sage Publications, London.

Payne N, Saul C. (1997). Variations in use of cardiology services in a health authority: comparison of coronary artery revascularisation rates with prevalence of angina and coronary mortality. *British Medical Journal*, **314**, 256–61.

Pencheon D. (2008). *The Good Indicators Guide: understanding how to use and choose indicators*. Available at: ✇ http://www.apho.org.uk/resource/item.aspx?RID=44584

Petts J, Wheeley S, Homan J, Niemeyer S. (2003). *Risk literacy and the public. MMR, air pollution and mobile phones*. Department of Health, London. Available at: ✇ http://www.dh.gov.uk/asset-Root/04/07/40/99/04074099.pdf (accessed 26 August 2010).

Pharoah PDP, Antoniou AC, Easton DF, Ponder BAJ. (2008). Polygenes, risk prediction, and targeted prevention of breast cancer. *New England Journal of Medicine*, **358**, 2796–803.

Picker Institute Europe (2011). Patient reviews. Available at: ✇ http://www.pickereurope.org/using-patientfeedback (accessed 17 May 2011).

Plsek PE,.Greenhalgh T. (2001). The challenge of complexity in health care. *British Medical Journal*, **323**, 625–8.

Popay J, Bennett S, Thomas C, *et al*. (2003b). Beyond beer, fags, egg and chips? Exploring lay understandings of social inequalities in health. *Social Health and Illness*, **25**, 1–23.

Popay J, Thomas C, Williams G, *et al*. (2003a). A proper place to live: health inequalities, agency and the normative dimensions of space. *Social Science and Medicine*, **57**, 55–69.

Porta ✇ (ed.) (2008). *A dictionary of epidemiology*, 5th edn. Oxford University Press, Oxford.

Porta M, Last J. (2008). *Dictionary of epidemiology*, 5th edn. Oxford University Press, Oxford.

Powell JE. (1976). *Medicine and politics: 1975 and after*. Pitman Medical, London. (How to work with full-time politicians and senior civil servants.)

Pozen A, Cutler DM. (2010). Medical spending differences in the United States and Canada: the role of prices, procedures, and administrative expenses. *Inquiry*, **47**, 124–34.

Prabhu VR, Hanley A, Kearney S (2008). Evaluation of a hospital volunteer programme in rural Australia. *Australian Health Review*. **32**, 265–70.

Pratt J. (1995). *Practitioners and practices. A conflict of values?* Radcliffe Medical Press, Oxford.

Preker AS, Harding A. (2003). *Innovations in health service delivery: the corporatization of public hospitals*. World Bank, Washington DC.

Price RH, Behrens T. (2003). Working Pasteur's quadrant: harnessing science and action for community change. *American Journal of Community Psychology*, **31**, 219–23.

Public Health Advisory Committee (2004). *A guide to health impact assessment: a policy tool for New Zealand*. Public Health Advisory Committee, National Advisory Committee on Health and Disability, Wellington. Available at: ✇ http://www.nhc.health.govt.nz/publications/phac-pre-2011/guide-health-impact-assessment-2nd-edition (accessed 24 May 2012).

Raffle A. (2010). Guest editorial: advertising private tests for well people. *Clinical Evidence*, **2**.

Raffle AE, Alden B, Quinn M, Babb PJ, Brett MT. (2003). Outcomes of screening to prevent cancer: analysis of cumulative incidence of cervical abnormality and modelling of cases and deaths prevented. *British Medical Journal* **326**, 901–4.

Rajaratnam JK, Marcus JR, Flaxman AD, *et al*. (2010). Neonatal, postnatal, childhood, and under-5 mortality for 187 countries, 1970–2010: a systematic analysis of progress towards Millennium Development Goal 4. *Lancet*, **375**, 1988–2008.

Ram KT, Klugman SD. (2010). Best practices: antenatal screening for common genetic conditions other than aneuploidy. *Current Opinion in Obstetrics and Gynecology*, **22**, 139–45.

Randolph, W., Viswanath K. (2004). Lessons Learned from public health mass media campaigns: marketing health in a crowded media world. *Annual Review of Public Health* **25**, 419–37.

Rawaf S, Bahl V. (1998). *Assessing health needs of people from minority ethnic groups*. Royal College of Physicians, London.

Rawls J. (1971). *A theory of justice*. Harvard University Press, Boston.

Reason P, Bradbury H. (2006). *Handbook of action research: participatory inquiry and practice*, concise edn. Sage Publications, London.

Rehm J, Mathers C, Popova S, Thavorncharoensap M, Teerawattananon Y, Patra J. (2009). Global burden of disease and injury and economic cost attributable to alcohol use and alcohol-use disorders. *Lancet*, **373**, 2223–33.

Reinhardt UE. (2011). The many different prices paid to providers and the flawed theory of cost shifting: is it time for a more rational all-payer system? *Health Affairs*, **30**, 2125–33.

Report of the Northern Territory Board of Inquiry into the Protection of Aboriginal Children from Sexual Abuse (2007).

Richardson A, Jackson C, Sykes W. (1992). *Audit guidelines in public health medicine: an introduction*. Nuffield Institute for Health Services Studies, University of Leeds, Leeds.

Rideout V, Foehr UG, Roberts DF. (2010). Generation M2: Media in the lives of 8- to 18-year-olds [Report on the Internet]. Henry J. Kaiser Family Foundation, Menlo Park. Available at: ℅ http://www.kff.org/entmedia/upload/8010.pdf

Rist RC. (1994). Influencing the policy process with qualitative research. In: Denzin NK, Lincoln YS, eds, *Handbook of qualitative research*, pp. 545–57. Sage, Thousand Oaks.

Robert Wood Johnson Foundation, The Pew Charitable Trust. *Health Impact Project*. Available at: ℅ http://www.healthimpactproject.org (accessed 26 August 2010).

Roberts H, Curtis K, Liabo K, et al. (2004). Putting public health evidence into practice: increasing the prevalence of working smoke alarms in disadvantaged inner city housing, *Journal of Epidemiology and Community Health*, **58**, 280–5.

Robinson R. (1993). Cost benefit analysis. *British Medical Journal*, **307**, 924–6.

Robinson R. (1993). Cost effectiveness analysis. *British Medical Journal*, **307**, 793–5.

Robinson R. (1993). Cost utility analysis. *British Medical Journal*, **307**, 859–62.

Robinson R. (1993). Costs and cost minimisation analysis. *British Medical Journal*, **307**, 726–8.

Robinson R. (1993). Economic evaluation and health care (a series of six articles in the BMJ). What does it mean? *British Medical Journal*, **307**, 670–3.

Robinson R. (1993). The policy context. *British Medical Journal*, **307**, 994–6.

Rose G. (1992). *The strategy of preventive medicine*. Oxford University Press, Oxford.

Rothenberg RB, Thacker SB. (1996). Guidelines for the investigation of clusters of adverse health events. In: Eliott P, Cuzick J, English D, Stern R, eds, *Geographical and environmental epidemiology methods for small-area studies*, pp. 264–77. Oxford University Press, Oxford.

Rothman KJ. (1990). A sobering start for the cluster busters' conference. *American Journal of Epidemiology*, **132(Suppl.1)**, S6–13.

Rothman KJ. (2002). *Epidemiology: an introduction*. Oxford University Press, Oxford.

Rothman KJ, Greenland S, Lash TL. (2008). *Modern epidemiology*, 3rd edn. Lippincott, Williams, & Wilkins. Philadelphia.

Rothman KJ, Greenland S, Poole C, Lash TL. (2008). Causation and causal inference. In: Rothman KJ, Greenland S, Lash TJ, eds, *Modern epidemiology*, 3rd edn, pp. 5–31. Lippincott Williams & Wilkins, Philadelphia .

Rouse A, Adab P. (2001). Is population coronary heart disease risk screening justified? A discussion of the national service framework for coronary heart disease (standard 4). *British Journal of General Practice*, **51**, 834–7.

Rowe L, Kidd ℅ (2010). *First do no harm: being a resilient doctor in the 21st century*. McGraw-Hill, London.

Royal Commission on Environmental Pollution. (2003). *Chemicals in products: safeguarding the environment and human health*, 24th Report of the Royal Commission on Environmental Pollution., Royal Commission on Environmental Pollution, London.

Royal Society of Medicine Press. *Effective health care bulletins*. Available at: ℅ http://www.york.ac.uk/inst/crd/ehcb_em.htm (accessed 24 May 2012). [Effective Health Care Bulletins are bimonthly publications for decision-makers, which examine the effectiveness of a variety of health care interventions. They are based on a systematic review and synthesis of research on the clinical effectiveness, cost-effectiveness, and acceptability of health service interventions. This is carried out by a research team using established methodological guidelines, with advice from expert consultants for each topic. The bulletins are subject to extensive and rigorous peer review.]

Royal Society Study Group. (1992). *Risk: analysis, perception and management*. Royal Society, London.

Rutstein D, Berenberg W, Chalmers T, et al. (1976). Measuring the quality of medical care. *New England Journal of Medicine*, **294**, 582–8.

Rychetnik L, Frommer M. (2002). A schema for evaluating evidence on public health interventions, version 4. National Public Health Partnership, Melbourne.

Rychetnik L, Wise M. (2004). Advocating evidence-based health promotion: reflections and a way forward. *Health Promotion International*, **19**, 247–57.

Sackett DL, Rosenber WM, Gray JA, Haynes RB, Richardson WS. (1996). Evidence based medicine: what it is and what it isn't. *British Medical Journal*, **312**, 71–2.

Saltman RB, Ferroussier-Davis O. (2000). The concept of stewardship in health policy. *Bulletin of the World Health Organization*, 732–9.

Salvatore AL, Krause N. (2010). Health and working conditions of restaurant workers in San Francisco's Chinatown: report of preliminary findings. *Public Health Reports*, **126(Suppl. 3)**, 62–9.

Sanderson C, Gruen R. (2006). *Analytical models for deci-sion-making.* Open University Press, Maidenhead.

Sandman PM. (1993). *Responding to community outrage: strategies for effective risk communication.* American Industrial Hygiene Association, Fairfax, VA.

Sandman PM, Lanard J. (2003). Fear is spreading faster than SARS—and so it should! ℘ http://www.psandman.com/col/SARS-1.htm (accessed 6 August 2010).

Scally G, Donaldson LJ. (1998). Clinical governance is here to stay. *British Medical Journal*, **317**, 61–5.

Schmid D, Schandl S, Pichler AM, *et al.* (2005). *Salmonella enteritidis* phage type 21 outbreak in Austria. *European Surveillance*, **11**, 67–9.

Schoen C, Osborn R, Huynh PT. (2004). Primary care and health system performance: adults' experiences in five countries. *Health affairs*, web exclusive, October 28, W4-497–503.

Schon D. (1983). *The reflective practitioner: how professionals think in action.* Temple Smith, London.

Schon DA, Rein M. (1994). *Frame reflection: toward the resolution of intractable policy controversies.* Basic Books: New York.

Scott A, Donaldson C. (1998). Clinical and cost effectiveness issues in health needs assessment. In: Wright J (ed.). *Health needs assessment in practice*, pp. 84–94. BMJ Books, London.

Scott-Samuel A. (1996). Health impact assessment—an idea whose time has come. *British Medical Journal*, **313**, 183–4.

Scott-Samuel A, O'Keefe E. (2007). Health impact assessment, human rights and global public policy: a critical appraisal. *Bulletin of the World Health* Organization, **85**, 212–17.

Seale C. (1999.) *The quality of qualitative research.* Sage, London.

Seaton A, Donaldson K. (2005) Nanoscience, nanotechnology, and the need to think small. *Lancet*, **365**, 923–4.

Secretary of State for Health. (2010). Equity and excellence: liberating the NHS. Department of Health, HMSO, London.

Seib KL, Dougan G, Rappuoli R. (2009). The key role of genomics in modern vaccine and drug design for emerging infectious diseases. *PLoS Genetics* **5**, e1000612.

Semenza JC, Rubin CH, Falter KH, *et al.* (1996). Heat-related deaths during the July 1995 heat wave in Chicago. *New England Journal of Medicine*, **335**, 84–90.

Shea B, Grimshaw J, Wells G, *et al.* (2007). Development of AMSTAR: a measurement tool to assess the methodological quality of systematic reviews. *BMC Medical Research Methodology*, **7**, 10.

Shekelle P. (2004). The appropriateness method. *Medical Decision-Making*; **24**, 228–31.

Shekelle PG, Lim Y-W, Mattke S, Damberg C. (2008). *Does public release of performance results improve quality of care? A systematic review* [online] Health Foundation London. Available at: ℘ www.health.org.uk

Shepperd S, Lewin S, Straus S, et al. (2009). Can We Systematically Review Studies That Evaluate Complex Interventions? PLoS Medicine, 6(8), e1000086.

Shojania KG, Grimshaw JM. (2005). Evidence-based quality improvement: the state of the science. *Health Affairs (Millwood)*, **24**, 138–50.

Shojania KG, Jennings A, Mayhew A, *et al.* (2010). Effect of point-of-care computer reminders on physician behaviour: a systematic review. *Canadian Medical Association Journal*, **182**, E216–25.

Shortell SM, Rundall TG, Hsu J (2007). Improving patient care by linking evidence-based medicine and evidence-based management. *Journal of the American Medical Association*, **298**, 673–6.

Shortliffe EH, Cimino JJ. (2006). *Medical informatics: computer applications in health care and biomedi-cine*, 3nd edn. Springer, New York.

Silvestri G, Pritchard R, Welch HG. (1998). Preferences for chemotherapy in patients with advanced non-small cell lung cancer: descriptive study based on scripted interviews. *British Medical Journal*, **317**, 771–5.

Smith A. (2010). *Americans and their Gadgets* [Report on the Internet]. Pew Research Center's Internet & American Life Project, Washington, DC Available at: ℘ http://www.pewinternet.org/Reports/2010/Gadgets.aspx

Smith KE, Fooks G, Collin J, et al. (2010). Is the increasing policy use of impact assessment in Europe likely to undermine efforts to achieve healthy public policy? *Journal of Epidemiology and Community Health*, **64**, 478–87.

Smith S, Newhouse JP, Freeland MS. (2009). Income, insurance, and technology: why does health spending outpace economic growth? *Health Affairs*, **28**, 276–1284.

Solutions for Public Health (2012). *Resources*. SPH, Oxford. Available at: ℘ www.sph.nhs.uk/sph-psu/resources

Sorian R, Baugh T. (2002). Power of information: closing the gap between research and policy. *Health Affairs*, **21**, 264–73.

Spiegelhalter D. (2002). Funnel plots for institutional comparison [comment]. *Quality and Safety in Health Care*, **11**, 390–1.

Spiegelhalter DJ, Abrams KR, Myles JP. (2004). *Bayesian approaches to clinical trials and health-care evaluation (Statistics in practice)*. Wiley Hoboken, New York.

Spiegelhalter DJ, Myles JP, Jones DR, Abrams KR. (1999). Methods in health service research: an introduction to Bayesian methods in health technology assessment. *British Medical Journal*, **319**, 508–12.

Squires DA. (2011). *The US Health System in perspective: a comparison of twelve industrialized nations, Commonwealth Fund*, July. Available at: ℘ http://www.commonwealthfund.org/~/media/Files/Publications/Issue%20Brief/2011/Jul/1532_Squires_US_hlt_sys_comparison_12_nations_intl_brief_v2.pdf

Standing Committee on Postgraduate Medical Education (SCOPME). (1999). *Doctors and dentists. The need for a process of review*, a working paper. SCOPME, London.

Starfield B. (1994). Is primary care essential? *Lancet*, **344**, 1129–33.

Statistics Canada, Canadian statistics. Available at: ℘ http://www40.statcan.ca/z01/cs0002_e.htm (accessed 8 September 2005).

Steel N, Bachmann M, Maisey S, et al. (2008). Self reported receipt of care consistent with 32 quality indicators: national population survey of adults aged 50 or more in England. *British Medical Journal*, **337**, a957.

Stevens A, Gillam S. (1998). *Needs assessment: from theory to practice*, BMJ series 3 **316:** 1448–51. Available at: ℘ http://www.bmj.com/content/316/7142/1448

Stevens A, Milne R, Burls A. (2003). Health technology assessment: history and demand. *Journal of Public Health Medicine*, **25**, 98–101.

Stevens A, Milne R. (2004). Health technology assessment in England and Wales. *International Journal of Technology Assessment in Health Care*, **20**, 11–24.

Stevens A, Raftery J (eds) (1997). *Health care needs assessment*, 2nd series. Radcliffe Medical Press, Oxford.

Stewart A, Burke W, Khoury MJ, Zimmern R. (2009). Genomics and public health. In: Detels R, Beaglehole R, Lansang MA, Gulliford M, eds, *Oxford Textbook of Public Health*, chapter 1.6. Oxford University Press, Oxford.

Stine NW, Chokshi DA. (2012). Opportunity in austerity — a common agenda for medicine and public health. *New England Journal of Medicine*, **366**, 395–7.

Stott R.Godlee F. (2006). What should we do about climate change? Health professionals need to act now, collectively and individually. *British Medical Journal*, **333**, 983–4.

Strasburger VC, The Council on Communications and Media, American Association of Pediatrics. (2006). Children, adolescents, substance abuse, and the media. *Pediatrics*, **126**, 791–9.

Straus S, Tetroe J, Graham I. (2009). *Knowledge translation in health care: moving from evidence to practice*. Wiley-Blackwell, Oxford.

Taylor A, Gostin L. (2010). International recruitment of health personnel. *Lancet*, **375**, 1673–5.

Taylor L, Gowman N, Quigley R. (2003). *Evaluating health impact assessment*. Health Development Agency, London. Available at: ℘ http://www.iaia.org/publicdocuments/pubs_ref_material/Evaluating%20HIA%20pdf.pdf (accessed 26 August 2010)

Tervalon M, Murray-Garcia J. (1998). Cultural humility versus cultural competence: a critical distinction in defining physician training outcomes in multicultural education. *Journal of Health Care for the Poor and Underserved*, **9**, 117–25.

The Cochrane Library. *The Cochrane Collaboration*. John Wiley & Sons, Ltd, Chichester. Available at: ℘ http://www.thecochranelibrary.com/ (accessed 27 August 2010).

The Lancet. (2009). *Health and Climate Change series*. Available at: ℘ www.thelancet.com (cited 29 August 2010).

The Presidential/Congressional Commission on Risk Assessment and Risk Management. (1997). *Framework for environmental health risk management*, Final report volume 1. Washington, DC.

Available at: ℬ http://www.riskworld.com/nreports/1997/riskrpt/pdf/epajan.pdf (accessed 6 August 2010).

The United States Agency for Healthcare Research and Quality. Available at: ℬ http://www.ahrq.gov/ (accessed 30 June 2005).

The World Bank Data Catalog. (2011). *Health, nutrition and population statistics*. Available at: ℳ http://data.worldbank.org/data-catalog/health-nutrition-and-population-statistics (accessed 30 July 2011).

Thistlethwaite JE, Spencer J (2008). *Professionalism in medicine*. Radcliffe, Oxford.

Thorpe KE, Florence CS, Howard DH, Joski P. (2004). The impact of obesity on rising medical spending. Health affairs, web exclusive, October 20, W4-480–6.

Tiplady P. (2002). *Public Health*, **116,** 384 .

Tobey JA. (1947). *Public health law*, 3rd edn. Commonwealth Fund, New York.

Tobias M, Jackson G. (2001). Avoidable mortality in New Zealand, 1981–6.

Trkman P. (2010). The critical success factors of business process management. *International Journal of Information Management*; **30,** 125–34.

Truckmann BC. (1965). Development sequence in small groups. *Psychology Bulletin*, **63,** 384–99.

Tudor Hart J. (1988). A new kind of doctor. Merlin Press, London.

Turning Point Model State Public Health Act. Available at: ℬ http://www.publichealthlaw.net/Resources/Modellaws.htm (accessed 13 August 2010).

Tuttle RM, Becker DV (2006). The Chernobyl accident and its consequences: update at the millennium. *Seminars in Nuclear Medicine*, **30,** 133–40.

Uhr J, Mackay K (ed.). (1996). *Evaluating policy advice: learning from Commonwealth experience*. Federalism Research Centre, Australian National University and Commonwealth Department of Finance, Canberra.

UK Association of Cancer Registries. *Guidelines on the release of confidential data*. Available at: ℳ http://www.ukacr.org/confidentiality/ (accessed 25 January 2010).

Umble KE, Diehl SJ, Gunn A, Haws S. (2007). *Developing leaders, building networks: an evaluation of the National Public Health Leadership Institute—1991–2006*. North Carolina Institute for Public Health, Chapel Hill. Available at: ℬ http://www.phli.org (accessed 20 August 2010).

UN Development Programme. (2011). *Multidimensional Poverty Index*. Available at: ℬ http://hdr.undp.org/en/statistics/mpi/ (accessed 30 May 2011).

UNICEF. (2011). *The $100 billion question: how do we secure a climate resilient future for the world's children?* UNICEF.

United Nations (2000). United Nations millennium declaration. United Nations, New York.

Urquhart J. (1996). Studies of disease clustering: problems of interpretation. In: Eliott P, Cuzick J, English D, Stern R, eds, *Geographical and environmental epidemiology methods for small-area studies*, pp. 278–85. Oxford University Press, Oxford.

Valdez R, Yoon PW, Qureshi N, Green RF, Khoury MJ. (2010). Family history in public health practice: a genomic tool for disease prevention and health promotion. *Annual Review of Public Health*, **31,** 69–87.

Van Wyk G. (2003). *A systems approach to social and organizational planning*. Trafford Publishing, Victoria, BC.

Vangen S, Huxham C. (2003). Nurturing collaborative relations. building trust in interorganizational collaboration. *Journal of Applied Behavioral Science*, **39,** 5–31.

Vieira V, Webster T, Weinberg J, Aschengrau A. (2009). Spatial analysis of bladder, kidney, and pancreatic cancer on upper Cape Cod: an application of generalized additive models to case-control data. *Environmental Health: A Global Access Science Source*, **8,** 3.

Virgil, Georgics, no 2, l 490 quoted in Wilson J. (2008). *Inverting the Pyramid*. Orion, London.

Viswanath K. (2005). Science and society: the communications revolution and cancer control. *Nature Reviews Cancer*, **5,** 828–35.

Viswanath K. (2006). Public communications and its role in reducing and eliminating health disparities. In: Thomson GE, Mitchell F, Williams MB, eds, *Examining the health disparities research plan of the National Institutes of Health: unfinished business*, pp. 215–53. Institute of Medicine, Washington DC.

Viswanath K, Blake KD, Meissner HI, et al. (2008). Occupational practices and the making of health news: a national survey of US health and medical science journalists. *Journal of Health Communication*, **13,** 759–77.

Wadsworth Y. (2010). *Building in research and evaluation: human enquiry for living systems*. Allen & Unwin, Sydney/Left Coast Press, San Francisco.

Wadsworth Y. (2011). *Do it yourself social research*, 3rd edn. Allen & Unwin, Sydney/Left Coast Press, San Francisco.

Wagenaar A, Salois M, Komor K. (2009). Effects of beverage alcohol price and tax levels on drinking: a meta-analysis of 1003 estimates from 112 studies. *Addiction*, **104**, 179–90.

Wakefield, MA, Loken B, Hornik RC. (2010). Use of mass media campaigns to change health behaviour. *Lancet* **376**, 1261–71.

Walker T. (2010). Why we should not set a minimum price per unit of alcohol. *Public Health Ethics*, **3**, 107–14.

Walshe K, Freeman T. (2002). Effectiveness of quality improvement: learning from evaluations. *Quality and Safety in Health Care*, **11**, 85–7.

Wanless D. (2004). *Securing good health for the whole population.* HM Treasury, London. Available at: ℘ http://www.dh.gov.uk/en/Publicationsandstatistics/Publications/PublicationsPolicyAndGuidance/DH_4074426 (accessed 21 August 2010).

We can end poverty 2015. *The Millennium Development Goals.* Available at: ℘ http://www.un.org/en/mdg/summit2010/ (accessed 30 May 2011).

Weiss CH. (1979). The many meanings of research utilization. *Public Administration Review*, **39**, 426–31.

Wells G, Shea B, O'Connell D, et al. The Newcastle-Ottawa Scale (NOS) for assessing the quality of non-randomized studies in meta-analyses. Available at: ℘ http://www.ohri.ca/programs/clinical_epidemiology/oxford.asp (accessed 29 March 2011)

West SL, O'Neal KK. (2004). Project DARE outcome effectiveness revisited. *American Journal of Public Health*, **94**, 1027–9.

Whitehead M, Petticrew M, Graham H, et al. (2004). Evidence for public health policy on inequalities: 2: assembling the evidence jigsaw. *Journal of Epidemiology and Community Health*, **58**, 817–21.

WHO European Centre for Health Policy. (1999). *Health impact assessment: main concepts and suggested approach*, Gothenburg consensus paper. ECHP, Brussels.

WHO. (2003). Special issue on HIA. *Bulletin of the World Health* Organization, **81**. Available at: ℘ http://www.who.int/bulletin/volumes/81/6/en/ (accessed 26 August 2010).

WHO. (2009).*Constraints to scaling up and costs*, background document for the Taskforce on Innovative International Financing for Health systems. Available at: M http://www.unicef.org/health/files/MBB_Technical_Background_Global_Costing_HLTF_Final_Draft_30_July.pdf (accessed 6 June 2011).

WHO. (2010). *10 facts on health financing.* Available at: ℘ http://www.who.int/features/factfiles/universal_health_coverage/en/index.html (accessed 30 May 2010).

WHO. (2011). *Global Status Report on Noncommunicable Diseases 2010.* WHO, Geneva. Available at: ℘ http://www.who.int/chp/ncd_global_status_report/en/index.html (accessed 30 May 2011).

WHO/FAO. (2003). *Diet, nutrition and the prevention of chronic diseases*, Report of the Joint WHO/FAO expert consultation, WHO Technical Report Series, No. 916 (TRS 916). WHO/Food and Agriculture Organization, Geneva.

WHO FCTC. (2010).*Framework Convention on Tobacco Control.* Geneva. WHO: Geneva. ℘ http://www.who.int/fctc/en/ [accessed 20 December 2010]

Whorton D, Krauss RM, Marshall S, Milby TH. (1977). Infertility in male pesticide workers. *Lancet*, **2**, 1259–61.

Wiki Public Health Available at: ℘ http://wikiph.org/index.php?title=Evidence_searches (accessed 30 May 2011).

Wikipedia. Available at: ℘ http://en.wikipedia.org/wiki/Incrementalism Accessed 30 May 2011.

Wikipedia. Available at: ℘ http://en.wikipedia.org/wiki/Satisficing (accessed 30 May 2011).

Wilkin D, Hallam L, Dogget M. (1992). *Measures of need and outcomes in primary health care.* Oxford Medical Publications, Oxford.

Wilkinson P. (2008). Climate change & health: the case for sustainable development. *Medical Conflict Survival*, **24(Suppl. 1)**, S26–35.

Will S, Ardern K, Spencely M, Watkins S. (1994). *A prospective health impact assessment of the proposed development of a second runway at Manchester International Airport*, written submission to the public inquiry. Manchester and Stockport Health Commissions, Manchester.

Williams G, Elliott E. (2010). Exploring social inequalities in health: the importance of thinking qualitatively. In: Bourgeault I, De Vries R Dingwall R, eds, *Handbook on Qualitative Health Research.* Sage, London.

Wismar M. Blau J. Ernst K, et al. (eds). (2007). *The effectiveness of. health impact assessment.* European Obserrvatory on Health Systems and Policies, WHO, Copenhagen. Available at: ℘ http://www.euro.who.int/__data/assets/pdf_file/0003/98283/E90794.pdf (accessed 26 August 2010).

W.K. Kellogg Community Health Scholars Program. (2001). *Stories of impact.* University of Michigan, School of Public Health, CHSP, National Program Office, Ann Arbor.

WK Kellogg Foundation (2004) Using logic models to bring together planning, evaluation, and action—logic model development guide, p. 3. Available at: ℗ http://www.wkkf.org/knowledge-center/resources/2006/02/WK-Kellogg-Foundation-Logic-Model-Development-Guide.aspx (accessed 18 November 2011).

Wolfstadt J, Gurwitz J, Field TS, *et al.* (2008). The effect of computerized order entry with decision support on the rates of adverse drug events: a systematic review. *Journal of General Internal Medicine*, **23**, 451–8.

World Bank. (2004). *Making services work for poor people*, World Development Report, The World Bank, Washington, DC. Available at: ℗ http://www-wds.worldbank.org/external/default/main?pagePK=64193027&piPK=64187937&theSitePK=523679&menuPK=64187510&searchMenuPK=64187283&siteName=WDS&entityID=000090341_20031007150121 (accessed 31 May 2011).

World Commission on Dams. (2000). *Dams and development: a new framework for decision-making.* Earthscan, London. Available at: ℗ http://pubs.iied.org/pdfs/9126IIED.pdf

World Health Assembly. (2005). *Revision of the International Health Regulations.* Available at: M http://www.who.int/csr/ihr/en/ (accessed 23 August 2010).

World Health Organization. (1978). *Primary health care,* Report of the International Conference on Primary Health Care, Alma-Ata, USSR, 6–12 September. WHO, Geneva.

World Health Organization. (1986). *Ottawa Charter for Health Promotion.* WHO, Geneva.

World Health Organization. (1998). *The new emergency health kit,* WHO document WHO/DAP/98.10. World Health Organization, Geneva.

World Health Organization (2000). *The World Health Report 2000. Health systems: improving performance.* World Health Organization, Geneva

World Health Organization. (2005). *Framework Convention on Tobacco Control,* WHO doc. A56/VR/4 (2003). Available at: ℗ http://www.who.int/tobacco/framework/WHO_FCTC_english.pdf (accessed 23 August 2010)

World Health Organization (2006). Guidelines for drinking water quality, 3rd ed. Available at: M http://www.who.int/water_sanitation_health/dwq/en/ (cited 3 August 2010).

World Health Organization. (2006). *Preparing a workforce for the 21st century: the challenge of chronic conditions.* WHO, Geneva.

World Health Organization. (2008). *Primary health care (now more than ever),* World Health Report. WHO, Geneva.

World Health organization (2009). *World Health Statistics Report 2009.* WHO, Geneva.

World Health Organization (2010). *Global Code of Practice on the International Recruitment of Health Personnel.* WHO, Geneva.

World Health Organization. (2010). *Obesity and overweight* [Report on Internet]. WHO, Geneva. Available at: ℗ http://www.who.int/mediacentre/factsheets/fs311/en/ / (accessed 31 May, 2012).

World Health Organization. (2011). *A prioritized research agenda for prevention and control of non-communicable disease.* WHO, Geneva.

World Health Organization. (2011). *Millennium development goals: progress towards the health-related millennium development goals.* Geneva. Available at: ℗ http://www.who.int/mediacentre/factsheets/fs290/en/index.html. (accessed on 27 May 2011).

World Health Organization. (2011). *World Health Statistics Report, 2011.* WHO, Geneva.

World Health Organization Sustainable Development and Healthy Environments. (1999). *Environmental health indicators: framework and methodologies,* Protection of the Human Environment Occupational and Environmental Health Series. WHO, Geneva.

World Health Organization. *Health systems performance.* Available at: ℗ http://www. who.int/health-systems-performance/ (accessed 21 March 2005).

World Health Organization . *The WHO family of international classifications.* Available at: ℗ http://www.who.int/classifications/en/ (accessed 20 March 2005).

World Health Organization. *WHO Statistical Information System (WHOSIS).* Available at: ℗ http://www.who.int/whosis/ (accessed 21 March 2005).

Wright J, Walley J, Philip A, *et al.* (2004). Direct observation for tuberculosis: a randomised controlled trial of community health workers versus family members. *Tropical Medicine & International Health* **9**, 559–65.

Wright J, Williams DRR, Wilkinson J. (1998). The development of health needs assessment. In: Wright J, ed., *Health needs assessment in practice,* pp. 1–11. BMJ Books, London.

Yawn BP, Suman VJ, Jacobsen SJ. (1998). Maternal recall of distant pregnancy events. *Journal of Clinical Epidemiology,* **51,** 399–405.

Index